ADVANCED HUMAN NUTRITION

ROBERT E.C. WILDMAN
DENIS M. MEDEIROS

CRC Press
Boca Raton London New York Washington, D.C.

From *Structure and Function of Domestic Animals* by W. Bruce Currie, CRC Press LLC, Boca Raton, Florida, 1992: Figures 1.2, 1.3, 1.6, 1.11, 1.12, 1.16, 1.17, 1.18, 1.19, 1.20, 1.21, 1.22, 1.23, 1.25, 1.27, 1.28, 3.2, 3.5, 4.4, 4.5, 5.1, 5.5, 5.7, 7.1, 7.2, 7.3, 10.8, 11.1, 11.2, 11.14, 13.1, 13.2, and 14.3.

From *Handbook of Molecular and Cellular Methods in Biology and Medicine* by Peter B. Kaufmann, William Wu, and Donghern Kim, CRC Press LLC, Boca Raton, Florida, 1995: Figures 16.1, 20.3, and 20.4.

From *The Concise Encyclopedia of Foods and Nutrition* by Audrey Ensminger and M. E. Ensminger, CRC Press LLC, Boca Raton, Florida, 1995: Figures 1.1, 1.7, 1.9b, 1.27, 2.2, 2.8, 2.11, 3.1, 3.3, 3.6, 3.8, 4.7, 10.2, 10.5, 10.7, 14.1, 14.2, 14.4, 15.1, 15.2, 16.2, 16.3, 17.1, 19.1, 19.2, and 20.1 and Appendices C, D, and E.

From *Handbook of Lipids in Human Nutrition* by Gene A. Spiller, CRC Press LLC, Boca Raton, Florida, 1995: Figures 5.2, 5.3, and 5.12.

From *Advanced Nutrition: Macronutrients* by Carolyn D. Berdanier, CRC Press LLC, Boca Raton, Florida, 1994: 1.8, 1.9a, 1.10, 1.14, 1.30. 2.3, 2.4, 2.5, 2.6, 2.7, 4.1, 4.2, 4.3, 4.6, 4.8, 4.9, 5.6, 5.8, 5.10, 5.11, 6.1, 6.2, 6.3, 6.4, 6.5, 6.6, 6.7, 6.8, 11.3, 11.4, 11.5, 11.6, 11.7, 11.8, 11.9, 11.11, 11.12, 11.13, 11.15, 11.16, 11.17, 13.5, 13.6, and 18.1.

From *Advanced Nutrition: Micronutrients* by Carolyn D. Berdanier, CRC Press LLC, Boca Raton, Florida, 1997: Figures 8.1, 8.2, 8.5, 8.6, 8.7, 8.8, 8.9, 8.10, 8.11, 8.12, 8.14, 8.15, 8.16, 8.17, 8.18, 8.19, 8.20, 8.21, 8.22, 8.23, 8.24, 8.25, 8.26, 8.27, 8.28, 8.29, 8.30, 8.31, 8.32, 8.33, 8.35, 8.36, 8.37, 8.38, 8.39, 8.40, 8.41, 9.1, 9.2, 10.1, 10.3, 10.4, 10.6, 10.9, 10.10, and 20.2.

CRC Desk Reference for Nutrition by Carolyn D. Berdanier, CRC Press LLC, Boca Raton, Florida, 1998: Figures 1.13, 11.10, and Appendices A, C, D, E, F, and G.

Library of Congress Cataloging-in-Publication Data

Catalog record is available from the Libray of Congress.

International Standard Book Number 0-8493-8566-?

CRC SERIES IN MODERN NUTRITION
Edited by Ira Wolinsky and James F. Hickson, Jr.

Published Titles

Manganese in Health and Disease, Dorothy J. Klimis-Tavantzis

Nutrition and AIDS: Effects and Treatments, Ronald R. Watson

Nutrition Care for HIV-Positive Persons: A Manual for Individuals and Their Caregivers,
  Saroj M. Bahl and James F. Hickson, Jr.

Calcium and Phosphorus in Health and Disease, John J.B. Anderson and
  Sanford C. Garner

Edited by Ira Wolinsky

Published Titles

Handbook of Nutrition in the Aged, Ronald R. Watson

Practical Handbook of Nutrition in Clinical Practice, Donald F. Kirby and
  Stanley J. Dudrick

Handbook of Dairy Foods and Nutrition, Gregory D. Miller, Judith K. Jarvis, and
  Lois D. McBean

Advanced Nutrition: Macronutrients, Carolyn D. Berdanier

Childhood Nutrition, Fima Lifschitz

Nutrition and Health: Topics and Controversies, Felix Bronner

Nutrition and Cancer Prevention, Ronald R. Watson and Siraj I. Mufti

Nutritional Concerns of Women, Ira Wolinsky and Dorothy J. Klimis-Tavantzis

Nutrients and Gene Expression: Clinical Aspects, Carolyn D. Berdanier

Antioxidants and Disease Prevention, Harinda S. Garewal

Advanced Nutrition: Micronutrients, Carolyn D. Berdanier

Nutrition and Women's Cancers, Barbara Pence and Dale M. Dunn

Nutrients and Foods in AIDS, Ronald R. Watson

Nutrition: Chemistry and Biology, Second Edition, Julian E. Spallholz,
  L. Mallory Boylan, and Judy A. Driskell

Melatonin in the Promotion of Health, Ronald R. Watson

Nutrition and the Eye, Allen Taylor

Laboratory Tests for the Assessment of Nutritional Status, Second Edition,
  H.E. Sauberlich

Advanced Human Nutrition, Robert E.C. Wildman and Denis M. Medeiros

Forthcoming Titles

Handbook of Diary Foods and Nutrition, Second Edition, Gregory D. Miller,
  Judith K. Jarvis, and Lois D. McBean

Management of Stress and Eating Disorders for Women and Children, Jacalyn J. Robert

Child Nutrition: An International Perspective, Noel W. Solomons

Childhood Obesity: Prevention and Treatment, Jana Parizkova and Andrew Hills

Alcohol and Substance Abuse in the Aging, Ronald R. Waston

Nutritional Anemias, Usha Ramakrishnan

Advances is Isotope Methods for the Analysis of Trace Elements in Man,
  Malcolm Jackson and Nicola Lowe

Forthcoming Titles Continued

Advanced Nutrition: Macronutrients, Second Edition, Carolyn D. Berdanier

Handbook of Nutrition for Vegetarians, Joan Sabate and Rosemary A. Ratzin-Tuner

Tryptophan: Biochemicals and Health Implications, Herschel Sidransky

Coenzyme Q: From Molecular Mechanisms to Nutrition and Health, Valerian E. Kagan and Peter J. Quinn

Nutraceuticals and Functional Foods, Robert E. C. Wildman

The Mediterranean Diet, Antonia L. Matalas, Antonios Zampelas, Vasilis Stavrinos, and Ira Wolinsky

Handbook of Nutrition and the Aged, Third Edition, Ronald R. Watson

Handbook of Nutraceuticals and Nutritional Supplements and Pharmaceuticals, Robert E. C. Wildman

Contents

Introduction xix

Chapter 1   Foundations of the Human Body 1
Elements and Molecules..1
Cell Structure and Organelles 2
The Nucleus and Genetic Aspects 10
Protein Synthesis 12
Electron Transport Chain and Oxidative Phosphorylation.....................15
Tissue 19
Organ Systems 21
Suggested Reading 35

Chapter 2   Food and the Human Body 37
Nutrients 38
Recommended Dietary Allowances...38
Dietary Reference Intakes 43
Food Sources of Nutrients..44
Food Components and Human Senses 50
Appetite...55
Suggested Reading 57

Chapter 3   Human Digestion and Absorption...................................59
Gastrointestinal Anatomy 59
Gastrointestinal Movement, Motility, and Neural Activity 64
Gastrointestinal Blood Supply and Flow Regulation 66
Gastrointestinal Endocrine and Paracrine Substances 67
Digestion and Absorption 69
    Oral Cavity..69
    Esophagus..71
    Stomach..72
    Small Intestine 74
Enterocyte Contributions to Digestion 76
Large Intestine 77

Chapter 4   Carbohydrates 79
Monosaccharides 80
Disaccharides and Oligosaccharides 84
Polysaccharides..85
Dietary Fiber Classification and Food Sources 88
Carbohydrate Digestion 91
INSIGHT: Physical and Physiological Properties of Fiber
    and Potential Benefits to Health 94

Chapter 5   Lipids 99
  General Properties and Nomenclature of Lipids 99
    Cis vs. *Trans* Fatty Acids..102
  Lipids in Food 106
  Dietary Lipid Requirements..109
  Digestion of Lipids 110
  Eicosanoids..113
  Steroids..114
  Lipoproteins 116
  INSIGHT: Health Implications and Interpretation
    of Lipoprotein-Cholesterol Levels 121

Chapter 6   Protein..123
  Amino Acids..123
  Protein Structures 127
  Dietary Protein, Digestion, and Absorption..129
  Dietary Protein Quality 132
  Roles of Amino Acids and Proteins in Metabolism 135
  Metabolism of Amino Acids..138
  Protein Requirements 143
  Amino Acid Requirements 146
  Determination of Protein Intakes by Food Source,
    Based on Limiting Amino Acids 147
  Excess Dietary Protein..148
  Protein Undernutrition..149
  INSIGHT: Causes of Global Protein Undernutrition 150

Chapter 7   Water 151
  Properties of Water 151
  Distribution of Water in the Human Body 152
  Sweat Water..153
  Urinary Water 155
  Water Balance..156
  Water Deficiency (Dehydration) and Intoxification............................158

Chapter 8   Vitamins..159
  Water Solubility 159
  Fat-Soluble Vitamins..160
    Vitamin A 160
    Vitamin D 167
    Vitamin E..173
    Vitamin K 178
  Water-Soluble Vitamins 182
    Vitamin C (Ascorbic Acid) 182
    Thiamin (Vitamin B_1) 186
    Riboflavin (Vitamin B_2)..191
    Niacin (Vitamin B_3) 195
    Vitamin B_6..200
    Folic Acid (Folate) 206

Vitamin B$_{12}$ 212
Biotin 216
Pantothenic Acid 218
Suggested Readings 224

Chapter 9   Major Minerals 225
Calcium 226
Phosphorus 232
Magnesium 235
Sodium, Chloride, and Potassium 238
Sulfur 243
Suggested Readings 244

Chapter 10   Minor Minerals 245
Iron 245
Zinc 254
Iodine 259
Copper 264
Selenium 269
Fluoride 273
Chromium 275
Manganese 277
Cobalt 278
Boron 278
Molybdenum 279
Vanadium 280
Nickel 281
Arsenic 282
Silicon 282

Chapter 11   Energy Metabolism 283
Total Energy Expenditure 283
Components of Energy Metabolism 285
Integrated Energy Metabolism 289
Major Metabolic Pathways 295
Energy Substrate Utilization 316

Chapter 12   Body Composition and Obesity 321
Methods for Assessing Body Composition 322
Variations in Body Composition 325
Adipocytes 327
Obesity 328
Regulation of Energy Intake, Storage, and Expenditure 333
Chemical Mediators of Energy Homeostasis 334
Neuro-Endocrine Influences 335
Obesity: Gender and Age 337
Obesity and Related Diseases 338
Diet Therapy 339
Pharmacological Treatment of Obesity 340

Surgical Treatment 342
Liposuction 342
Suggested Readings 342

Chapter 13   Nutrition and Activity 343
Muscle and Fiber Types 343
Muscle Adaptations to Strength Training 346
Muscle Adaptations to Endurance Exercise 346
Hormonal Adaptation to Acute and Chronic Exercise 347
Carbohydrate Metabolism and Exercise 349
Triglyceride and Fatty Acid Metabolism and Exercise 352
Protein and Amino Acid Metabolism and Exercise 354
Coordinated Energy Metabolism During Exercise 355
Vitamins, Minerals, and Exercise 357
Water and Exercise 359
Common Nutrition Practices Used in Attempts to Enhance Performance 360
Suggested Readings 364

Chapter 14   Nutrition Supplements and Nutraceuticals 367
Herbs 368
Arginine 369
Aspartic Acid 369
Boron 370
Carnitine 370
Carotenoids 371
Chondroitin Sulfate 372
Chromium 372
Creatine 374
Coenzyme Q10 (Ubiquinone) 375
Choline 376
DHEA 377
Echinacea 379
Flavonoids 379
Garlic (*Allium sativum*) 380
Ginger 380
Ginkgo 381
Glycerol 382
HMB (β-hydroxy-β-methylbutyrate) 383
Laetrile 383
Licorice 384
Ornithine 384
Phytoestrogens 385
Pyruvate 385
Saponins 386
Saw Palmetto 387
Soy Products 387
St. John's Wort 388
Vanadium 388
Valerian 389

Yohimbine 390
References and Suggested Readings..390

Chapter 15   Nutrition and Human Reproduction 399
Pregnancy..399
Lactation..403
Infancy...405
Suggested Readings..409

Chapter 16   Cardiovascular Disease and Nutrition 411
General Energy Metabolism in Myocardial Tissue 412
Cardiac Energy Metabolism During Reduced O_2 Delivery (Ischemia)...............414
Cardiac Energy Metabolism During Hypertrophy 415
Cardiac Hypertrophy...415
Risk Factors for Heart Disease 417
Hypertension 417
Cholesterol 420
Atherosclerosis..421
Clinical Intervention..423
Dietary Guidance..425
Other Nutritional Factors and Cardiovascular Disease 429

Chapter 17   Cancer and Nutrition...433
Tumors and Cancer..433
Genetic Alterations Causing Cancer......................................435
Inheritance 436
Stages of Cancer Formation 436
Cancer Treatment..437
Cancer Risk Factors 439
Chemoprevention 440
Dietary and Behavioral Influences on Cancer.........................440
Unproven Oral Treatment Options 449
Nutritional Concerns of Conventional Therapies....................450
Suggested Readings..450

Chapter 18   Diabetes and Nutrition 451
Definition, Etiology and Classification....................................451
Insulin Resistance 454
Pathophysiology of Insulin Resistance...................................455
Other Specific Types of Diabetes Mellitus...............................455
Diagnostic Criteria for Diabetes Mellitus................................456
Medical Complications Associated with Diabetes Mellitus.........457
Medical Nutritional Therapy for Diabetes Mellitus 459
Non-Nutritional Medical Therapy..465
Suggested Readings..467

Chapter 19   Osteoporosis and Nutrition 469
Bone Tissue..469
Osteoporosis..473

Menopause and Estrogen 474
Medical, Nutritional, and Behavioral Prevention
    and Treatment of Osteoporosis 475
Suggested Readings..480

Chapter 20   Nutrition Research: Past, Present, and Future 483
Nutrition Research in the 20th Century 483
Determination of Nutrient Requirements 485
Nutrition Laboratory Research 487
Laboratory Tools 487
Suggested Readings..496

Chapter 21   Nutrition in the 21st Century 497
Nutrition Past..497
Suggested Readings..501

Appendix A.   Common Food Additives..503

Appendix B.   Growth Charts 511

Appendix C.   Vitamins 517

Appendix D.   Minerals 527

Appendix E.   Sweetening Agents, Sugar Substitutes 535

Appendix F.   Normal Clinical Values for Blood 541

Appendix G.   Some Common Medicinal Plants................................543

Index..559

Series Preface

The CRC Series in Modern Nutrition is dedicated to providing the widest possible coverage of topics in nutrition. Nutrition is an interdisciplinary, interprofessional field par excellence. It is noted by its broad range and diversity. We trust the titles and authorship in this series will reflect that range and diversity.

Published for a broad audience, the volumes in the CRC Series in Modern Nutrition are designed to explain, review, and explore present knowledge and recent trends, developments, and advances in nutrition. As such, they will appeal to professionals as well as the educated layman. The format for the series will vary with the needs of the author and the topic, including, but not limited to, edited volumes, monographs, handbooks, and texts.

Contributors from any bonafide area of nutrition, including the controversial, are welcome.

I welcome the contribution of the book Advanced Human Nutrition written by Robert Wildman and Denis Medeiros. They have had first hand knowledge and exposure to the subject in their past and present roles of students, teachers, and researchers. The book will not only be useful as a text, but also as a reference and research resource.

Ira Wolinsky, Ph.D.
University of Houston
Series Editor

The Authors

Robert E. C. Wildman, Ph.D. R.D. received his B.S. degree in Clinical Dietetics and Nutrition from the University of Pittsburgh in 1988. After a couple years of clinical training, Dr. Wildman completed a M.S. degree in Foods and Nutrition in 1991 at The Florida State University followed by his Ph.D. in Human Nutrition with an emphasis in Cardiac Physiology in 1994 at The Ohio State University. He is currently on the faculty in the Department of Nutrition and Dietetics at the University of Southwestern Louisiana.

Dr. Wildman is a member of the American Society of Nutrition Sciences, the American Society for Clinical Nutrition, and the National Strength and Conditioning Association. He is the Nutrition Editor for Rodale Press as well as the Series Editor for the CRC Press Series entitled Nutraceuticals. Dr. Wildman also cofounded Columbus Fitness Consultants, Inc.

Denis Medeiros, Ph.D., R.D. received his B.S. degree from Central Connecticut State University Biology in 1976, his M.S. from Illinois State University in Physiology in 1976, and his Ph.D. in Nutrition from Clemson University in 1981. He has been on the faculties of Mississippi State University and The University of Wyoming and currently is a Full Professor of Human Nutrition at Ohio State University. Dr. Medeiros is a former Associate Dean for Research and Dean of the College of Human Ecology at Ohio State University. He has also spent time studying at the Medical University of South Carolina in Charlestown and the Washington University School of Medicine in St. Louis, Missouri. Dr. Medeiros is Chair-elect of the Department of Human Nutrition at Kansas State University.

Dr. Medeiros' major research area has focused upon the role of trace elements, particularly copper, on the integrity of the cardiovascular system. He has received approximately $2 million in grants to support his research endeavors and has authored or co-authored more than 90 peer-reviewed research articles. He has taught classes both at the introductory and advanced levels for undergraduate students and has taught graduate level courses throughout his career. Dr. Medeiros has received various outstanding teaching awards for his efforts.

Acknowledgments

Drs. Robert Wildman and Denis Medeiros would like to thank the following individuals for their efforts and assistance in the completion of this book:

Research Assistants Colleen Naccarato, M.S., R.D.; Beth Halloran Webb, M.S., R.D.; Jennifer Greenley, M.S. R.D.; Richard Bruno, M.S.; Jennifer Tucker, B.S.; Sheila Quickel, B.S.; and Dessa Hartz, R.D., C.D.E.

Scholarly contributors: Dr. Thunder Jalili and Richard Bruno, M.S.

Graphic design and artistic assistance: Richard Bruno, M.S.; Tam Tran, B.S.; and Evan Grunbaum, B.S.

The authors would also like to express their most sincere appreciation to Drs. Carolyn Berdanier and Bruce Currie for permission to utilize graphics derived from their books published by CRC Press entitled *Advanced Nutrition: Macronutrients, Advanced Nutrition: Micronutrients, CRC Desk Reference for Nutrition,* and *Structure and Function of Domestic Animals.* Many graphics in this textbook are derived from these works as well as the CRC Press *Foods and Nutrition* and *The Concise Encyclopedia of Foods and Nutrition.*

Introduction

From the dawning instance of conception to the waning moments of senescence, the human body exists in a continuum to nourish itself. Man, as a living entity, is in reality a reflection of the compilative and coordinated efforts of trillions of microscopic metabolic units, which came to be known as cells. To support their operations, human cells require a homeostatic environment and a continuous supply of energy. Energy is derived from either dietary consumption or the utilization of internal stores of carbohydrate, amino acids, and triglycerides. Ethyl alcohol or ethanol ingested as a constituent of alcoholic beverages can also be a source of energy. These molecules are ultimately metabolized to carbon dioxide and water and a portion of their released energy captured within adenosine triphosphate (ATP) molecules. ATP can then be applied to power cellular operations.

Beyond the energy nutrients, human cells require the availability of other vital substances such as vitamins and minerals. Vitamins include a class of organic-based molecules that are involved in multiple aspects of cellular operations. Vitamins are broadly classified into two groups based upon their properties relating to water solubility: nine water-soluble and four lipid-soluble (fat-soluble) vitamins can function in antioxidation and other redox operations, and coenzymatic and cofactor mechanisms. While all vitamins are stored within the human body, the location and degree of storage capability will vary greatly from vitamin to vitamin. With the exception of organ meats, plant-derived foods such as whole grains, fruits, and vegetables, appear to be among the better natural sources for most vitamins. The most outstanding contradiction to this general rule is vitamin B_{12} which is only available in animal-based foods.

Minerals dissolved throughout intracellular and extracellular fluids and as structural components of tissue are involved in a variety of human operations. Of the 23 or so minerals involved in human operations, 7 are considered major minerals because of their relatively greater contribution to body mass, as well as their greater quantity requirement in our diet. The remaining minerals contribute significantly less to human mass and are needed to be supplied by the diet in relatively lesser amounts. However, dietary need and contribution to body mass cannot be confused with physiological importance. For instance, an animal raised on either a copper- or iron-deficient diet will perish within weeks.

Water provides the medium of the human body as it provides the basis of intracellular and extracellular fluids. Water also provides the fluid basis for secretory events and a means of waste removal. The human body is approximately 60% water and while appreciable quantities are created within the human body, it cannot balance the substantial loss of water on a daily basis. Signs of water deficiency or dehydration are perhaps the most rapid occurring manifestations of nutrient imbalance and is an extremely important performance concern for athletes.

While dietary triglycerides are often viewed primarily as an energy substrate for human cells, they must also be recognized as providers of essential fatty acids. Essential fatty acids belong to the ω3 and ω6 polyunsaturated fatty acid (PUFA) families. The importance of these fatty acids is to serve as the precursor molecule for the synthesis of eicosanoid molecules, which includes prostaglandins, leukotrienes, and thromboxanes. Eicosanoids function largely as messengers released by a variety of tissue and elicit a local response such as vasodilation and increased platelet aggregation.

As an adjunct to conventional medical practices, many ancient civilizations utilized certain foods including vegetables, roots, and spices for the prevention and treatment of various ailments. For many cultures these nutritional applications endured time and continue today. However, in many other cultures, especially Western societies, many of these nutritional practices were forsaken in light of the advent of the pharmaceutical industry. Today however, health practitioners are revamping interest into food components with pharmaceutical properties or nutraceuticals and evolving their role in modern medicine. Plant-derived substances with purported health benefits include carotenoids, flavonoids, organosulfur compounds, terpenoids, fiber, ubiquinone, capsaicin, and herbs. Oils from fish and plants are good sources of specialized polyunsaturated fatty acids utilized by human cells to make eicosanoid structures, as discussed above.

As with all complex structures and systems, the human body is vulnerable to injury and imperfection. While the response to injury is fundamental to human existence, it can also be the basis of disease. For example, atherosclerosis has been discussed as an excessive inflammatory-fibroproliferative response to endothelial insults to the arterial wall. Atherosclerosis evolves from an initial injury to vascular tissue as the result of mechanical or chemical insults. Disease can also arise from the very foundation of multicellular life itself — cell proliferation. The development of a tumorous cell involves mutations to certain cell-proliferation regulatory genes. Thus, a cell loses tight control of its own proliferation. Its daughter cells are then destined to carry the same mutated genes and reproduce in the same uncontrolled manner as well. As most diseases are processes, or more interestingly normal processes that have gone awry, nutrition can be highly involved in various aspects related to process. This includes initial injury or pathogenesis as well as the progression and treatment of a disease. For example, certain dietary factors augment cellular antioxidant potential and lessen the risk of genetic mutations induced by free-radicals. Furthermore, nutritional factors can influence the rate of proliferation of tumorous cells, as well as the ability of cancerous tumors to spread. In another example, caloric imbalance ultimately leads to obesity which is highly associated with certain cancers, heart disease, diabetes, and other disease states. Also, diet influences blood lipid profiles and blood pressure which are pivotal in the initiation and progression of heart disease.

Nutrition as an area of study relies upon an understanding of its parent sciences: chemistry and biology. This text has been written with the assumption that the reader possesses a basic understanding of inorganic and organic chemistry, biology, and biochemistry. Therefore, many aspects directly related to these areas will be presented as part of the discussion without introductory details. The first unit of this text will provide a general review of basic human anatomy and physiology in light of the significant application of nutrition aspects to these areas.

1

Foundations of the Human Body

Undeniably, nutrition is of primary importance to the anatomical and physiological development and maintenance of the human body. This complex multicellular entity consists of organ systems and tissue working in synthium to support growth, maturation, defense, and reproduction. From an evolutionary perspective, humans developed into bipedal primates endowed with enormously expanded cerebral hemispheres, particularly the frontal lobes, which are responsible for intelligent behavior and muscular dexterity. These characteristics allow humans to move agilely in various directions, investigate their environment, and understand and learn complex behaviors. Unlike other animals, these characteristics also allow humans the potential to investigate and comprehend the importance of their own nutrition. In a general sense, humans are inhalation units and food processors, combustion units for energy molecules, as well as storage facilities for excessive energy, waste removing and defensive, internally and externally communicative, locomotive, and reproduction capable. All of these functions are founded and/or influenced by nutritional intake.

Comprehension as to how to nourish the human body demands at the very least a basic understanding of just what it is that needs to be nourished. But where does one begin this understanding? Perhaps the most obvious starting point would be at the cellular level. While it is indeed easier for humans to think of themselves as a single unit, the truth of the matter is that they are a compilation of some 60 to 100 trillion *cells*. Every one of those cells is a living entity, engaging in homeostatic operations to support self-preservation, while in some manner concurrently engaging in homeostatic mechanisms for the human body as a whole. Each cell is metabolically active, and thus requires nourishment, while at the same time producing waste. Therefore, nutrition can not merely be defined as the study of the nourishment of the human body, but even more so as the nourishment of individual cells and the tissue and organs they make up as well. However, an understanding of nutrition needs to go beyond the living or viable portions of the body to recognize the "building blocks" of cells themselves, namely, elements and molecules.

Elements and Molecules

Of the more than 100 elements known at this time, the human body employs about 27 or so. Oxygen is the most abundant element in the human body, accounting for about 63% of its mass. Carbon (18%), hydrogen (9%), and nitrogen (3%) follow oxygen, in decreasing order of abundance (Table 1.1). Carbon, hydrogen, oxygen, and nitrogen atoms are foundations for the most abundant types of molecules in the body, namely, water, proteins, lipids, carbohydrates, and nucleic acids. Water typically accounts for about 55 to 65% of human mass, while proteins and lipids collectively may contribute about 30 to 45% or so. Last,

TABLE 1.1
Elements of the Human Body

Major Elements (%) [a]		Trace Elements [b]
Oxygen	63.0	Silicon
Carbon	18.0	Aluminum
Hydrogen	9.0	Iron
Nitrogen	3.0	Manganese
Calcium	1.5	Fluorine
Phosphorus	1.0	Vanadium
Potassium	0.4	Iodine
Sulfur	0.3	Tin
Sodium	0.2	Boron
Chloride	0.1	Selenium
Magnesium	0.1	Chromium
		Cobolt
		Arsenic
		Molybdenum
		Zinc

[a] Element (% of body mass).
[b] Each trace element contributes less than 0.01% to total body mass.

TABLE 1.2
Theoretical Contributors to Body
Weight for a Lean Man and Woman

Component	Man (%)	Woman (%)
Water	62	59
Fat	16	22
Protein	16	14
Minerals	6	5
Carbohydrate	<1	<1
	100	100

nucleic acids, carbohydrates, and other organic molecules contribute about 1% or so to human mass. The remaining portion of the body, about 5%, is largely minerals (Table 1.2).

With the exception of water, the major molecule types of the human body are complex and largely constructed of simpler molecules. For example, proteins are comprised of amino acids linked by peptide bonds. Deoxyribonucleic acid (DNA) and ribonucleic acid (RNA) are assembled from nucleotides which themselves are constructed from smaller molecules, namely, purine and pyrimidine bases, phosphoric acid, and a carbohydrate, 2-deoxy-D-ribose and D-ribose for DNA and RNA, respectively. Triglycerides (triacylglycerol) are comprised of three fatty acids esterified to a glycerol molecule, while glucose molecules can be linked together by anhydride bonds to form the carbohydrate storage polymer, glycogen.

Cell Structure and Organelles

While there are over 200 different types of cells in the human body, each performing a unique or somewhat enhanced function, most of the basic structural and operational

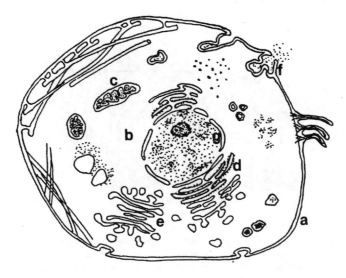

FIGURE 1.1
General cell structure featuring the plasma membrane (a), cytoplasm (b), mitochondria (c), endoplasmic reticulum (d), Golgi apparatus (e), secretory release of substances (f), and the nucleus (g).

features are conserved among all cells. This means that while skeletal muscle cells and adipocytes (fat storage cells) may seem very different in many respects, including primary purpose, color, and shape, the most basic structures and functions of both cell types are virtually the same. This allows us to discuss cells initially as a single entity, and then to expound in later discussion to recognize unique and/or highly specialized functions of specific cells (Figure 1.1).

Human cells have an average size of 5 to 10 micrometers (μm) and were first described using light microscopy. Light microscopy allows an imaging magnification of about 1500×. However, it was not until the advent of electron microscopy that the finer detail of cell organelles and ultrastructural aspects were scrutinized. Electron microscopy has the potential to expand the imaging magnification up to 250,000×.

Enveloped in a fluid plasma membrane, the cell can be divided into two major parts—the nucleus and the cytoplasm. The plasma membrane is approximately 7.5 to 10 nanometers (nm) thick, and its approximate composition by mass is proteins, 55%; phospholipids, 25%; cholesterol, 13%; other lipids 4%; and carbohydrates, 3%. The plasma membrane is arranged in a lipid bilayer structure, thus making the membrane merely two molecules thick (Figure 1.2). Phospholipids and cholesterol make up most of the lipid bilayer and are oriented so that their hydrophilic (water-soluble) portion faces the watery medium of the intracellular and extracellular fluids and their hydrophobic (water-insoluble) portion faces the internal aspect of the bilayer. The major phospholipids in the plasma membrane can vary among cell types; however, they will generally include phosphatidylcholine (lecithin), phosphatidylethanolamine, phosphatidylserine, and sphingomyelin (Figure 1.3). Inositol phospholipids are functionally important in cell signaling operations; however, their quantitative contribution to plasma membrane lipid mass is relatively small. The hydrophobic inner region of the bilayer provides a transit barrier impermeable to hydrophilic substances such as ions, glucose, and urea.

The plasma membrane of a small human cell may contain 10^9 lipid molecules, about half of which are phospholipids. Cholesterol and glycolipids account for most of the remaining lipid. The planar cholesterol molecule is oriented so that its hydrophilic hydroxyl group is directed towards the polar ends of phospholipids, and their hydrophobic steroid rings and

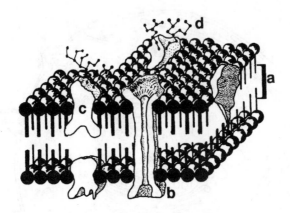

FIGURE 1.2

Membrane structure: the fluid mosaic. A phospholipid bilayer (a) with associated proteins. Transmembrane proteins (b) can extend all the way through the membrane, as in the ion channel displayed. Peripheral proteins (c) are associated with only one side of the bilayer. Carbohydrate extensions (d) from membrane structures form the glycocalyx.

hydrocarbon tail are directed towards the hydrophobic middle region of the plasma membrane bilayer (Figure 1.4). The concentration of cholesterol adds stability to the plasma membrane by preventing phospholipid fatty acid hydrocarbon chains from crystallizing.

Proteins are a major component of plasma membrane, accounting for about 50% of its mass. However, with respect to the molecular size differential between membrane proteins and lipids, the ratio of lipid to protein molecules is about 50 to 1. Cell membrane proteins occur either as peripheral or integral proteins that float within the bilayer. Integral or transmembrane proteins extend through the plasma membrane and function primarily as ion channels, carriers, active transporters, receptor bases, and enzymes. Typically, the portion of these proteins that extends through the hydrophobic core of the plasma membrane is composed mostly of amino acids with nonpolar side chains. Transmembrane proteins are mostly glycoproteins with their carbohydrate moiety extending into the extracellular fluid. Peripheral proteins are typically associated with integral membrane proteins on the intracellular side of the plasma membrane, and their function is mostly enzymatic.

Carbohydrates, in the form of polysaccharides, attached to plasma membrane proteins (glycoproteins) and lipids (glycolipids), along with proteoglycans make up the glycocalyx (Figure 1.2). The glycocalyx provides a carbohydrate coat on the extracellular face of plasma membrane which appears to be involved in receptor activities and cell-to-cell adhesion.

The plasma membrane encloses the cytoplasm, which is comprised of the cytosol and organelles. The cytosol is the clear intracellular fluid containing several substances dissolved, suspended, or anchored within the watery medium. These substances include electrolytes, proteins, glucose and glycogen, amino acids, and lipids. The concentration of these intracellular substances can differ tremendously from the extracellular fluid (Table 1.3). For example, the extracellular fluid may be 14 times more concentrated with sodium and 10 times less concentrated with potassium in comparison to the intracellular fluid. One function of integral membrane proteins is to pump certain substances against their concentration or diffusion gradients to maintain these differences for physiological purposes.

Many of the highly specialized operations that take place inside cells occur within membrane-contained organelles. Organelles include the *endoplasmic reticulum, Golgi apparatus, lysosomes, peroxisomes,* and *mitochondria*. While most types of cells will contain all of these organelles or a highly specialized version of them, their contribution to the total cell

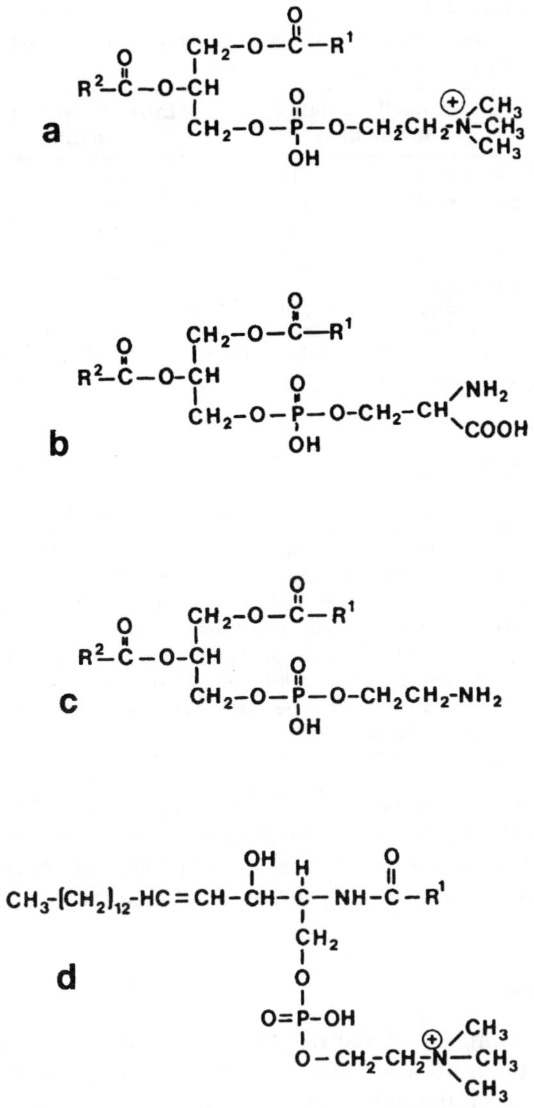

FIGURE 1.3
Phospholipid molecular structures: phosphatidylcholine or lecithin (a), phosphatidylserine (b), phosphatidylethanolamine (c), and sphingomyelin (d). The R indicates the position of fatty acids.

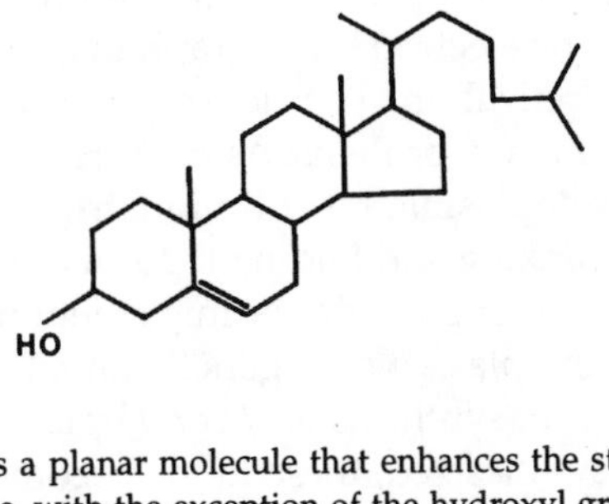

FIGURE 1.4
Cholesterol molecule. Cholesterol is a planar molecule that enhances the stability of the plasma membrane. It is generally a hydrophobic molecule, with the exception of the hydroxyl group (–OH).

TABLE 1.3

Concentration Differences of General Solutes across the Plasma Membrane[a]

	Intracellular fluid (mmol/liter)	Extracellular fluid (mmol/liter)
Sodium (Na+)	12	145
Potassium (K+)	155	4
Hydrogen (H+)	13×10^{-5}	3.8×10^{-5}
Chloride (Cl−)	3.8	120
Bicarbonate (HCO3−)	8	27
Organic anions	155	0

[a] Electrolyte concentration across the skeletal muscle plasma membrane.

TABLE 1.4

Overview of Organelle Function

Organelle	Function and Features
Nucleus	Site of most DNA and transcription; site of rRNA production
Mitochondria	Site of most ATP synthesis in cells; some DNA
Lysosomes	Contains acid hydroxylases for digesting most biomolecule types
Endoplasmic reticulum	Synthesizes proteins and lipid substances destined to be exported from cell; site of glucose 6-phosphatase; participates in ethanol metabolism
Golgi apparatus	Further processes molecules synthesized in the endoplasmic reticulum: packaging site for exocytosis-destined molecules; synthesizes some carbohydrates
Peroxisomes	Contain oxidases; participates in ethanol metabolism

volume can vary. For example, myocytes (muscle cells) contain a rich complement of mitochondria, while the total surface area of endoplasmic reticulum in a hepatocyte (liver cell) is 30 to 40 times greater than the surface area of the plasma membrane. General functions associated with different organelles are presented in Table 1.4.

Endoplasmic Reticulum

The endoplasmic reticulum is a tubular network that is situated adjacent to nuclei. In fact, the space inside the tubular network containing the endoplasmic reticulum matrix is connected to the space between the two membranes of the nuclear envelope (Figure 1.1). The membrane of the endoplasmic reticulum is very similar to the plasma membrane, thus consisting of a lipid bilayer densely embedded with proteins. The endoplasmic reticulum is a major site of molecule formation and metabolic operations within cells.

Visually the endoplasmic reticulum can be separated into the rough (granular) and smooth (agranular) endoplasmic reticulum due to the presence of ribosomal complexes attached to its outer surface. The electron micrograph in Figure 1.5 displays the ribosomal studding of the endoplasmic reticulum. The ribosomes of the rough endoplasmic reticulum are the site of synthesis for many proteins. As they are being synthesized, growing protein chains thread into the endoplasmic reticulum matrix where they can undergo rapid glycosylation as well as cross-linking and folding to form more compact molecules. In general, proteins synthesized by the rough endoplasmic reticulum are destined for either exocytosis or to become part of the plasma or organelle membranes. Contrarily, the smooth endoplasmic reticulum is a site of synthesis of several lipid molecules including phospholipids and cholesterol. Once synthesized, these lipids become incorporated into the endoplasmic reticulum membrane, allowing for regeneration of the membrane lost in the form

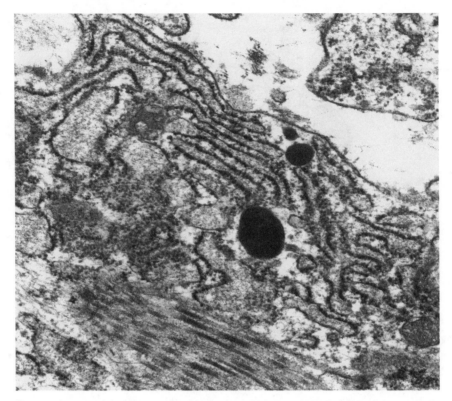

FIGURE 1.5
Rough endoplasmic reticulum. Electron micrograph of rough endoplasmic reticulum (28,000×) presenting the ribosomal studding.

of transport vesicles destined for the Golgi apparatus. Last, the endoplasmic reticulum engages in other significant cellular operations. First, the endoplasmic reticulum of specific cells, such as parenchyma of the liver and kidneys, contains glucose 6-phosphatase which liberates glucose from glucose 6-phosphate generated by gluconeogenesis as well as glycogen breakdown. Also, the endoplasmic reticulum is the site of detoxification of potentially harmful substances such as drugs as well as alcohol. The cytochrome P_{450} system is the primary site of endoplasmic reticulum detoxification operations.

Golgi Apparatus

The Golgi apparatus is composed of several stacked layers of thin, flat, enclosed vesicles and is located in close proximity to both nuclei and endoplasmic reticulum. It functions both in the processing of substances produced by the endoplasmic reticulum as well as synthesizing some carbohydrates. The carbohydrates include sialic acid and galactose as well as more complex polysaccharide–protein-based molecules such as hyaluronic acid and chondroitin sulfate, which are part of the proteoglycan component of mucus and glandular secretions as well as being primary components of the organic matrix of connective tissue such as bone, cartilage, and tendons. However, it is the molecule-processing and vesicle-formation activities of the Golgi apparatus that are without doubt its most famous attributes. As molecules, especially proteins, are manufactured in the endoplasmic reticulum, they are transported throughout the tubular system destined to reach

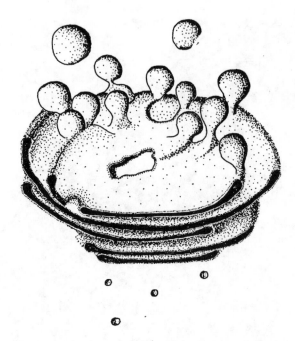

FIGURE 1.6
Golgi apparatus. Budding of vesicles from the plasma membrane face of the Golgi apparatus. The vesicles generally contain substances that will be secreted from the cell.

the agranular portion in closest proximity to the Golgi apparatus. At this location small transport vesicles pinch off and transport these substances to the Golgi apparatus (Figure 1.6). The vesicles introduce their cargo to the Golgi apparatus by fusing with its membrane.

Once inside the Golgi apparatus, endoplasmic reticulum-derived molecules, which are primarily proteins, can have more carbohydrate moieties added and become incorporated into highly concentrated packets. Eventually the packets will bud off of the Golgi apparatus and diffuse into the cytosol. The packets are then ready to fuse with the plasma membrane and release their contents into the extracellular space in an exocytotic process. In light of this activity, these packets are often referred to as secretory vesicles or secretory granules. Cells with greater endocrine, exocrine, paracrine, and autocrine activities, such as the pancreas, adrenal glands, and anterior pituitary gland, will present more secretory vesicles when observed with electron microscopy. Thus, contents of these packets may be hormones, neurotransmitters, eicosanoids, or ductal secretions. Contrarily, some of the concentrated packets are not destined for exocytosis as highly specialized buds from the Golgi apparatus become lysosomes.

Lysosomes and Peroxisomes

Lysosomes, usually between 250 to 750 nm in diameter and loaded with hydrolytic enzyme-containing granules, function as an intracellular digestive system. More than 50 different acid hydroxylases have been determined in lysosomes and are involved in digesting various proteins, nucleic acids, mucopolysaccharides, lipids, and glycogen. Lysosomes are very important in cells such as macrophages. Meanwhile, peroxisomes appear to be produced by specialized buddings of the smooth endoplasmic reticulum and contain oxidases which help detoxify potentially harmful substances. Peroxisomes will

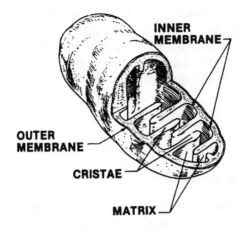

INNER MEMBRANE

OUTER MEMBRANE

CRISTAE

MATRIX

FIGURE 1.7
Mitochondria. Note the inner and outer mitochondrial membranes.

also participate to some degree in ethanol (alcohol) and the oxidation of long-chain fatty acids.

Mitochondria

Aerobic adenosine triphosphate (ATP) generation takes place in mitochondria, which are self-replicating organelles found in almost every cell type in the human body (Figure 1.1). Mitochondria can vary in size within the different types of cells. In some cells, mitochondria may be only a few hundred nm in diameter, while in others they may be as large as 1 μm in diameter and as long as 7 μm in length. The shape of mitochondria can also vary among cell types. For instance, mitochondria are spherical in brown adipose cells, sausage-shaped in muscle cells, and more oval in hepatocytes. The density of mitochondria within a cell type depends primarily upon the oxidative energy demands of that cell. For instance, in light of their dedication to the synthesis of chemical compounds, hepatocytes contains about 800 mitochondria per cell. Likewise the high ATP demands of muscle cells require a rich complement of mitochondria as well. Mitochondria account for about 25 to 35 and 12 to 15% of cardiac and skeletal myocyte volume, respectively.

Mitochondria tend to be located within cells in areas near organelles of high energy demands. Thus, mitochondria would typically appear in close proximity to the nucleus and ribosomes where protein synthesis occurs or near contractile myofibrils in muscle cells. Also, triglyceride-rich lipid droplets are typically visualized adjacent to or at least in close proximity to mitochondria.

Mitochondria contain two lipid/protein bilayer membranes which are commonly called the outer membrane and the inner membrane (Figure 1.7). The outer membrane is very porous and is largely unfolded, while the inner membrane is relatively impermeable and highly folded, which greatly expands its surface area. Along with the other phospholipids common to cellular membranes, diphosphatidylglycerol or cardiolipin is found in mitochondrial membranes, particularly in the inner membrane. Enzymes such as monoamine oxidase, acyl CoA synthetase, glycerophosphate acyltransferase, and phospholipase A_2 are associated with the outer membrane, while adenylate kinase and creatine kinase are found in the intermembrane space.

The inner mitochondrial membrane is the site of oxidative phosphorylation and contains enzymes and cytochrome complexes of the electron transport chain. It also provides a barrier enclosing the mitochondria matrix. The mitochondrial matrix is concentrated with enzymes, largely involved in energy nutrient oxidation, and some DNA. For instance, the enzymes associated with fatty acid oxidation as well as the Krebs cycle are found within the mitochondrial matrix. Oxidative phosphorylation produces mainly ATP, utilizing a series of oxidative enzyme complexes known as the electron-transport or respiratory chain.

The Nucleus and Genetic Aspects

The nucleus provides a storage and processing facility for DNA. It is enclosed by the porous nuclear envelope which is actually two separate membranes, the outer and inner (Figure 1.1). At certain regions, the outer nuclear membrane is connected with the membrane of the endoplasmic reticulum. This allows the space between the two nuclear membranes to be continuous with the matrix of the endoplasmic reticulum. Very large protein-associated pores penetrate the nuclear envelope, allowing molecules having a molecular weight up to 44,000 to move through the envelope with relative ease.

DNA, RNA, and Genes

By and large the deoxyribonucleic acid (DNA) contained within human cells is localized in the nucleus. Small amounts of DNA are also found in mitochondria. All mature human cells, with the exception of erythrocytes (red blood cells; RBCs), will contain one or more nuclei. As a rule, cells beget cells; therefore all nucleated cells will contain the same DNA. Each DNA molecule contains a myriad of regions (*genes*) which code for proteins. Since digestion breaks down ingested food proteins into amino acids prior to absorption into the body, proteins must be constructed within cells from their building blocks — amino acids. Genes contain the instructions for the synthesis of all human proteins. This includes structural proteins, enzymes, contractile proteins, and protein hormones. Proteins will then be involved, either directly or indirectly, in the metabolism of all other molecules in the human body.

DNA molecules are extremely long. It has been estimated that the longest human chromosome is over 7.2 cm long. Human cells contain 23 pairs of chromosomes (22 autosomal and 1 sex-linked), with the exception of sperm and eggs which only have one of each 23 chromosomes. It has been estimated that the DNA in human chromosomes collectively codes for as many as 100,000 proteins.

Despite the fact that human DNA are polymers consisting of billions of *nucleotides* linked together, there are only four nucleotide monomers (Figure 1.8). *Adenine* and *guanine* are *purine* bases while *thymine* and *cytosine* are *pyrimidine* bases. The 5-carbon carbohydrate, deoxyribose, is added to the bases to form adenosine (A), thymidine (T), guanosine (G), and cytosine (C). These structures, which are called *nucleosides,* are found in DNA in a phosphorylated form referred to as nucleotides. DNA links of nucleotides can be written in shorthand format, for example, ATGGATC.

DNA exists in human cells as double-stranded chains arranged in an antiparallel manner. This is to say that one DNA polymer runs in a 3′ to 5′ direction, while the complementary strand runs in a 5′ to 3′ orientation. The strands are held together by complementary base-pairing whereby adenosine on one-strand hydrogen bonds with thymidine on the

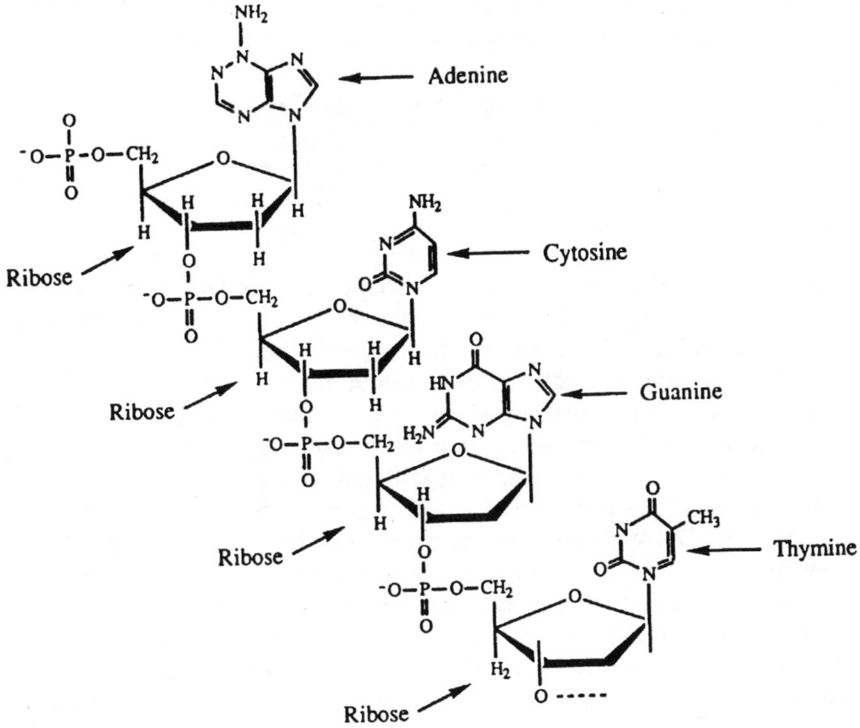

FIGURE 1.8
DNA bases linked by phosphodiester bonds.

other chain, and guanine base-pairs with cytosine (Figure 1.9). The average length of human genes is about 20,000 base-pairs.

Whereas DNA in the nucleus is substantial in quantity and strongly associated with histone proteins to form complex chromosomal structures, the DNA in mitochondrial, contains less than 17,000 base pairs and a very limited number of coding regions. Mitochondrial DNA contains genes for 13 of the 67 or so protein subunits of the electron transport chain as well as for *ribosomal RNA* (rRNA) and *transfer RNA* (tRNA).

The process of protein synthesis has to overcome a few obstacles. First, genes coding for proteins are located primarily within the nucleus. Meanwhile, ribosomal complexes which are the apparatus of protein synthesis exist either within the cytosol or studding the endoplasmic reticulum. Thus, the information inherent in DNA must be delivered from one location to another. This obstacle is overcome by *mRNA* (messenger RNA). Second, the amino acids necessary to synthesize proteins must be made available at the site of protein synthesis. This obstacle is overcome by tRNA. Amino acids are delivered to ribosomal complexes by tRNA and correctly oriented to allow the incorporation in growing protein chains (Figure 1.10).

Protein synthesis begins with *transcription,* the process of producing a strand of mRNA that is complementary to the DNA gene being expressed. First the double-stranded DNA is temporarily opened at the site of the gene and then ribonucleotides are sequentially base-paired to the DNA template. The process is catalyzed by RNA polymerase II and influenced and regulated by promoter and enhancer sequences of DNA occurring either prior to or after the coding region. The formation of the DNA–RNA complementary base-pairing is the same as for DNA–DNA base-pairing, with one exception: the pyrimidine base *uracil* (U) substitutes for thymine in base-pairing with adenine. Other than the substitution of a uracil base for thymine, the molecular structure of RNA is the same as DNA with the exception that the nucleotides contain ribose instead of deoxyribose.

Base-Pairing of Nucleic Acid Bases

DNA–DNA	DNA–RNA
A–T	A–U
C–G	C–G

The initial RNA strand created during transcription, called *hetergeneous nuclear RNA* (hnRNA), is relatively large and generally unusable in this state. Therefore the newly created hnRNA strand must undergo *posttranscriptional* modification. Segments of the hnRNA strand that do not code for the final protein must be removed and the remaining segments that do code for the final protein must be joined together. This process is called *splicing*, while the removed segments are referred to as *introns* and the remaining segments are *exons*. Furthermore, the RNA strand is modified at both ends.

The ribosomal complexes providing the site of protein synthesis must be constructed from RNA subunits. DNA contains specific regions which, when transcribed, produce RNA strands that are not used in instructing protein amino acid sequencing but rather are used to construct ribosomal complexes. The enzyme RNA polymerase I, transcribes the rRNA 45S precursor which undergoes a number of cleavages and ultimately produces the 18S and 28S rRNA. The latter rRNA is hydrogen-bonded to a 5.8S rRNA molecule. Last, a 5S rRNA is produced by RNA polymerase III. The 18S rRNA complexes with proteins to form the 40S ribosomal subunit, while the 28S, 5.8S, and 5S rRNA complex with proteins to form the 60S ribosomal subunit. The 40S and the 60S ribosomal subunits migrate through the nuclear pores and ultimately condense to form the 80S ribosome which, once situated, becomes a site of protein synthesis.

Protein Synthesis

In order for proteins to be constructed, the abstruse genetic nucleotide language must be translated into amino acid chains. This led to the coining of the term *translation*. Amino acids are specifically linked together as dictated by the sequencing of RNA in the finalized version of mRNA. Messenger RNA contains a series of triplets of bases coding for a given amino acid. These coding triplets, or *codons*, are the complimentary base triplets originally transcribed in DNA (Table 1.5). RNA codons in mRNA either indicate a specific amino acid or they are signals for either the initiation or termination of the synthesis of a protein. Certain amino acids will have more than one RNA triplet; for example, alanine has four codons while arginine has six. Contrarily, some amino acids will only have a single codon; for example methionine and tryptophan both only have one codon apiece. Codons are nearly universal, meaning that they will code for the same amino acids in most species; however, some differences have been found in codons translated in mitochondria.

Transfer RNAs are small cytosolic RNA molecules of about 80 nucleotides in length. They attach to specific amino acids and deliver them to ribosomal complexes. Transfer RNA is then able to recognize when to include its amino acid into growing protein chain by codon–antiocodon recognition. Each tRNA contains a triplet of bases that will interact with its complimentary codon on the mRNA strand being translated. This allows the sequencing of amino acids into growing protein chains to be a very accurate process.

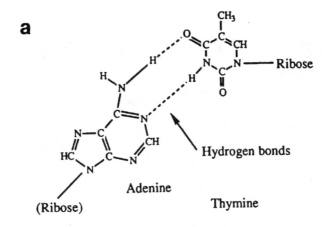

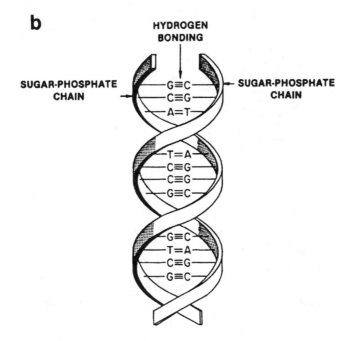

FIGURE 1.9
Hydrogen bonding between complimentary nucleotide bases. The hydrogen bond link between adenine and thymine (a); and hydrogen bonding between the double helical DNA strands (b).

Proteins that are synthesized on ribosomal complexes studding the endoplasmic reticulum thread into the endoplasmic reticulum matrix. As mentioned previously, these proteins are often modified by the addition of carbohydrate moieties to form glycoproteins. In contrast, proteins formed in association with cytosolic ribosomal complexes mostly remain as free proteins. Again, the free proteins formed in the cytosol remain mostly within the cell, while most of the protein formed in association with the endoplasmic reticulum is destined for exocytosis from the cells or to become part of cell membranes.

From an energy standpoint, protein synthesis is a very ATP-expensive operation. To begin with, amino acids must be activated before they can attach to their corresponding

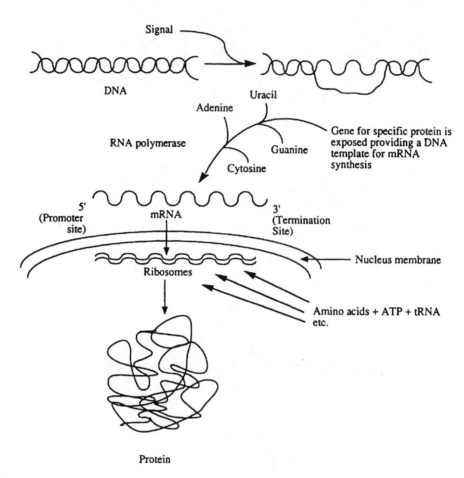

FIGURE 1.10
Protein synthesis.

TABLE 1.5
Genetic Code

First Base (5′)	Second Base				Third Base (3′)
	U	C	A	G	
U	Phe	Ser	Tyr	Cys	U
	Phe	Ser	Tyr	Cys	C
	Leu	Ser	Term	Term	A
	Leu	Ser	Term	Trp	G
C	Leu	Pro	His	Arg	U
	Leu	Pro	His	Arg	C
	Leu	Pro	Gln	Arg	A
	Leu	Pro	Gln	Arg	G
A	Ile	Thr	Asn	Ser	U
	Ile	Thr	Asn	Ser	C
	Ile	Thr	Lys	Arg	A
	Met	Thr	Lys	Arg	G
G	Val	Ala	Asp	Gly	U
	Val	Ala	Asp	Gly	C
	Val	Ala	Glu	Gly	A
	Val	Ala	Glu	Gly	G

tRNA. Thus, if a synthesized protein contains 500 amino acids, then 500 ATP molecules must be utilized simply in forming amino acid-tRNA associations. Furthermore, the initiation of translation as well as protein elongation requires even more energy. A portion of the energy demands is provided by the hydrolysis of guanosine triphosphate (GTP). It is estimated that every amino acid–amino acid linkage in a protein requires the energy contribution made by the hydrolysis of four high-energy bonds, provided by ATP and GTP.

Electron Transport Chain and Oxidative Phosphorylation

Perhaps the most important function of any cell in the human body is the formation of ATP. ATP is then used by cells to promote three major categories of function: membrane transport, synthesis of molecules, and mechanical work. Substances either directly or indirectly transported by *active* or ATP-requiring processes include sodium, potassium, chloride, urate, and hydrogen ions as well as other ions and organic substances (Figure 1.11). The cost of active transportation can be extremely heavy in some cells. For example, tubular cells in the kidneys attribute as much as 80% of their ATP expenditure to active transportation. Meanwhile, the synthesis in cells of chemical compounds such as proteins, purines, pyrimidines, cholesterol, phospholipids, and a whole host of other compounds is also extremely energy costly. Some cells may dedicate as much as 75% of their produced ATP to synthetic processes. With regard to mechanical work performed by cells, muscle fiber contraction accounts for most of the ATP utilized for these specialized processes. The balance comes mostly from the minimal contribution of ameboid and ciliary motion performed by certain cells.

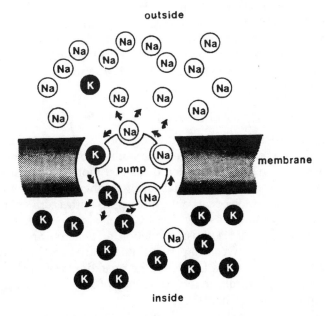

FIGURE 1.11
Sodium/potassium ATPase pump. ATP is hydrolyzed to provide the energy necessary to concomitantly pump sodium and potassium across the plasma membrane against their concentration gradients.

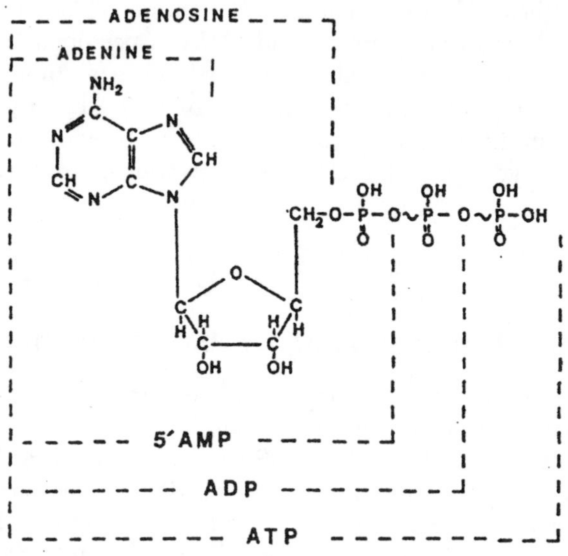

FIGURE 1.12
Adenosine triphosphate. ATP is the primary high-energy molecule produced in human cells. Bonds between the phosphate groups are hydrolyzed to liberate energy which is applied to cellular processes.

ATP is constantly consumed and regenerated in human cells. The structure of ATP, which is depicted in Figure 1.12, reveals an adenine base linked to ribose which itself has a tail of three phosphates linked in series by anhydride bonds. The free energy derived from ATP comes from the hydrolytic splitting of anhydride bonds. These bonds thus became known as *high-energy bonds*. When ATP is hydrolyzed the $\Delta G^{\circ\prime} = -7.3$ kcal/mole. The free energy released when ATP is hydrolyzed is used to drive reactions that require energy. Generally, adenosine diphosphate (ADP) is formed, along with inorganic phosphate (P_i) or adenosine monophosphate (AMP) and pyrophosphate (PP_i). Furthermore, ATP can transfer a phosphate group to compounds such as glucose. ATP, ADP, and AMP are interconvertable by the adenylate kinase reaction.

$$ATP + AMP \leftrightarrow 2\,ADP$$

Carbohydrates, amino acids, triglycerides, ethanol, and their intermediates, derived directly from the diet or mobilized from cellular stores, provide the substrates for ATP formation. As discussed in greater detail later, these fuel molecules must engage in various chemical reaction series or *pathways* in order for their inherent energy to be utilized in the formation of ATP. The utilization of carbohydrate begins with a series of chemical reactions occurring in the cytosol, known as *glycolysis*. Glycolysis generates a net production of 2 ATP molecules by substrate-level phosphorylation, an anaerobic process. Glycolysis also generates pyruvate molecules which can enter mitochondria and be converted to the activated 2-carbon residue acetyl CoA. Likewise, the breakdown of fatty acids, some amino acids, as well as ethanol also results in the production of acetyl CoA. These metabolic pathways are discussed in detail in Chapter 11.

Mitochondrial acetyl CoA condenses with oxaloacetate to form citrate, which then enters the Krebs cycle (Figure 1.13). The Krebs cycle, also known as the citric acid cycle and the tricarboxylic acid (TCA) cycle, is a series of seven main chemical reactions in which the final reaction regenerates oxaloacetate. Therefore, this pathway is considered cyclic. The net result of these reactions is the production of reduced cofactors which will then transfer the electrons to the electron transport chain. NADH and $FADH_2$ are the reduced forms of

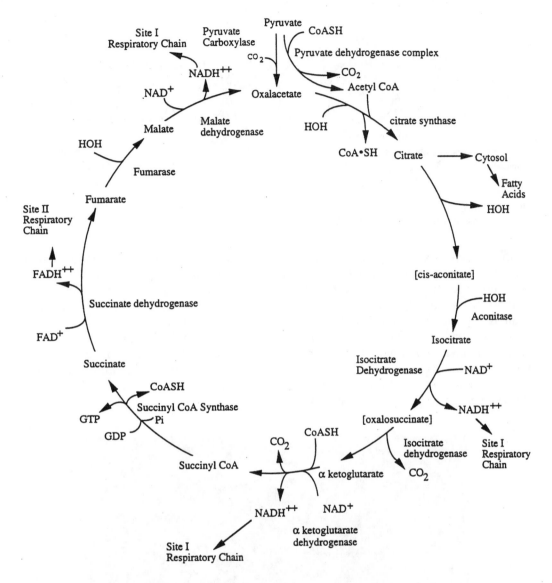

FIGURE 1.13
The Krebs cycle. Reduced electron carriers (NADH and FADH$_2$) transfer electrons to the electron transport chain (respiratory chain).

NAD$^+$ and FAD, respectively. Reactions in the Krebs cycle produce 3 NADH and 1 FADH$_2$. Fatty acid oxidation (β-oxidation) also creates NADH and FADH$_2$, and how many of these reduced cofactors are produced depends upon the length of a particular fatty acid. Furthermore, NADH is also produced in the conversion of pyruvate to acetyl CoA in the mitochondria as well as by glycolysis in the cytosol.

Carbon dioxide is produced in the conversion of pyruvate to acetyl CoA as well as in two reactions in the Krebs cycle. These reactions are the primary producers of this metabolic waste molecule in cells. Guanosine triphosphate (GTP) is also generated by a reaction in the Krebs cycle and functions to drive certain biochemical reactions, such as translation.

As mentioned above, ATP is generated anaerobically in one chemical reaction of glycolysis. This is an important source of ATP for all cells and is the sole source of ATP for

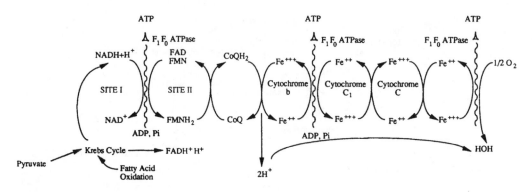

FIGURE 1.14

Electron transport chain. Note that O_2 is the final electron acceptor.

erythrocytes (RBCs), which lack mitochondria. However, most of the ATP generated within cells occurs via oxidative phosphorylation by the electron transport chain. Oxygen is required for operation of the electron transport chain as the final acceptor of electrons. Without the availability of oxygen, the flow of electrons through the electron transport chain is halted and mitochondrial ATP generation ceases (Figure 1.14).

The electron transport chain is a series of protein-based complexes stitched into the mitochondrial inner membrane. The inner membrane is highly folded, which increases its surface area and thus the number of electron transport chains per mitochondrion. The folds are known as *cristae* and mitochondria of certain cells, such as cardiac muscle cells, are densely packed with cristae (Figure 1.15).

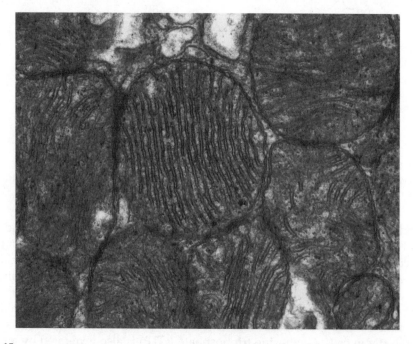

FIGURE 1.15

Electron micrograph of cardiac myocyte mitochondria (25,000×). Note the densely packed inner membrane or cristae.

Reduced cofactors, NADH and $FADH_2$, transfer electrons to the electron transport chain. NADH is viewed as free floating within the mitochondrial matrix as well as the cytosol. Thus, when NAD^+ becomes reduced to NADH, it can diffuse to electron transport chains. This certainly seems true of NADH generated within the mitochondria. However, NADH produced in the cytosol probably must rely on an electron-translocation system for its electrons to reach the electron transport chain. On the other hand, FAD is bound tightly to enzymes in the mitochondrial inner membrane. Thus, FAD reduced to $FADH_2$ will not need to endure diffusion and is in theory immediately available to the electron transport chain.

Electrons move forward through the electron transport chain towards O_2 because of the large $\Delta G^{\circ\prime}$ gradient. The transfer of electron from NADH to O_2 occurs in three stages, each of which is associated with the production of one ATP. Meanwhile, the transfer of electrons from $FADH_2$ to O_2 occurs in two principal steps, both of which are associated with the production of one ATP. Therefore 3 ATP will be created for each NADH oxidized and 2 ATP will be created for each oxidized $FADH_2$.

Electrons are passed from NADH to flavin mononucleotide (FMN) as catalyzed by NADH dehydrogenase. FMN then passes the electrons through a series of iron–sulfur (Fe-S) complexes to coenzyme Q (CoQ). Coenzyme Q accepts the electrons one at a time, first forming semiquinone and then ubiquinol. The energy liberated by the transfer of electrons at this point is adequate to pump protons to the cytosolic side of the mitochondrial inner membrane. The pumping of electrons at this and other points of the electron transport chain establishes a chemoelectrical potential or proton-motive force. As the mitochondrial inner membrane is generally impermeable to proton diffusion, movement of protons back into the matrix occurs through highly specialized ATP-synthase complexes (F_0-F_1/ATPase). F_0 proteins form a physical channel allowing proton passage through the membrane and are also connected to the F_1 (ATP-synthesizing head) proteins. This is the site of ATP formation. $FADH_2$ also passes its electrons to coenzyme Q. However, since the FMN stage was bypassed, there is not an associated pumping of a proton across the mitochondrial inner membrane.

Electrons are transferred from coenzyme Q to cytochrome b and c_1 and then to cytochrome c via the actions of cytochrome reductase. These cytochromes along with others in the electron transport chain consist of an iron-containing heme prosthetic group associated with a protein. Enough energy is liberated in the transfer of electrons from coenzyme Q to cytochrome c to pump a proton across the inner membrane.

Cytochrome c transfers electrons to the cytochrome aa_3 complex, which then transfers the electrons to molecular oxygen and creates water. Cytochrome c oxidase is the enzyme involved with the transfer of electrons to oxygen, and again the energy liberated is significant enough to pump another proton across the mitochondrial inner membrane.

Tissue

Similar cells performing similar or supportive tasks constitute tissue. All of the 200 or so cell types in the human body are generally classified as belonging to four basic kinds of tissue. *Epithelial* tissue lines surfaces such as blood vessels, reproductive, digestive, and urinary tracts, ducts, and skin. It is subclassified into three types of epithelial cells: squamous, cuboidal, and columnar (Figure 1.16). *Muscle* tissue is comprised of contractile muscle cells (myocytes) and includes skeletal, cardiac, and smooth muscle cell types (Figure 1.17).

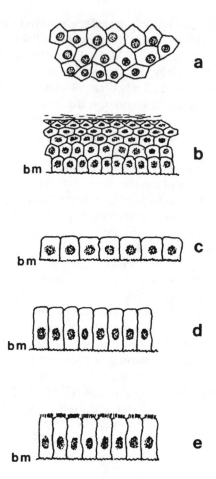

FIGURE 1.16

Epithelia. Different types of epithelia include: (a) squamous, (b) stratified squamous, (c) cuboidal, (d) columnar, and (e) ciliated columnar. Squamous epithelium tends to be flat. Basal membranes (bm) are indicated.

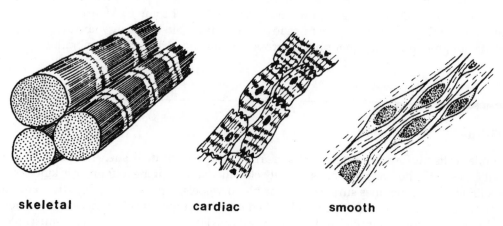

skeletal   **cardiac**   **smooth**

FIGURE 1.17

Muscle cell types.

While the general purpose of muscle tissue is to contract, the different types of muscle have structural and physiological differences. *Nervous* tissue, such as in the central and autonomic nervous systems and other nerves, allows for communication and sensory perception. Last, *connective* tissue is the most abundant, widely distributed, and varied tissue type. It exists as a thin mesh or webbing that helps hold tissue and organs together as well as providing strong fibers for bones, cartilage, and tendons. Blood is also considered a form of connective tissue.

Organ Systems

Organs are structures that are made up of two or more kinds of tissue. The contributing tissue is organized in such a way that they can perform more functions than the independent tissue alone. Organ systems are groups of organs arranged in a manner that they can perform a function more complex than any of the organs independently. The 11 organ systems in the human body and their component organs are presented on Table 1.6.

TABLE 1.6
Organ Systems

Organ System	Tissue/Organ(s) Involved
Integumentary	Skin, hair, nails, sense receptors, oil glands
Skeletal	Bones and joints
Muscular	Muscles
Nervous	Brain, spinal cord, nerves
Circulatory	Heart, blood vessels
Lymphatic	Lymph nodes, lymph vessels, thymus, spleen, tonsils
Respiratory	Nose, pharynx, larynx, trachea, bronchi, lungs
Digestive	Mouth, pharynx, esophagus, stomach, small intestine large intestine, rectum, anal canal, salivary glands, tongue, liver, gall bladder, pancreas, teeth
Urinary	Kidneys, ureters, urinary bladder, urethra
Reproductive (male)	Testes, ductas deferens, urethra, prostate, penis, scrotum
Reproductive (female)	Ovaries, uterus, uterine (fallopian) tubes, vagina, vulva, breasts

Bone and the Skeleton

The human skeleton is a combination of 206 separate bones and supporting ligaments and cartilage. The bones of the skeleton are attached to muscles, allowing for locomotion. Bones are also utilized for protection. The skull and the vertebrae enclose the brain and spinal cord, respectively, thereby protecting the central nervous system. Twelve pairs of ribs extend from the vertebrae and protect the organs of the chest. Bone also serves as a storage site for several minerals, such as calcium and phosphorus, and is the site of formation for red blood cells (*erythropoesis*).

By approximately 6 weeks of pregnancy, the skeleton is rapidly developing and is visually noticeable with imaging instrumentation. Bone continues to grow until early adulthood, complementing the growth of other body tissue. Up until this point bones grow in both length and diameter. However, around this time, the growth of longer bones, such as the femur, humerus, tibia, and fibula, ceases and the adult height is realized. Some of the bones of the lower jaw and nose continue to grow throughout an individual's life, although the rate of growth slows dramatically.

The longest, heaviest, and strongest bone in the human body is the femur. Its length in an adult is about one fourth of their total height, and it is designed to handle physical stresses, such as vigorous jumping, greater than 280 kg/cm² (approximately 2 tons/in.²). Meanwhile the three small bones in the inner ear are among the smallest bones and the tiny pisiform bone of the wrist is very small as well, having the approximate size of a pea.

Bone contains several different types of cells which are supported by a thick fluid called the *organic matrix*. The organic matrix is about 90 to 95% collagen protein and the remainder is a homogeneous medium called *ground substance*. The collagen fibers are typically oriented along lines of tensile force which provides bone with its tensile strength. The ground substance contains extracellular fluid with proteoglycans, especially chondroitin sulfate and hyaluronic acid. Also deposited within the organic matrix are mineral deposits called *hydroxyapatite* ($Ca_{10}(PO_4)_6(OH)_2$). Hydroxyapatite are calcium and phosphate salt crystals. A typical crystal is about 400 Å (angstroms) long, 100 Å wide, and 10 to 30 Å thick. These crystals have the geometric shape of a long thin plate. Magnesium, sodium, potassium, and carbonate ions are associated with hydroxyappatite crystals. Small blood vessels also run throughout bone and deliver substances to and away from it.

Bone is constantly being *turned over*. This is to say that specific cells are constantly remodeling bone by absorbing and depositing bone components. *Osteoclasts*, which are large phagocytic cells, secrete proteolytic enzymes that digest proteins in the organic matrix and acids (i.e., lactic and citric acids) that solubilize the minerals. On the other hand, *osteoblasts*, found on the surfaces of bone, secretes bone components. Turnover allows bone to adapt or be remodeled according to the demands placed upon it. For example, one of the benefits of weight-training is an increased stress placed on bone, which then adapts by increasing its density. Contrarily, prolonged exposure to zero gravity in space travel decreases the stress on bone and results in a loss of bone density. An expanded discussion of the anatomy and physiology of bone will be presented in Chapter 19.

Nervous Tissue

Nervous tissue is comprised mostly of nerve cells (*neurons*) which serve as a very rapid communication system in the human body (Figure 1.18). The central nervous system (CNS) includes the brain and spinal cord and represents the thinking and responsive portion of human nervous tissue. Links of neurons extend from the CNS to various organs and other tissue, thereby allowing for regulation of their function. Also, links of neurons extend to all skeletal muscle, allowing the CNS to initiate and control movement. Special neurons function as sensory receptors and are located in the skin and in sensory organs (i.e., tongue, nose, ears, eyes) and inside the body. These receptors send afferent impulses to the brain to provide information (i.e., pain, smell, taste, temperature) regarding the external and internal environment. Neurons are *excitable cells* which are able to respond to a stimulus by changing the electrical properties of their plasma membrane. Only muscle and nerve cells possess this ability and thus are deemed excitable.

Electrolytes are dissolved in extracellular and intracellular fluids. However, their concentrations are equal across the plasma membrane (Table 1.3). The concentrations of sodium (Na^+), chloride (Cl^-), and calcium (Ca^{2+}) are greater in the extracellular fluid, while the concentration of potassium (K^+) is greater in the intracellular fluid. For instance, the concentration of sodium in the extracellular fluid is about 14 times greater than in the intracellular fluid, while potassium is about 10 times more concentrated in the intracellular fluid relative to the extracellular fluid. The concentration differences provide the potential for

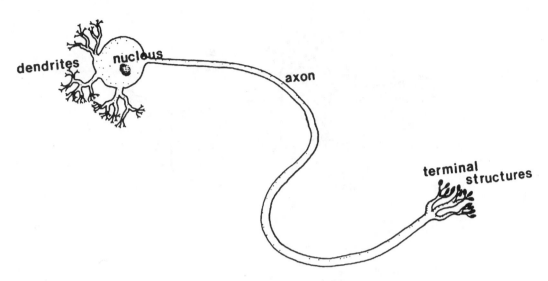

FIGURE 1.18
General neuron structure.

electrolytes to diffuse across the plasma membrane through their respective ion channels when opened (Figure 1.19). At rest, a leaking of potassium ions through channels allows for the development of a net negative charge associated with the intracellular fluid in the vicinity of the plasma membrane and a positive charge associated with the extracellular fluid associated with the plasma membrane. This polarizes the membrane, and the charge difference is referred to as the *resting potential* which is –90 mV as measured in the intracellular fluid. When neurons, like muscle, are stimulated, the resting potential cell is rapidly and transiently reversed and then returns to the resting state. This event, named an *action potential*, is propagated along the plasma membrane like a ripple on a pond.

Although some neurons are very long and may extend several meters or so, the trek of a neural impulse traveling either from a sensory neuron to the brain or from the brain to skeletal muscle or organs, or simply within the brain itself, requires the transmission of the impulse along several neurons linked together. An impulse reaching the end of one neuron is transferred to the next neuron by way of *neurotransmitter* molecules. There are numerous neurotransmitters employed by nervous tissue, including serotonin, norepinephrine, dopamine, histamine, and acetylcholine. Terminal branches of neurons come in close contact with other neurons or tissue such as skeletal or various organs (Figure 1.20). This near connection is the *synapse*, and neurotransmitters are released from the signaling neuron and interact with receptors on the receiving cell as depicted in Figure 1.21. This can initiate or inhibit the firing of an action potential on that cell.

The brain is an organ that is very densely packed with neurons. It weighs about 1600 g in an adult man and about 1450 g in an adult woman and is protected by the skull. It is so designed as to interpret sensory input and decipher other incoming information, to develop both short- and long-term memory, to originate and coordinate most muscular movement, and to regulate the function of many organs. The brain can be subdivided into (1) cerebral hemispheres, (2) diencephalon (thalamus, hypothalamus, epithalamus), (3) brain stem (midbrain, pons, medulla), and (4) the cerebellum. While nutrition is directly involved in the proper development and function of all these regions, certain locations will be especially important. For example, the hypothalamus will be discussed to a greater extent than other regions with respect to its involvement in appetite regulation.

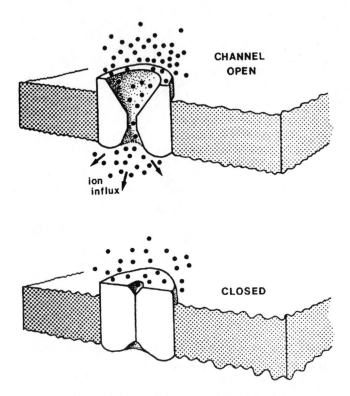

FIGURE 1.19
Ion channel. The regulated opening of ion channels allows for rapid diffusion across the membrane.

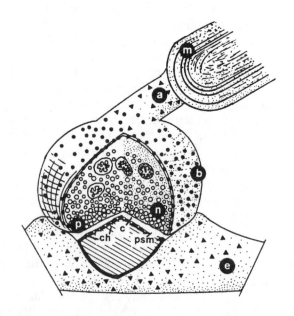

FIGURE 1.20
Axon terminal synapsing with target cell. Displayed is the axon (a), terminal bouton (b), insulating myelin sheathing (m), neurotransmitter-containing vesicles (n) ready to fuse with the presynaptic membrane (p), contacted cell (e), synaptic cleft (c), and ion channels (ch) on the postsynaptic membrane (psm).

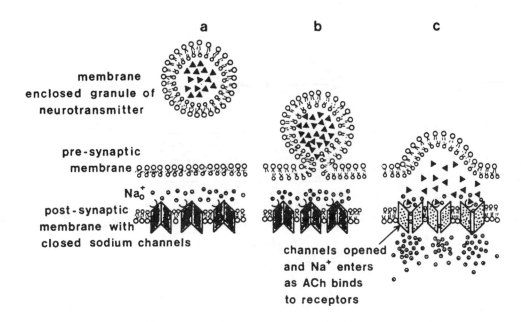

FIGURE 1.21
Neurotransmitter release and action on adjacent cell. Here the nurotransmitter is acetylcholine (Ach), which will open sodium channels on skeletal muscle cells and elicit and action potential.

The spinal cord is about 42 cm (17 in.) and extends from the foramen magnum of the skull; it is continuous with the medulla of the brain stem, and reaches the level of the first lumbar vertebra. The spinal cord in essence is a two-way neural impulse conduction pathway to and from the brain. It is encased by protective vertebrae.

Skeletal Muscle

Skeletal muscle is comprised mostly of very specialized cells that have the ability to shorten or contract upon command by the motor cortex of the brain. Because these cells are very long they are often referred to as *muscle fibers*. Each muscle fiber is encased in a fine sheath of connective tissue called the endomesium and several fibers are themselves bundled up in parallel and encased in a connective tissue sheathing and called fascicles. The fascicles are themselves bundled within dense, coarse connective tissue called the epimysium. Skeletal muscle is so named because it is anchored at both ends to different bones of the skeleton. One anchoring site is called the origin, whereby the bone is generally immobile, whereas the other attachment is called the insertion, in which the pulled bone is moved.

Like neurons, skeletal muscle fibers are excitable as well. In fact, the excitability of skeletal muscle fibers is very similar to that of neurons. However, the end result of excitability in muscle fibers is the contraction or shortening of that cell. There are two principal types of muscle fibers: type I or slow-twitch fibers and type II fast-twitch fibers. The outstanding characteristics of these fiber types will be discussed in Chapter 13.

Light and electron microscopy provide insight to the structural differences between muscle fibers and other cells. Each muscle fiber contains hundreds to thousands of small

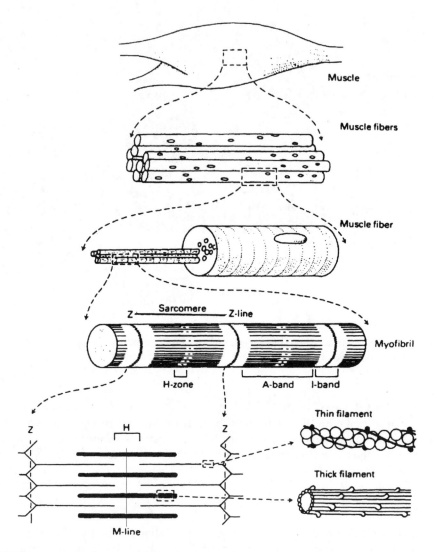

FIGURE 1.22
Gross to fine organization of skeletal muscle components.

fiber-like units called *myofibrils*. Myofibrils can account for as much as 80% of a skeletal muscle cell's volume. Each myofibril is a stalk-like collection of protein (Figure 1.22). The predominant proteins are *actin* and *myosin* which are referred to as thin and thick filaments, respectively. They are organized into a tiny contraction region called a *sarcomere*, which sits next to adjacent and connected sarcomeres (Figures 1.22, 1.23, and 1.24). Other proteins associated with the sarcomeres are *troponins* and *tropomysosin*. These proteins are involved in regulating the contraction of sarcomeres.

When skeletal muscle cells are stimulated, calcium (Ca^{2+}) ion channels open and calcium floods into the region of myofibrils and bathes the sarcomeres. Calcium enters the intracellular fluid from either the extracellular fluid or from storage within an organelle called *sarcoplasmic reticulum*. However, most of the calcium enters from the sarcoplasmic reticulum, which is a modified version of the smooth endoplasmic reticulum. Calcium then interacts with troponin proteins and initiates contraction by removing tropomyosin from the

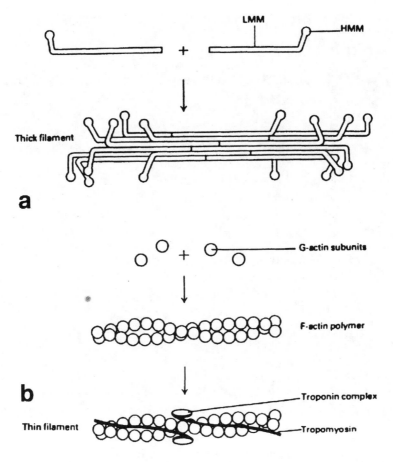

FIGURE 1.23
Components of thick and thin filaments. Thick filaments (a) are comprised of stalks of myosin, which is sectioned into light meromyosin and heavy meromyosin. Thin filaments are comprised of G-actin proteins, which are polymerized into a filament (F-actin). Troponin and tropomyosin proteins are associated with F-actin filaments.

actin-myosin binding site (Figure 1.25). Myosin then slides actin fibers towards the center of the sarcomere, thereby shortening the sarcomere. Furthermore, there is a concomitant shortening of adjacent sarcomeres within a myofibril. Myofibrils in parallel shorten, thereby shortening a myofiber. The shortening of bundled myofibers allows for the shortening of a muscle as a whole.

In order for muscle fibers to contract, a lot of ATP must be utilized and some of the released energy is harnessed to power the contraction. ATP is also necessary for a contracted muscle cell to relax. When the stimulus is removed, ATP is needed to pump calcium out of intracellular fluid of muscle fiber into the sarcoplasmic reticulum or across the plasma membrane.

Heart, Blood, and Circulation

The adult heart is about the size of the carrier's fist and weighs about 250 to 350 g. It serves to pump blood through about 100,000 miles of blood vessels to all regions of the human body. Blood leaves the heart through the "great arteries," namely, the aorta and pulmonary trunk, which feed into arteries that feed into smaller arterioles and subsequently tiny

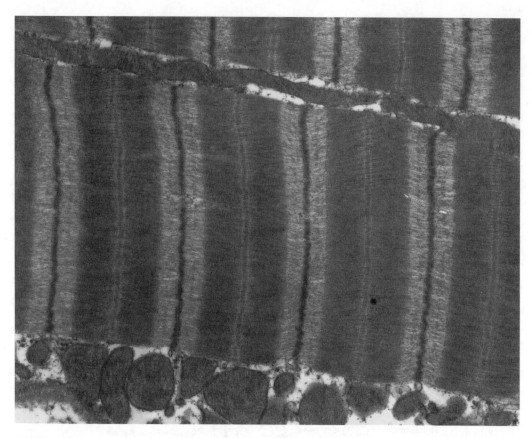

FIGURE 1.24
Electron micrograph of adjacent sarcomeres (27,000×). Note the banding arrangement as well as the presence of adjacent mitochondia.

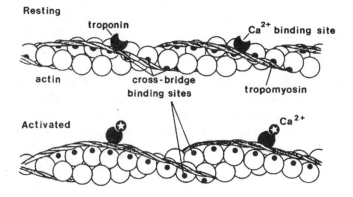

FIGURE 1.25
Calcium binding to troponin results in the movement of tropomyosin and the revealing of myosin binding sites on actin. This allows myosin to bind and myofibrils to contract.

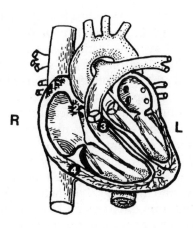

FIGURE 1.26
Human heart. Displayed are the right (R) and left (L) sides of the heart as well as the AV node (1), right atrium (2), aortic valve (3), and right ventricular wall with specialized Purkinje fibers that function to stimulate heart muscle cells to contract.

capillaries that thoroughly infiltrate tissue. Blood drains from capillaries into larger venules, which themselves drain into larger veins that ultimately return blood to the heart. The blood is a delivery system. It delivers oxygen, nutrients, and other substances to cells throughout the human body. At the same time, blood also serves to remove the waste products of cell metabolism such as CO_2 and heat from tissue. Capillaries are the actual site of exchange of substances and heat between cells and the blood.

The heart consists of four chambers (two atria and two ventricles) and can be divided into a left and right half (Figure 1.26). The left half, consisting of the left atrium and ventricle, serves to receive oxygen-rich blood returning from the lungs and pump it to all tissue throughout the body. The right half of the heart, consisting of the right atrium and ventricle, serves to receive oxygen-poor blood returning from tissue throughout the body and to pump it to the lungs. Therefore, the heart functions as a relay station for moving blood throughout the body in one large loop.

The heart is composed primarily of muscle cells that are mostly similar to skeletal muscle cells, yet retain certain fundamental differences. Although most of the events involved in contraction of cardiac muscle are the same as skeletal muscle, the heart is not attached to bone. Furthermore, the heart does not require stimulus from the motor cortex to initiate contraction. The stimulus invoking excitability in the heart comes from a specialized pacemaker region called the *atrioventricular node* or simply the AV node. The heart may beat in excess of 2 billion times throughout human life.

The blood is comprised of two main parts, the *hematocrit* and the *plasma*. *Erythrocytes* (RBCs) are the sole component of the hematocrit and function primarily as a shuttle transport for oxygen. Hematocrit is the percentage of the blood volume that is RBCs. A typical adult hematocrit may be 40 to 45%. Plasma is about 55% of the blood. About 92% of the plasma is water, while the remaining 8% includes over 100 different dissolved or suspended substances such as nutrients, gases, electrolytes, hormones, and proteins such as albumin and clotting factors.

The remaining components of blood are the *leukocytes* (white blood cells) and *platelets*, which collectively make up about 1% of blood. White blood cells are the principal component of the immune system and provide a line of defense against bacteria, viruses, and other intruders, whereas platelets participate in blood clotting.

RBCs have the responsibility of transporting oxygen throughout the human body. About 33% of the weight of a RBC is attributed to a specialized protein called *hemoglobin*. Hemoglobin is a large molecule that contains four atoms of iron. Hemoglobin's job is to bind to oxygen so that it can be transported in the blood. There are about 42 to 52 million RBCs per cubic millimeter of blood, and each healthy cell contains about 250 million hemoglobin molecules. Since each hemoglobin molecule can carry four O_2 molecules, there is the potential to transport one billion molecules of O_2 in each RBC.

When the heart pumps, blood is propelled from the right ventricle into the *pulmonary arteries* for transport to the lungs. Upon reaching the lungs and the pulmonary capillaries, CO_2 exits the blood and enters into the lungs. It is then removed during exhalation. At the same time, O_2 enters the blood from the lungs and binds with hemoglobin in RBCs. The oxygen-containing blood leaves the lungs and travels back to the heart.

Also as the heart contracts, blood is pumped from the left ventricle into the *aorta*. Blood moves from the aorta into the arteries, then arterioles, and finally tiny capillaries in tissue. Blood that has perfused tissue is drained into small venules which drain into larger veins and subsequently the vena cava. The blood leaving the heart is rich with oxygen, while the blood returning to the heart from tissue is relatively poor in O_2. Carbon dioxide from tissue dissolves into the blood with some being converted to carbonic acid via erythrocyte carbonic anhydrase. The venous blood is then pumped by the heart to the lungs to reload with O_2 and release CO_2. Measurement of the blood pumped out of the heart, directed towards either the lungs or body tissue during one heart beat is *stroke volume*. By multiplying stroke volume by heart rate *cardiac output* is determined.

$$\text{cardiac output} = \text{stroke volume (milliliters)} \times \text{heart rate (beats/minute)}$$

Cardiac output is the volume of blood pumped out of the heart, either to the lungs or towards body tissue, in a minute's time. It should not matter as to which of the two destinations one considers as they occur simultaneously and will have a similar stroke volume. Adults have a cardiac output of 5 l/min. During exercise, both heart rate and stroke volume increase, which consequently increases cardiac output. In some, cardiac output may increase as much as 5 to 6 times during heavy exercise. This allows for more oxygen rich blood to be delivered to working skeletal muscle.

Under resting and comfortable environmental conditions, about 13% of the left ventricular cardiac output goes to the brain, 4% to the heart, 20 to 25% to the kidneys, 10% to the skin, and the rest to the remaining tissue in the body, such as the digestive tract, liver, and pancreas. During heavy exercise, a greater proportion of this cardiac output is routed to working skeletal muscle. This requires some redistribution of blood routed to other, less active, areas at that time, such as the digestive tract. On the other hand, during a big meal and for a few hours afterward, a greater proportion of this cardiac output is routed to the digestive tract, which steals a portion of the blood directed to areas having no immediate need, like skeletal muscle.

Blood Pressure

Whether or not blood is in the heart or in blood vessels, it has a certain pressure associated with it. In fact, blood moves through circulation from an area of greater blood pressure to an area of lower blood pressure. When the heart contracts, the pressure of the blood in the heart increases enough to drive the movement of blood throughout circulation. Pressure is

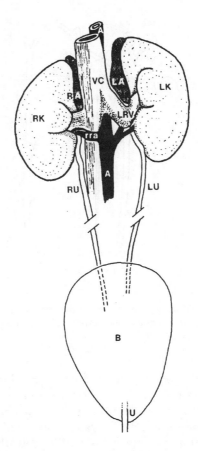

FIGURE 1.27
The urinary system. Displayed are the right (RK) and left (LK) kidneys, the abdominal aorta (A) from which branch the right (rra) and left renal arteries (rra) and right and left (LRV) renal vein and vena cava (VC). Also shown are the positioning of the right (RA) and left (LA) adrenal glands.

the force exerted upon a surface and it is measured in millimeters of mercury (mmHg). Blood pressure is typically measured in a large artery, such as the brachial artery in the arm, and is expressed as systolic pressure over diastolic pressure. For instance, when blood pressure is measured at 120/80 or "120 over 80" the pressure exerted by systemic arterial blood is 120 mmHg during left ventricular contraction and 80 mmHg when the left ventricle is relaxing between beats.

Renal System

Typically understated in function, the kidneys regulate the composition and volume of the extracellular fluid, which includes the blood. The two kidneys, along with their corresponding ureters, the bladder, and urethra, make up the urinary or renal system (Figure 1.27). Although the kidneys are less than 1% of total body weight, they receive about 20 to 25% of the left ventriclur cardiac output. Together the kidneys will filter and process approximately 180 liters of blood-derived fluid daily.

Each kidney contains about one million *nephrons*, which are the blood-processing units (Figure 1.28). Each nephron engages in two basic operations: (1) it filters plasma into a

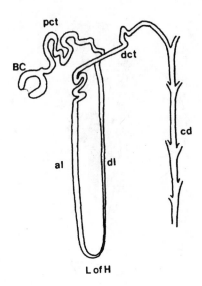

FIGURE 1.28

The nephron. Distinct regions of the tubule system include Bowman's capsule (BC), the proximal convoluted tubule (pct), the descending (dl) and ascending (al) portions of the loop of Henle (L of H), and the distal convoluted tubule (dct) and collecting duct (cd).

series of tubes; and (2) it processes the filtered fluid, reabsorbing needed substances while excreting unwanted or extra substances as urine. A relatively high capillary pressure (60 mmHg) in the glomerulus drives the formation of plasma-derived fluid (*ultrafiltrate*) into the first aspect of the nephron tubule system, Bowman's capsule. Ultrafiltrate is a water-based solution containing electrolytes, sulfites, bicarbonate, phosphates, amino acids, glucose, urea, creatinine, and other substances. Blood cells and most plasma proteins are too large and are not filtered.

There are two possible fates for the components of the ultrafiltrate—they are either reabsorbed back into the blood or become part of urine. Normally the reabsorption of substances such as glucose and amino acids is extremely efficient. On the other hand, the reabsorption of water and electrolytes involves hormonal regulation (i.e., aldosterone and antidiuretic hormone). The active processes in the renal tubule system engaged in reabsorbing glucose, amino acids, and some electrolytes require a significant amount of energy.

Of the 180 liters of fluid filtered and processed by the nephrons daily, less than 1% actually becomes urine. Thus, the reabsorptive processes of the kidneys are extremely powerful. Beyond regulating the composition of the extracellular fluid, the kidneys engage in other homeostatic operations. The kidneys are very sensitive to hypoxia and secrete the endocrine factor *erythropoietin* which stimulates erythropoeisis in bone marrow. Furthermore, renal parenchyma contains a vitamin D metabolizing enzyme which converts a less active form of vitamin D to its most active form.

Hormones

There are two ways that one region of the human body can communicate with the other. The first is by way of nerve impulses and the second is by way of hormones. Hormones are

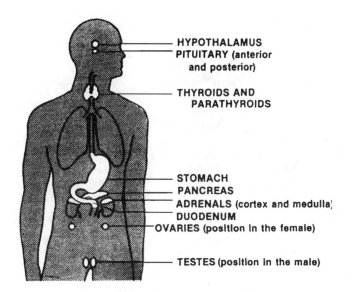

HYPOTHALAMUS
PITUITARY (anterior
and posterior)

THYROIDS AND
PARATHYROIDS

STOMACH
PANCREAS
ADRENALS (cortex and medulla)
DUODENUM
OVARIES (position in the female)

TESTES (position in the male)

FIGURE 1.29
Endocrine organs.

synthesized by endocrine glands of various organs including the pituitary gland, parathyroid gland, thyroid gland, hypothalamus, pancreas, stomach, small intestine, adrenal glands, placenta, and gonads (ovaries and testicles) (Figure 1.29). They are largely protein and protein-based (i.e., glycoproteins), amino acid-based, or cholesterol-derived steroid molecules. Examples of protein hormones include insulin, growth hormone, glucagon, and antidiuretic hormone. Examples of hormones made from the amino acid tyrosine are epinephrine (adrenalin), and thyroid hormone (T_3/T_4). Steroid hormones are made from cholesterol and include testosterone, estrogens, cortisol, progesterone, and aldosterone. Hormones are released into circulation and interact with specific receptor complexes on one or more tissues. Only those cells that have a specific receptor for a given hormone will respond to that hormone. Some cell receptors are located on the plasma membrane and are typically part of a larger complex that has an associated intracellular event upon binding. For instance, the binding of the pancreatic hormone glucagon to glucagon receptors on tissue such as the liver results in an increase in cytosolic cAMP levels. Because cAMP is then responsible for initiating glucagon-intended cellular events, cAMP has been called a second messenger. Other second messengers include Ca^{2+}, cGMP, inositol triphosphate, and diacylglycerol (Figure 1.30). Other hormones, such as thyroid hormone and steroid-based hormones have nuclear receptors. These hormones exert their activity by influencing gene expression (Table 1.7).

Some hormones may have receptors on cells of only one kind of tissue, while other hormones may have receptors on cells of many tissues. For example, the hormone prolactin stimulates milk production in female breasts. Therefore, the cells associated with the milk-producing mammary glands will have receptors for prolactin, while cells of most other kinds of tissue will not have prolactin receptors. Contrarily, growth hormone receptors will be found on cells of many kinds of tissue in the body.

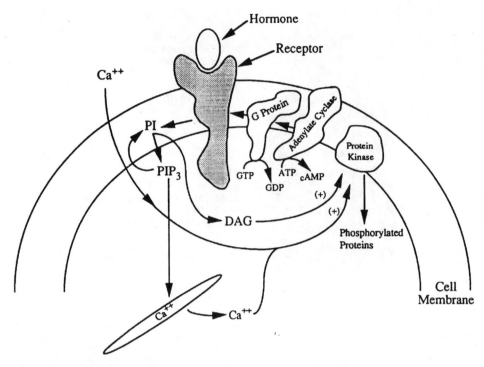

FIGURE 1.30
Second messenger system. The binding of a hormone to its receptor results in an increased intracellular presence of active substances (second messengers) such as calcium (Ca^{2+}), diacylglycerol (DAG), and inositol triphosphate (PIP_3).

TABLE 1.7
Relation of Some Hormones to Nutrition and Metabolism and Their General Function

Source	Hormone	Principal Activity
Pituitary gland	Growth hormone	↑ Growth of most tissue by ↑ protein synthesis and ↑ fat utilization for energy
	Prolactin	↑ Mammary milk formation during lactation
	Antidiuretic hormone	↓ H_2O loss by kidneys by ↑ H_2O reabsorption in nephrons
Thyroid gland	Thyroid hormone	↑ Rate of metabolism
	Calcitonin	↓ Blood calcium levels by ↑ kidney loss and ↓ digestive absorption of calcium
Parathyroid gland	Parathyroid hormone	↑ Blood calcium levels by increasing bone resorption
Adrenal glands	Aldosterone	↑ Sodium reabsorption in kidneys
	Cortisol	↑ Glucose release into blood from liver by breaking down glycogen (stored glucose); ↑ protein catabolism in muscle
	Epinephrine (adrenalin)	↑ Heart rate and stroke volume; ↑ glucose release into blood from liver
		↑ Glycogen breakdown in liver and muscle
		↑ Fat mobilization from fat cells
Pancreas	Insulin	↑ Glucose uptake by fat cells and skeletal muscle
		↑ Processes of fat and glycogen production and storage
		↑ Amino acid uptake and protein production
	Glucagon	↑ Fat release from fat cells
		↑ Liver glycogen breakdown
		↑ Glucose production in liver

Suggested Reading

Guyton, A.C., *Textbook of Medical Physiology*, 8th ed., W.B. Saunders, Philadelphia, PA, 1991.

Marks, D.B., *Biochemistry*, 2nd ed., Harwell Publishing, Philadelphia, PA, 1994.

Murray, R.K., Granner, D.K., Mayes, P.A., and Rodwell, V.W., *Harper's Biochemistry*, 24th ed., Appleton & Lange, Stamford, CT, 1996.

2

Food and the Human Body

Food is any material that is taken into the human body for the purpose of satisfying hunger, growth, maintenance, tissue repair, reproduction, work, or pleasure. As a general rule, humans must eat other forms of life, their derivatives, or synthetically created versions of these things to subsist. Not all forms of life follow this rule. For example, plants largely exist without consuming other forms of life. They are able to absorb water and minerals from the soil in which they grow. At the same time, nitrogen compounds are also extracted from the soil and utilized in the production of amino acids and proteins. Plants can also harness solar electromagnetic radiation for the synthesis of carbohydrates and also produce lipid structures, including a variety of fatty acids. Plants also participate in symbiotic relationships with microorganisms. This can be said for humans and other animals as well. For example, the microflora of the human lower gastrointestinal tract produce small, yet nutritionally significant, quantities of biotin and vitamin K.

Plants exist at the lower end of the food chain, thus serving as food for other life forms. Many animals consume plants to obtain their nourishing substances and are referred to as *herbivores. Carnivorous* animals will eat other animals, while *omnivores* will eat both plants and animals. Humans are omnivorous by nature and exist at the highest end of the food chain.

The ability of food to nourish the human body is indeed the very essence of nutrition science. At this time there are about 40 or so substances that are absolutely required components of the human diet. These substances include several amino acids, a couple of fatty acids, water, vitamins, and minerals. In addition there are several other food-endowed factors that are not necessarily required but are recognized at this time as highly beneficial in the promotion of a healthier existence. These substances include plant fibers and a long list of molecules recently called *nutraceuticals*. The term "nutraceutical" is derived from the concept that these food factors may have somewhat of a pharmaceutical impact in the human body—that they may be beneficial in the prevention, treatment, or recovery of disease. For example, some of these factors have antioxidant properties, while others may increase the activity of detoxifying systems in human cells. The term "nutraceutical" is more encompassing in comparison to terms such as "phytochemicals" and "medicinal botanicals," which imply only plant sources.

Food is consumed by humans for several reasons beyond simple nourishment. Many social, psychological, and philosophical factors can also be involved. A food's sensory characteristics, such as its taste, mouth-feel, sound, and smell, also influence its consumption. For example, several food items, such as soda and snack foods are relatively nutrient void; however, their physical and sensory characteristics make them very appealing and popular.

The isolation of certain food substances or the synthetic creation of those substances in laboratories has allowed for the practice of nutrition supplementation to expand tremendously. It is now a multibillion dollar industry worldwide. A discussion of nutrition supplements along with an expanded discussion of nutraceuticals can be found in Chapter 14.

Nutrients

A nutrient nourishes the human body in one or perhaps several ways. This is to say that a substance provides a function that is considered to be beneficial to human life. For example, vitamin B_6 is important in the metabolism of amino acids, while iron is a key component of hemoglobin, myoglobin, and cytochromes. Typically, nutrients have either been classified as *essential* or *nonessential*. Essential nutrients are said to be those substances absolutely necessary for growth, development, and maintenance, and are not made in the body either at all or in sufficient quantity to meet physiological needs. The list of essential nutrients includes 9 amino acids, 2 polyunsaturated fatty acids, 13 vitamins, about 12 minerals, and water (Table 2.1). On the other hand, the nonessential nutrients are those substances that are either synthesized in the body in adequate quantity or not necessarily essential for growth, development, and maintenance. The list of nonessential nutrients is longer than the list of essential nutrients and has many discrepancies.

TABLE 2.1
Essential Nutrients for Humans

Energy Nutrients	Vitamins	Minerals	Other
Protein[a]	A, D, E, K	Calcium, iron, phosphorus,	Water
Carbohydrates[a]	C, thiamin, riboflavin,	zinc, magnesium, copper,	
Fat[a]	niacin, folate, B_6, B_{12},	iodide, selenium,	
	biotin, pantothenic acid.	manganese, fluoride,	
		chromium, molybdenum,	
		sodium, potassium,	
		chloride.	

[a] Considerations for essentiality will be addressed in later chapters.

Recommended Dietary Allowances

In the U.S., the *recommended dietary allowances* (RDAs) are the recommended average levels of intake for essential nutrients that have been determined by the Food and Nutrition Board to be adequate to meet the known needs of practically all healthy persons (Table 2.2). Several other countries (i.e., Canada) have similar recommendations. They are based on the most current scientific literature. First published in 1943, the RDAs have been revised several times, with the most recent publication (10th edition) having been released in 1989. The nutrient recommendations are ingestion amounts and are intended to be part of a normal diet. The RDAs take into account factors that influence the absorption and utilization of the given nutrients. For instance, the digestion and absorption of several nutrients is incomplete, and the recommendation takes this into account. Also, if a nutrient has one or more precursor substances, the recommendation is adjusted for the efficiency of conversion from the precursor substance(s) to the essential nutrient. This is the case with the conversion of carotenoids to vitamin A and the amino acid tryptophan to niacin.

TABLE 2.2

The Recommended Dietary Allowances

Median Heights and Weights

		Weight		Height		Average Energy Allowance (kcal)	
	Age (years) or Condition	(kg)	(lb)	(cm)	(in)	(kg)	Per Day
Infants	0.0–0.5	6	13	60	24	108	650
	0.5–1.0	9	20	71	28	98	850
Children	1.0–3.0	13	29	90	35	102	1,300
	4.0–6.0	20	44	112	44	90	1,800
	7.0–10	28	62	132	52	70	2,000
Males	11.0–14	45	99	157	62	55	2,500
	15–18	66	145	176	69	45	3,000
	19–24	72	160	177	70	40	2,900
	25–50	79	174	176	70	37	2,900
	51+	77	170	173	68	30	2,300
Females	11.0–14	46	101	157	62	47	2,200
	15–18	55	120	163	64	40	2,200
	19–24	58	128	164	65	38	2,200
	25–50	63	138	163	64	36	2,200
	51+	65	143	160	63	30	1,900
Pregnant	1st trimester						Plus 0
	2nd trimester						Plus 300
	3rd trimester						Plus 300
Lactating	1st 6 months						Plus 500
	2nd 6 months						Plus 500

(continues)

TABLE 2.2 (continued)

Fat-Soluble Vitamins

	Age (years) or Condition	Protein (g)	Vitamin A (m RE)[a]	Vitamin D (mg)	Vitamin E (mg-a TE)[b]	Vitamin K (mg)
Infants	0.0–0.5	13	375	7.5	3	5
	0.5–1.0	14	375	10	4	10
Children	1.0–3.0	16	400	10	6	15
	4.0–6.0	24	500	10	7	20
	7.0–10	28	700	10	7	30
Males	11.0–14	45	1,000	10	10	45
	15–18	59	1,000	10	10	65
	19–24	58	1,000	10	10	70
	25–50	63	1,000	5	10	80
	51+	63	1,000	5	10	80
Females	11.0–14	46	800	10	8	45
	15–18	44	800	10	8	55
	19–24	46	800	10	8	60
	25–50	50	800	5	8	65
	51+	50	800	5	8	65
Pregnant		60	800	10	10	65
Lactating	1st 6 months	65	1,300	10	12	65
	2nd 6 months	62	1,200	10	11	65

TABLE 2.2 (continued)

Water-Soluble Vitamins

	Age (years) or Condition	Vitamin C (mg)	Thiamin (mg)	Riboflavin (mg)	Niacin (mg NE)	Vitamin B$_6$ (mg)	Folate (mg)	Vitamin B$_{12}$ (mg)
Infants	0.0–0.5	30	0.3	0.4	5	0.3	25	0.3
	0.5–1.0	35	0.04	0.5	6	0.6	35	0.5
Children	1.0–3.0	40	0.7	0.8	9	1	50	0.7
	4.0–6.0	45	0.9	1.1	12	1.1	75	1
	7.0–10	45	1	1.2	13	1.4	100	1.1
Males	11.0–14	50	1.3	1.5	17	1.7	150	1.4
	15–18	60	1.5	1.8	20	2	200	1.7
	19–24	60	1.5	1.7	19	2	200	2
	25–50	60	1.5	1.7	19	2	200	2
	51+	60	1.2	1.4	15	2	200	2
Females	11.0–14	50	1.1	1.3	15	1.4	150	2
	15–18	60	1.1	1.3	15	1.5	180	2
	19–24	60	1.1	1.3	15	1.6	180	2
	25–50	60	1.1	1.3	15	1.6	180	2
	51+	60	1	1.2	13	1.6	180	2
Pregnant		70	1.5	1.6	17	2.2	400	2.2
Lactating	1st 6 months	95	1.6	1.8	20	2.1	280	2.6
	2nd 6 months	90	1.6	1.7	20	2.1	260	2.6

(continues)

TABLE 2.2 (continued)

Minerals

	Age (years) or Condition	Calcium (mg)	Phosphorus (mg)	Magnesium (mg)	Iron (mg)	Zinc (mg)	Iodine (m)	Selenium (m)
Infants	0.0–0.5	400	300	40	6	5	40	10
	0.5–1.0	600	500	60	10	5	50	15
Children	1.0–3.0	800	800	80	10	10	70	20
	4.0–6.0	800	800	120	10	10	90	20
	7.0–10	800	800	170	10	10	120	30
Males	11.0–14	1,200	1,200	270	12	15	150	40
	15–18	1,200	1,200	400	12	15	150	50
	19–24	1,200	1,200	350	10	15	150	70
	25–50	800	800	350	10	15	150	70
	51+	800	800	350	10	15	150	70
Females	11.0–14	1,200	1,200	280	15	12	150	45
	15–18	1,200	1,200	300	15	12	150	50
	19–24	1,200	1,200	280	15	12	150	55
	25–50	800	800	280	15	12	150	55
	51+	800	800	280	10	12	150	55
Pregnant		1,200	1,200	320	30	15	175	65
Lactating	1st 6 months	1,200	1,200	355	15	19	200	75
	2nd 6 months	1,200	1,200	340	15	16	200	75

Estimated Safe and Adequate Daily Dietary Intakes of Vitamins and Minerals

	Age (years)	Biotin (mg)	Pant. Acid (mg)	Copper (mg)	Manganese (mg)	Fluoride (mg)	Chromium (mg)	Molybdenum (mg)
Infants	0.0–0.5	10	2	0.4–0.6	0.3–0.6	0.1–0.5	10.0–40	15–30
	0.5–1.0	15	3	0.6–0.7	0.6–1.0	0.2–1.0	20–60	20–40
Children	1.0–3.0	20	3	0.7–1.0	1.0–1.5	0.5–1.5	20–80	25–50
and	4.0–6.0	25	3.0–4.0	1.0–1.5	1.5–2.0	1.0–2.5	30–120	30–75
Adolescents	7.0–10	30	4.0–5.0	1.0–2.0	2.0–3.0	1.5–2.5	50–200	50–150
	11+	30–100	4.0–7.0	1.5–2.5	2.0–5.0	1.5–2.5	50–200	75–250
Adults		30–100	4.0–7.0	1.5–3.0	2.0–5.0	1.5–4.0	50–200	75–250

[a] Retinol equivalents: 1 retinol equivalent = 1 m retinol equivalent or 6 m β-carotene.

[b] α-Tocopherol equivalents. 1 mg d-α-tocopherol =1aTE.

In a different scenario, protein has an RDA and is therefore considered essential as a single entity. However, it is certain amino acids found within protein that are the true essential nutrients, not protein as a whole. The allowance for protein is the sum of the different requirements for several amino acids that occur in different proportions in various food proteins.

The determination of a physiological requirement level for the essential nutrients has been an area of some debate and is not uniform throughout the recommendations. For example, the physiological need of a nutrient by an infant is often equated with the amount necessary to maintain satisfactory growth and maturation. However, for an adult the physiological need of certain substances may be equated to the intake level necessary to maintain body weight and to prevent depletion of the nutrient from the body as determined by balance studies and the maintenance of acceptable blood and tissue concentrations and indices. Or, the physiological need for certain nutrients may be determined as the amount necessary to prevent failure of a specific function or the development of signs of deficiency. This amount may differ greatly for an amount necessary to maintain adequate stores of that nutrient. Therefore, there is not an absolute set of criteria used to determine physiological need used for all essential nutrients.

The RDAs are determined through:

- Nutrient balance studies
- Studies of the physiological impact of absolute and marginal deficiency and repletion
- Measurements of tissue saturation or adequacy of molecular function in relation to intake
- Nutrient intakes of fully breast-fed infants and healthy people from their food supply
- Epidemiological observations of nutrient status in populations in relation to intake
- Extrapolation of data from animal studies.

Once criteria are determined to establish the physiological need for a specific nutrient, then an average intake requirement can be obtained for healthy representative groups of people classified by gender and age. Assuming that population requirements follow a Gaussian pattern of distribution (normal, bell-shaped distribution) the group average intake requirement plus two standard deviations would include approximately 98% of the individuals within that group (Figure 2.1). However, in reality, the requirements for most essential nutrients are not normally distributed. The recommendations for energy are based upon the group mean requirement for weight maintenance, not two standard deviations above the mean, which would theoretically promote weight gain for most individuals within the group.

Dietary Reference Intakes

Just recently, the Food and Nutrition Board in the U.S. developed the *dietary reference intakes* (RDI) that serve as reference values that are quantitative estimates of nutrient intakes to be

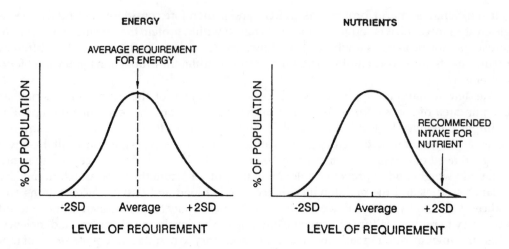

FIGURE 2.1
Two bell-shaped curves for nutrient requirements of a given nutrient. The recommendation (RDA) for nutrients (except energy) is based on two stardard deviations (SD) above the population mean or estimated average requirement (EAR).

used for planning and assessing diets for healthy people. Included in this set of reference values are the RDAs, along with three other types of values. Thus, the development of the DRIs is really an expansion of the RDAs. As mentioned above, the RDA is the average daily dietary intake level that has been determined to meet the nutrient requirement of about 98% of the population of healthy individuals. They are based upon the *estimated average requirement* (EAR) and are set at two standard deviations above the EAR (Figure 2.1). The RDA and the EAR are two of the four RDI values. The remaining two RDI reference values are the *adequate intake* (AI) and *tolerable upper intake level* (UL).

The AI is set instead of an RDA if sufficient evidence is not available to calculate an EAR. These values are based on observed or experimentally determined estimates of nutrient intake by a group(s) of healthy individuals. An RDA and an AI can differ in that an RDA is set to meet the needs of 98% of a given population (age, gender, and reproductive condition). Contrarily, if the EAR is unknown, as the case when the AI is set, it is difficult to estimate what percentage of a given population's requirement would be met by the AI level. The UL is the highest level of daily nutrient intake that is not likely to pose a health threat. Most individuals in the general population are included in this group. As intake of a nutrient climbs above the UL, the risk of toxicity effects increases as well.

Food Sources of Nutrients

In general, the nourishment of the human body can be accomplished by consuming other forms of life and their derivatives or laboratory-created versions of their components. As different forms of life can have vastly different structural and functional aspects, it is logical to think that nutrient density will differ among foods. For example, since the primary tissue type in mammals is skeletal muscle, meats will be among the better food sources of factors found within skeletal muscle. This includes protein and creatine. Contrarily, plants which do not have self-locomotive properties, do not contain skeletal muscle and logically would not be a better source of protein or creatine. However, plants produce several factors that improve the smell, taste, and coloring of their seed-carrying offspring. This allows fruits and vegetables to be more attractive to animals that might consume them and ultimately transport and release the seeds in new locations after they have traversed their gastrointestinal systems. Thus, plant-derived foods may be unique in their ability to provide such substances as carotenoids.

Water

Water is ingested in two forms: in drinking water and foods and beverages. Water is found in almost every food source. In animals and plants it provides the basis for the intracellular and extracellular fluids. In other food sources it can function as a dispersing medium or solvent or as the dispersed phase in some emulsified products such as butter and margarine. Many fruits and vegetables have a water content of greater than 75 to 80% of their mass. For example, tomatoes and lettuce are approximately 95% water, while cabbage, oranges, and bananas are 92, 87, and 75% water, respectively. Milk is about 87% water, while most meats are about two thirds water. On the other hand, rice is only 12% water and oils and shortening are basically void of water.

Protein

Proteins are amino acid-based polymers found in all forms of life. In many well-developed countries such as the U.S., individuals may derive a greater portion of their protein from the ingestion of animal products. Meanwhile, in other parts of the world, individuals may obtain the majority of their dietary protein from plant-based foods.

The protein derived from animal sources is primarily milk proteins, muscle cell proteins, connective tissue proteins, and egg proteins. Milk proteins are casein, which make up 78% of milk's nitrogen-based mass, and the serum proteins, which contribute about 17% to the mass. The remaining 5% is largely nonprotein nitrogen-containing substances, which include amino acids and peptides. Casein is a heterogeneous family of phosphoproteins which exist in milk as relatively large, nearly spherical particles of 30 to 300 nm in diameter. Casein can be separated by electrophoresis into three major components, α-, β-, and γ-casein, so designated in decreasing order of mobility. The serum proteins or whey proteins consist largely of β-lactoglobulin, lactalbumin, immune globulins, and other albumins. β-Lactoglobulin, having a molecular weight of 36,000, is the most abundant whey protein. It is rich in the amino acids, lysine, leucine, glutamic acid, and aspartic acid and consists of two subunits. It is the only milk protein to contain the sulfur-containing amino acid cysteine, which plays a role in the development of the flavor of cooked milk. The immune globulins are largely IgM, IgA, and IgG (1 and 2). The concentration of these factors is greater in colostrum.

The protein in animal flesh (meat) is about 70% structural or fibrillar proteins and about 30% water-soluble proteins. Myosin (~38%), actin (~17%), and tropomyosin (~7%) are the predominant fibrillar proteins, along with stroma (connective tissue) proteins (~6%). The myosin has a molecular weight of about 500,000 and is about two thirds alpha-helical in structure. It has two general functions, structural and enzymatic (ATPase), and is divided into two subunit types, heavy meromyosin (HMM) and light meromyosin (LMM). Actin occurs in two forms, G-actin which is spherical in shape and has a molecular weight of about 47,000, and F-actin which is a large polymer of G-actin.

Meat skeletal muscle contractile portions are covered in layers of connective tissue. The amount and nature of the connective tissue greatly influences the toughness or tenderness of a meat. The predominant connective tissue protein type is collagen. Collagen is arranged in a triple helix called tropocollagen in which molecules are arranged in parallel to form fibrils. The presence of hydroxyproline and hydroxylysine is very important in the cross-linking of adjacent molecules.

Fish proteins are similar to mammalian meat proteins; however, there are some differences. In fish, skeletal muscle is organized so that shorter fibers are arranged between connective tissue sheets. Microscopically the striated appearance of fish myofibrils is similar to mammals and contains the same proteins. The soluble fraction of fish protein is predominantly enzymes and is recognized as about 22% of the total protein content in fish.

Egg proteins can be divided into egg white proteins and egg yolk proteins. Egg white contains at least eight proteins, including ovalbumin, conalbumin, ovomucoid, avidin, flavoprotein-apoprotein, "proteinase inhibitor," ovomucin, and globulins. These proteins, which collectively make up about 11% of liquid egg white, vary greatly in purpose. For example, ovomucoid is a trypsin inhibitor, avidin binds biotin, conalbumin binds iron, and ovomucin inhibits hemagglutination. Hemagglutination is the agglutination of red bloods cells, which is often caused by viruses. The phosphoprotein ovalbumin, which has a molecular weight of 45,000, is the most abundant protein.

As egg yolk contains a considerable amount of lipid, much of the protein found in egg yolk is in the form of emulsifying lipoproteins. Lipoproteins such as lipovitellin and lipovitellenin are excellent emulsifiers, thus explaining why egg yolk is often utilized as emulsifying entities in recipes.

Wheat proteins contain unique properties not only relative to animal proteins but to other plant proteins as well. Some of these properties allow for bread making. There are four main protein fractions in wheat proteins: albumin, globulin, gliadin, and glutelin. When the latter two proteins, as part of flour, are mixed with water they form gluten. Gluten's elastic properties allow for a structural network that holds together other bread components such as starch and air, giving bread structure. Gluten proteins are relatively high in the amino acid glutamine and relatively low in lysine, methionine, and tryptophan.

Soy proteins are a good source of all essential amino acids except methionine and tryptophan. Soy proteins do not include gliadin or glutelin; therefore soy flour can not be used in bread-making without special additives to enhance bread volume. Soy proteins appear to be mostly complex multiprotein globulins. Isolated soy protein (ISP) is used commercially in drinks mixed with fruit and water, coffee whiteners, liquid whipped toppings, and sour cream dressings.

Carbohydrates

As will be discussed in greater detail in Chapter 4, carbohydrates are a molecular class that includes sugars, starch, and fiber. The sugars include both monosaccharides (i.e., glucose, galactose, and fructose) and disaccharides (i.e., sucrose, lactose, and maltose). Starch consists mainly of straight and branching polymers of the monosaccharide glucose. While fibers are also polymers of monosaccharide, they are not limited to glucose. Fibers are generally undigestable by human digestive enzymes; however, bacterial fermentation of several types of fibers occurs in the lower portion of the human digestive tract.

While animal flesh will contain glycogen, much of this carbohydrate is rapidly depleted during slaughter. Therefore, carbohydrate moieties, as part of molecules such as glycolipids and glycoproteins along with minimal amounts of remaining glycogen, provide the small amount of carbohydrate in animal flesh. Unlike in animal flesh, mammalian milk is a good source of carbohydrate. The predominant carbohydrate in milk is the sugar lactose.

Plant sources, on the other hand, are rich in carbohydrates. Carbohydrates are found in fruits, vegetables, legumes, and grains and their flours. Sweeteners derived from plants, such as corn starch, also provide carbohydrate. Corn starch can be partially hydrolyzed to yield smaller carbohydrate fragments to provide a sweet taste. The addition of fructose, forming high-fructose corn-syrup (HFCS) is a popular sweetener especially in the soda industry.

Plant starch occurs in small granules that vary among different species. Starch occurs as either straight chains, amylose or branching chains called amylopectin (Figure 2.2). The number of glucose units can vary from a few hundred to several thousand. Some starch sources, such as peas, may have as much as 75% amylose. Meanwhile, other starch sources, such as corn, rice, and potatoes, amylose is but a minor component (17 to 30%) of total starch. Starch is largely an energy reserve for plant operations.

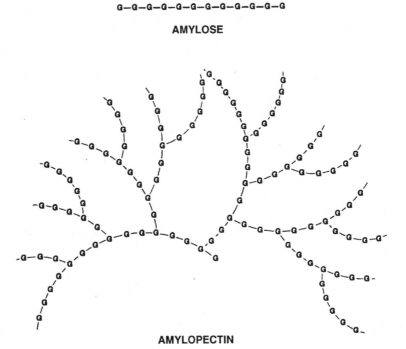

FIGURE 2.2
Starch. Amylose is a straight glucose polymer, while amylopectin contains polymer branch points.

Fiberous carbohydrate molecules or *fiber* include cellulose, hemicellulose, gums, mucilages, algal polysaccharides, and pectic substances. Fiber is often referred to as *nonstarch polysaccharides* (NSP). Lignin is also considered a fiber although it is not truly a polysaccharide. Fibers are mostly structural components of plants, found in cell walls and other regions. For example, cellulose is a long fibrous molecule that is relatively rigid, even in solution. Adjacent cellulose molecules tend to hydrogen-bond, resulting in cellulose crystals that are stalk-like. Heating cellulose-containing foods decreases the crystalinity of cellulose complexes, which decreases the toughness of the food. While fibers are generally recognized for their structural properties, some fibers such as gums and mucilages may have more nonstructural roles in plants.

Lipids

As much as 99% of all lipids in the foods we eat (plants and animals) are in esterified forms. Triglycerides or fat consists of three fatty acids esterified to glycerol, while phospholipids contain two fatty acids. Almost all of the cholesterol in the foods humans eat is esterified to a single fatty acid. Nearly all of the cholesterol in the human diet will come by way of animal-based foods.

As will be discussed in greater detail in Chapter 5, fatty acids vary not only in their length but also in their degree of unsaturation and the nature of their unsaturation. Typical fatty acid length in foods and in the human body generally vary between 2 to 24 carbons. Fatty acids can contain a single point of unsaturation or double bond (monounsaturated fatty acid) or multiple double bonds (polyunsaturated fatty acid). Furthermore, while it is more common to find double bonds in the *cis* configuration they may also be present in the *trans* configuration.

Foods not only vary in the amount of fat they contain but also in the types of fatty acids. For example, fat stores of higher animals contain mostly palmitic, oleic, and stearic acids and tend to be rich in saturated fats. The fatty acid profile of depot fat in animals can be influenced by the feed they consume. Ruminant milk fats have a greater variety of fatty acids, including various shorter chain fatty acids (butyric acid, caproic, caprylic, and capric acid). However, the majority of the fatty acids are palmitic, oleic, and stearic acids. Marine oils are generally lower in saturated fatty acids and higher in unsaturated fatty acids and in remarkably longer-chain unsaturated fatty acids such as eicosapentaenoic and docosahexaenoic acids, which are utilized in eicosanoid synthesis in humans. Fruit seed fats contain primarily palmitic, oleic, and at times linoleic acid. Seed fats tend to have relatively low content of saturated fatty acids, with the exception of palmitic acid.

While most of the double bonds of unsaturated fatty acids in the human body as well as food are of the *cis* configuration, there is the presence of *trans* configurated double bonds as well. In the gut of ruminant animals, microbes produce *trans* fatty acids which are then absorbed. This leads to the deposition of small quantities of *trans* fatty acid in their flesh and also in their milk. For instance, the level of *trans* fatty acid isomers in cow's milk is about 2 to 4% of total fatty acids. Dairy products thus become one of the most significant dietary sources of *trans* fatty acids. Another significant dietary source of *trans* fatty acids are snack foods that include hydrogenated oils in their recipes. The catalytic hydrogenation of oils by the food industry leads to the production of *trans* fatty acids.

Vitamins

Vitamins vary in their general solubility in water. Vitamins A, D, E, and K are considered water-insoluble or fat-soluble, while vitamins C, B_6, B_{12}, thiamin, riboflavin, niacin, folic acid, pantothenic acid, and biotin are water soluble. The solubility of the vitamins can certainly influence their availability within foods. Furthermore, vitamin B_{12} is only found in animal foods, while certain vitamins are produced by bacteria in the human colon. Also, some foods provide vitamin precursor substances, which can be converted to the active vitamin form in the human body. Meanwhile, other vitamins are added to food products in a process called *fortification*. Last, some vitamins have naturally occurring antagonists that can bind to them in the gut and limit their availability for absorption. Meanwhile, other vitamins must either interact with other substances produced in human digestive juices or have molecules attached to them for efficient absorption. These qualities are listed in Table 2.3 and will be discussed in greater detail in Chapter 8.

TABLE 2.3

Selected Characteristics of Vitamins

Only Found in Animal Sources	Commonly Used in Fortification	Have Precursor Molecules	Made by Gut Microflora	Have Natural Antagonists	Require Other Molecules for Efficient Absorption
Vitamin B_{12}	Vitamin A	Vitamin A	Biotin	Thiamin	
Vitamin D	Vitamin D	Niacin	Vitamin K	Biotin	Vitamin B_{12}
Vitamin A	Vitamin C				
	B-Vitamins				

Minerals

The presence of minerals in foods is a combination of minerals, present in the form of inorganic and organic salts or combined with organic molecules such as phosphorus in phospholipids and high-energy phosphate molecules (i.e., ATP) or zinc, copper, iron, magnesium, selenium, etc. as metalloenzymes. The mineral content of foods is determined by ashing or incinerating. However, this process underestimates nitrogen and is not entirely accurate in other regards as well. One of the most influential factors with regard to the mineral content of plants is the respective soil content in which they were grown. For herbivores, carnivores, and omnivores the availability of minerals in plants, especially trace minerals, will ultimately influence the mineral nutriture in a respective species.

Many of the major minerals found in the human body are components of salts and are present in their ionized form, either independent or part of a larger complex. For instance, sodium, potassium, magnesium, and calcium are found as cations, while chloride and sulfates are found as anions. Minerals are also present in foods in the form of *chelates*, which are larger metal complexes formed by coordinate covalent bonding between a ligand and a metal.

Like some of the vitamins, natural components of foods can impact the availability of several minerals for absorption. *Phytates*, a component of plants and associated with fibrous entities, can form insoluble complexes with trace metals such as iron and zinc in the digestive tract. Furthermore, minerals may be provided in different forms, which affects the efficiency of their absorption. Perhaps the most significant example is iron. Much of the iron present in animal flesh is in the form of heme. Heme iron demonstrates a greater efficiency of absorption in comparison to iron otherwise present in animals and plants as non-heme iron.

It should go without mentioning that the total mineral content as well as the relative presence of the various minerals will differ among food sources. For instance, the sodium, potassium, and magnesium content of cow's milk (skim) are 50, 145, and 13 mg/100 ml, respectively. Meanwhile the total calcium and phosphorus content of cow's milk are approximately 115 and 70 mg/100 ml. Animal flesh (muscle) contains much more magnesium relative to calcium and much more potassium relative to sodium. In general, most plants have a high potassium-to-sodium ratio. In fact, sodium is present in wheat only at about 80 parts per million (ppm) and thus can be considered a trace mineral component.

Food Components and Human Senses

Taste

The ability of a food to elicit a smell (olfaction) or taste (gustation) is physiologically significant as it evokes decision-making processes of the central nervous system. Taste and olfactory senses are among the oldest and most influential of the human senses. Taste is elicited
primarily by the function of *taste buds* and is strongly influenced by olfactory events. Both
taste and olfactory sensation involves chemoreception of food components. Other sensory
information detected in the oral cavity, such as the detection of a food's texture by mechanoreceptors and the presence of food components, as in chili peppers, which elicit propri-
oception (pain) also contribute to the perception of taste.

Taste receptors or buds are located primarily within proturbances called papillae on the
surface of the tongue (Figure 2.3). Additional taste buds can be found on the palate, throat,
and epiglottis. Adults have about 10,000 total taste buds, but this number seems to wane
after the age of 45. Taste buds will vary in their chemoreceptive sensitivity to different types
of substances. Taste is a coordinated perception involving four primary taste qualities:
sweet, sour, bitter, and salty, and a limited number of secondary tastes. While a single taste
bud may register more than one of these basic tastes, it will be exceptionally sensitive to
one, perhaps two, primary tastes vs. the others. Furthermore, taste buds with similar taste
sensitivities are localized in specific regions of the tongue. As Figure 2.4 depicts, the middle
tip of the tongue is more sensitive to sweet. Also, the proximal lateral surfaces of the tongue
are more sensitive to salty, while the lateral surface more distal is more sensitive to food
components providing a sour taste. Last, the more distal medial aspect of the tongue is
more sensitive to bitter food substances.

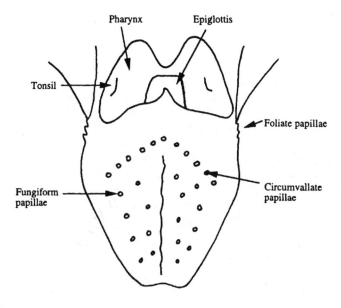

FIGURE 2.3
Papillae of the tongue.

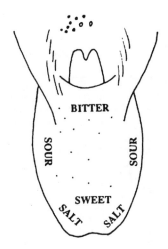

FIGURE 2.4
Locations on the tongue associated with different tastes.

Each taste bud is composed of about 40 specialized epithelial cells and has a total length of about 1/16 of a millimeter and a diameter of about 1/30 of a millimeter. The general design of a taste bud is presented in Figure 2.5. There are two general types of cells in taste buds, taste cells, which are continuously turned over (days), and sustentacular cells, which appear to be more supportive in nature. The outer tips of taste cells are arranged around a small opening called a taste pore. Microvilli, providing the site of chemoreception, extend from the surface of the taste cells exposed to the oral cavities. Taste nerve fibers are interwoven among the taste cells.

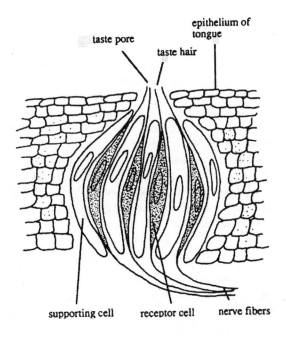

FIGURE 2.5
Taste bud.

TABLE 2.4

Molecules and Characteristics Related to Taste

Taste	Characteristics
Sweet	Property of sugars such as glucose, sucrose, fructose, lactose, and related substances; also lead acetate, beryllium salts, alanine, chloroform, and artifical sweetners such as saccharin and aspartyl-phenylalanine methylester (Nutrasweet)
Salty	Generally sodium chloride and other salts such as potassium chloride, sodium fluoride, calcium chloride, will have a salty taste; however, as the component atoms get larger in size the taste can change to bitter (example, potassium bromide is both salty and bitter and potassium iodide is mostly bitter)
Bitter	Alkaloid substances such as quinine, picric acid, strychnine, nicotine, caffeine, cocaine, and heavy metal salts (Figure 2.6)
Sour	Recognized as the property of hydrogen ions; therefore acids in general will have a sour taste; the nature of the acid group will allow for fluctuations in sour intensity (for example, organic acids will typically have a stronger effect than inorganic acids at the same pH)

When receptors on taste cells interact with specific substances, membrane ion (perhaps calcium) channels open, and the membrane becomes depolarized. The depolarization then spreads to the synaptic surface between the taste cell and the taste nerve fiber. The influx of calcium in this area, and subsequent membrane depolarization, evokes the release of norepinephrine which evokes an action potential on the taste nerve fiber. Taste impulses from the anterior two thirds of the tongue first traverse the fifth cranial nerve and then the chorda tympani into the facial nerve. Taste sensations from the posterior tongue as well as the back of the oral cavity are transmitted via the glossopharyngeal nerve. Smaller pathways are also recognized. Table 2.4 presents the characteristics associated with the four basic taste perceptions, while Figure 2.6 presents molecules associated with a bitter taste.

Smell

Receptors sensitive to substances evoking the sense of smell are located in olfactory epithelium in the upper region of the nasal cavity. Odoriferous substances interact with epithelial cell receptors whose cilia extensions allow for a surface area of 600 cm^2. These substances must dissolve into the mucus coating of the nasal epithelium to interact with cilia receptors. The interaction of odoriferous substances and cilia receptors appears to activate G-proteins and inositol triphosphate-induced calcium release. The release of a neurotransmitter evokes an action potential on an associated neuron which synapses in a glomerulus with second order neurons. From there, neurons pass through the olfactory tract to the inferior frontal lobe of the cortex and on to the other areas of the brain, including the limbic system, to evoke a memory-based emotional and behavioral response (Figure 2.7). There may be as many as 2000 different odors detectable.

Color

Color is a general name applied for all sensations derived from retinal activity. Light is a form of electromagnetic radiation with a wavelength between 400 and 800 nm. Food substances that elicit color are present both naturally or as additives utilized by food manufacturers to enhance the asthetic characteristics of an item. In addition to color, another important visual characteristic of food is *gloss*. Gloss is a reflecting property of a food surface. Naturally occurring food colorants can be largely subdivided into four main groups:

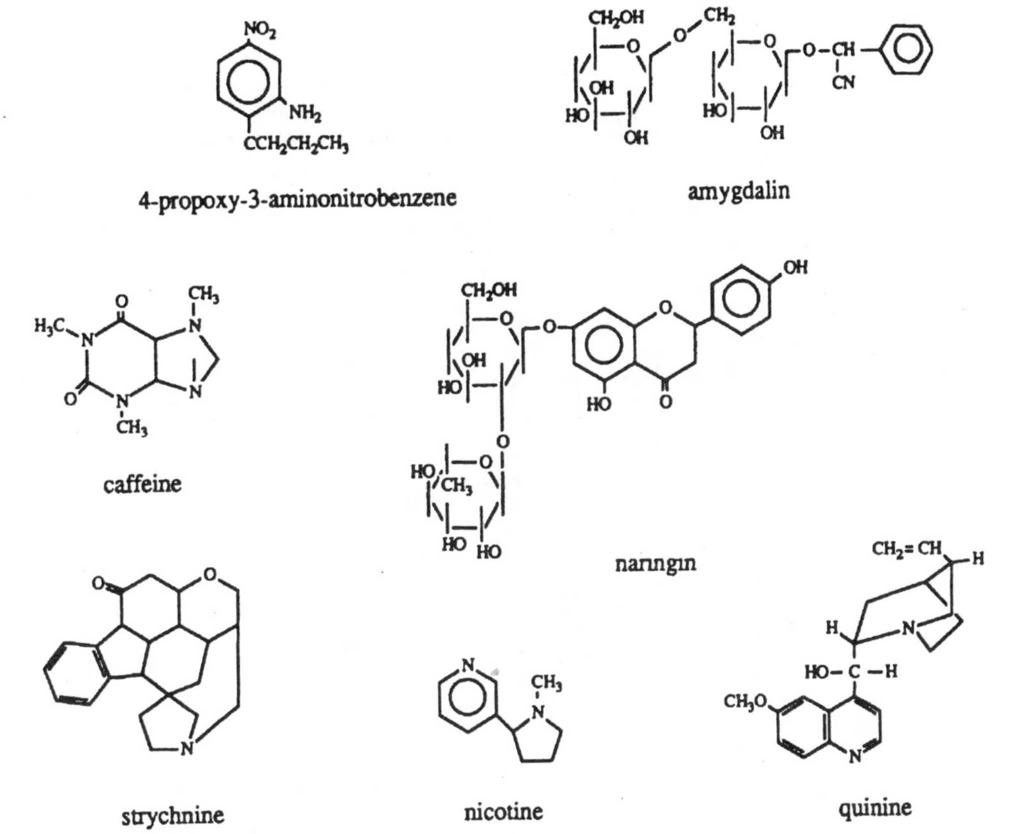

4-propoxy-3-aminonitrobenzene

amygdalin

caffeine

naringin

strychnine

nicotine

quinine

FIGURE 2.6
Molecules that elicit a bitter taste.

(1) *tetrapyrrole* compounds such as chorophyll in green vegetables and leaves, hemes in meat and fish, and bilins; (2) *isoprenoid* derivatives such as the carotenoids widely found in fruits, vegetables, crustaceans, eggs, cereals, etc.; (3) *benzopyran* derivatives such as anthrocyanins and flavonoids, found in root vegetables and fruits such as berries and grapes; and (4) *artifacts* such as melanoidins and caramels, found in syrups and cereal products, especially after heat treatment.

Tetrapyrole (four pyroles) pigments comprise most of the basic structure of heme pigments, which are basic components of hemoglobin and myoglobin in animals. Heme contains a central iron atom that provides the anchoring point for each of the four individual pyrole moities. Fresh meat contains very little hemoglobin; therefore most of the reddish-purple color is attributable to the presence of myoglobin. When myoglobin is bound to oxygen, the pigment produces a red color; however, as the central irons in heme molecules become oxidized with time, forming metmyoglobin, the reddish color gives way to brown.

Chlorophyll is the green pigment that provides the characteristic color to many vegetables and leafy plants. chlorophylls may also provide color to unripe fruits; however, during the ripening process, chlorophyll fades and other pigments dictate the color. In plants chlorophyll is located in chloroplasts and is a large tetrapyrole-based molecule like heme. However, magnesium, not iron, occupies the central position in chlorophyll.

The carotenoids (carotenes and xanthophylls), whose name is derived from carrots (*Daucus carota*), are perhaps the recognizable form of coloring pigment within the isoprenoid class. Carotenes and xanthophylls differ only slightly in that true carotenes are

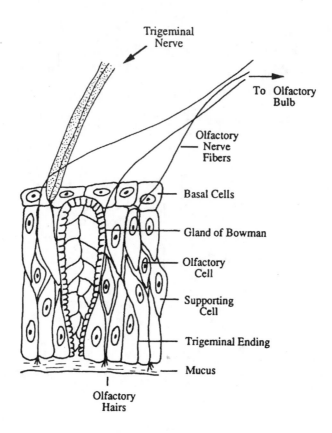

FIGURE 2.7
Olfactory cells.

purely hydrocarbon molecules (i.e., lycopene, α-carotene, β-carotene, γ-carotene), the xanthophylls (i.e., lutein, capsanthin, cryptoxanthin, zeaxanthin, astaxanthin) contain oxygen in the form of a hydroxyl, methoxyl, carboxyl, keto, or epoxy group. The structure of β-carotene is presented in Figure 2.8. With the exception of crocetin and bixin, naturally occurring carotenoids are tetraterpenoids. In general, carotenoids have a basic structure of 40 carbons with unique modifications; however, a notable exception is *bixin*. Bixin is a 24-carbon food color additive and is derived from the seed coat of a tropical brush fruit, *Bixa orellana*. The carotenoids are pigments that generally produce colors of yellow, orange, and red.

Different foods will have different kinds and relative amounts of carotenoids. Also the carotenoid content can vary seasonally and during the ripening process. For instance, peaches contain violaxanthin, cryptoxanthin, β-carotene, persicaxanthin, neoxanthin, and as many as 25 other carotenoids. Apricots, on the other hand, contain mostly β-carotene, γ-carotene, and lycopene, while carrots contain about 50 to 55 ppm of carotene total, mostly α-carotene, β-carotene, and γ-carotene, as well as lycopene. Many vegetable oils also contain carotenoids, with palm oil containing the most. For instance, crude palm oil contains up to 0.2% carotenoids.

While animals can not synthesize carotenoids, animal foods will contain these substances if the animal ingested carotenoid-containing plants. For instance, it is not uncommon for egg yolk to contain lutein, zeaxanthin, and cryptoxanthin. Also, an animal can alter an ingested carotenoid. For instance, crustaceans contain protein-bound carotenoids that allow for a blue or blue-gray coloring.

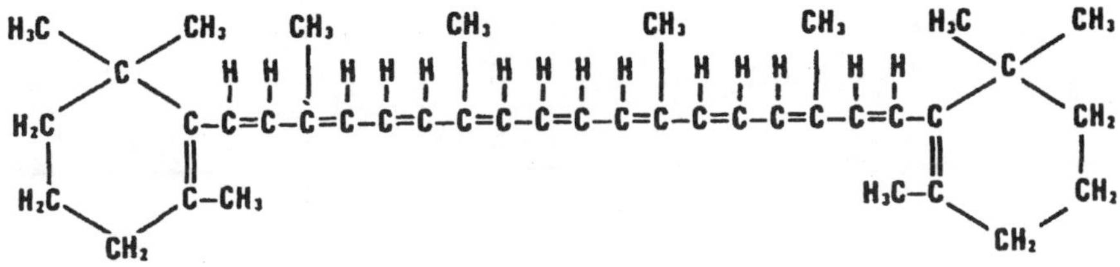

FIGURE 2.8
β-Carotene.

During the ripening process of fruits and vegetables, the content of carotenoids can change. The content of chlorophyll decreases as the content of carotenoids increase. For instance, in the ripening tomato, which changes from green to red, the content of lycopene and carotenes, increase as the content of chlorophyll decreases; also, the ratio of carotenoids to xanthophylls tends to also increase.

There are a few synthetic carotenoids, including β-carotene, β-apo-8′-carotenal (apocarotenal), and canthaxanthin. β-Carotene has a light yellow to orange color; β-apo-8′-carotenal (apocarotenal) imparts a light reddish orange color; and canthaxanthin imparts an orange-red to red color.

Anthocyanins are present in the sap of plant cells, and their basic structure consists of a phenyl-benzopyrylium (flavylium) with a number of hydroxy or methoxy substituents. They are responsible for the red, blue, and violet coloring of many fruits and vegetables. Anthocyanins occur in numerous fruits and vegetables, including blueberries, apples, red cabbage, cherries, grapes, oranges, peaches, plums, radishes, raspberries, and strawberries. Only about 16 anthocyanidins have been identified in plants, including pelargonidin, cyanidin, delphinidin, peonidin, malvidin, and petunidin, which are the most common (Figure 2.9). Cyanidin-based molecules provide much of the characteristic color to bing cherries, red Delicious apples, and cranberries.

The *flavonoids* or *anthoxanthins* are glycosides that have a benzopyrone foundation. The flavonoids by themselves impart little color; however when they bind with iron, blue and green color is revealed. Furthermore, flavonoids can serve as a enzymatic substrate for the browning process. Perhaps the most ubiquitous flavonoid is quercetin (Figure 2.10). Hesperidin is also a common flavoinoid, especially in citrus fruits (Figure 2.11).

Appetite

The factors that appear to influence human appetite and satiety appear to include external cues as well as internal factors. The mere sight of food or the interaction between volatile food molecules and olfactory senses can initiate hunger. The taste and texture of food, along with other sensory perceptions, can evoke either positive or negative signals that allow for continuation of eating or slowing down or terminating ingestion of a substance. For example, appetite can be enhanced with the sight, smell, or initial taste of a delightful food for one individual, while that same food may be avoided or purged if ingested by another. Afferent signals associated with a food are processed and integrated into the central learning system and processed in memory.

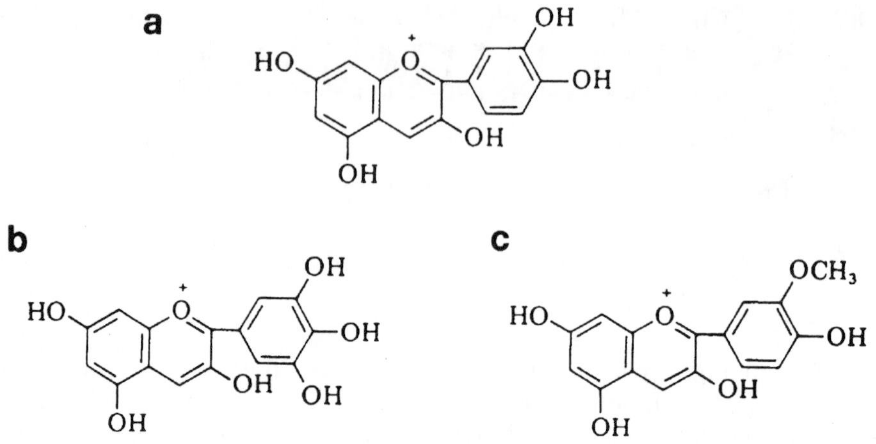

FIGURE 2.9
The anthocyanidins: cyanidin (a), delphinidin (b) and peonidin (c).

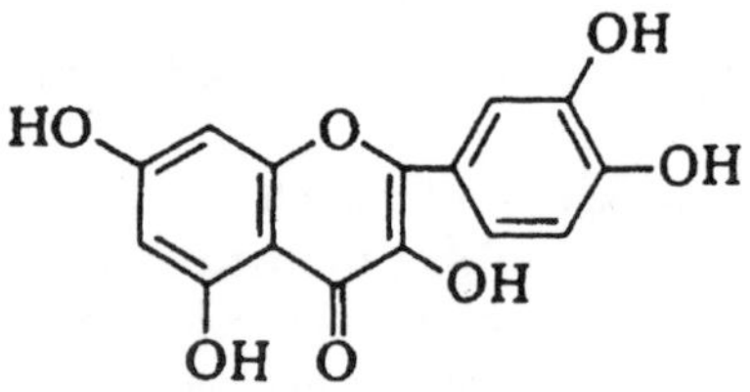

FIGURE 2.10
Quercetin.

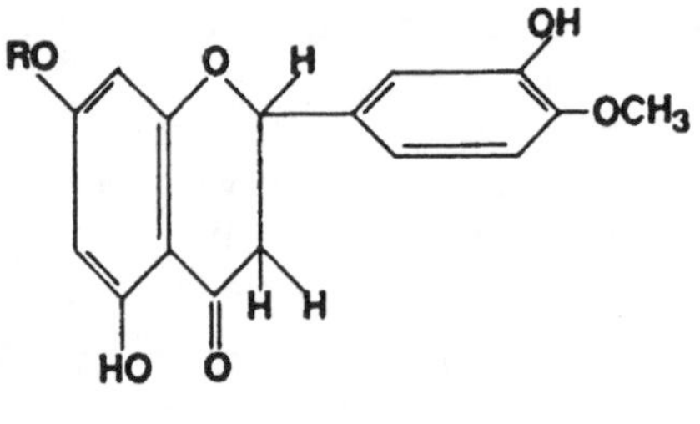

FIGURE 2.11
Hesperidin.

Events associated with the gastrointestinal system that influence appetite include distention of various GI compartments, hormones, and effects of substances within the ingested food. Distention of the pharynx, esophagus, stomach, and intestines is associated with events negatively influencing appetite. Cholecystokinin (CCK) is the hormone most studied in relation to appetite. For example, studies have demonstrated that intraperitoneal infusion of CCK decreases appetite in hungry rats. Other gastrointestinal hormones impacting hunger include somatostatin (via the pancreas) and bombesin. Insulin and glucagon also influence appetite.

The area of the brain most associated with hunger and satiety is the hypothalamus. More specifically, certain regions of the hypothalamus have been regarded as "control centers" for hunger and satiety. The lateral and a medial aspect of the ventromedial nucleus have been identified as the "feeding" and "satiety" centers, respectively. Appetite and hormonal and neuropeptide influences, food consumption, and body weight and composition will be discussed more thoroughly in Chapter 11.

Food Additives

Food additives are substances added to food to enhance its flavor, texture, or appearance or to retard spoilage or augment its nutritional value. Food additives can be either incidental additives or intentional additives. In the U.S., the law governing additives to foods is the Food Additives Amendment to the Federal Food, Drug and Cosmetic Act of 1958. See Appendix A for a listing of common food additives.

Suggested Readings

deMan, J. M., *Principles of Food Chemistry*, 2nd ed., Van Nostrand Reinhold, New York, 1990.
Ensminger, A. H., Ensminger, M. E., Konlande, J. E., and Robson, J. R. K., *Concise Encyclopedia of Foods and Nutrition.* CRC Press, Boca Raton, FL, 1995.

3

Human Digestion and Absorption

With the exception of intravenous infusion, nutrient entry into the body takes place by way of the gastrointestinal or alimentary tract. This tract is in essence a tube extending from the mouth to the anus, whose lumen is considered to be outside of the body (Figure 3.1). The gastrointestinal tract, or simply "the gut," along with organs such as the salivary glands, pancreas, liver, and gall bladder that empty supportive substances into the gut, make up the gastrointestinal system. The primary objectives of the gastrointestinal system are to break down complex food components into substances appropriate for absorption into the body as well as to provide a means of waste removal from digestive and metabolic operations. To meet these objectives the gastrointestinal system must engage in digestive, motility, secretory, and absorptive operations.

Gastrointestinal Anatomy

Histologically the wall of the gastrointestinal tract is fairly consistant throughout its length (Figure 3.2). While some variation does exist allowing the specialized operations inherent to different segments of the gastrointestinal tract, the structure of the wall can be discussed in a general manner. The gastrointestinal tract wall is characterized by several distinct layers. The layer closest to the lumen is the *mucosa*. The outermost region of the mucosa, the *muscularis mucosae*, is composed of mostly smooth muscle. Adjacent to the muscularis mucosae is the *submucosa*. Situated outside the submucosa is a layer of circular smooth muscle which is covered by a layer of longitudinal smooth muscle. The outermost layer of the gastrointestinal wall is the *serosa*. Buried within the different layers of the gastrointestinal tract wall are blood vessels, which transport nutrients, oxygen, and hormones to and from the wall, as well as nerve plexuses which control wall activity.

The *mouth* and the *pharynx* provide entry to the gastrointestinal tract. Several secretory glands (Figure 3.3) located in the mouth release *saliva*, which begins the chemical digestion of food while also supporting chewing or *mastication* and swallowing or *deglutination* mechanisms. Swallowed content enters the *stomach* by traversing the 25 cm (10 in) muscular *esophagus*. The stomach is also approximately 25 cm in length and is J-shaped with its curvature towards the right (Figure 3.4). It is situated just beneath the diaphram and is separated from the esophagus by a thickened muscular ring at the distal esophagus called the *lower esophageal sphincter* (LES) or *cardiac sphincter*, with respect to its close anatomical proximity to the heart. Distally, the stomach is separated from the small intestine by another smooth muscular ring called the *pyloric sphincter*. The volume of an empty adult stomach is only about 50 ml or about 1 2/3 oz; however, it can accommodate as much as 1.5 l (52 oz) or more during a meal. The stomach is subdivided into three segments: the *fundus, body,* and *antrum,* whose walls are characterized by the presence of several exocrine and

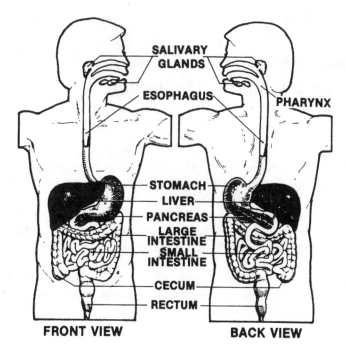

FIGURE 3.1
The human digestive system.

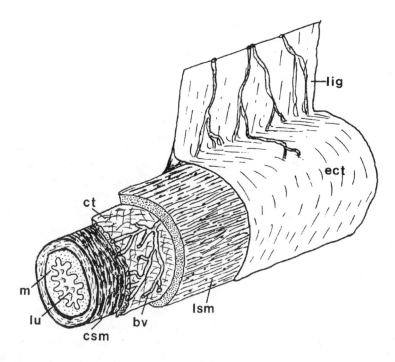

FIGURE 3.2
General anatomical structure of the digestive tract wall. Here the lumen (lu), mucosa (m), circular smooth muscle (csm), longitudinal smooth muscle (lsm), connective tissue (ct, ect), blood vessels (bv), and supporting ligaments (lig) are indicated.

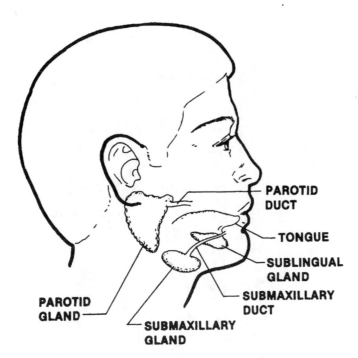

**PAROTID
DUCT**

TONGUE

**SUBLINGUAL
GLAND**

**SUBMAXILLARY
DUCT**

**PAROTID
GLAND**

**SUBMAXILLARY
GLAND**

FIGURE 3.3
Location of primary salivary glands.

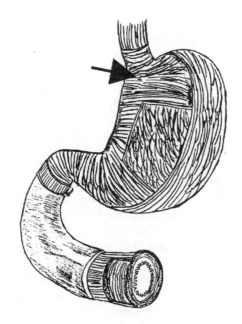

FIGURE 3.4
The stomach. The arrow indicates the layers of smooth muscle.

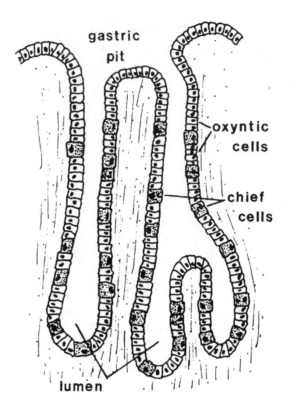

FIGURE 3.5

Oxyntic glands. The oxyntic glands of the stomach secrete HCl, pepsinogen, intrinsic factor, mucus, and other substances into the lumen of the stomach.

endocrine glands. The *oxyntic* glands are the primary type of gastric gland, and these structures contain exocrine cells that secrete a HCl solution, pepsinogen, intrinsic factor, mucus and other substances (Figure 3.5). The density of the glands along with the histology can vary regionally in the stomach.

The contents of the stomach are slowly released into the small intestine, which is approximately 3 m (10 ft) in length and can be divided into three segments. The *duodenum* is the most proximal segment to the stomach and is typically about 30 cm (~1 ft) in length. Secretions from the liver and gall bladder, via the hepatic bile ducts and cystic duct, respectively, combine in the common bile duct, which empties into the duodenum through the *sphincter of Oddi*. Secretions from the pancreas, via the pancreatic duct, flow into the terminal aspect of the common bile duct and subsequently flow into the duodenum via the sphincter of Oddi. In order, the *jejunum* and the *ileum* are the distal segments of the small intestine and combine for approximately 2.75 m (~9 ft) in length.

The small intestine is the primary site of digestion and absorption in the gastrointestinal tract. In an effort to optimize digestive and absorptive operations, the surface area of the small intestine wall is greatly enhanced by three mucosal modifications. First, the small intestine wall is thrown into folds (*rugae*) called *valvulae conniventes* (folds of Kerckring). These circular folds, which extend as much as 8 mm into the lumen, increase the surface area of the small intestine wall 3-fold (Figure 3.6). Next, millions of finger-like projections called *villi* protrude from the small intestine wall and enhance the surface

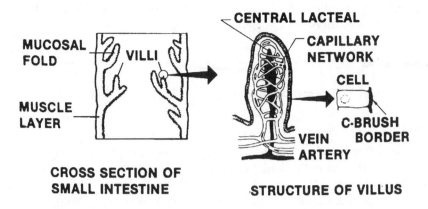

MUCOSAL FOLD

VILLI

MUSCLE LAYER

CROSS SECTION OF SMALL INTESTINE

CENTRAL LACTEAL

CAPILLARY NETWORK

CELL

C-BRUSH BORDER

VEIN

ARTERY

STRUCTURE OF VILLUS

FIGURE 3.6

Three levels of folding of the small intestine. The folds of Kerkring are merely folding of the mucosa. Extending from the folds of Kerkring are finger-like projections (villi) which are lined with enterocytes. The lumenal face of the plasma membrane of enterocytes has thousands of bristle-like extentions called microvilli.

area another 10-fold. The villi themselves are lined primarily with small intestine epithelial cells called *enterocytes*, which are highly specialized for digestive and absorptive operations. Last, the plasma membranes of the enterocytes contain fine evaginations called *microvilli* on their luminal surface. A single enterocyte may contain about 1700 microvilli, each typically being about 1 μm in length and 0.1 μm in diameter. Microscopically, this gives the lining of the small intestine a *brush border* appearance. Microvilli expand the surface area another 20-fold. Cumulatively, the folds of Kerckring, villi, and microvilli enhance the surface area of the small intestine about 600 times to approximately 300 m², or roughly the size of a tennis court.

In the gastrointestinal tract, villi are unique to the small intestine and are specifically designed to provide nutrients entrance to the body. Internally, each villus contains a capillary and a central lacteal, which together provide the means for nutrient absorption (Figure 3.6). In general, small absorbed water-soluble substances will enter the systemic circulation by crossing the capillary wall. On the other hand, most absorbed lipid-soluble substances are destined to enter the blood indirectly by first draining into the central lacteal as part of a lipoprotein (chylomicron) and flowing through the lymphatic circulation.

In the depths between villi are the *crypts of Lieberkühn*. The cells found in these crypts undergo rapid mitosis and the new cells then migrate up the villi to allow continuous replacement of enterocytes that are being sloughed off the tip of the villi. Enterocyte turnover is approximately 3 to 5 days. Other cells in the crypts include protein-secreting *paneth cells*, mucus-secreting *goblet cells*, and *enterochromaffin cells*, which perform endocrine activities. Last, lymphoid tissue, called *Peyer's patches*, is also found in the wall of the small intestine and contains both T lymphocytes and B lymphocytes. Peyer's patches provide a line of defense against bacteria and other ingested foreign substances.

The small intestine is separated from the *large intestine* or *colon* by the ileocecal valve. The large intestine is approximately 1.5 to 1.8 m (5 to 6 ft) long with an average diameter of 6 cm (~2.5 in.), with the diameter decreasing moving distally. The large intestine can be segmented in order into the cecum, colon, rectum, and anal canal. Also, with respect to directional movement of contents through the colon in an upright human, regions of the colon are often referred to as ascending, transverse, and descending. The large intestine is the site of a rich bacterial population and is involved in absorbing water and some electrolytes as well as in the activities involved in defecation.

Gastrointestinal Movement, Motility, and Neural Activity

Smooth Muscle

The motility of substance throughout the length of the gastrointestinal tract is provided by the smooth muscle found in the wall. Longitudinal smooth muscle fibers extend along the length of the gastrointestinal tract, while the circular smooth muscle fibers wrap around the tract. Individual muscle fibers, approximately 200 to 500 μm in length and 2 to 10 μm in diameter, are arranged in bundles containing up to 1000 fibers each. While adjacent bundles of smooth muscle fibers are separated by a thin region of connective tissue, they are fused together at several points which allows for muscle bundle contraction to occur as a syncytium. Therefore, when an action potential is fired anywhere within the muscle mass, it has the potential to be conducted throughout the mass, which then can contract as a unit.

Contraction of the smooth muscle in the gastrointestinal tract wall appears to occur rhythymically and is associated with the presence of waves in the smooth muscle membrane potentials. Two types of electrical waves occur in smooth muscle cells: slow waves and spikes. Slow waves, which assumedly are caused by undulating activity of Na^+/K^+ pumps, alter the membrane potential by 5 to 15 mV. Their frequency can vary, depending largely upon the location in the gastrointestinal tract. For instance, slow waves occur at a frequency of about 3/min in stomach, while occuring at a rate of 12/min in the duodenum.

Slow waves are not actually action potentials and therefore do not directly evoke contraction of smooth muscle. However, when slow waves exceed –40 mV they give rise to spikes which are indeed true action potentials and thus stimulate muscle contraction. Spikes or spike potentials differ from the action potentials characteristic of neurons in at least two ways. First, spike potentials, which last 10 to 20 msec, are about 10 to 40 times longer than neuron action potentials. Second, the ion channels involved in the spike potential are unique as well. Spike potentials appear to be caused by slow-opening/-closing Ca^{2+}/Na^+ channels, which is different than the rapid-opening/-closing Na^+ channels involved in the action potentials of neurons. Spike potentials can also be distinguished from slow waves based upon ion channel activity. Slow waves are not associated with an increase in intracellular calcium and therefore do not evoke fiber contraction. Like other muscle fibers, smooth muscle cells of the gastrointestinal tract wall contract in response to an increase in intracellular calcium concentration acting through a calmodulin-controlled mechanism.

In addition to rhythmic contraction, gut smooth muscle also exhibits tonic contraction. While demonstrating fluctuations in intensity, tonic contractions are continuous and protracted, lasting as long as several minutes to hours. The origin of tonic contraction may be the result of a repetitive series of spike potentials or the influence of certain hormones or other factors that allow for continuous depolarization of the membrane potential.

Enteric Nervous System

The gastrointestinal tract is endowed with the *enteric nervous system* (ENS) which is functionly distinct, yet interconnected to the CNS. This means that while the ENS can function on its own, its activity is still influenced by the autonomic extensions of the CNS. Furthermore, sensory neurons originating in the intestinal wall epithelium communicate with both the enteric and CNS.

The ENS extends from the esophagus to the anus, contains approximately 100,000,000 neurons, and is characterized by two main plexuses. The myenteric plexus or Auerbach's plexus is the outer plexus and is located between the longitudinal and circular smooth muscle layers; it runs the entire length of the ENS. The proximity of this complex relative to smooth muscle layers makes the myenteric plexus ideal to control motor activity along the length of the gastrointestinal tract. Stimulation of the myenteric plexus generally results in increased wall tone, rate and intensity of rhythmic contractions, and velocity of excitatory wave conduction along the wall of the gastrointestinal tract. Contrasting these operations, stimulation of the myenteric plexus can also result in some inhibitory activity as well. For instance, some of its neurons release inhibitory neurotransmitters, such as vasoactive inhibitory polypeptide (VIP), when stimulated. The significance of this activity includes relaxation of intestinal sphincter muscles such as the pyloric sphincter and the ileocecal valve, thus allowing passage of intestinal contents to move from one gut segment into another. The second plexus, known as the submucosa plexus or Meissner's plexus, is situated within the submocosa and is mainly involved in gastrointestinal secretions and local blood flow regulation.

The gastrointestinal tract is extrinsically innervated by both the sympathetic and parasympathetic systems. Both systems indirectly elicit a response in the gastrointestinal system by first synapsing with neurons of the ENS. Furthermore, chemoreceptors and mechanoreceptors in the mucosa of the gastrointestinal tract can relay afferent impulses to the CNS or elicit a reflex by way of ENS plexuses. Since the activities of the ENS and the sympathetic and parasympathetic nervous systems are not under conscious control, these systems are collectively referred to as the autonomic nervous system.

The *vagus* nerve supplies almost all of the parasympathetic activity down to the level of the transverse colon, while fibers supplied by the pelvic nerve innervate the decending colon, sigmoid colon, rectum, and the anal canal. Furthermore, cholinergic fibers innervating the striated muscle in the upper third of the esophagus and external anal canal are also delivered by the vagal and pelvic nerves, respectively. Parasympathetic fibers are especially dense in the orad (oral cavity) and most analward segments of the gastrointestinal tract, while not being particularly as dense in the small intestine. Parasympathetic stimulation generally increases gastrointestinal activity, while some inhibitory processes do result.

Unlike parasympatheic innervation, the density of sympathetic innervation is more consistant throughout the length of the gut. Sympathetic fibers originate in the T-5 through L-2 regions of the spinal cord, and preganlionic fibers synapse in the celiac, superior or inferior mesenteric, or hypogastric ganglia. From there, postganglionic fibers innervate regions of the myenteric and submucosal plexuses. Neurons of the ENS then relay signals to smooth muscle, secretory, and endocrine cells of the gastrointestinal tract and generally elicit a response that decreases gastrointestinal activity.

Neurons of the ENS produce a variety of potential neurotransmitter substances, including acetylcholine, epinephrine, ATP, dopamine, serotonin, VIP, γ-aminobutyric acid (GABA), glycine, cholecystokinin (CCK), leu-enkephalin and met-enkephalin, substance P, secretin, neurotensin, motilin, and gastric-releasing peptide (GRP), which is the mammalian analog of amphibian peptide bombesin. While the roles of a few of these substances in ENS activity are well established, the presence of other substances have not necessarily been linked to physiological function.

Acetylcholine mediates contraction of the smooth muscle in the gut as well as secretions from the salvary glands, stomach, pancreas, and small intestine. On the other hand, norepinephrine generally inhibits smooth contraction, secretion, and blood flow. GRP is a 27-amino acid peptide released from neurons in the gastric antrum and fundus, as well as the pancreas, and stimulates the release of gastrin, CCK, pancreatic polypeptide, insulin, glucagon, and somatostatin. VIP is a 28-amino acid peptide and is produced by neurons throughout the gastrointestinal tract, salivary glands, and pancreas. VIP release causes relaxation of the LES, the proximal stomach, and internal anal sphincter.

Movements of the Gastrointestinal Tract

The gastrointestinal tract exhibits two basic types of movement. *Propulsive movements* move contents forward while *mixing movements* allow for a thorough blending of gastrointestinal contents. *Peristalsis* is the basic propulsive movement. A ring of muscular constriction encircling the gut is initiated and then begins to move forward or analward by pushing the intestinal matter in front of the ring forward. Distention is a strong stimulus for the origin of a peristaltic wave. For instance, if intestinal matter stretches the gut wall, a contractile ring is initiated about 2 to 3 cm behind the point of distention and peristalsis is propagated in the direction of the anus. In addition, the gut can relax several centimeters on the anus side of the distention to ease transit of matter into that area. Parasympathetic signals can also initiate peritalsis along with irritation of the mucosal lining of the gut. Futhermore, an intact myenteric plexus is necessary for effectual peristaltic waves in the associated area.

Mixing movements differ from one segment of the gastrointestinal tract to another. In areas just prior to a sphincter closure, forward movement of intestinal matter is blocked and thus peristaltic waves take on a more distinctive mixing role. In other regions, local constrictive contractions occur approximately every several centimeters in a regimented fashion to help chop and blend intestinal contents.

Gastrointestinal Blood Supply and Flow Regulation

Gastrointestinal Vasculature

The gastrointestinal tract receives blood from several arterial branches of the abdominal aorta. For instance, the celiac artery delivers blood to the stomach; the superior mesenteric artery delivers blood to the small intestine and proximal portion of the large intestine; and the inferior mesenteric artery supplies blood to the more distal aspects of the large intestine. Small arterial branches of the superior mesenteric artery ultimately serve individual villi as a capillary network is centralized inside each of these mucosal projections (Figure 3.6).

Once blood has perfused these regions, it drains into its respective veins, which then drain into the hepatic portal vein. By design, blood that has perfused the gut, as well as the pancreas and spleen, is destined to flow to the liver before returning to the heart. This allows the liver to have "first shot" at substances absorbed into intestinal wall capillaries.

Furthermore, as the blood courses through hepatic sinusoids, gut-derived bacteria and other debris can be removed by reticuloendothelial cells, often called Kupfer cells, before entering circulation at large.

Gastrin (G-17)

Glu-Gly-Pro-Trp-Leu-Glu-Glu-Glu-Glu-Glu-Ala-Tyr-Gly-Trp-Met-Asp-Phe-NH₂

$$HSO_3$$

Cholecystokinin

Lys-(Ala, Gly, Pro, Ser)-Arg-Val-(Ile, Met,Ser)-Lys-Asn-(Asn,Gln,His,Leu₂,Pro,Ser₂)-Arg-Ile-(Asp,Ser)-Arg-Asp-Tyr-Gly-Trp-Met-Asp-Phe-NH₂

$$HSO_3$$

Secretin

His-Ser-Asp-Gly-Thr-Phe-Thr-Ser-Glu-Leu-Ser-Arg-Leu-Arg-Asp-Ser-Ala-Arg-Leu-Gln-Arg-Leu-Leu-Gln-Gly-Leu-Val-NH₂

FIGURE 3.7
Amino acid composition of gastrin, CCK, and secretin.

Gastrointestinal Endocrine and Paracrine Substances

Distributed throughout the gastrointestinal tract are cells possessing endocrine and/or paracrine function. These cells manufacture and secrete substances such as *5-hydroxytryptophan* (serotonin), *cholecystokinin, gastrin, secretin, gastric inhibitory polypeptide* (GIP), *motilin, neurotensin,* and *somatostatin.* Interesting is the finding that many of these substances are also found in the neural ending of the enteric nervous system.

Gastrin is secreted by gastrin cells (G-cells) which are located primarily in the glands of the gastric antrum and also in the mucosa of the duodenum. Several polypeptides of varying lengths possess gastrin activity. All of these polypeptides possess an identical COOH-terminal amino acid sequence (-Tyr-Met-Asp-Phe-NH₂) with the terminal phenylalanine (Phe) residue being amidated (-NH₂). The most abundant forms are G-17 (I and II) and G-34 (big gastrin) with the number denoting the quantity of amino acids in the polypeptide. Figure 3.7 presents the amino acid sequence of G-17. G-14 (minigastrin) is also physiologically active, while pentagastrin (G-5) is a synthetic form of gastrin. During interdigestive periods or fasting, gastrin levels in the plasma are on the order of 50 to 100 pg/ml and are mostly attributable to G-34. However, when G-cells are stimulated during a meal, more G-17 is released. G-17 and G-34 are equipotent. However, the half-life of G-34 is approximately 38 min, whereas the half-life of G-17 is only 7 min.

The stimulus for gastrin release from G-cells includes the presence of small peptides, certain amino acids (especially phenylalanine and tryptophan), and calcium in the lumen of the stomach. In addition, neural stimulation, either mediated directly by the vagus or indirectly by gastric distention-initiated ENS reflexes, evokes gastrin release. Gastrin-releasing peptide (GRP) appears to be the neurotransmitter released as a result of vagal stimulation. The primary role of gastrin is to regulate gastric acid secretion while also mediating pepsinogen and intrinsic factor secretion. Gastrin is approximately 1500 times more potent than histamine in stimulating acid release from oxyntic glands. Gastrin also stimulates the growth of the oxyntic glands as well. Gastrin release is reduced relative to increasing acidity in the lumen of the stomach.

Similar to gastrin, the polypeptide cholecystokinin (Figure 3.7) is also present in multiple forms and is secreted from cells located in the mucosa of the duodenum and jejunum. Also, molecules exhibiting CCK activity have the same active COOH-terminal tetrapeptide sequence as gastrin. Isolated forms of CCK include CCK-58, CCK-39, CCK-33, CCK-22, and CCK-8. CCK release is stimulated by the presence of intraluminal fatty acids having a chain length of nine or more carbons and their corresponding monoglycerides. Further, partially digested proteins and individual amino acids such as phenylalanine and tryptophan as well as intraluminal glucose promote CCK release. GRP also seems to stimulate the release of CCK. Among the well-established roles of CCK are to stimulate the release of pancreatic enzyme secretion, gall bladder contraction, and relaxation of the sphinctor of Oddi. CCK also has an effect on gastric and intestinal motility and a trophic effect on the pancreas. CCK also appears to be invloved in appetite suppression, which will be discussed in more detail in Chapter 12.

Contrasting gastrin and CCK, secretin has only one circulating form, a 27-amino acid polypeptide (Figure 3.7). It is released from secretin-containing cells located in the mucosa of the duodenum and jejunum when the hydrogen ion content of the proximal small intestine increases. Circulating levels of secretin increase when intraluminal pH falls below 4.5. Also, intraluminal fatty acids may evoke the release of secretin. The major function of secretin is to stimulate the pancreas to release a bicarbonate-rich alkaline solution into the pancreatic duct. Also, secretin promotes water and bicarbonate secretion from the biliary system. Secretin also exhibits other functions such as inhibition of gastric emptying and inhibition of gastric acid secretion and release of pepsinogen in the stomach. However, whether or not these functions are physiologically significant remains uncertain.

Beyond mucosa cells throughout the intestinal tract, somatostatin is also manufactured and released from D-cells in the pancreatic islets of Langerhans as well as nerve fibers in both the central and enteric nervous systems. Somatostatin occurs as either SS-14 or SS-28, and circulatory levels are increased due to the presence of fat and protein in the intestines and to some degree by an acidic pH in the antrum region of the stomach, as well as in the duodenum. While having many functions outside of digestive physiology, somatostatin is involved in inhibiting gastrin release from G-cells and pancreatic enzyme release, as well as the secretion of stomach acid. Beyond these roles, somatostatin may also be involved in inhibiting secretin and CCK release as well as inhibiting the absorption of amino acids, water, and electrolytes, and gut motility.

Gastric inhibitory peptide (GIP) is produced and released from cells located primarily in the duodenum and jejunum. GIP is a 42-amino acid polypeptide released in response to an intraluminal presence of several substances including glucose, amino acids, and hydrolyzed triglycerides as well as being released in response to an increase in duodenal hydrogen ion concentration. While its name suggests a regulatory role in gastric acid secretion, this function has not been proven to be physiological. However, GIP does have a physiological role in intensifying the glucose-stimulated release of insulin.

Motilin, a 22-amino acid linear polypeptide, is released from mucosal cells of the upper small intestine. The level of motilin increases during interdigestive periods. Motilin is believed to initiate myoelectric migrating complexes (MMC) in the duodenum, which occur every 90 min or so during interdigestive periods and function as a sweeping mechanism moving digestive residue analward. Other peptide mediators of digestive activity include neurotensin, pancreatic polypeptide, and peptide YY. The understanding of the function of these regulatory peptides is still unclear. It has been suggested that neurotensin, a 13-amino acid molecule secreted by ileal mucosal cells in response to the presence of intraluminal fat, may contribute to the inhibition of gastric acid release. The 36-amino acid pancreatic polypeptide and peptide YY molecules have been suggested to be involved in regulation of pancreatic exocrine secretion and gastric acid secretion. Pancreatic polypeptide and peptide YY are produced by the islets cells of the pancreas and mucosal cells of the ileum and colon, respectively.

Histamine is not a protein but is derived from the amino acid histidine by the actions of histidine decarboxylase. In addition to its established activities as a neurotransmitter, histamine is also secreted from gastric mast cells. While the mechanisms leading to the release of histamine from these cells is relatively unclear, the paracrine function of histamine in evoking gastric acid secretion is well known. Therapeutically, histamine-H_2-receptor antagonists, such as cimetidine, inhibit parietal cell hydrochloric acid secretion as stimulated by gastrin, acetylcholine and histamine analogs.

Digestion and Absorption

The foundation of human nourishment is the consumption of other living entities or their products. From within these other life forms, humans obtain elements and molecules common to both. As mentioned in the preceding chapter, essential nutrients are substances that humans are unable to produce, either at all or in adequate quantities, and that thus must be provided by the diet. Due to the complex nature of food digestive activities are necessary to liberate nutrients, such as freeing minerals for proteins, reducing the size of nutrients, such as breaking down complex proteins to amino acids or complex starch to monosaccharides, and/or to modify a nutrient so that it can be recognized by transport systems involved in its absorption.

Oral Cavity

Once food enters the mouth it is chewed or masticated and bathed in salivary juice. Incisors are more anterior in the mouth and provide a strong cutting action, while more posteriorally the molars provide a grinding mechanism. Figure 3.8 presents the structure of a tooth. Chewing is controlled by nuclei in the brain stem which innervates the muscles of the jaw via the 5th cranial nerve. A coordinated effort by all muscles in the jaw can generate a force of 55 pounds on the incisors and 200 pounds on the molars. Chewing physically tears food

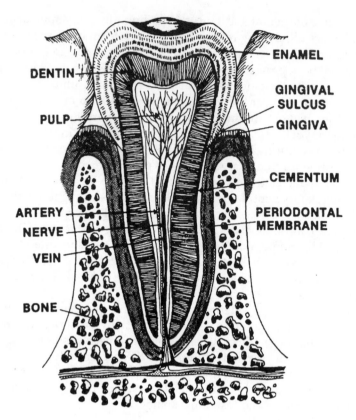

FIGURE 3.8
Structure of a tooth.

apart, while the actions of the tongue help position food between teeth and both actions together mix food with saliva.

Saliva helps to lubricate food for easier swallowing, solubilization of food components for taste perception, for cleaning the mouth and teeth to prevent caries, and to initiate chemical digestion. About 1 to 1.5 l of saliva are produced daily by the glands of the oral cavity. The *parotid*, *submandibular*, and *sublingual* glands, along with well-distributed *buccal* glands, are the principal glands involved in producing a complex compilation of enzymes, mucus, R-proteins, growth factors, antibacterial and antiviral factors, ions, and water (Figure 3.3). Last, saliva contains the blood group substances A, B, AB, and O.

Two types of protein secretions are found in saliva. First, the *serous* type of protein secretion, which is secreted by the parotid, submandibular, and sublingual glands contains *phytalin* (α-amylase). In addition, *lingual lipase* is secreted by the sublingual glands. α-Amylase begins the chemical digestion of starches by cleaving α1-4 links between glucose monomers. Lingual lipase hydrolyzes certain ester bonds of triglycerides and is of particular significance in infants. Another salivary enzyme, named *kallikrein*, does not have catabolic properties but supports the digestive process by converting a plasma protein into bradykinin, which increases blood flow to salivary glands. Second, the *mucous* type of protein secretion contains the lubricating glycoprotein *mucin*. Along with the submandibular and sublingual glands, the buccal glands also secrete mucus.

The inorganic component of saliva includes sodium, potassium, chloride, bicarbonate, calcium, magnesium, and phosphate. At rest, saliva is hypotonic; however the potassium concentration (30 mEq/l) is greater than plasma. Opposingly, the concentration of sodium, chloride, and bicarbonate, all about 15 mEq/l, are below plasma levels. For sodium and chloride their concentration in saliva at rest may only be about 10 to 15% of their levels in plasma. When saliva flow is stimulated, the concentration of potassium decreases, although not below plasma levels. Contrarily, the concentration of sodium, chloride, and bicarbonate increase, with the latter rising above plasma concentration. This increases salivary pH to approximately 7.8 from a resting pH of 6.0 to 7.0.

Saliva is also very important for oral hygiene. With the exception of periods of sleep, saliva is secreted at a basal rate of about 0.5 ml/min and the protein is predominately of the mucous type. The secretion of saliva helps wash away pathogenic bacteria and residual food particles from teeth. Saliva also contains antibacterial factors such as thiocyanate ions, several proteolytic enzymes, including *lysozyme*, and antibodies which collectively destroy a significant quantity of bacteria in the oral cavity.

While the concentration of sodium and potassium can be influenced by aldosterone and antidiuretic hormone, the rate of salivary flow is controlled autonomically. This is to say that hormones that influence the release of other digestive secretions have little effect on salivary flow. Furthermore, the autonomic control of salivary secretion is unique from many other organs in that both parasympathetic and sympathetic activity will elicit flow. However, parasympathetic activity has a far greater influence on flow.

Esophagus

The act of swallowing involves both voluntary and involuntary activity. Three overlapping layers of striated muscle, the *superior, middle,* and *inferior pharyngeal constrictors*, make up the musclar wall of the pharynx. The inferior constrictor also thickens at a point to form a muscular ring that constitutes the *upper esophageal sphincter*. The striated muscle continues down about one third of the length of the esophagus and gives way to circular and longitudinal smooth muscle. Circular smooth muscle thickens at the distal aspect of the esophagus, forming the lower esophageal sphincter.

The act of swallowing is complex and involves coordinated and unvarying efforts of both voluntary and involuntary actions. At rest the upper esophageal sphincter is contracted to close the esophageal inlet. In contrast, the pharyngeal muscle exhibits only a low level of tone. The act of swallowing involves a series of voluntary and even some involuntary motions occurring in sequence, beginning with the clenching down of the jaws. Subsequently the tongue is elevated against the hard palate and elevation of the soft palate allows the nasopharynx to separate from the oropharynx. Next, there is a voluntary and then involuntary contraction of the pharyngeal muscles that moves in the direction of the esophageal inlet. Concomitantly, strap muscles in the neck move the pharyngeosophageal junction, thereby properly aligning the esophageal inlet with the pharynx. The 1 to 2-sec relaxation of the upper esophageal sphincter allows the bolus of food to pass into the esophagus as forced through the mouth by the tongue and through the pharynx by its peristaltic contraction.

A powerful re-contraction of the upper esophageal sphincter is associated with the initiation of a peristaltic wave that propels food along the length of the esophagus. There is no delay in the transition from striated muscle to smooth muscle contraction, and a bolus of food can smoothly traverse the length of the esophagus in about 6 to 9 seconds. Relaxation of the lower esophageal sphincter occurs as the peristaltic wave is initiated and propagates to the length of the esophagus. It remains relaxed until the peristaltic wave meets the sphincter, and then after a brief interlude to allow the bolus to move into the stomach, it contracts forcefully.

Stomach

The primary operations of the stomach are to (1) provide a depot for ingested food and regulate its release into the small intestine; (2) provide an acidic environment supportive of protein digestion and bacteriocidal activities; (3) secrete a proteolytic enzyme; and (4) secrete substances that assist in vitamin B_{12} absorption. The *outer longitudinal, middle circular,* and *inner oblique* layers of smooth muscle in the wall of the stomach can relax and allow for the accommodation of approximately 1.5 liters of content without significantly increasing intragastric pressure. Furthermore, the musculature of the stomach wall provides both mixing movements as well as the propulsive movements which allows for a regulated release of gastric contents into the small intestine. These layers (Figure 3.4) can differ from one another with regard to distribution throughout the stomach as well as their own thickness in different regions of the stomach. For instance, while the circular layer is for the most part complete throughout the stomach wall, the longitudinal layer is absent from the anterior and posterior surfaces. Also, the thicknesses of both the circular and longitudinal layers increases in a proximal to distal stomach manner.

Oxyntic glands (Figure 3.5), located largely in the body and fundus, contain a variety of exocrine cell types which include *parietal* (oxyntic) cells that secrete HCl and intrinsic factor; *peptic* cells, which secrete mainly pepsinogen; and *mucous neck* and *surface* cells which produce large amounts of mucus. Some endocrine cells can also be found lining the oxyntic gland. Quantitatively, parietal cells make up approximately one third of the cells lining the gland, while chief cells contribute about 20 to 25% and mucous neck and surface cells contribute about 20% and 10%, respectively.

The release of hydrochloric acid solution by parietal cells, which has a pH of 0.8, creates an acidic environment in the stomach, is important in the denaturing of complex three-dimensional proteins, pepsin activation, liberating various nutrients from organic complexes, and destruction of ingested microbes. The pH of stomach juice is about 1.5 to 2.5. The mixture of ingested material and gastric secretions is known as *chyme*.

During interdigestive periods, basal acid secretion is approximately 10% of maximum and exhibits circadian rhythym with the output during evening being significantly higher than morning. The stimulation of gastric acid release in response to a meal is divided into three phases, the *cephalic* phase which accounts for approximately 30% of gastric acid secretion and the *gastric* and *intestinal* phases which produce 60% and 10% of the gastric acid secretion, respectively. Other aspects of digestion demonstrate phasic periods as well.

The cephalic phase occurs when food stimulates pressure-sensitive mechanoreceptors in the mouth and chemoreceptors in the mouth and nasal cavity. Also, the mere thought of food can trigger central pathways that relay impulses to vagal efferent nerves that reach the stomach. Therefore, the cephalic phase can be completely blocked by vagotomy. Vagal innervation can increase gastric acid secretion by directly stimulating parietal cells via acetylcholine as well as indirectly by stimulating the release of gastrin via GRP. The cephalic phase release of gastric acid can be inhibited by low stomach pH. Because the pH of stomach juice is about 2.0, acid release is impeded until food proteins reach the stomach and buffer the acid, thus causing the pH to climb above 3.0. This allows the cephalic phase to have its most significant impact on gastric acid secretion.

The gastric phase begins when distension of the stomach wall stimulates mechanorecep-tors. This action elicits vagovagal and intramural reflexes, which stimulate both gastrin release and acid secretion. The vagovagal reflex stimulates acid secretion by the same means as the cephalic phase. Furthermore, distention of the mucosa around oxyntic glands increases acid release by a local reflex mechanism. As mentioned previously, the release of gastrin is inhibited by a low gastric intraluminal pH. However, without regard to intralu-minal pH, distention will still result in acid release by reflex and local mechanisms.

The intestinal phase of gastric acid secretion is relatively minor and is not exactly clear. Duodenal luminal distention increases acid secretion by way of a hormone named *enterooxyntin*. Furthermore, the uptake of amino acids into duodenal mucosal cells also appears to be associated with increased acid release.

As mentioned above, pepsin is an endopeptidase and is manufactured and stored in an inactive pepsinogen proenzyme or *zymogen* form which has a molecular weight of approx-imately 42,500. There are two primary pepsinogen molecules, denoted as I and II. Recently, a third class of pepsinogen, called slow-moving protease because of its slow migration rate in an electrophoretic field, has also been identified. Pepsinogens are converted to active pepsins at a low pH by the loss of a portion of their NH_2-terminus amino acid sequence. They then function optimally at a pH < 3.5 and hydrolyze interior peptide bonds, espe-cially those involving aromatic amino acids. The α-amylase derived from salivary secre-tions continues to digest complex carbohydrates in the stomach; however, it becomes inactivated in the highly acidic environment.

Intrinsic factor, which is a mucoprotein with a molecular weight of 55,000, is required for efficient absorption of vitamin B_{12} in the small intestine. Once vitamin B_{12} is released from polypeptides in foods via gastric pepsin, it can combine with intrinsic factor. However, most of the vitamin B_{12} in the stomach will initially combine with R-proteins which are also secreted by gastric glands. Vitamin B_{12} has a greater affinity for R proteins. The "R" denotes the rapid transit of these proteins in an electrophoretic field.

The general release of gastric secretions is primarily under the control of of acetylcholine, gastrin, and histamine, all of which elicit their function by first binding with their respec-tive receptor on secretory cells. Acetylcholine stimulates the release of secretions from all gastric secretory cell types. This includes pepsinogen from peptic cells, hydrochloric acid from parietal cells, mucus from mucous neck cells, and gastrin from G-cells. By contrast, gastrin and histamine strongly stimulate the release of hydrochloric acid from parietal cells, but have little stimulatory impact on other secretory cell types.

Gastric emptying occurs as a result of intense peristaltic contractions in the antrum. For the most part, antral peristaltic contractions are weak and function as a mixing mechanism for food and gastric secretions. However, approximately 20% of the time when food is present, the peristaltic waves are about 6 times more intense than mixing waves and the constricting rings propel food powerfully towards the pylorus. Each intense wave forces or pumps about 1 to 3 ml of chyme into the duodenum.

Release of gastric contents into the small intestine occurs intermittantly and is regulated by several stimulatory and inhibitory factors which originate in both the stomach and small intestine. The degree of filling and the excitatory effect of gastrin on gastric peristalsis com-pete with duodenal signals such as enterogastric feedback reflexes and hormonal feedback. Generally, the greater the gastric distention, the more rapid the emptying. Furthermore, liq-uids seem to be emptied more rapidly than solids. Perhaps the most rapidly emptied sub-stance is an isotopic saline solution. Its emptying rate decreases as the solution is modified to a more hypotonic or hypertonic concentration. The presence of fat substances in the duodenum slows gastric emptying by stimulating the release of CCK which inhibits emp-tying. Acid in the duodenum also decreases gastric emptying by a neural reflex mechanism.

TABLE 3.1
Pancreatic Digestive Enzymes

Proteolytic	Lipolytic	Amylolytic	Nucleases	Others
Trypsinogen	Lipase	α-Amylase	Deoxyribonuclease	Procolipase
Chymotrypsinogen	Prophospholipase A_1		Ribonuclease	Trypsin Inhibitor
Proelastase	Prophospholipase A_2			
Procarboxypeptidase A	Nonspecific esterase			
Procarboxypeptidase B				

Small Intestine

In the small intestine, chyme is mixed with pancreatic secretions and bile by way of segmentation or mixing contractions of circular smooth muscle and sleeve contractions of longitudinal smooth muscle. Meanwhile, peristaltic waves serve to propel food analward through the small intestine. The low pH of entering chyme is quickly neutralized by bicarbonate and H_2O secretions of both the pancreas as well as *Brunner's glands* located in the mucosa of the first few centimeters of the duodenum.

The digestive secretions of the pancreas (Table 3.1) and bile from the liver are complex composites of digestive entities as well as some metabolic waste. Pancreatic *acini* and associated duct cells secrete a juice that is clear, colorless, alkaline, and isotonic. It contains both organic and inorganic components which ultimately reach the duodenum via the pancreatic duct and subsequently the common bile duct. Total pancreatic juice secretion for an adult is approximately 1 to 2 liters daily. The organic components include protein. In fact, the pancreas produces and secretes more protein per gram of tissue than any other tissue. Digestive enzymes are produced and stored as inactive zymogen molecules to prevent autolysis of acini cells. As mentioned above, activation of digestive zyomogen enzymes takes place in the duodenum and is initiated by the brush border enzyme enterokinase (*enteropeptidase*). Enterokinase activates trypsinogen by cleaving an NH_2-terminal portion of the molecule. Trypsin, the active form of trypsinogen, is then able to activate other digestive zymogens including other trypsinogen molecules.

Trypsin inhibitor and colipase should not necessarily be considered digestive enzymes. Trypsin inhibitor appears to be active in pancreatic acini secretory vesicles. Its purpose is to protect pancreatic parenchyma by binding to trypsin molecules formed in premature autocatalysis. Procolipase, once activated, is a cofactor for lipase activity. In addition, other proteins, such as immunoglobins, kallikrein, lysosomal enzymes, alkaline phosphatase, and albumin, are part of pancreatic secretions although in relatively small quantities.

The inorganic component of pancreatic secretions includes water, sodium, potassium, chloride, calcium, magnesium, and bicarbonate. Calcium and magnesium are present in concentrations approximating 25-35% of their plasma concentration. The large production of bicarbonate in ductal epithelium is attributed to intracellular conversion of CO_2 and H_2O via the enzyme carbonic anhydrase. The release of bicarbonate into the duct lumen utilizes a HCO_3^-/Cl^- antiport mechanism.

Basal secretion of the aqueous component of pancreatic juice, which is largely H_2O and bicarbonate, is about 2 to 3% of the maximal rate, while the basal secretion of the enzymatic component is approximately 10 to 15% of maximal. While the mechanisms responsible for basal secretions are undetermined, the mechanisms involved in stimulated secretion are well understood. The release of the aqueous portion of pancreatic secretion is largely related to duodenal intraluminal pH while the enzymatic component secretion is attributed primarily to the presence of fat and protein. Therefore, the stimulus is strongest during the intestinal phase of digestion; however, secretion will also occur to a lesser extent during the cephalic and gastric phases. During the cephalic phase, vagal efferents to the pancreas release acetylcholine at both ductule and acinar cells with a stronger response being evoked within acinar cells. The result is a relatively low volume of pancreatic juice with a relatively high concentration of enzymes. Subsequently, distention on the stomach stimulates pancreatic secretion via a vagovagal reflex. The contribution of the cephalic and gastric phases to total pancreatic juice production may be approximately 20% and 5 to 10%, respectively.

The intestinal phase accounts for as much as 70 to 80% of pancreatic secretory response as the presence of protein and fat in an acidic chyme mixture elicit the release of secretin and CCK. In addition, products of protein and fat digestion, as well as acid, also stimulate pancreatic enzyme release as they interact with duodenal wall receptors. This results in a vagovagal reflex, with acetylcholine being released at the synapses with both ductule and acinar cells. Acetylcholine and CCK, both independently and combined, have little stimulatory impact on ductule cells; however, they can potentiate the effects of secretin.

As much as 1200 ml of bile is secreted by the liver daily. Bile is produced almost continuously in hepatocytes, which are epithelial cells arranged in plates in liver lobules. Bile is secreted into tiny bile canaliculi ("little canals") that run between the hepatocyte plates and drain into a series of larger ducts and ultimately to the hepatic duct and then the common bile duct. Bile flowing through the common bile duct can then either be released into the duodenum or drain into the gall bladder. During fasting periods as much as half of the hepatic bile enters the gall bladder, while the remaining bile continues through to the small intestine. More than 90% of the bile acids (bile salts) emptied into the small intestine is reabsorbed in the distal ileum. Via the portal vein they are returned to the liver and resecreted into bile, where again approximately half will drain into the gall bladder. As fasting becomes more protracted, bile storage in the gall bladder is increased. The recirculation of bile acids is called *enterohepatic circulation* and a single bile acid molecule may make as many as 18 circuits before being eliminated in the feces.

Bile is a watery composite of substances such as bile acids, bilirubin, cholesterol, fatty acids, phospholipids, electrolytes, and bicarbonate. During interdigestive periods, bile is routed into the cystic duct for storage in the gall bladder. While the maximal volume of the gall bladder is approximately 20 to 60 ml, the equivalent of 450 ml can be stored within the gall bladder due to concentrating efforts of its wall mucosal cells. Bile is normally concentrated 5-fold. However, mucosal efforts can produce a stored bile solution concentrated 12-fold to 20-fold. Water, sodium, chloride, and other electrolytes are absorbed by the mucosal cells, thereby concentrating the remaining substances such as bile salts, cholesterol, phospholipids, and bilirubin as displayed in Table 3.2. Even though bile acids and other components are concentrated in the gall bladder, the stored solution is still isotonic while the pH is lowered.

When stimulated, such as during the presence of a meal, the smooth muscle within the wall of the gall bladder contracts and bile is propelled towards the small intestine. The most potent stimulus for emptying the gall bladder during intradigestive periods is CCK. The emptying of the gall bladder can also be stimulated by cholinergic nerve fibers from both the vagal nerve and the ENS. It is likely that vagal discharges actually initiate gall bladder contraction and combined stimuli maintain gall bladder contraction during digestion. This would discourage retrograde flow of bile back into the gall bladder as well as the draining of bile coming from the liver during periods of digestion. The gall bladder releases

TABLE 3.2
Concentration Differences: Hepatic and Gall Bladder
Bile

	Hepatic Bile	Gall Bladder Bile	Unit
Water	9.75	9.2	g/l
Bile salts	0.11	0.6	g/l
Bilirubin	0.004	0.03	g/l
Cholesterol	0.01	0.03–0.09	g/l
Fatty acids	0.012	0.03–0.12	g/l
Lecithin	0.004	0.03	mEq/l
Na^+	145	130	mEq/l
K^+	5	12	mEq/l
Ca^{2+}	5	23	mEq/l
Cl^-	100	25	mEq/l
HCO_3^-	28	10	mEq/l

about two thirds of its bile within the first hour of digestion. CCK also evokes relaxation of the sphincter of Oddi, thus allowing bile to flow into the duodenum.

Bile is important not only to supply several substances essential for lipid digestion, but also to provide an avenue for the elimination of some substances that are inappropriate for urinary excretion. In general, these substances are organic and relatively large (molecular weight >300). Also, their hydrophobicity results in their binding to plasma albumin, which decreases their filtration into the renal tubular system. The most significant of these substances is bilirubin, which is a metabolite of hemoglobin produced by reticuloendothelial cells of tissue such as the spleen. Bilirubin is released into the blood and binds with albumin. Hepatocytes remove bilirubin and conjugate it to glucuronic acid forming bilirubin glucuroninde, which is then added to bile. Because cholesterol circulates within lipoprotein complexes and is not filtered by the kidneys, its presence in bile may also be interpreted as an excretory mechanism.

In addition to the water entering the body in foods, water forms the basis for digestive secretions as well. Thus digestion occurs within a water-based medium. Bile acids act as detergents to solubilize small lipid droplets in the watery medium. With the assistance of colipase the coating of lipid droplets with bile acids allows the interaction of pancreatic lipase and cholesterol esterase with their substrates.

Enterocyte Contributions to Digestion

Enterocytes not only provide the entry site for nutrient absorption, but will also play an integral part in nutrient digestion. Several carbohydrate-digesting enzymes (disaccharidases and α-1-6 dextrinase) as well as enterokinase are associated with the brush border. Furthermore, proteases specific for short-chain length peptides are located within enterocytes and play a significant role in finalizing protein digestion. Several transport proteins are located on the luminal surface, as well as the basolateral surfaces, of enterocytes and facilitate absorptive operations. For example, the absorption of glucose first involves a Na^+-dependent symport carrier system, which translocates glucose and sodium inside the enterocyte. Glucose can then cross the basolateral membrane by facilative diffusion.

Meanwhile, sodium is actively pumped across the basolateral membrane by a Na^+/K^+ ATPase. The continual absorption of glucose through enterocytes is dependent upon an electrochemical gradient for sodium.

In addition to undergoing rapid mitosis, cells in the crypts of Lieberkühn secrete approximately 1800 ml of fluid per day. The composition of this fluid is similar to extracellular fluid with a slightly alkaline pH. The fluid provides a medium for nutrient absorption and is subsequently reabsorbed by enterocytes. These cells are particularly sensitive to toxins such as thus produced by cholera. Once small water-soluble substances, such as amino acids, monosaccharides, and certain vitamins and minerals, traverse the enterocyte lining they can enter the circulation by entering the capillary within the villus center (Figure 3.6). Contrarily, lipid-soluble substances such as cholesterol-esters, triglycerides, and lipid-soluble vitamins are primarily encorporated into chylomicron lipoproteins within enterocytes which then enter the lacteal in the central region of the villus. The small intestine will absorb the bulk of the nutrients while some absorption occurs in the stomach and colon. The finer details of the digestion and absorption of nutrients will be discussed throughout the text.

Large Intestine

The large intestine engages in two primary operations. First, it absorbs water and electrolytes from the entering contents which happens predominantly in the proximal half, and second, it stores fecal matter till defecation which occurs in the distal half. The large intestine can absorb as much as 5 to 7 liters of fluid and electrolytes in a day, if so challenged. Despite lacking villi, the mucosa of the large intestine is amply supplied with crypts of Lieberkühn whose cells secrete copious amounts of mucus. The large intestine is inhabited by more than 400 different species of bacteria. Some bacteria produce nutrients that can be absorbed, including vitamin K, biotin, and short-chain fatty acids (acetic, propionic, butyric acids). The composition of feces is approximately 30% bacteria, 10 to 20% fat, 10 to 20% inorganic matter, 2 to 3% protein, and 30% undigested fibers and dried components of digestive juices such as bilirubin and its metabolites. The coloring of feces is primarily attributable to the presence of stercobilin and urobilin which are metabolites of bilirubin. Meanwhile, the odorous characteristics of feces are due to the presence of bacterial by-products such as indoles, skatole, mercaptans, and hydrogen sulfide, and are highly individualized based upon diet and colonic bacterial profile.

4

Carbohydrates

For many individuals there is often a lot of consideration given with regard to dietary carbohydrates. For instance, some weight loss diet programs may restrict carbohydrates as an energy source, while other programs will provide carbohydrates as more than 65% of total energy. Furthermore, endurance athletes may dedicate a large portion of their total energy consumption to carbohydrates to optimize performance. While there are both myths and truths to some of these theories, on a percentage basis, carbohydrates provide the greatest part of human energy intake, both in developed and underdeveloped countries worldwide. Also, the involvement of carbohydrates, both in food and in human physiology, is not limited to just the provision of energy. Most dietary fibers are classified as carbohydrates, and, while dietary fiber does indeed provide a limited amount of energy to the human body, its role in digestive operations and perhaps disease prevention is much more significant.

To create energy-providing carbohydrates from the nonenergy-providing molecules H_2O and CO_2 is a talent bestowed upon plants. In photosynthesis, plants couple H_2O and CO_2 by harnessing solar energy. Along with carbohydrates, molecular oxygen (O_2) is also a product of this reaction.

$$6\,CO_2 + 6\,H_2O \longrightarrow C_6H_{12}O_6 + 6\,O_2$$

During man's preagricultural existence, carbohydrate intake largely came by way of fruits, vegetables, leaves, and roots. Today, industrial processing has increased the consumption of cereal grains, especially milled grains, as well as refined sugar cane, producing the "table sugar," sucrose. Within many developed countries, the last century has shown not only changes in the types of carbohydrates consumed but also in the carbohydrate contribution to total energy intake. For instance, the total consumption of carbohydrate in the U.S. has declined, now providing about one half of total energy. Sucrose consumption, which has increased over the last century, now accounts for about $1/4$ of carbohydrate energy and about $1/8$ of the total American energy intake. The average consumption of sucrose, either by adding sucrose at home or by consuming manufactured foods and beverages containing sucrose, was about 20 kg (45 lb) per American in 1990. The carbohydrate content of selected foods is listed in Table 4.1.

Carbohydrate does not have an established RDA quantity, although as part of the RDA recommendations, the National Research Council has suggested that more than one half of total dietary energy be derived from carbohydrate. There does appear to be a minimal requirement of 50 to 100 g of dietary carbohydrate to prevent the formation of excessive ketone bodies. It is also recommended that dietary carbohydrate be derived primarily from fruits, vegetables, whole grains, and their products, as well as lower-fat milks and dairy products.

TABLE 4.1
Carbohydrate Content of Selected Foods[a]

Food	Carbohydrate (%)
Table sugar	100%
Ice cream, cake, pie	40-50%
Fruits/vegetables	5-20%
Nuts	<10%
Peanut butter	<10%
Milk	5%
Cheese	1%
Shellfish	<1%
Fish	<1%
Butter	0%
Oil	0%

[a] Percentage based on weight.

The term *carbohydrate* was coined long ago as scientists observed a consistent pattern in the chemical formula of most carbohydrates. Not only were they composed of only carbon, hydrogen and oxygen, but also the ratio of carbon to water is typically one to one ($C:H_2O$). Thus, carbohydrate literally means carbon with water. Chemical carbohydrates are defined as polyhydroxyl aldehydes and ketones and their derivatives. Carbohydrates can vary from simpler 3- to 7-carbon single unit molecules to very complex branching polymers. While hundreds of different carbohydrates exist in nature, this text will take the simplest approach and group them into just a few broad categories: *monosaccharides, disaccharides, oligosaccharides,* and *polysaccharides.*

Monosaccharides

The monosaccharides that are relevant to human nutrition may be classified based on carbon number and include the trioses, tetroses, pentoses, and hexoses. Both aldoses (aldehydes) and ketoses (ketones) are present (Figure 4.1). Hexoses are the more common form of monosaccharides in the human diet. These include *glucose, galactose,* and *fructose.* Glucose is found in some foods in a free form, especially ripened fruits and vegetables, while the majority of the glucose in the human diet is derived from the digestion of disaccharides and starch. Glucose is also the principal carbohydrate found in human circulation and is often referred to as *blood sugar.* Galactose is also found free in some foods, but to a relatively small degree. Most of the galactose in the human diet is derived from the digestion of the disaccharide lactose, which is found in milk and dairy foods. Fructose is found naturally in fruits and honey and is also derived from the disaccharide sucrose. Fructose is also provided in the human diet in the form of the popular food sweetening agent high-fructose corn syrup (HFCS).

Trioses such as glyceraldehyde and dihydroxyacetone are found as intermediary products of metabolic pathways (i.e., glycolysis). Tetroses include erythrose, threose, and erythrulose. The pentoses include the aldoses: xylose, ribose, and arabinose and the ketoses xylulose and ribulose. Ribose, for instance, is a component of the nucleic acids (DNA and RNA). The alcohol derivative of ribose, ribitol, is found as a component of the water-soluble

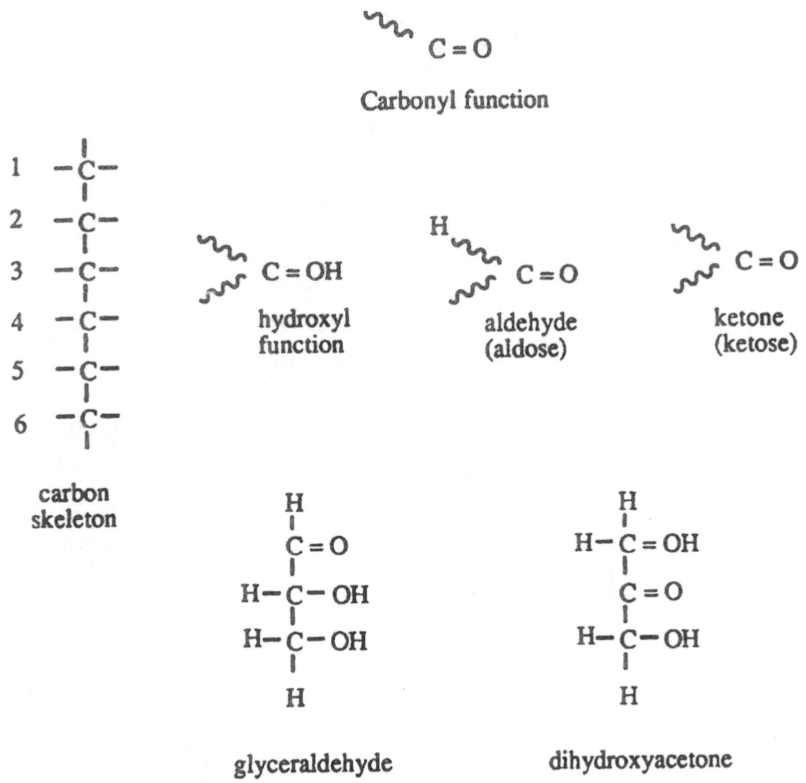

FIGURE 4.1
Basic structures of monosaccharides.

vitamin, riboflavin. Also, high energy phosphate compounds such as ATP, ADP, and AMP, plus the dinucleotides such as NAD and NADP all contain ribose as part of their chemical makeup. The other pentoses, especially xylose, are common in some fiber types such as hemicellulose. Many of the more common monosaccharides are presented in Figures 4.2 and 4.3.

While it is common to represent monosaccharides as straight-chain structures, in an aqueous environment there is a reaction between the aldehyde group of carbon 1 and the alcohol group from carbon 5. This produces a hemiacetal group, which gives the typical cyclic structural appearance. The numbering of straight and cyclic carbohydrates is presented in Figure 4.4. The position of the hydroxyl group on the asymmetric carbon farthest away from the carbonyl group (C=O) when designated in the straight-chain fashion is used to designate the D and L isomer series of the carbohydrates. If the OH group is on the right, then the monosaccharide is classified within the D series as in Figures 4.2 and 4.3. Conversely, if it is on the left side, the monosaccharide is classified within the L series. The D series is the naturally occurring form, whereas the L series results from chemical synthesis.

"*Epimers*" in sugars refer to differences in the configuration around one carbon. A good illustration of this is the difference between glucose and galactose, where the composition and molecular weights are the same, but the OH group on carbon 4 is different between the two compounds (Figure 4.5). Another example of carbohydrate epimers is the difference in configuration around the carbonyl carbon, which are referred to as *anomers*. In the cyclic method of depicting monosaccharides, if the OH group around the carbonyl carbon is in

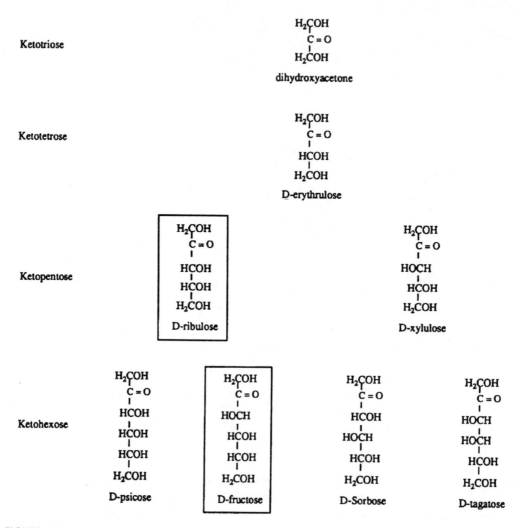

FIGURE 4.2

D-Ketoses having three to six carbons. Those ketoses of nutritional significance are enclosed in boxes.

the "down" position, this is referred to as the α designation. If the carbonyl carbon is in the "up" position, this is termed the β position. This α and β epimer difference becomes especially important in the bonding nature between monosaccharides and has a profound effect upon the ability of humans to digest these carbohydrates.

In order for a monosaccharide to become metabolically active it must become phosphorylated. Not only will phosphorylation activate the carbohydrate, but it also "locks" it within the cell. One example is glucose 6-phosphate which is created in the first step of glycolysis. Once created, glucose 6-phosphate, like other phosphorylated carbohydrates, is readily active and will not accumulate within a cell. In fact, almost all of the carbohydrates present within cells, or as components of cellular structure, are in the form of more complex carbohydrates. Some other monosaccharide derivatives are present within cells, and include amino sugars, acetyl amino sugars, uronic acids, glyconic acids, and sugar alcohols.

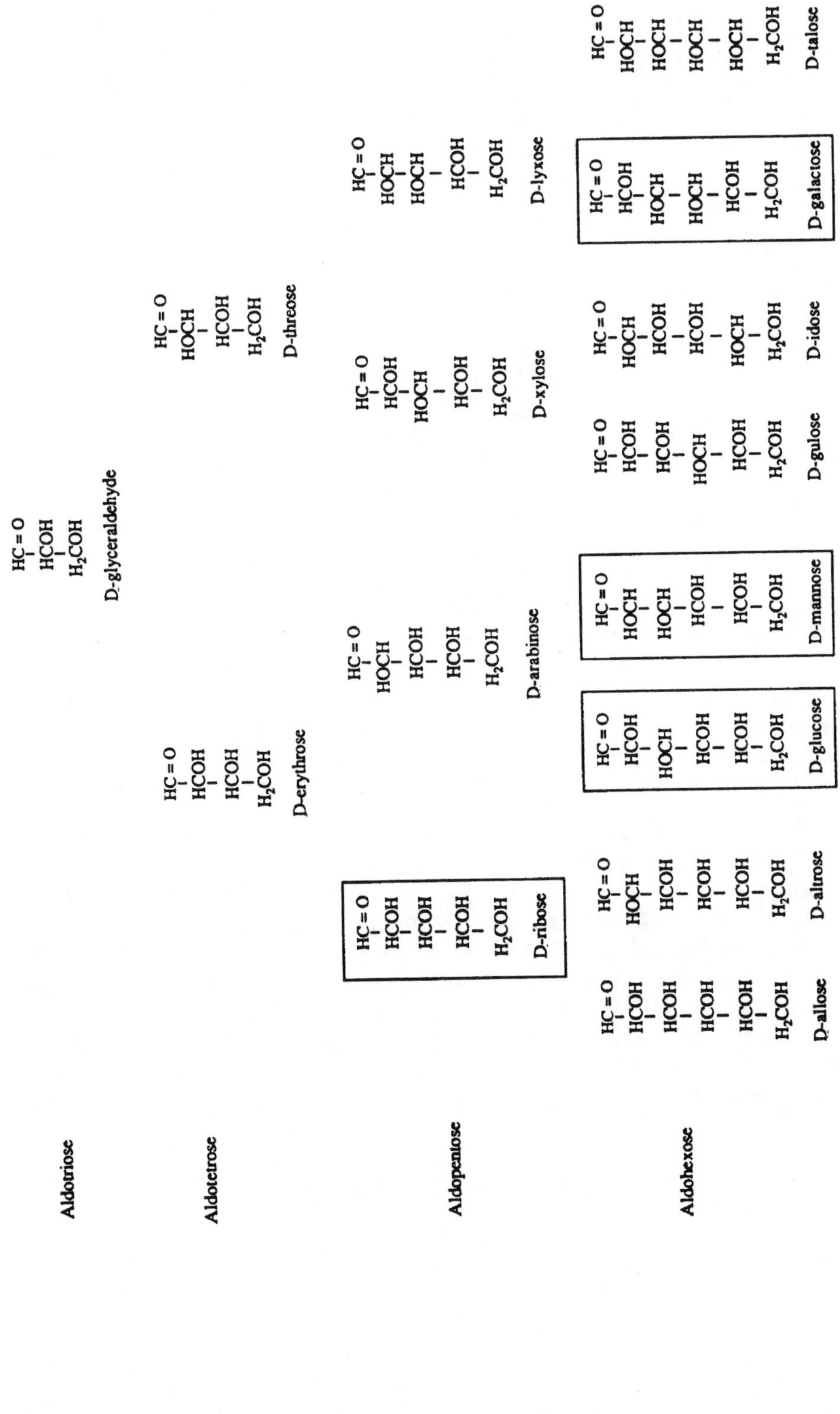

Aldotriose

HC=O
HCOH
H₂COH

D-glyceraldehyde

Aldotetrose

HC=O
HCOH
HCOH
H₂COH

D-erythrose

HC=O
HOCH
HCOH
H₂COH

D-threose

Aldopentose

HC=O
HCOH
HCOH
HCOH
H₂COH

D-ribose

HC=O
HOCH
HCOH
HCOH
H₂COH

D-arabinose

HC=O
HCOH
HOCH
HCOH
H₂COH

D-xylose

HC=O
HOCH
HOCH
HCOH
H₂COH

D-lyxose

Aldohexose

HC=O
HCOH
HCOH
HCOH
HCOH
H₂COH

D-allose

HC=O
HOCH
HCOH
HCOH
HCOH
H₂COH

D-altrose

HC=O
HCOH
HOCH
HCOH
HCOH
H₂COH

D-glucose

HC=O
HOCH
HOCH
HCOH
HCOH
H₂COH

D-mannose

HC=O
HCOH
HCOH
HOCH
HCOH
H₂COH

D-gulose

HC=O
HOCH
HCOH
HOCH
HCOH
H₂COH

D-idose

HC=O
HCOH
HOCH
HOCH
HCOH
H₂COH

D-galactose

HC=O
HOCH
HOCH
HOCH
HCOH
H₂COH

D-talose

FIGURE 4.3
D-Aldoses having three to six carbons. Those ketoses of nutritional significance are enclosed in boxes.

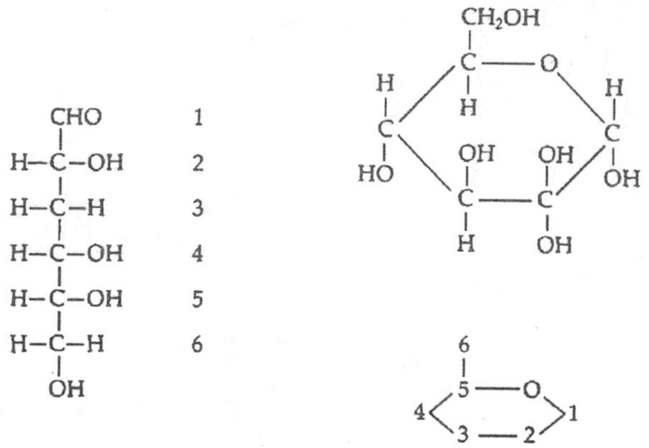

FIGURE 4.4
Carbon numbering of straight and cyclic hexose carbohydrates.

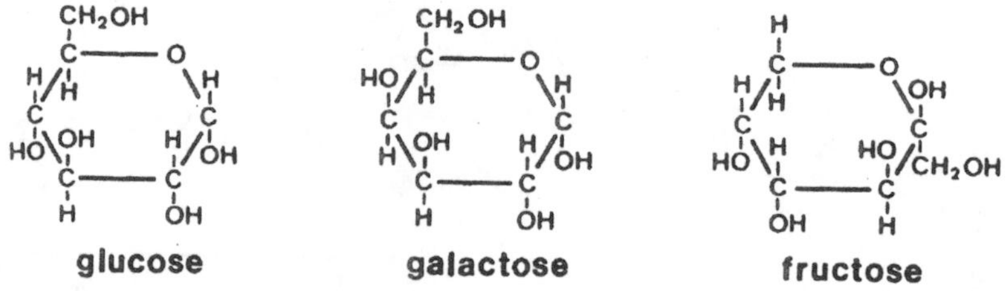

FIGURE 4.5
Monosaccharides: glucose, fructose and galactose.

Disaccharides and Oligosaccharides

Oligosaccharides are composed of 2 to 10 monosaccharides linked together by *glycosidic* bond linking of the OH groups of adjacent monomeric units. Disaccharides are the most common examples of oligosaccharides. They are composed of two monosaccharides covalently linked together. The three most common disaccharides are *sucrose, lactose,* and *maltose.* Sucrose, which is composed of fructose and glucose, is commonly referred to as cane sugar or table sugar, as mentioned above. Lactose or milk sugar, which is composed of glucose and galactose, will aid in the absorption of dietary calcium and is thought to promote the growth of beneficial bacteria in the large intestine. Maltose is composed of two glucose units. Maltose is found only for a brief time in the life of a plant, usually in the seed. It is also an intermediate product of the digestion of more complex carbohydrates (starch) in the gut.

Disaccharide	Monosaccharide Components
Lactose	Glucose + Galactose
Sucrose	Glucose + Fructose
Maltose	Glucose + Glucose

Of the carbohydrates mentioned above, only lactose is derived from animals. The remaining two disaccharides are derived from plants. The term *sugar* is often applied to monosaccharides and disaccharides. These carbohydrates elicit a sweet taste, with fructose being the most sweet. The relative sweetness of the sugars along with common artificial sweeteners is presented in Table 4.2.

TABLE 4.2
Sweetness Ratings of Sugars and Alternatives

Type of Sweetener	Relative Sweetness to Sucrose	Typical Sources
Sugars		
Lactose	0.2	Dairy
Maltose	0.4	Sprouted seeds
Glucose	0.7	Corn syrup
Sucrose	1.0	Table sugar
Fructose	1.7	Fruit, honey, soft drinks
Sugar Alcohols		
Sorbitol	0.6	Dietetic candies, sugarless gum
Mannitol	0.7	Dietetic candies
Xylitol	0.9	Sugarless gum
Artificial Sweeteners		
Aspartame (Nutrasweet)	200	Diet soft drinks and fruit drinks, powdered sweetener
Acesulfame-K	200	Sugarless gum, diet drink mixes, powdered, diet sweetener, gelatin and puddings
Saccharin	500	Diet soft drinks

Stachyose, verbacose, and *raffinose* are oligosaccharides whose metabolic fate is somewhat unique from other oligosaccharides in that they are primarily fermented by bacteria in the colon. This gives rise to their known claim to fame as flatulence producers. Legumes (beans) have appreciable levels of these monosaccharides. In beans, these sugars range from 2 to 4% of the dry weight. These are referred to as the raffinose family of sugars and are galactosyl-sucrose derivatives. For example, raffinose is sucrose linked with galactose. Stachyose is raffinose bonded to a second galactose monomer. Verbacose, which is composed of five monosaccharides, is stachyose with a third galactose monomer bonded to it.

Polysaccharides

Polysaccharides are composed of repeating monosaccharide units, most commonly glucose. While the length may vary, they are rather long, and the covalent bonds in the primary structure are found between carbons 1 and 4. For branched polysaccharides, a bond is typically found between carbons 1 and 6, if hexoses are the monosaccharides involved. These bond types are depicted in Figure 4.6. The position of the bonds, known as either the α or β configuration, will determine the properties and digestive fate of these compounds due to the ability of digestive enzymes to recognize only a particular configuration.

There are several types of polysaccharides. One of the most common is starch, which serves primarily as a storage form of carbohydrate in plants. Starch can be one long chain

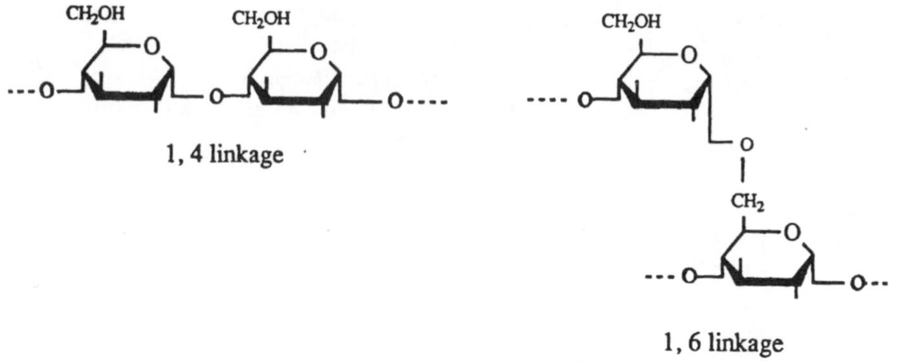

CH₂OH   CH₂OH   CH₂OH

1, 4 linkage

1, 6 linkage

FIGURE 4.6
Diagrams of α1-4 and α1-6 links between glucose molecules.

or it can be branched. Grains are among the richest sources of starch, as are legumes. For cereal grains most of the starch is found within the endosperm compartment, as depicted in Figure 4.7. Starch is referred to as a homopolysaccharide as it contains only glucose monomers linked via α1-4 and α1-6 glycosidic linkages. Starch is often referred to as a *glucan* as it yields only glucose when it is broken down. About 15 to 20% of the starch in the American diet is attributed to *amylose*. This polysaccharide is a straight-chain glucose polymer with α1-4 linkages which are depicted in Figure 4.6. It is present as a helical coil and forms hydrated micelles. *Amylopectin* (Figure 4.8) comprises about 80 to 85% of the starch in the American diet, and is a branched-chain polymer. The α1-6 branches occur at approximately every 24 to 30 glucose monomers. All other bonds between glucose monomers are α1-4 links. It does not coil effectively and tends to form colloidal suspensions in water. *Glycogen* in animal tissue is also a homopolysaccharide. It is often referred to as "animal starch" as it contains repeating glucose units. However, glycogen differs from starch in that the branching occurs every 8 to 12 residues. Animal flesh glycogen is not a significant source of dietary carbohydrate as it becomes depleted shortly after slaughter. However, it

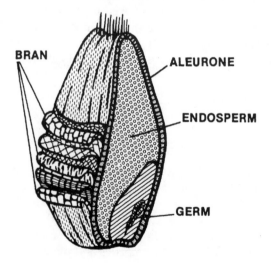

FIGURE 4.7
Structure of a grain of wheat.

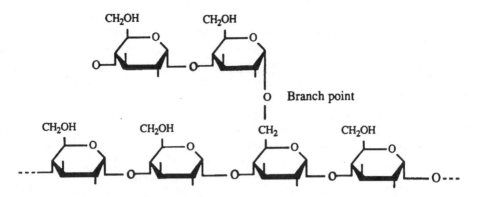

FIGURE 4.8
Diagram of α1-6 links between glucose monomers in amylopectin.

is very important as a carbohydrate storage form in humans, particularly in the liver and muscle tissue. The glycogen concentration in skeletal muscle is 1 to 2% of muscle wet weight and in liver can reach up to 8 to 10% of liver wet weight. Adipose tissue has just under 1% glycogen, by weight.

Several polysaccharides are involved in structural roles. For instance, *cellulose* is a structural polysaccharide found within plant cell walls. It is composed of repeating glucose monomers. *Hemicellulose* is another structural polysaccharide and is also a component of plant cell walls. It is composed of a mixture of both straight-chain and highly branched polysaccharides containing pentoses, hexoses, and uronic acids. Pentoses such as xylans, mannans, galactans, and arabicans are found in relatively higher abundance. Hemicelluloses are somewhat different from cellulose in that they are not limited to glucose and that they are also more vulnerable to hydrolysis by bacterial degradation. Another homopolysaccharide is *pectin*, in which the repeating subunits are methylgalacturonic acid units. It is a jelly-like material that acts as a cellular cement in plants. The linkage between the subunits is a β1-4 linkage. The carboxyl groups become methylated in a seemingly random manner as fruit ripens. Chemically related to pectin is *chitin*. Chitin is not a plant polysaccharide, but is found within the animal kingdom, but not necessarily humans. It is a β1-4 homopolymer of *N*-acetylglucosamine found in shells or exoskeletons of insects and crustacea.

Another class of polysaccharides are *glycosaminoglycans*. Glycosaminoglycans, which are sometimes called mucopolysaccharides, are characterized by their content of amino sugars and uronic acids which occur in combination with proteins in body secretions and structures. These polysaccharides are responsible for the viscosity of body mucus secretions. They are components of extracellular amorphous ground substances surrounding collagen and elastin fibers and cells of connective tissues such as bone, tendons, and ligaments. These molecules hold onto large amounts of water and they occupy space which allows for some cushioning and lubrication. Also, in combination with glycoproteins and glycolipids, the glycosaminoglycans form the cell coat or carbohydrate-dense glycocalyx present in animal cells..

Some examples of glycosaminoglycans are *hyaluronic acid* and *chondroitin sulfate*. Hyaluronic acid is a component of the ground substance found in most connective tissue, including synovial fluid of joints. It is a jelly-like substance composed of repeating disaccharides of β-glucuronic acid and *N*-acetyl-ᴅ-glucosamine. Hyuronic acid can contain several thousand disaccharide residues and is unique, differing from the other glycoaminoglycans in that it will not interact with proteins to form *proteoglycans*.

Chondroitin sulfate is composed of β-glucuronic acid and *N*-acetylgalactosamine sulfate. This molecule has a relatively high viscosity and capability to bind water. It is the major organic component of the ground substance of cartilage and bone. Both of these polysaccharides have β1-3 linkage between uronic acid and acetylated amino sugars, but are linked by β1-4 covalent bonds to other polysaccharide units. Unlike hyaluronic acid, chondroitin sulfate will bind to proteins to form proteoglycans.

Heparin is a naturally occurring anticoagulant and serves as another example of a glycosaminoglycan. It is produced by mast cells of connective tissue and is stored as granules within these cells. Mast cells are located around the inner portion of capillaries of connective tissue. Chemically, heparin is composed of sulfate-glucosamine and glucuronic acid. It has an α1-4 linkage between the disaccharide repeating units. Heparin inhibits the action of thrombin upon fibrinogen and prevents the formation of fibrin threads and clot formation. Heparin also interferes with prothrombin activator that converts prothrombin to thrombin.

Dietary Fiber Classification and Food Sources

Dietary fiber is plant material, both polysaccharide and lignin, that is resistant to human digestive enzymes. Another descriptor used for these molecules is *nonstarch polysaccharides* (NSP); however, this would not include lignin. Lignin is not considered a polysaccharide or a carbohydrate, although it is considered a fiber. Table 4.3 provides the percentage of the total weight of a food attributable to fiber.

TABLE 4.3
Fiber Content of Selected Foods

Food	Fiber (% weight)
Almonds	3
Apples	1
Lima beans	2
String beans	1
Broccoli	1
Carrots	1
Flour, whole wheat	2
Flour, white wheat	<1
Oat flakes	2
Pears	2
Pecans	2
Popcorn	2
Strawberries	1
Walnuts	2
Wheat germ	3

Dietary fiber is classified as either *soluble* or *insoluble*, based on its propensity to dissolve in water. Soluble fibers include pectin (pectic substances), gums, and mucilages. Insoluble fibers are composed of cellulose, hemicellulose, lignin, and modified cellulose. Table 4.4 classifies fiber and gives food sources for each type. Foods vary in the levels of total fiber and the contribution of different fiber types. Foods that tend to be better sources of soluble fibers are fruits, legumes, oats, and some vegetables. Meanwhile, richer sources of insoluble fibers include cereals, grains, legumes, and vegetables, especially those with a mature cell wall. The amount of fiber present within the human diet can vary geographically, as well as by gender. In some developed countries, such as the U.S., fiber consumption is relatively lower than in other societies. The average intake of fiber in America is only about 12 to 15 g daily, which is well below recommendations of the World Health Organization of 25 to 40 g daily. Americans consume a diet in which less than one half of their carbohydrate intake comes from fruits, vegetables, and whole grains. Some African societies consume as much as 50 g of fiber daily.

TABLE 4.4
Fiber Types and Characteristics, Food Sources, and Bacterial Degradation

Types of Fiber	Food Sources	Degradation
Soluble		
Pectins	Whole wheat flour, bran, cabbage, beans, apples, root vegetables	+
Gums	Oatmeal, dried beans, other legumes	+++
Mucilages	Food additives	+++
Insoluble		
Cellulose	Whole wheat flour, bran, cabbage family, peas, beans, apples, root vegetables	+
Hemicellulose	Bran, cereals, whole grains	+
Lignin	Mature vegetables, wheat	0

Note: + Denotes the degree of bacterial fermentation.

As remarked above, starch and glycogen have repeating monomeric subunits covalently bonded with α1-4 linkages. The human digestive enzyme amylase can only hydrolyze the α1-4 linkages. In addition, there is an α1-6 dextrinase (isomaltase) that can hydrolyze the branch points. Amylase is not able to hydrolyze the β1-4 covalent bonds found in such fibers as cellulose. However, the microflora of the human colon are able to metabolize some fibers and produce short-chain fatty acids (acetic, propionic, and butyric acids) as metabolites. These short-chain (sometimes called volatile) fatty acids are potentially an energy source for colonic mucosal cells or may be absorbed into the hepatic portal vein. Thus, the classic idea that fiber does not impart energy to the human diet may not be true, as the resulting volatile fatty acid by-products of fermentation can be absorbed by the lumen of the colon and subsequently utilized for energy.

Cellulose is the most abundant organic molecule on the earth. It is easily recognizable in terms of its structure with repeating glucose units, similar to amylose, but with the β1-4 linkage described above. Cellulose is synthesized on the plant cell wall by an enzyme complex called cellulose synthase. Almost as soon as nascent cellulose chains are formed they assemble with other cellulose molecules and form microfibrils that strengthen the cell wall. Cellulose, along with certain other fibers (hemicellulose and pectin) and proteins, are found within the matrix between the cell wall layers. This concept is not too unlike human connective tissue matrix, such as within bone, tendons, and ligaments.

Hemicellulose is quite different from cellulose. It is rather heterogeneous and is composed of a lot of pentoses and hexoses covalently bonded in a β1-4 linkage with side chains. The monosaccharides found in hemicelluloses include xylose, mannose, and galactose.

These sugars are referred to as xylans, mannans, and galactans when they are in the form of polymers composing the hemicelluloses. Other monosaccharide subunits include arabinose and 4-O-methyl glucuronic acids. Lignin is not a carbohydrate but is considered an insoluble dietary fiber. It is composed of aromatic polymers of chemicals from plant cell walls and provides plants with their "woody" characteristics. Lignins are highly complex and variable polymers. While there is no specific organizational structure, they are composed of three major aromatic alcohols: coumaryl, coniferyl, sinapyl. These units are often modified, allowing for as many as 40 different lignin structures.

The soluble fibers such as pectin are composed mostly of galactouronic acid that has been methylated. The units are connected by β1-4 linkages. The degree of methylation normally increases during the ripening of fruit and allows for gel properties. Gums and mucilages are similar to pectin in structure and properties, with hexoses and pentoses monomers making up these soluble fiber types. For instance, guar gum is a linear mannan with galactose side chains. Gums are polysaccharides that are synthesized by plants at the site of an injury and may function like scar tissue in humans. Mucilages are produced by secretory cells of plants to prevent excess transpiration.

The soluble fibers are thought to exert a preventive role against heart disease as they appear to have the ability to lower serum cholesterol levels. Oat bran is a good example of a fiber source with an appreciable level of soluble fiber that may demonstrate these physiological effects under controlled conditions. Also, soluble fibers can slow the rate of glucose absorption from the small intestine, although the true significance of this property is still debated.

Analysis of Fiber

Historically, there has been a lot of confusion as to how much fiber is present in a particular food. This early misinformation was likely due to the methods employed to quantify fiber in food items. Much of the early fiber analysis work used the *crude fiber method* as this was the primary method used to determine the quantity of fiber for ruminant animals. The method is essentially a sequential extraction of the material analyzed with hot dilute acid followed by dilute alkali. The crude fiber method is good for analyzing the fiber content for cattle, but not for humans. What is fiber to a human is not fiber to cattle and this system underestimated the soluble and insoluble fiber content of foods for humans.

Newer methods came into existence once the limitations of the crude fiber method became apparent. The *acid detergent method*, so-called because the analysis protocol involved boiling samples in sulfuric acid, was used to estimate the fiber component of cellulose and lignin. This method was developed for feeds and forages and was not very good for soluble fiber determination. Alternatively, the *neutral fiber method* involved boiling the material in sodium lauryl sulfate and EDTA-borate at a pH of 7.0. It adequately determined plant cell wall components, such as cellulose, lignin, and hemicellulose, but again was not good for the soluble components of dietary fiber. The neutral fiber method was modified for the analysis of human foods since these foods are often high in starch and fat. The modification allowed for fat extraction, followed by treatment with amylase to break down the starch.

In the years that followed, a newer method was developed that combined the acid detergent and the neutral detergent methods. Termed the *Van Soest method*, it provided a better estimation of all insoluble fiber components than either of the two methods just mentioned. However, this methodology, too, was limited by its inability to quantify the soluble fibers.

The best method to be developed for the complete analysis of dietary fiber, both soluble and insoluble, is the *Southgate fractionation system*. This became the "bench reference" method or state-of-the-art method. It allowed for an accurate estimation of pectic substances, hemicellulose, cellulose, and lignin, using a sequential extraction procedure. Nonfibrous material is removed first, followed by removal of pectic substances with hot water and a chelator. Hemicellulose is then extracted in several fractions by first adding dilute sodium hydroxide (NaOH) under nitrogen to precipitate the material. This step is repeated with alcohol added to get a second component of hemicellulose. Finally, under the influence of strong sodium hydroxide and nitrogen, the final fraction of hemicellulose can be obtained (hemicellulose fractions A, B, and C). Cellulose is extracted by precipitation in 17.5% NaOH. Finally, lignin is extracted by the addition of 72% sulfuric acid. While this method obtained accurate estimations of individual fiber components, this method is indeed time consuming and laborious. Laboratories wanting to analyze large numbers of food samples found this method relatively expensive and rather impractical.

With respect to simply determining total fiber content of a food sample, the greatest breakthrough came with the development of the *"enzymatic method"* or the *"Prosky method."* This method provides the most complete assessment of fiber content, including soluble and insoluble components. Here enzymatic removal of protein and starch from fat-extracted food occurs first. Then 95% ethanol is used to precipitate the soluble dietary fiber. Residual protein is then quantified and the sample is corrected for ash and protein content; finally, fiber is determined gravimetrically. Some soluble fibers may still be lost, but this system provides the best estimate of total dietary fiber. However, unlike the Southgate fractionation system, this method does not break down fiber into the individual components. In fact, it may actually overestimate fiber by not completely removing some of the nonfibrous material from a sample. Table 4.5 reviews each of these fiber analysis methods, including which fiber components each estimates as well as their practical and application limitations.

TABLE 4.5
Methods of Fiber Analysis

Method	Comments	Accuracy
Crude	Analysis for cellulose, hemicellulose, and lignin	Underestimates fiber
Acid detergent	Good for cellulose and lignin, but marginal for hemicellulose and pectin	Underestimates fiber
Neutral detergent	Good for cellulose, hemicellulose and lignin, but not for soluble fibers	Underestimates fiber
VanSoest	Combination of acid and neutral detergent; not good for soluble fibers	Underestimates fiber
Southgate	A fractionation method of analysis; all fractionation fiber components, including both insoluble and soluble; the best reference method; very time-consuming	Accurate
Enzymatic or Prosky	Very good method for analyzing all components of fiber, does not break them down into individual fiber types; rapid	Overestimates fiber

Carbohydrate Digestion

The objective of carbohydrate digestion is to liberate monosaccharides from disacchrides and more complex polymers. This activity begins in the mouth, as salivary secretions contain amylase. The digestive impact of salivary amylase is short-lived, yet significant. Oral contents are swallowed, traverse the esophagus, and deposit in the stomach. The optimal pH range for amylase activity is approximately 6.6 to 6.8. Therefore, once the swallowed contents are thoroughly mixed with the highly acidic gastric juice, amylase activity ceases. There is virtually no carbohydrate digestion in the gastric juice. While some acid hydrolysis of sucrose may occur, it is not considered of physiological significance.

In the small intestine, the major carbohydrate digestive enzyme is α-amylase, which is secreted by acinar cells of the pancreas. Both the salivary and pancreatic amylase will hydrolyze the α1-4 glycosidic linkages such that the starches consumed in a diet are converted sequentially to maltose, maltotrisoses, α-dextrins, and some trace glucose. With respect to branched starch, a mixture of dextrins, averaging six glucose residues per molecule and containing α1-6 linkages, will be generated. These linkages will be hydrolyzed by a brush border enzyme referred to as α1-6-dextrinase or isomaltase.

The reactions which break down starch into α-dextrins, maltose, and maltotrioses occurs in the intestinal lumen. The remainder of carbohydrate digestion is believed to occur along the intestinal surface. When the sugars are hydrolyzed to monosaccharides, the products are therefore in close proximity to the transport proteins. Enterocytes lining the villi of the small intestine contain disaccharidases, namely, *maltase, lactase*, and *sucrase*. These enzymes are associated with microvillus plasma membranes. These disaccharidases may not always be present in sufficient amounts to handle the digestion of disaccharides in the gut. This leads to an accumulation of the undigested disaccharide. This may produce a disaccharide intolerance, with symptoms including diarrhea resulting from the increased osmotic pressure in the lumen of the gut. Furthermore, bacterial fermentation of the disaccharides can result in common symptoms such as flatulence, nausea, and bloating. Any medical situation that damages the intestinal mucosa by preventing cell proliferation of the enterocytes, such as protein energy malnutrition or celiac disease, can produce a brush border enzyme deficiency.

The most well-known and wide-spread disaccharidase deficiency condition is a lactase deficiency which produces a *lactose intolerance*. Lactase deficiency has been reported in 55% of Mexican-American males, 73.8% of adult Mexicans from rural Mexico, 44.7% of Greeks, 56% of Cretans, 66% of Greek Cypriots, 68.8% of Jewish individuals living in North America, 50% of Indian adults and 20% of Indian children, 45% of African American children, and 80% of Alaskan Eskimos. Caucasians and those of Scandinavian descent normally have a lower prevalence of lactose intolerance than do Asian adults. There are more individuals who are lactose intolerant than tolerant. Lactase begins to be synthesized in fetal life and is at its maximal activity at birth. At the time of weaning, lactase activity may have dropped to about 90% of the level of activity at birth. The decline in lactase activity is not influenced by the level of lactose in the diet as once popularly promoted. It is more likely a genetically controlled event. Individuals who are tolerant are thought to have inherited the gene from a genetic mutation and as a dominant gene. Those individuals who have the enzyme are descendants of some African and Middle Eastern tribes and Northern Europeans. The genetic adaptation is thought to be related to the development of dairying in these regions.

Despite the problem of lactose intolerance, milk consumption need not be discouraged in those susceptible populations. In most studies, 250 ml (~1 cup) of milk, which normally contains 12 g of lactose, will not cause adverse effects. The drinking of milk by children should not be discouraged unless it causes severe diarrhea. Dairy products, where the lactose is prehydrolyzed or where *Lactobacillus acidophilus* can be added to milk during processing to hydrolyze the lactose, are available. Lactase enzyme tablets can be added to milk to digest the lactose. Fermented foods such as yogurt have bacteria that can digest lactose. Foods such as cottage cheese and aged cheddar cheese contain low levels of lactose and are not likely to produce problems.

As mentioned above, stachyose and raffinose are be found in most legumes and these shorter links of monosaccharides are generally resistant to human carbohydrate digestive enzymes. Legumes are plants that have a single row of seeds in their pods. What are commonly called legumes, such as peas, green beans, lima beans, pinto beans, black-eyed peas, garbanzo beans, lentils, and soybeans, are often the seeds of legume plants. So, like lactose, these carbohydrates will stay intact in the intestinal lumen. Once in the colon, these carbohydrates are subject to bacterial fermentation. Similar by-products are produced as with lactose as well as similar symptoms. Commercially available products (i.e., Beano) are enzyme preparations that enhance digestion of these carbohydrates when consumed just prior to the legume-containing meal.

Absorption of Monosaccharides

The absorptive cells of the small intestinal lining will absorb some hexoses at a greater rate than others. Galactose and glucose are known to be actively absorbed against a concentration gradient, whereas others, such as fructose, are not. Apparently, the basic requirement for active transport is based on the presence of the 6-carbon structure and an intact OH group at position 2. Oxygen and sodium are required, and selective metabolic inhibitors can block the active transport. The transport is selective, with some sugars transported at a greater rate than others. With glucose transport (1.0) serving as the reference standard, the rate of galactose transport appears to be slightly greater (1.1), while the transport rates of fructose (0.4), mannose (0.2), xylose (0.15), and arabinose (0.10) are lower.

Glucose and galactose seem to compete with one another for absorption aboard a common carrier. And, as mentioned, both of these monosaccharides are absorbed by active transport. However, fructose is absorbed by facilitative diffusion. Thus, fructose needs to bind to a membrane protein carrier, as well as to move down a concentration gradient. Mannose, xylose, and arabinose are absorbed by passive diffusion.

A protein carrier, sodium, and energy in the form of ATP are required for active transport of glucose and galactose. The sodium gradient hypothesis states that glucose or galactose will associate with a protein carrier on the microvillus membrane which will also have a binding site for sodium (Figure 4.9). The energy released by sodium moving down its concentration gradient into the cell is sufficient to also move glucose into the cell against its concentration gradient. Sodium is subsequently pumped out of the cell by an ATPase to maintain the gradient. Two sodium ions for each monosaccharide transported are needed. Once it is inside the cell, 15% of the monosaccharide leaks back out through the brush border, 25% diffuses through the basolateral membrane, and 60% leaves on the serosal side through a carrier mechanism, all of which are independent of sodium. Due to these multiple exit avenues, monosaccharides such as glucose and galactose do not accumulate to significant levels within enterocytes. Most of the absorption of monosaccharides occurs in the upper portion of the small intestine. The trioses and tetrasaccharides are absorbed through passive diffusion.

Nondigestible Starch

There is a growing body of evidence to suggest that some starches are incompletely hydrolyzed as well. This enzyme-resistant starch may be in the form of insoluble, semicrystalline granules. If starch granules are heated to over 100°C, the granularity is lost and starch is gelatinized or the granules swell. This increases the availability of the starch to digestive

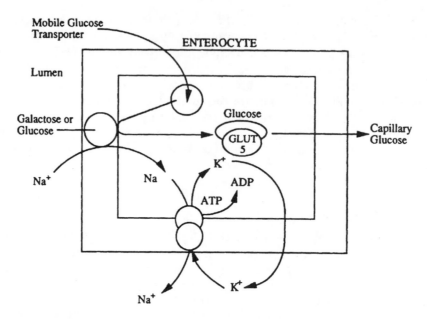

FIGURE 4.9

Absorption of glucose and galactose across the small intestinal mucosa. Glucose or galactose both bind to a transmembrane protein that also binds sodium. The energy from sodium moving down its concentration gradient is sufficient to transport glucose into the cell against its concentration gradient. Sodium is then pumped out of the cell by an ATPase.

enzymes. However, when the starch cools, there is some recrystallization of the starch. This is called "retrogradation" and is resistant to α-amylase hydrolysis. Uncooked starch, such as that present in bananas, is also resistant to hydrolysis for similar reasons in the crystalline structure. This implies that the metabolizable energy is decreased from such food sources. The undigested starch will most likely be fermented in the colon by bacteria and the short-chain fatty acids that result (e.g., acetate, butyrate) will be absorbed and contribute about 3 kcal/g. The glycemic effect of starch is therefore lowered and this decreases insulin secretion.

INSIGHT: Physical and Physiological Properties of Fiber and Potential Benefits to Health

The physiological attributes of fiber largely depend upon their physical characteristics, namely, molecular design and solubility. While most of the physiological interaction of dietary fibers was once thought to be limited to within the digestive tract, newer evidence suggests that derivatives of intestinal fiber metabolism can influence internal operations as well. The physical characteristics of dietary fiber can evoke different gastrointestinal responses, depending upon the segment of the digestive tract. These responses include gastric distention, influence upon emptying rate, augmentation of residue quantity and moisture content, and fermentation by bacteria in the lower digestive tract, as well as influencing the turnover of specific bacteria species present. The bacterial population of the

TABLE 4.6

Changes in Fecal Bulk Due to Various
Dietary Fiber Sources

Food Item	% Increase in Fecal Weight
Bran	127
Cabbage	69
Carrots	59
Apple	40
Guar gum	20

colon will likely increase due to fiber fermentation and may contribute as much as 45% to the fecal dry weight. The influence of fiber upon fecal mass is presented in Table 4.6.

Fiber is subject to bacterial degradation in the colon, as presented in Table 4.4. Pectins, mucilages, and gums appear to be almost completely fermented, while cellulose is only partly degraded. Also, because of its unique molecular design, lignin virtually goes unfermented. The degradation of food fibers by intestinal bacteria may be related to the physical structure of the plant itself as fibers derived from fruits and vegetables appear to be, in general, more fermentable than those from cereal grains. Volatile fatty acids, namely, acetic, proprionic and butyric acids, are produced during bacterial fermentation. These fatty acids can be utilized as an energy source for colon mucosal cells as well as be absorbed into the portal circulation. Hydrogen gas, carbon dioxide, and methane are also produced during bacterial metabolism of fiberous material.

A clinical estimation of bacterial fermentation of fibrous material is the *hydrogen breath test*. Hydrogen gas produced by bacterial fermentation can dissolve into the blood and circulate to the lungs whereby it diffuses into alveoli and is subsequently exhaled. However, it must be recognized that bacterial fermentation of other digestive residues, such as lactose, will also produce hydrogen gas. Thus, this must be considered if quantification of expired hydrogen gas is to be used as an indicator of fiber fermentation. The opposite is true as well. Bacterial fermentation of fiber must be controlled if the hydrogen breath test is to be applied to estimate lactose intolerance.

There are several physical properties of fiber and each type of fiber is somewhat unique (Table 4.7). The water-holding capacity or the *hydration* of fiber is one of the more interesting physical properties. A given fiber's ability to hold onto water is enhanced by the presence of monomers that have free polar groups, such as OH, COOH, SO_4, and C=O groups. Pectic substances, mucilages, and hemicellulose have the greatest water-holding capacity. Cellulose and lignin also have a propensity to hold onto water. However, since soluble fibers tend to be more fermentable, the water is normally released in the colon and absorbed. Therefore, in a practical sense, it is the insoluble fibers that hold onto water throughout the total length of the intestinal tract and give the fecal mass greater water content.

In the small intestine, the hydration of fiber will contribute to the formation of a gel matrix. This can increase viscosity of the contents within the small intestine and slow the rate of absorption of nutrients. It has been suggested that a slowing of the rate of carbohydrate absorption may be beneficial to individuals with diabetes by potentially decreasing the glycemic index of a food.

Another physical property of dietary fiber is that it may bind intestinal material such as bile acids, cholesterol, and toxic compounds. For instance, lignin seems to be very efficient

TABLE 4.7
Physical Properties of Some Fiber Types

Type	Action
Cellulose	Holds water; reduced colonic pressure; reduced trace mineral excretion; reduced transit time; reduced trace mineral absorption
Hemicellulose	Holds water; increased stool bulk; may bind bile acids; reduced colonic pressure; reduced transit time
Pectins, gums, mucilages	Slow gastric emptying; binds bile acids; decreased trace mineral excretion; reduced trace mineral absorption
Lignin	Holds water; may bind trace minerals; binds fecal steroids

in binding bile acids present in the digestive tract. Pectin and other acidic polysaccharides also appear to bind bile acids. However, cellulose has little ability to bind bile acids. The ability of soluble fibers and lignin to bind bile acids is believed to be responsible for some of the hypocholesterolemic effect of dietary fiber. When more bile acids are complexed to fiber components, less bile acid is reabsorbed by the intestine. Thus, the enterohepatic circulation of bile acids is decreased and more bile acids are excreted in the feces. This is believed to result in the dedication of more hepatic cholesterol to the synthesis of new bile acids. Thus, less cholesterol may be available for incorporation into VLDL and export into circulation. As VLDL becomes LDL, the effect is a reduction in total cholesterol and LDL cholesterol levels.

Cation exchange or metal binding capacity of fiber is also recognized as a physical property of fiber. This can have potential consequences in terms of nutrient absorption and requirements. Minerals such as calcium, zinc, copper, iron, cadmium, and mercury may bind to fiber and be made less available for absorption. The number of free carboxyl groups on fiber components and the uronic acid content of the fibers will increase metal binding. Lignin also has this property. The soluble fibers are very efficient metal chelators in the digestive tract.

Dietary fiber is also known to interact with other components of the diet, particularly protein and carbohydrate. Cellulose and hemicellulose, composed primarily of xylans, can reduce the *in vitro* proteolytic activity of human pancreatic trypsin. Amylase and lipase activities are also depressed. A low protein diet will give a more positive mineral balance with a high fiber diet. With regard to free radical scavenging, lignin appears to have some capability. It is likely that the phenolic groups within lignin facilitate this activity, and it has been speculated that this may be a contributing factor in the prophylactic properties of fiber with regard to certain cancers.

The physical attributes of fiber contribute to perhaps their most renowned effect, the ability to alter the bulk and composition of feces as well as its transit time. Increased fecal bulk from a high dietary fiber intake is due to (1) the presence of undegraded fiber residue, (2) increase in fecal water, (3) increase in bacterial cell mass caused by fiber fermentation, and (4) fiber type. Noncellulose polysaccharides, such as gums, mucilages, and pectin, are ineffective bulking agents largely due to the almost complete degradation via bacterial fermentation (Table 4.6). Conversely, cellulose, hemicellulose, and lignin are more efficient bulking agents. Transit time is increased on a low dietary fiber diet, and vice versa. Normal transit time for cultures living in a high-fiber consuming society is 24 to 48 hours. In Western cultures, where the dietary fiber content is considerably less, it is not unusual for transit time to be as high as 72 h or greater. With respect to intestinal motility, a higher fiber diet is a standard recommendation for the prevention and alleviation of constipation.

While plasma cholesterol and glycemic index may be reduced as discussed above, there may be some negative consequences to too much dietary fiber consumed. It has been suggested that higher fiber intakes (>30 g/d) may facilitate the intestinal chelation and subsequent removal of essential elements, especially polyvalent cations such iron, zinc, copper, magnesium, and calcium. Also, excessive dietary fiber may produce *phytobezoars*, potentially resulting in gastrointestinal obstruction. Furthermore, a reduction in the efficiency of energy nutrient digestion may also be experienced, although this notion has been considered a positive from certain health perspectives such as therapeutic weight loss.

Soluble fiber may have some negative consequences with respect to turnover of colon crypt cells. Feeding diets high in soluble fiber to rodents, for instance, does result in increase cellular proliferation of colon cells. It has been suggested that this situation might place an organism at increased risk for colon tumors. In contrast, insoluble fibers do not have this propensity. Table 4.8 provides the total fiber and soluble fiber content of select foods.

TABLE 4.8
Total and Soluble Fiber Content of Selected Cereal Brans

Crude Bran Source (100 g)	Total Dietary Fiber (g)	Soluble Fiber (g)
Wheat bran (1-2/3 cups)	42	3
Oat bran (2/3 cups)	16	7
Rice bran (1 cup)	22–24	3–9
Corn bran (1-1/4 cups)	85	2–3

Controlled human studies have demonstrated that feeding wheat bran and cellulose to subjects with high fecal mutagens lowers the mutagen counts and also the toxic secondary bile acids, such as lithocholic and deoxycholic acids. This was in comparison with a more typical diet supplemented with oat bran which is endowed with more soluble fiber. Thus, in this sense, insoluble fibers may be protective against colon cancer, while soluble fibers may afford protection against coronary heart disease via decreases in blood cholesterol levels. Therefore, unless medically warranted, fiber consumption should include a mixture of fiber types from a variety of foods.

5

Lipids

Classically, lipids have been defined as substances that are generally insoluble in water but soluble in organic solvents such as ether, acetone, and chloroform. There are a variety of different kinds of lipids applicable to human structure and function including fatty acids, triglycerides (triacylglycerols), phospholipids, and sterols (i.e., cholesterol). All too often lipids are viewed only from an energy perspective. For instance, fatty acids are oxidized to form ATP in almost all human cells and are the principal source of energy during periods of fasting. Furthermore, the storage of triglycerides, can represent as much as 90,000 to 100,000 kcal of energy for an average adult male. Further still, triglycerides, or more commonly, fat, account for as much as a third or more of the total energy consumed in many countries and is the focus of many body weight reduction efforts. However, to view lipids only from an energy perspective would greatly understate their unique properties and physiological significance. Body fat has excellent insulating properties, thereby guarding against heat loss. Also, body fat deposits provide internal padding to protect visceral organs. Dietary essential fatty acids (EFA), linoleic acid and linolenic acid, are converted into local-acting eicosanoid factors. These factors are fundamentally involved in the regulation of numerous cellular and tissue operations such as blood pressure, platelet aggregation, bronchial constriction, chemotaxis, and inflammation. Diglycerides are the basis of phospholipids, which are the foundational component of cellular membranes and lipoproteins. Glycolipids and cholesterol are also key components of cell membrane. Cholesterol also serves as the precursor molecule for a variety of steroid molecules such as testosterone, DHEA, estrogens, cortisol, and aldosterone.

General Properties and Nomenclature of Lipids

Fatty Acids

Fatty acids (Figure 5.1) are unique in a molecular sense in that they have a polar carboxyl end and a nonpolar methyl end. The two ends of a fatty acid are separated by a hydrocarbon region of varying length. Fatty acids do not cyclize; therefore they exist as chains of hydrocarbon. The carboxyl end has water-soluble properties, while the hydrocarbon tail, which includes the methyl end, is insoluble. Thus, shorter fatty acids tend to be more water-soluble than longer fatty acids. For instance, fatty acids containing six carbons or less are very miscible in water while those with ten or more carbons are not miscible. The fatty acids of relevance to human nutrition are monocarboxylic and have an even number of carbons. Odd-chain length fatty acids do occur in the diet as well as within human tissue, but to a significantly lesser degree. Table 5.1 provides a listing of common fatty acids.

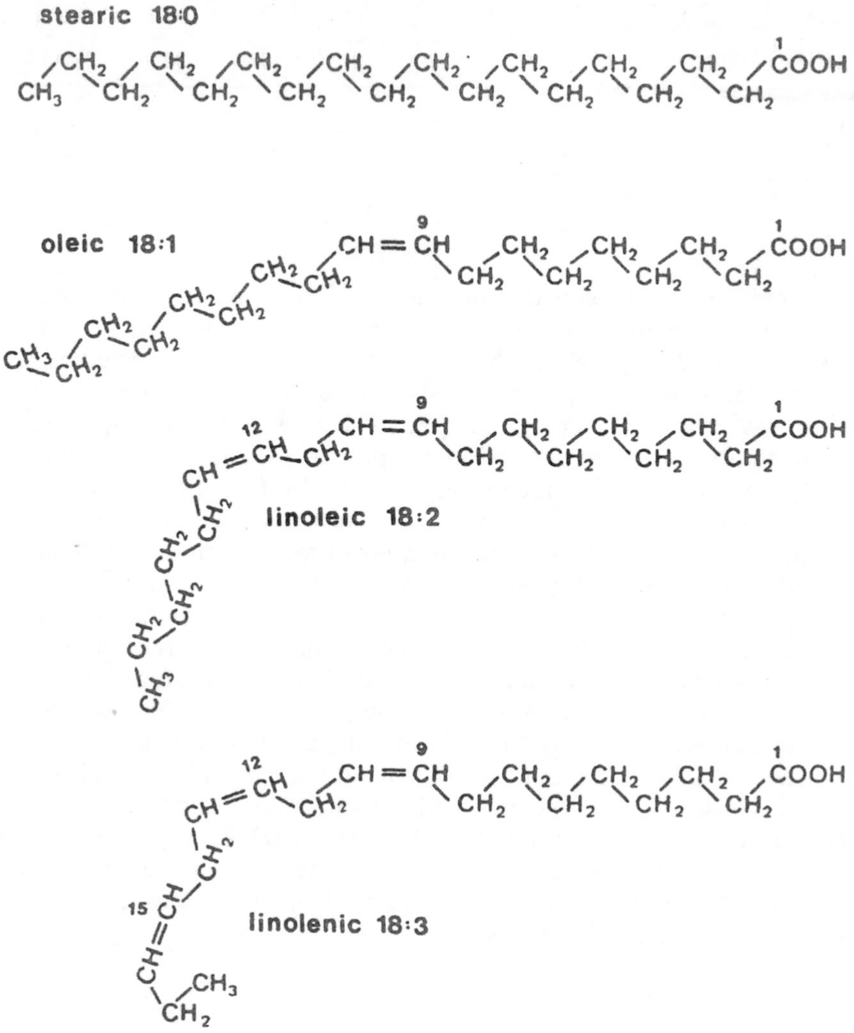

stearic 18:0

oleic 18:1

linoleic 18:2

linolenic 18:3

FIGURE 5.1

Fatty Acids. Stearic acid is saturated and oleic acid is monounsaturated. Linoleic and linolenic acids are polyunsaturated fatty acids.

Fatty acid chain length is easily determined by counting the total number of carbon atoms. Acetic acid is the smallest fatty acid, having only 2 carbons, and arachidic acid is one of the longer fatty acids, consisting of 20 carbons. Fatty acids are often subclassified in terms of their length. Short-chain fatty acids contain 2 to 4 carbons, while medium-chain and long-chain fatty acids contain 6 to 12 and 14 to 26 carbons, respectively. However, there does seem to be some variation in the designation of fatty acids by scientists into these three categories.

Beyond length, fatty acids can vary in their degree of *saturation*. This is in reference to whether or not the hydrocarbon tail contains the maximal number of hydrogen atoms. Locations along the fatty acid hydrocarbon chain whereby a double covalent bond is present are sometimes referred as *points of unsaturation*. The terms *saturated*, *monounsaturated*, and *polyunsaturated* are applied to fatty acids containing no double bonds, a single double bond, or more than one double bond, respectively. Examples of a saturated fatty

TABLE 5.1
Common Fatty Acids

Saturated Fatty Acids	Nomenclature	Unsaturated Fatty Acid	Nomenclature
Acetic acid	2:0	Palmitoleic acid	16:1 ω-9
Butyric acid	4:0	Oleic acid	18:1 ω-9
Caproic acid	6:0	Linoleic acid	18:2 ω-6
Caprylic acid	8:0	Linolenic acid	18:3 ω-3
Capric acid	10:0	Arachidonic acid	20:4 ω-6
Lauric acid	12:0	Eicosapentaenoic acid	20:5 ω-3
Myristic acid	14:0	Docosahexaenoic acid	22:6 ω-3
Palmitic acid	16:0		
Stearic acid	18:0		
Arachidic acid	20:0		

acid (SFA), monounsaturated fatty acid (MUFA), and a polyunsaturated fatty acid (PUFA) are presented in Figure 5.1.

Identifying the position of double bonds can be accomplished by counting from either end of the fatty acid molecule. Starting at the carboxyl end and counting the carbons to the double bonds applies the delta (Δ) system. Counting from the methyl end is referred to as the omega (ω) system. ("n" is often used in substitution of "ω".) The latter system derives its nomenclature from the Greek alphabet as omega is the last letter. For instance, the fatty acid in Figure 5.2 can be identified as either $18:3\Delta^{9,12,15}$ or $18:3\omega3$. Here the "18" indicates the total number of carbon atoms while the "3" following the colon indicates the total number of double bonds. The first carbon of the three double bonds can be found at carbon 9 when counting from the carboxylic end, according to the delta system. When applying the omega system, and thus counting from the methyl end, only the position of the 1st carbon of the initial double bond is indicated, as the ensuing double bond will occur following a methylene group.

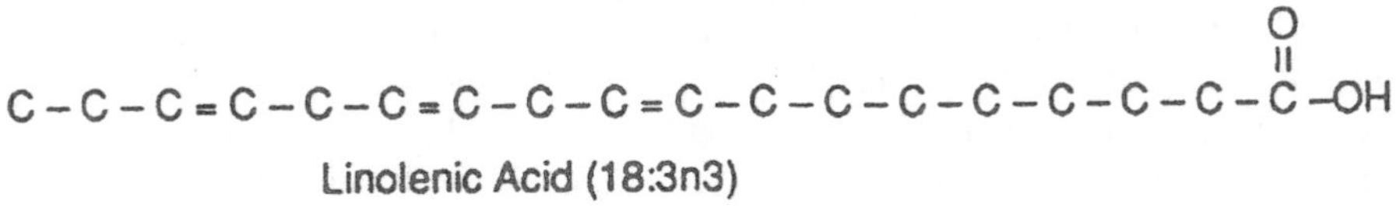

$$C-C-C=C-C-C=C-C-C=C-C-C-C-C-C-C-C-\overset{\overset{\displaystyle O}{\|}}{C}-OH$$

Linolenic Acid (18:3n3)

FIGURE 5.2
Linolenic acid.

As the length of a fatty acid influences its solubility properties, so will its degree of unsaturation. The greater the number of double bonds, the greater the polarity of a fatty acid and thus its solubility in water. Melting point is also influenced by chain length and the number of double bonds in a manner similar to solubility. Thus, in general, the greater the chain length and the more saturated a fatty acid, the higher its melting point. All of the common unsaturated fatty acids are liquid at room temperature except for oleic acid.

Fatty Acid Synthesis, Elongation, and Desaturation

Many human cells can synthesize fatty acids; however the liver and to a lesser degree adipose tissue are the primary sites of synthesis. Other tissue possessing a recognizable ability to synthesize fatty acids are the kidneys, mammary glands, lung, and the brain. Acetyl

CoA, which is an intermediate of carbohydrate, amino acid, and ethanol metabolism, is the building block for the cytosolic fatty acid synthesis. *Acetyl CoA carboxylase* and *fatty acid synthase* are the key regulatory enzymes involved. The latter enzyme is actually a complex system of several enzymatic and nonenzymatic protein subunits, all coded by the same gene. The process of making fatty acids is referred to simply as fatty acid synthesis or *de novo lipogenesis*. Palmitic acid (16:0) is the product fatty acid and the metabolic pathway will be discussed in greater detail in Chapter 11.

Several factors, such as diet and genetic considerations, are known to significantly influence human fatty acid synthesis. For instance, when humans eat a very high-carbohydrate, especially sucrose-based carbohydrate, fatty acid synthesis increases relative to consuming an isocaloric, lower-carbohydrate diet. Also, in many obese individuals it is believed that significant fatty acid synthesis may occur despite the consumption of a high-fat diet. Fatty acid synthesis seems to be regulated at several levels. For instance, expression of the acetyl CoA carboxylase gene may be induced by insulin, while insulin and cytosolic citrate also increase its activity. Long-chain acyl-CoA (activated fatty acids), cAMP, and glucagon all decrease acetyl CoA carboxylase activity. Many of the same influences upon acetyl CoA carboxylase also exist for fatty acid synthase. Interestingly, it appears that there may be a nuclear protein that selectively binds ω-3 and ω-6 PUFA. These PUFAs decrease the expression of the FAS gene. It seems that ω-3 PUFAs are more potent at this task. Also, increasing levels of plasma FFA are associated with decreased lipogenesis.

NADPH provides the reducing hydrogens for fatty acid synthesis. Most of the NADPH is derived from the *pentose phosphate pathway* or *hexose monophosphate shunt*, which will be explained in more detail in Chapter 11. Cytosolic malic enzyme and isocitrate dehydrogenase are also sources of NADPH; however, the significance of the latter enzyme is believed to be minor.

Human cells can also elongate and desaturate existing fatty acids. The cellular organelles responsible for elongation are either the endoplasmic reticulum or mitochondria, with the former being more significant. In the endoplasmic reticulum the sequence of elongation reactions is similar to fatty acid synthesis in which the source of the two-carbon unit is malonyl CoA and the reducing power is provided by NADPH. The *fatty acid elongase* system of enzymes catalyzes the reactions. Fatty acids that can act as primers for elongation include saturated fatty acids containing 10 carbons or more as well as unsaturated fatty acid. Elongation of stearic acid is elevated during the myelination of brain tissue, thereby providing 22- and 24-carbon fatty acids. Fatty acids of this length are found in sphingolipids. Elongation of fatty acids appears to be depressed during caloric deprivation.

Double bonds may be added to fatty acids, via desaturating enzymes. This occurs within the endoplasmic reticulum. Desaturating enzymes were named with the delta system in mind. Certain human cells express Δ-5 *desaturase*, Δ-6 *desaturase*, or Δ-9 *desaturase*. For instance, desaturation of stearic acid (18:0) by Δ-9 desaturase results in oleic acid (18:1 ω-9). Because humans lack enzymes to desaturate beyond the 9th carbon of a fatty acid, the vital unsaturated fatty acids linoleic acid (18:2 ω-6) and linolenic acid (18-2 ω-3) are dietary essentials.

Cis vs. Trans Fatty Acids

The orientation of hydrogen atoms about a double bond influences the structure and thus physical properties of a fatty acid. If the hydrogen associated with the carbons of a double bond is positioned on the same side it is a *cis* arrangement. On the other hand, if the hydrogens bonded to the carbons are on opposite sides of the double bond, it is referred to as a *trans* arrangement and the fatty acid is called a *trans* fatty acid. Fatty acids with the same length and position of double bonds, yet differing in the orientation of the hydrogen atoms, will have different chemical names. For instance, 18:1 ω-9 with a *cis* arrangement is called oleic acid, while 18:1 ω-9 with a *trans* arrangement is called elaidic acid.

Cis-Configured double bonds tend to kink or bend a fatty acid chain, while *trans* fatty acids maintains more of a straight chain similar to saturated fatty acids (Figure 5.3). This influences the physical properties of cellular membranes. Quite simply, with an increased presence of *cis*-configured bonding, there is more fluid in the membrane. Conversely, a membrane with an increased amount of saturated or *trans*-bonded fatty acids will have a less fluid membrane. The *cis* arrangment is by far the more prevalent arrangements of double bonds in fatty acids in foods and the human body.

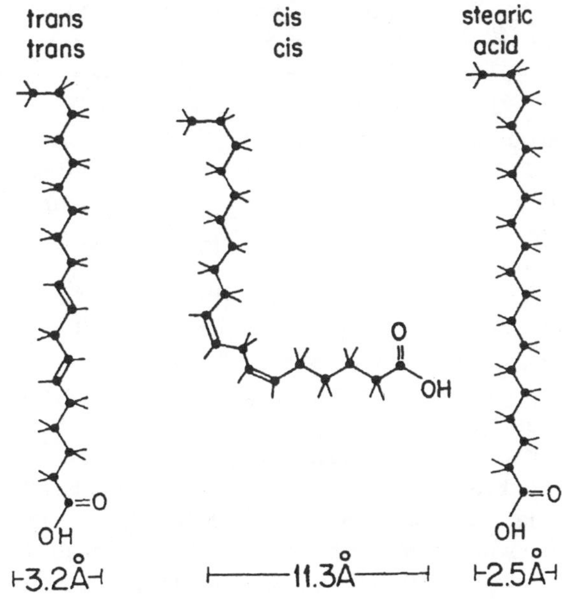

FIGURE 5.3
Cis vs. *trans arrangements* and their effect upon kinking or bending of the hydrocarbon tail.

Trans fatty acids also influence several metabolic operations by influencing the operation of several lipid enzymes. *Trans* isomers of 18:2 ω-6 decrease prostaglandin synthesis, thereby increasing the requirement for linoleic acid for prostaglandin functions. *Trans* isomers of 18:2 ω-6 (*cis, trans* and *trans, trans*) are also devoid of essential fatty acid activity. Also, the *trans* isomer of 18:1 ω-9 (elaidic acid) may decrease the activity of Δ-6 desaturase and Δ-9 desaturase. Studies involving human fibroblasts have shown that *trans* fatty acids impair the microsomal desaturation and chain elongation of both linoleic and linolenic acid (essential fatty acids) to their longer chain metabolites, especially *arachidonic acid* and *docosahexaenoic acid*. The ramifications of these effects may be most significant during the gestational development of humans. Thus, it has been recommended that pregnant women decrease their *trans* fatty acid consumption. *Trans* fatty acids do appear to cross the placental barrier and are probably also secreted into human milk.

Essential Fatty Acids

For decades, it was believed that dietary fatty acids served only to provide fuel and had no essential physiological function. However, in the 1920s research began to reveal the fact that there was an essential role for fatty acids, as animals fed a fat-free diet demonstrated poor growth and impaired reproduction. Scientists suggested that fat contained an essential factor which at the time they called vitamin F; however, the structure and function were still unknown. Linoleic acid (18:2 ω-6 PUFA) was soon identified and suggested to be an EFA. Some even referred to linoleic acid as vitamin F. However, in the 1970s scientists also began to recognize the essentiality of ω-3 PUFA as well. Humans do not have Δ-12 desaturase and Δ-15 desaturase; therefore 18-carbon ω-3 and ω-6 PUFAs are by nature dietary essentials to man.

The true essential fatty acids for humans are linoleic acid (18:2 ω-6) and linolenic acid (18:3 ω-3). These fatty acids are presented in Figure 5.1. Other longer-chain PUFAs such as arachidonic acid (AA) (20:4 ω-6) and eicosapentenoic acid (EPA) (20:5 ω-3) and docosahexaenoic acid (DHA) (22:6 ω-3) can be made from available linoleic and linolenic acids by a series of elongations and desaturations (Figure 5.4). Thus, to make 20:4 ω-6 from 18:2 ω-6 and 20:5 ω-3 from 18:3 ω-3 requires first the activity of Δ-6 desaturase, then elongation, and then Δ-5 desaturase. The formation of 22:6 ω-3 (DHA) is a little more involved. First, 20:5 ω-3 is elongated to 22:5 ω-3 and then 24:5 ω-3, followed by Δ-6 desaturation to yield 24:6 ω-3 and then partial β-oxidation to 22:6 ω-3 (DHA). Alternatively, to seemingly go backwards and create 20:5 ω-3 (EPA) from 22:6 ω-3 (DHA) requires peroxisomal and endoplasmic reticulum enzyme assistance. The endoplasmic reticulum membrane is the site of the desaturating enzymes and can be found in various tissues such as the liver, intestinal mucosa, retina, and brain.

Interestingly, the activity of Δ-6 desaturase is known to be regulated by several hormonal and dietary factors. For instance, insulin and the presence of EFA tend to increase its activity, while glucose, epinephrine, and glucagon tend to decrease its enzymatic activity. While both ω-3 and ω-6 PUFA compete for the same desaturating enzymes, both Δ-5 desaturase and Δ-6 desaturase prefer ω-3 over ω-6 PUFA. However, an increased diet ω-6:ω-3 PUFA ratio, as typical of the Western diet, will slow down the conversion of linolenic acid to EPA and DHA. The activity of Δ-6 desaturase seems to decline relative to age. Also, premature infants are limited in their ability to produce EPA and DHA from linolenic acid, as are some hypertensive individuals and some diabetics. Individuals consuming a diet rich in DHA and EPA, typically from fish, tend to have higher levels of these fatty acids in plasma and tissue phospholipids and lesser amounts of arachidonic acid.

Linolenic acid is found mostly in triglycerides and cholesterol esters and in only small amounts in phospholipids. Conversely, EPA is found mostly in phospholipids and in cholesterol esters and only in smaller amounts in triglycerides. DHA is also found mostly in phospholipids. The cerebral cortex, retina, testis, and sperm contain higher concentrations of DHA.

It is believed that paleolithic man consumed a diet with an essential fatty acid (ω-6:ω-3) ratio of approximately 1:1. Today, most developed societies consume a diet lower in ω-3 PUFA and higher in ω-6 PUFA. This is largely attributed to the domestication of animals and the increased consumption of vegetable oils. For instance, wild game as consumed by human ancestors is very lean (3 to 4% total fat) and contains a respectable quantity of ω-3 PUFA. However, today domesticated animals such as cattle contain much more fat, which is relatively high in hypercholesterolemic saturated fatty acids and lower in ω-3 PUFA. A wild chicken egg, for instance, may have a ω-6:ω-3 PUFA ratio of 1.3:1. However, a domesticated chicken egg, as available in most supermarkets, may have a ratio of 19:1. Furthermore, selective hydrogenation of ω-3 PUFA in soybean oil, which is used in the production of many food recipes (i.e., snack foods), has further increased the ω-6:ω:3 PUFA.

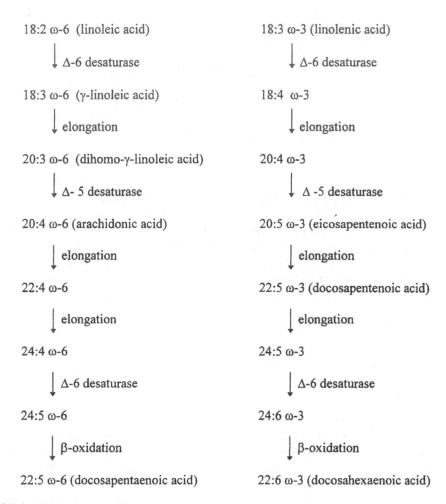

FIGURE 5.4
Synthetic pathways for eicosanoids.

Phospholipids

Phospholipids are lipid compounds that contain phosphatidic acid, which is composed of glycerol, 2 fatty acids, and a phosphate (PO_4) group (Figure 5.5). They are amphiphylic by nature, able to attract both water-soluble and fat-soluble substances, thereby making them ideal for cellular membranes and lipoprotein shells. Generally phospholipids are unavailable as an energy source. The various phospholipids differ from each other by what is attached to the PO_4 group. The sn-1 or α carbon of the glycerol backbone is usually esterified to a saturated fatty acid while the sn-2 or β carbon usually is esterifed to an unsaturated fatty acid which can be an EFA or a derivative on an EFA. The sn-3 carbon is attached to a phosphate group, again by an ester bond. Phosphatidyl choline (lecithin), phosphatidyl ethanolamine (cephaline), phosphatidyl serine, and phosphatidyl inositol are the most common types of phospholipids, as depicted in Figure 1.3. All of these phospholipids are found in abundance in the cell membranes of various tissues.

Plasmogens are compounds in which one of the fatty acids, usually at the sn-1 carbon of ethanolamine, is replaced by a long-chain ether group. Other compounds related to

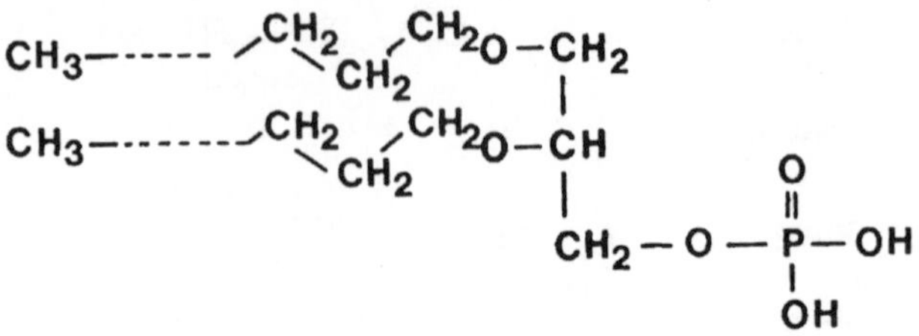

FIGURE 5.5
Phosphatidic acid.

phospholipids are sphingolipids. These compounds do not contain glycerol but instead contain sphingosine, an 18-carbon monounsaturated alcohol. Sphingomyelin is found in large amounts in the myelin sheath of nerve tissue. It contains phosphatidyl choline at the terminal carbon and a fatty acid at the sn-2 position. In a rare inherited condition, termed *Niemann-Pick disease*, individuals lack the enzyme sphygomylinase, which is the enzyme responsible for sphingomyelin cleavage. This disease is characterized by the deposition of sphingomyelin in almost every organ and tissue of the body and is usually fatal before the third year of life.

Lipids in Food

While the diet will provide lipids other than triglycerides and cholesterol, most attention is focused upon these forms of lipids. Food triglycerides are often referred to as either fat or oil, with fat having a more solid consistency at room temperature and oils being more fluid. Food triglycerides will contain a variety of fatty acid types (Table 5.2) As mentioned above, it is the contribution proportions of different fatty acids in a triglyceride source that dictate its phase, either liquid or solid, at a given temperature. Again, longer-chain fatty acids with a lesser degree of unsaturation will allow for a more solidified triglyceride source.

Oil is a natural component of plants and their seeds. It became available after the invention of the continuous screw press, named Expeller®, and the steam-vacuum deodorization process by D. Wesson. Later, solvent extraction methods were developed, further increasing the availability of vegetable oils. Common plant oils include sunflower, safflower, corn, olive, coconut, and palm oil. Butter is made from the fat in milk, while lard is hog fat and tallow is the fat of cattle or sheep. As plants are generally cholesterol free, the cholesterol intake of humans is solely attributed to the consumption of animal foods or foods that use animal products in their recipe. It is found in animal tissue primarily in the form of cholesterol esters and a smaller proportion of free cholesterol. Table 5.3 provides a list of foods and their compositional mass of both triglyceride and cholesterol.

If a triglyceride contains the same fatty acid esterified at all three positions on glycerol, it is called a *simple triglyceride*. Examples are tripalmitate or tributyrate. However, it is more common to find more than one type of fatty acid in the same triglyceride. These molecules are called *mixed triglycerides*. If a fat source contains a greater percentage of saturated fatty acids it is often referred to as a "saturated fat," despite the presence of other types of fatty acids. The same applies for MUFAs and PUFAs. Oftentimes food fat is expressed as a ratio of PUFA/SFA, or more simply, the P/S ratio. Animal foods have a lower P/S ratio while

TABLE 5.2

Approximate Fatty Acid Composition of Common
Triglyceride Sources (%)

Triglyceride Source	SFA	MUFA	PUFA
Butter fat	66	30	4
Beef fat	52	44	4
Lard	41	47	12
Coconut oil	87	6	2
Palm kernel oil	81	11	2
Palm oil	49	37	9
Vegetable shortening	28	44	28
Peanut oil	18	49	33
Margarine	17	49	34
Soybean oil	15	24	61
Olive oil	14	77	9
Corn oil	13	25	62
Sunflower oil	11	20	69
Safflower oil	10	13	77
Canola oil	6	62	32

Note: SFA = saturated fatty acids; MUFA = monounsaturated fatty acids; PUFA = polyunsaturated fatty acids.

most oils have a higher P/S ratio. Notable exceptions are tropical plant oils (coconut, palm, and palm kernel oils) that have a lower P/S ratio due to a relatively high content of medium-chain length saturated fatty acids. Even though they are solid at room temperature they are considered oils because they still have much lower melting points then animal fats.

The most prevalent saturated fatty acids in the Western diet are palmitic (16:0) and stearic acid (18:0), while the most prevalent unsaturated fatty acids are oleic acid (18:1 ω-9) and linoleic (18:2 ω-6). Collectively, these four fatty acids account for over 90% of the fatty acids in the typical American diet. Most of the fatty acids consumed by Americans have an even number of carbons, which generally ranges between 14 to 26 carbons. A notable exception is butyric acid (4:0) found in dairy products. Quite simply, foods contain very little odd-chain length fatty acids. For instance, less than 0.5% of the total fatty acids in olive oil contain an odd number of carbons. Lard contains less than 1% of its fatty acids as odd-chain length.

The major sources of the essential fatty acids are PUFA-rich vegetable oils and marine oils. Linoleic acid is particularly high in sunflower, corn, safflower, and soybean oils. Canola, lin-seed, and soybean oils all contain respectable amounts of linolenic acid; however, only lin-seed oil contains more linolenic acid than linoleic acid (Table 5.4). It is estimated that soybean oil contributes as much as two thirds of the oil used to make shortening by manufacturers in the U.S. and as much as 84% of the fat used in margarines. However, selective hydrogenation processing reduces more of the linolenic acid than the linoleic acid, further increasing the linoleic/linolenic acid ratio of the oil. Linolenic acid is especially concentrated in marine oils. Therefore, the consumption of fish is the primary provider of this essential fatty acid.

Human milk contains both ω-3 and ω-6 PUFA, which is probably indicative of their essentiality for growth and development. Maternal dietary fat composition can affect the EFA content of the milk. For instance, lactating mothers who consume fish have a higher DHA content of their breast milk than lactating vegetarian mothers.

In recent times, concern has been expressed as to the content of dietary *trans* fatty acids and their impact upon human health. *Trans* fatty acids can be found in most natural fat

TABLE 5.3
Approximate Fat and Cholesterol Content of Selected Foods

Food	Fat	Cholesterol

By Weight (%)

Animal products

Food	Fat	Cholesterol
Beef	32	<1
Bologna	29	1
Butter	82	2
Chicken, white meat	4	<1
Cheese, cheddar	32	1
Cheese, cottage (4%)	4	<1
Codfish	<1	Trace
Egg, whole	12	4
Egg, white	<1	Trace
Halibut	3	Trace
Hamburger	13	<1
Lamb chops	36	1
Mackerel	6	Trace
Margarine	82	—
Milk, whole	3	<1
Milk, skim	Trace	Trace
Pork chops	21	1
Pork sausage	46	1
Salmon	3	Trace

Plant products

Food	Fat	Cholesterol
Avocado	13	—
Bread, white	4	<1
Cereals and grains	1–2	—
Crackers	1	—
Fruits	<1	—
Leafy vegetables	<1	—
Legumes	<1	—
Margarine	82	—
Root vegetables	<1	—

By Grams

Animal products

Food	Fat	Cholesterol
Beef (4 oz)	36	101
Bologna (1 slice)	7	13
Butter (1 pat)	4	11
Chicken, white meat (3 oz)	7	41
Cheese, cheddar (1 c)	37	139
Cheese, cottage (4%) (1 c)	10	31
Codfish (4 oz)	7	35
Egg, whole (1 ea)	5	213
Egg, white (1 ea)	—	Trace
Halibut (4 oz)	5	131
Hamburger (4 oz)	14	58
Lamb chops (2.5 oz)	18	84
Mackerel (4 oz)	16	78
Margarine (1 pat)	3	—
Milk, whole (1 c)	8	33
Milk, skim (1 c)	Trace	Trace
Pork chops (2.5 oz)	12	18
Pork sausage (1)	6	11
Salmon (4 oz)	4	Trace

TABLE 5.3 (continued)
Approximate Fat and Cholesterol Content of Selected Foods

Food	Fat	Cholesterol
By Grams		
Plant products		
Avocado (1)	27	—
Bread, white (1 slice)	1	Trace
Cereals and grains (1 c)	1	—
Crackers (4)	2	—
Fruits (1 ea)	<1	—
Leafy vegetables (1/2 c)	<1	—
Legumes (1/2 c)	<1	—
Margarine (1 pat)	6	—
Root vegetables (1/2 c)	<1	—

sources, although their prevalence is generally low. Beef, butter, and milk triglycerides may contain 2 to 8% *trans* fatty acids. *Trans* fatty acids are created by microbes in the rumen and then absorbed and circulated to mammary glands and other tissue. Additionally, *trans* fatty acids can be created during the processing of oils (i.e., margarine and other hydrogenated oils). Salad oils may contain 8 to 17% *trans* fatty acids, while shortenings contain 14 to 60%. Typically, about one half of the *trans* fatty acids in the Western diet, which may include 3 to 7% of their total fatty acids as *trans* fatty acids, is derived from animal sources. The remaining one half of the *trans* fatty acids is derived from processed oils, either consumed plain or used in recipes (i.e., snack foods). Also, the substitution of hydrogenated oils for tropical oils by many food manufacturers has further increased the consumption of *trans* fatty acids.

TABLE 5.4
Linoleic and Linolenic Acid Composition
of Common Oils (% of Total Fatty Acids)

Oil	Linoleic Acid	Linolenic Acid
Soybean	54	7
Safflower	76	0.5
Sunflower	68	1
Corn	54	1
Olive	10	1
Canola	22	10
Palm	10	1
Cottonseed	54	1
Peanut	32	—
Linseed	16	54

Dietary Lipid Requirements

Efficient cholesterol synthesis in hepatocytes, and to a lesser degree in other tissue, eliminates the dietary need for cholesterol. Similarly, the ability to make and modify fatty acids nearly eliminates the absolute need for fat in the human diet. However, as they are needed to make eicosanoids, ω-3 and ω-6 PUFA are indeed dietary essentials. It has been estimated that as long as humans receive 2 to 3% of their fat from a variety of natural sources, they will meet their minimal EFA requirements. The optimal intake for linolenic acid is estimated to be 800 to 1100 mg/d and that of EPA and DHA, to be 300 to 400 mg daily.

Deficiency of EFA results in several anatomical and physiological anomalies. For instance, 18:2 ω-6 is critical to dermal integrity as a component of *o*-linoleoyl-ceramides. These molecules help form the lipid bilayers that fill the intercellular spaces in the outer epidermis (stratum corneum). In light of an EFA deficiency, 18:2 ω-6 is replaced by 18:1 ω-9, which decreases epidermal water barrier integrity and also results in cell hyperproliferation. Also, some of the growth and anomalies associated with EFA deficiency may be related to eicosanoid involvement in pituitary and hypothalmic hormone release.

Digestion of Lipids

Fat digestion begins in the mouth with the secretion of lingual lipase, which is a component of the secretion derived from a salivary gland at the base of the tongue. Lingual lipase activity increases as the food–saliva mixture enters the stomach and the pH becomes more acidic. Furthermore, this enzyme does not require the emulsifying effect of bile to penetrate fat droplets. Thus, the contribution of lingual lipase to total fat digestion is significant, yet still quantitatively minor in comparison to the small intestinal digestion. There are also gastric and intestinal mucosal-secreted lipases, but, collectively, these lipases contribute very little to overall lipid digestion. The gastric lipase is usually more active in the duodenum. The simplest approach to detail lipid digestion is to discuss the process in three phases: *intraluminal, mucosal,* and *secretory.*

Intralumenal Phase

The most active site of lipid digestion is the upper jejunum. Emulsification of lipids by bile salts is a prerequisite prior to enzymatic hydrolysis. The process begins by mechanical action in the stomach to form a coarse emulsion of chyme. Chyme then mixes with pancreatic secretions of the small intestine as the stomach empties. The release of lecithin from the bile and the production of monoglycerides from earlier digestion facilitate the emulsification process. The polar nature of these compounds allows for the formation of micelles within an aqueous environment of the small intestine (Figure 5.6). As emulsification proceeds, the pancreatic lipases hydrolyze the lipid. This will release polar lipids and further enhance the emulsification process and micellular formation.

There are three types of pancreatic lipases and one coenzyme that are active in the small intestine. The release of the pancreatic lipases is under the control of the hormone cholecystokinin (CCK), produced by the intestinal mucosal cells. Not only does this hormone control pancreatic secretion, but it facilitates the release of bile from the gallbladder by stimulating the gallbladder to contract. Also, CCK produces a relaxation of the sphincter muscle at the neck of the gallbladder as well as the sphincter of Oddi.

Pancreatic lipase is responsible for most of the triglyceride hydrolysis and cleaves the fatty acids preferentially at sn-1 and secondarily at sn-3 (Figure 5.7). Less than half of the triglycerides are completely hydrolyzed to fatty acids and glycerol. However, most of the

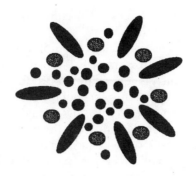

= Bile salt
= Phospholipids
= Glycerides and cholesterol

FIGURE 5.6
Structure of a micelle.

fatty acids liberated will have more than ten carbons. The enzyme acts on the surface of micelles that have the triglycerides exposed. The pancreatic coenzyme, colipase, promotes the formation of a lipase–colipase bile salt complex that allows for hydrolysis. Colipase is composed of about 100 amino acids and has distinct properties of hydrophobicity. It has been speculated that colipase associates strongly with pancreatic lipase molecules, while at the same time anchoring itself to the lipid globule. As the result of lipase activity, monoglycerides, fatty acids, and glycerol are released into the aqueous environment of the intestinal lumen and are continually solubilized by the bile salts. These products are brought into contact with the surface of the microvilli.

Cholesterol esterase is another pancreatic enzyme. Cholesterol esters in the small intestine comprise about 15% of the total cholesterol. The esterified form cannot be absorbed intact, so it must be hydrolyzed. If the ester linkage is not broken, the cholesterol ester passes into the colon.

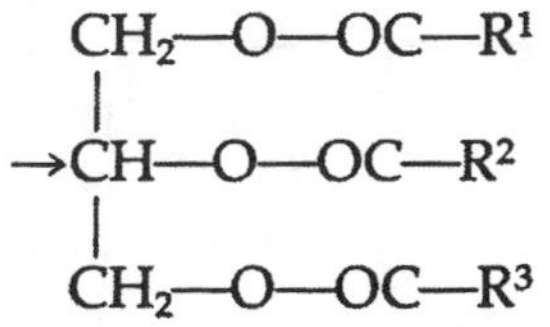

$$CH_2\!-\!O\!-\!OC\!-\!R^1$$
$$\rightarrow CH\!-\!O\!-\!OC\!-\!R^2$$
$$CH_2\!-\!O\!-\!OC\!-\!R^3$$

FIGURE 5.7
sn Positioning on a glycerol backbone of a triglyceride. The arrow indicates the sn-2 position.

Another pancreatic lipid-digesting enzyme is phospholipase, which as an energy source hydrolyzes fatty acids from phospholipids. In actuality, this is of rather minor importance since the average Western diet averages only about 2 g of phospholipids daily. Most of this is phosphatidyl choline (lecithin), which is poorly absorbed. There are actually two forms of phospholipase: A-1 and A-2. Phospholipase A-2 will hydrolyze the sn-2 fatty acid of lecithin to produce lysolecithin and a free fatty acid. Lysolecithin and fatty acids are readily absorbed. Within mucosal enterocytes, some of the lysolecithin is reesterified with a fatty acid by the enzyme lysophophatidyl choline acyltransferase. The phospholipid is needed for chylomicron formation. The remaining lysolecithin has the sn-1 fatty acid removed by the A-1 phospholipase within the mucosal cell.

Bile is a major factor in lipid digestion. Bile is a complex composite, as discussed in Chapter 3. Along with its emulsifying factors, namely bile salts, phospholipids, and cholesterol, bile also contains bilirubin, which is a breakdown product of hemoglobin. When bile is secreted by the liver and is deposited into the gall bladder in between meals it is concentrated about 5- to 10-fold or even greater. Bile salts should also be considered an excretory mechanism for the elimination of cholesterol from the body.

Cholic acid and chenodeoxycholic acid are formed from cholesterol and are the primary bile salts. Cholesterol has a hydroxyl (-OH) group on carbon 3 (see Figure 1.4). In hepatocytes, cholesterol is hydroxylated at carbon 7 to produce chenodeoxycholic acid, and further hydroxylation at carbon 12 yields cholic acid. After these compounds have been formed, another enzyme conjugates the bile acids with an amino acid. Conjugation with glycine forms glycocholic or glycochenodeoxycholic acid, while conjugation of bile salts to taurine forms taurocholic or taurochenodeoxycholic acids. Once these bile acids are secreted into the small intestine, they may be further modified in the ileum or colon by intestinal bacteria. For instance, cholic acid may be deconjugated and dehydroxylated at carbon 7 to produce deoxycholic acid (Figure 5.8). Chenodeoxycholic acid may have the same reaction to produce lithocholic acid. Collectively these two derivative bile acids are referred to as secondary bile acids. The primary and secondary bile acids are absorbed by the ileum and colon and are passed into the portal circulation for recirculation via an energy-dependent process. The bile acids return to the liver to be recycled again. About 94% of the bile acids secreted into the intestine are reabsorbed and this process is referred to as the *enterohepatic circulation*. In the blood, the bile acids are normally complexed to albumin. Of the approximately 18 g of bile acids secreted each day, less than one-half of a gram is lost via the feces.

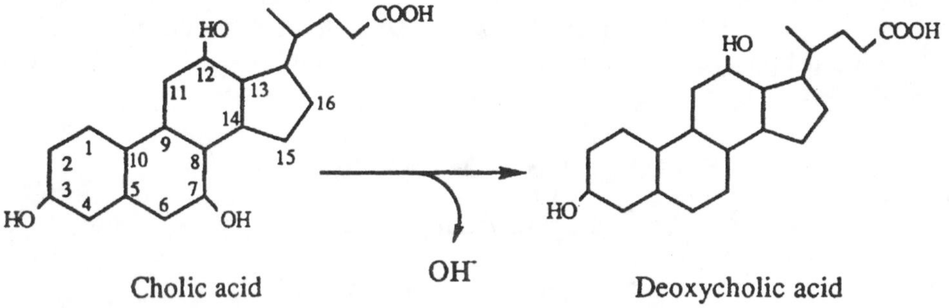

FIGURE 5.8
Conversion of cholic acid to deoxycholic acid.

Mucosal Phase

The micelle allows the lipid breakdown products to diffuse to the surface of the intestinal epithelium. Absorption of micelle-associated substances occurs through the partitioning from the micelle into the aqueous phase, followed by uptake by the plasma membrane. The free fatty acids and monoglycerides are transported across the microvillus membrane by a passive process due to the lipid solubility of these products in the membrane. Glycerol is absorbed by a carrier-mediated mechanism. Most of the absorption occurs in the first half of the intestine.

A low-molecular weight protein in the mucosal cell cytoplasm called *fatty acid binding protein* (FABP) functions to transport longer-chain fatty acids (>12 carbons) to the smooth endoplasmic reticulum where triglycerides can be resynthesized. With respect to cholesterol, some of it may be reesterified either by acyl-CoA-cholesterol acyltransferase (ACAT) or mucosal cholesterol esterase. Cholesterol is reesterified primarily to unsaturated fatty acids. The resynthesized triglycerides are incorporated into a lipoprotein by the addition of phospholipid, cholesterol, cholesterol esters, and apoprotein B. Chylomicrons then migrate to the Golgi apparatus where glycoproteins may be added. Those fatty acids with ten carbons or less are transported unesterified and leave the mucosa through the portal blood system. These are generally bound to albumin. There are no free fatty acids found within the lymph.

Secretory Phase

This phase is relatively simple. Formed chylomicrons are discharged, via exocytosis, through the lateral portion of the mucosal cells into the extracellular space and enter the lacteal, a blind-ended lymph vessel. As mentioned above, the shorter-chain fatty acids leave directly through the portal vein.

Eicosanoids

Essential fatty acids are precursors for eicosanoids, a large group of physiologically and pharmacologically active compounds that include prostaglandins (PG), thromboxanes (TX) and leukotrienes (LT). However, not all of the physiological properties associated with ω-3 and ω-6 PUFAs are related to their conversion to eicosanoids.

Eicosanoids are derived from 20-carbon PUFAs, namely, 20:3 ω-6 (dihomo γ-linolenate, DL), 20:4 ω-6 (AA), and 20:5 ω-3 (EPA). The preliminary enzymes that initiate their conversion to eicosanoids are *lipoxygenase* and *cyclooxygenase* systems. However, AA can undergo a variety of enzymatic processing by the cytochrome P_{450} system in the endoplasmic reticulum to form metabolites with interesting biological properties. This occurs mainly in the liver and kidney. For instance, epoxygenase metabolites of AA have renal vasoconstricting properties and are involved in ion transport. Also, free radical-mediated peroxidation of AA leads to the creation of a series of prostaglandin-like compounds called *isoprostanes* which may have potent vasoconstriction properties. Free radicals may attack AA as part of lipoproteins or cellular membranes creating these derivatives. Measurement of isoprostane levels in the urine and plasma has been suggested as a reliable indicator of *in vivo* lipid peroxidation. Enhanced urinary isoprostane levels have been identified in smokers.

EFAs are primarily stored as fatty acids esterified to phospholipids at the sn-2 position of glycerol. Liberation of the EFA from this location is accomplished by cleavage via phospholipase A_2. This enzyme can be inhibited by certain steroid drugs used as antiinflammatory agents. The EFA composition of the diet can influence the concentration amounts of the various EFAs and derivatives in membrane phospholipids. Thus, dietary fat composition can influence eicosanoid function by manipulating the pool of available eicosanoid precursors.

Different prostaglandin, leukotriene, and thromboxane structures can be derived from different EFA or derivatives and are designated within *series* or *groups*. In series 1, 2 and 3 eicosanoids are derived from 20:3 ω-6 (LN), 20:4 ω-6 (AA), and 20-5 ω-3 (EPA), respectively (i.e., PGE_1, PGI_2, PGI_3), where the subscript number indicates the series. Arachidonic acid is also the precursor for series 4 leukotrienes (leukotrienes and lipoxins), while 20:5 ω-3 (EPA) is also a precursor for series 5 leukotrienes. One notable exception is that the series 3 leukotrienes are derived from DL, not EPA. Furthermore, DL is converted to AA. See Figure 5.9 for an eicosanoid synthesis flow diagram. In several situations, eicosanoids derived from 20:4 ω-6 work in opposition to those derived from 20:5 ω-3.

Prostaglandins may be derived from each of the above three groups via the cyclooxygenase pathway. Thromboxanes, which have significant effects on blood platelet function, are also synthesized via this pathway. Leukotrienes are synthesized by the lipoxygenase pathway. The involvement of these enzymes is indicated in Figure 5.9. Regarding the cyclooxygenase pathway, this involves the consumption of two molecules of molecular oxygen catalyzed by prostaglandin endoperoxide synthases (G/H), which is really two separate enzyme activities: (1) cyclooxygenase and (2) peroxidase. Aspirin and nonsteroidal antiinflammatory drugs can inhibit cyclooxygenase activity. The end product of the cyclooxygenase activity associated with AA is prostaglandin PGH_2, which is converted to PGD_2, PGE_2, and PGF_2, as well as to TXA_2 and PGI_2. The production of these eicosanoids depends upon the needs of the cell type. For instance, PGD_2 is a major AA metabolite produced in the brain (involved in sleep and thermoregulation), platelets, mast cells, uterus, skin, skeletal muscle, and renal medulla. PGE_2 formation occurs in many tissues including blood vessels, intestines, prostate, uterus, and ovarian tubes. Thomboxane A synthase, a primary eicosanoid-converting enzyme in platelets, converts PGH_2 to TXA_2. TXA_2 is a potent vasoconstrictor and platelet aggregation agent which is critical in hemorrhagic response. Overproduction of TXA_2 has been suggested as a pivotal factor in myocardial infarction associated with atheromas. It has a half-life of 30 sec. PGI_2, with a half-life of a few minutes, is produced in the aorta and has vasodilation and platelet antiaggregation effects.

The different prostaglandins differ only slightly in their molecular composition. For instance, E is designated when there is a C=O group at carbon 9, whereas F is the designation when the OH group is at carbon 9.

Steroids

Steroids are a class of lipid molecules that are derived from the basic sterol structure of cholesterol (see Figure 1.4). Steroids include estrogens, androgens, DHEA, adrenocorticoid hormones, and cholesterol itself. Also, vitamin D and bile salts are derived from cholesterol. Because cholesterol is a amphipathic lipid, it is employed as a structural component of cell membranes and lipoprotein shells. Cholesterol-based hormones tend to have intracellular receptors and exert much of their effect by influencing gene expression. See Figure 5.10 for an overview of biologically important steroids.

For an adult, about 700 mg of cholesterol is synthesized daily, and the liver and the intestines each synthesize about 10% of the total. Virtually all nucleated cells have the ability to synthesize cholesterol, a process that takes place within the endoplasmic reticulum and cytosol. Acetyl CoA is the source of all carbon atoms in cholesterol. In the initial reaction, two molecules of acetyl CoA condense to form acetoacetyl CoA, a reaction catalyzed by cytosolic thiolase enzyme (Figure 5.11). Acetoacetyl CoA condenses with another molecule of acetyl CoA to form 3-hydroxy-3-methylglutaryl (HMG). This reaction is catalyzed by

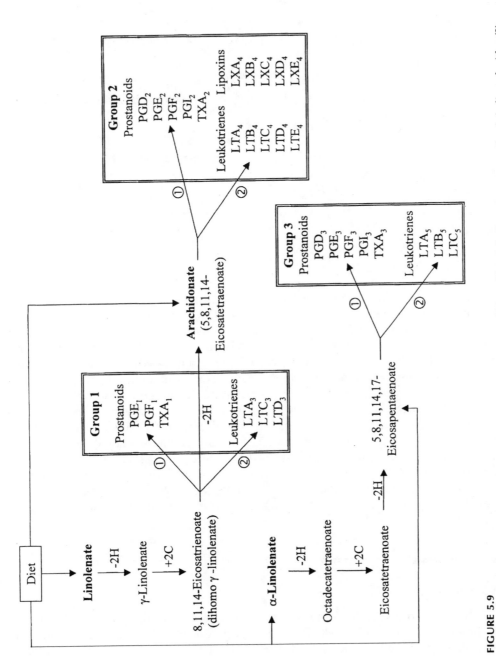

FIGURE 5.9

Eicosanoid formation pathways. The cyclooxygenase reaction is indicated by a (1) and the lipoxygenase reaction is indicated with a (2).

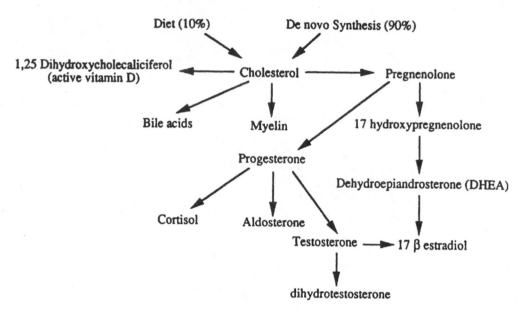

FIGURE 5.10
Biologically important cholesterol derivatives.

HMG-CoA synthase. The next reaction is the rate-limiting step and the target of many drugs prescribed to lower blood cholesterol levels. HMG is converted to mevalonate in a two-stage reduction by NADPH by HMG-CoA reductase, an enzyme of the endoplasmic reticulum. Mevalonate is then activated by three ATPs in a series of kinase reactions to form mevalonate 3-phospho-5-pyrophosphate, which is susequently decarboxylated to form the active isoprenoid unit isopentenyl pyrophosphate. Six isopentenyl pyrophosphate molecules form squalene, which is then converted to lanosterol and ultimately cholesterol.

Cholesterol synthesis is influenced by several factors and primarily involves the regulation of HMG-CoA reductase. Fasting seems to significantly reduce the activity of HMG-CoA reductase. Also, there is a negative feedback mechanism applied by the intermediate mevalonate and the final product, cholesterol. Cholesterol synthesis is also influenced by dietary consumption of cholesterol. While most of the research in this area was performed on rodents, it seems that as the dietary level of cholesterol increases, the level of endogenous cholesterol production decreases. However, this effect mainly takes place in the liver.

Lipoproteins

Within the blood, triglycerides and cholesterol esters are transported within a phospholipid, cholesterol, and protein shell. These transport vesicles, called lipoproteins, are produced primarily within hepatocytes and enterocytes. The core of the typical lipoprotein is composed of cholesterol, which is almost entirely esterified, and triglycerides. Some diglycerides and monoglycerides may be present as well.

Phospholipids contribute most of the molecules found as part of the outer shell. Their polar phosphate group is oriented towards the outer aqueous environment of the blood

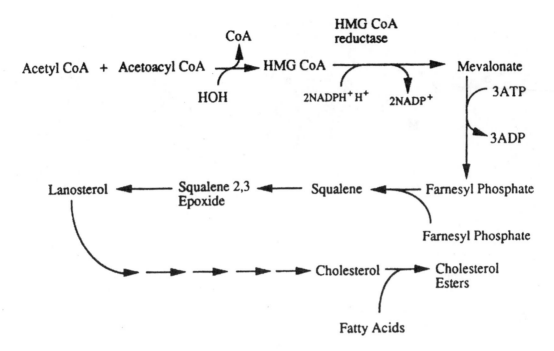

FIGURE 5.11
Cholesterol synthesis.

while their two fatty acids are oriented toward the hydrophobic core. Also in the shell are specialized proteins (*apoproteins* or *apolipoproteins*). While some of the significance of these proteins is to enhance the miscible properties of lipoproteins, perhaps more important are their other properties. As described in greater detail below, apoproteins have enzymatic and receptor-associated activities.

The composition of the lipoproteins differs depending on type, origin, and physiological function. The four basic types are chylomicrons, very-low-density lipoproteins (VLDL), low-density lipoproteins (LDL), and high-density lipoproteins (HDL). There are often intermediate types, such as intermediate-density lipoprotein (IDL), and various subtypes of HDL (1, 2, C, and apoE rich). Figures 5.12 and 5.13 provide a good summary as to the chemical and physical characteristics of these basic lipoprotein types.

Chylomicrons are produced in the small intestine where their primary function is the absorption of diet-derived triglycerides and cholesterol and their transportation in the blood. VLDL is produced in the liver and transports both endogenously produced triglycerides and cholesterol as well as that derived from chylomicrons to peripheral tissues. LDLs are formed as a metabolic product from VLDLs. The change is the result of successive hydrolysis of VLDL core triglycerides by *lipoprotein lipase*. Fatty acids are translocated into peripheral tissue, while glycerol dissolves into circulation. With the removal of triglyceride from its core, VLDL become more dense, and the relative mass of cholesterol in the core increases. VLDL becomes IDL and then cholesterol-rich LDL. Cholesterol from LDL is delivered to selective cell types. HDL may be produced both in the small intestine and the liver. However, about 80% of the HDL is of hepatic origin. Within the framework of lipoprotein metabolism is the exchange of apoproteins between certain lipoproteins, as discussed below.

Lipoproteins differ in density, chylomicrons being the least dense, but the greatest in diameter, and vice versa (Figure 5.11). The opposite situation can be said to apply to HDLs.

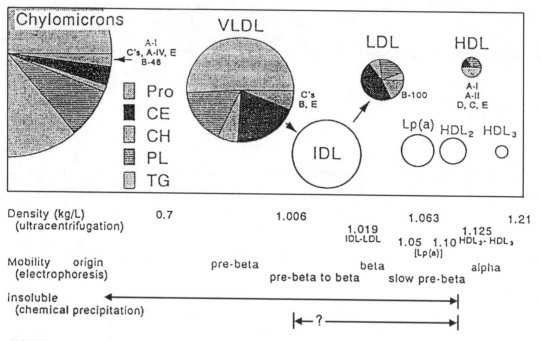

FIGURE 5.12
Lipoprotein characteristics.

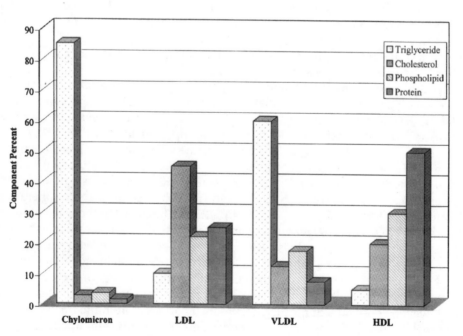

FIGURE 5.13
Lipoprotein composition.

The various classes of lipoproteins may be separated by a variety of means, including ultra-centrifugation, various types of chromatography, electrophoresis, and chemical precipitation techniques. Often used is sequential ultracentrifugation where the plasma is layered with a salt such as sodium chloride (NaCl), sodium bromide (NaBr), or potassium bromide (KBr) at a particular density. For example, if KBr is the salt of choice and its density is 1.006 g/ml, VLDL will float to the top because it is less dense than the salt solution. If the lipoprotein beneath the salt layer is carefully removed and again layered with KBr or another substance with a slightly higher density, then floatation of LDL will occur. Electrophoresis is an older method originally used to separate the lipoproteins. Since this approach separates proteins based on mass or size, HDLs will migrate the furthest and the chylomicrons will often remain at the origin.

Using gel permeation chromatography, the lipoproteins are placed on top of a column (usually 1 m in length) and traverse a collection of agarose beads of varying pore sizes. Smaller particles, such as HDL, will move through the pores of the beads and will thus be retarded and exit from the opposite end of the column last. Conversely, larger lipoproteins, such as chylomicrons and VLDL will navigate around the beads and so will more quickly through the column and be eluted first.

The apoprotein portions of lipoproteins have several types and designations. HDL has apoproteins A-I and A-II. Chylomicrons also have some apoprotein A-II. LDL has apoprotein B-100. Chylomicrons contain a protein closely related to B-100, called B-48, which is smaller than the B-100. B-48 is synthesized in the small intestine, and B-100 is synthesized in the liver; however, both apoproteins are expressed from the same gene. B-48 is the product of post-translational modification of B-100. Apoproteins C-I, C-II, and C-III are smaller polypeptides found in VLDL, HDL, and chylomicrons. An arginine-rich apoprotein, designated Apo E, is found scattered among the VLDL, chylomicrons, and HDL. As alluded to earlier, some of these apoproteins are activators of certain key enzymes or they may serve as binding sites for cell membrane receptors. For instance, lipoprotein lipase requires apoprotein C-II as an activator or cofactor.

Metabolism of Lipoproteins

Chylomicrons are formed in the small intestine, and the enzyme lipoprotein lipase plays an important role in the hydrolysis of its core triglycerides. Lipoprotein lipase is located attached to the endothelial lining of tissue capillaries, primarily muscle, adipocytes, and lactating mammary glands, and secondarily in the spleen, lungs, renal medulla, aorta, and diaphram. Lipoprotein lipase has a specific phospholipid binding site that anchors chylomicrons to the enzyme. The actions of lipoprotein lipase reduce the quantity of triglycerides in circulating chylomicrons by 90%. The remaining triglyceride ultimately enters the liver as chylomicron remnants are transported into hepatocytes.

Apoprotein A and B-48 are present in just-released or *nascent* chylomicrons. As they circulate, chylomicrons must pick up apoproteins C-II and E. Apoproteins A and C-II eventually dissociate from chylomicrons and associate with HDL as chylomicrons become smaller through the successive hydrolysis of the triglycerides. The chylomicron remnant is taken up by the liver by an apoprotein E receptor-mediated site.

The liver is the site origin for VLDL; however it should be noted that very small amounts of VLDL-like particles are released from the small intestine in between meals. VLDLs transport triglycerides and cholesterol from the liver to extrahepatic tissue. VLDLs are initially constructed within the smooth endoplasmic reticulum. Apoprotein B-100, which is synthesized by ribosomal complexes in the rough endoplasmic reticulum, is incorporated into

VLDL within the smooth endoplasmic reticulum. Apoprotein B-100 is perhaps the largest protein in the human body. The smooth endoplasmic reticulum is also the site of triglyceride formation utilizing phosphatidic acid as the base. Semideveloped VLDL particles are then passed to the Golgi apparatus, whereby more lipids and carbohydrate residues are added. This formation is very similar to the synthesis of chylomicrons. VLDL, and chylomicrons are released from their synthesizing cell into the extracellular fluid by reverse pinocytosis. In the liver, VLDL gain access to the blood by entering sinusoids or channels flowing between rows of hepatocytes. Chylomicrons, on the other hand, must enter a lacteal, located in the center of the villus (Figure 3.6), and navigate the lymphatic circulation, eventually gaining access to the general circulation via the thoracic duct.

In some individuals, the ability to construct apoprotein B is genetically obstructed. This results in the inability to synthesize both chylomicrons and VLDL. Large fat droplets are observed in liver and small intestinal parenchyma in these individuals. This condition is referred to as *abetalipoproteinemia*.

While traces of apoproteins A and C can be found in nascent VLDL, by and large VLDL do not receive these apoproteins until they encounter HDL in the bloodstream. VLDL breakdown occurs in a manner similar to chylomicron breakdown. Triglycerides are digested by the actions of LPL, and VLDL shrink in size and change in composition. VLDL become IDL and then LDL. In the process, apoprotein C is transferred back to HDL, thereby generally limiting further triglyceride removal.

There are specific binding sites for apoprotein B-100 in various tissues, such as the liver, arterial smooth muscle, fibroblasts, lymphocytes, and other tissue. The liver removes about 70% of circulating LDL and the remaining 30% is removed by all other tissue combined. The receptor is referred to as the LDL (B-100, E) receptor, as not only will it recognize apoprotein B-100-rich LDL but also apoprotein E-rich lipoproteins. The entire complex binds to the receptor and is engulfed by pinocytosis. Apoprotein B-100 is broken down by lysosomes. Cholesteryl esters are hydrolyzed, but later are reesterified. The buildup of cholesterol in the cell will inhibit the key cholesterol-producing regulatory enzyme 3-hydroxyl-3-methylglutaryl CoA reductase (HMG-CoA reductase). However, the oversupply of cholesterol by this process will also inhibit the synthesis of LDL-receptors. If too much cholesterol accumulates in the cells, the receptor synthesis decreases and LDL-cholesterol cannot enter the cell. This results in a buildup of cholesterol within the blood, increasing the risk of heart disease.

HDL is synthesized by both small intestine and liver. Intestinal HDL lacks apoprotein C and E, but has apoprotein A. Apoprotein C and E are synthesized only in the liver and later transferred to intestinal HDL by interaction with hepatic HDL. The initially synthesized lipoprotein by either tissue (nascent HDL) contains phospholipid bilayers composed of apoproteins and free cholesterol and is disc-shaped. It is often called discoidal HDL. The plasma enzyme *lecithin-cholesterol acyltransferase (LCAT)* binds with the surface of HDL. This enzyme is activated by apoprotein A-I and converts HDL shell phospholipid and free cholesterol into cholesterol esters and lysolecithin. Cholesterol esters enter the HDL core, while lysolecithin is transferred to plasma albumin. The result is a more spherically shaped HDL particle. LCAT also esterifies cholesterol from other lipoproteins and extrahepatic tissue as well. HDL is eventually removed from circulation by HDL receptors in the liver. The presence of apoprotein A-I on HDL greatly enhances its removal.

Cholesterol ester transfer protein or apoprotein D is another component of HDL. It will transfer the esterified cholesterol on HDL to the other lipoproteins. Thus, the cholesterol endowed to HDL can be transported to the liver and removed via a HDL receptor, or it can be transferred to other lipoproteins (i.e., chylomicron remnants and LDL) which themselves are subject to removal from the circulation. The removal and transportation of cholesterol from extrahepatic tissue by HDL and its delivery to the liver have been called *reverse cholesterol transport*.

As HDL acquires more cholesterol esters in its core, its size and density changes. The uptake of cholesterol by HDL_3 increases its diameter about twofold and its density decreases from about 1.125 to 1.210 g/ml to about 1.063 to 1.125 g/ml, forming HDL_2. The hydrolyzation of HDL phospholipid and triglyceride by *hepatic lipase* allows HDL_2 to reduce its size and regain some of its density, thereby regaining some of its HDL_3 qualities. HDL_3 then reenters circulation. HDL_2 concentrations are inversely related to the incidence of coronary artery disease, as discussed below and in Chapter 16.

INSIGHT: Health Implications and Interpretation of Lipoprotein-Cholesterol Levels

The ability to control plasma cholesterol levels, in particular LDL-cholesterol, is partly genetic as it relates to the apoprotein B-100 receptor density on hepatocyte membranes. The decreased ability to produce this receptor could be due to a genetic anomaly resulting in decreased mRNA synthesis of the apoprotein B-100 transcript. The result is elevated plasma cholesterol levels, a strong risk factor for heart disease. A decreased level of HDL-cholesterol, especially HDL_2, is also a risk factor. Other factors such as cigarette smoking, hypertension, diabetes, obesity, decreased physical activity levels, and even male gender increase the risk of heart disease.

Serum cholesterol levels demonstrate a linear relationship with the percent arterial intimal surface covered with raised lesions, but the relationship with coronary heart disease risk ratio is curvilinear. How can this discrepancy be resolved? The key lies in that a critical percent area of the surface of blood vessels must be covered with raised lesions before a statistical effect is observed. When 60% or greater of the surface area of blood vessels is covered with lesions, a linear response with respect to mortality rate from coronary heart disease is observed.

Defining from a clinical perspective who is at risk for heart disease has undergone revision over the years. One such scheme uses a screening approach. Desirable total blood cholesterol levels are below 200 mg/100 ml plasma; borderline is 200 to 239 mg/100 ml, and high blood cholesterol or hypercholesterolemia is greater than 240 mg/100 ml. Total blood cholesterol represents the sum of the cholesterol distributed in all lipoprotein fractions. This should be a fasting measure, thereby removing the presence of chylomicrons.

If an individual is below 200 mg/100 ml, the recommended follow-up is simply to repeat the measurement within 5 years. If the levels are borderline and without any two other heart disease risk factors or presence of heart disease, then dietary information and annual recheck of level is recommended. However, if there is presence of coronary heart disease or two other risk factors for heart disease, one of which may be male gender, then a lipoprotein analysis is recommended and further clinical action, guided by the LDL-cholesterol level. LDL-cholesterol levels defined as desirable are levels below 130 mg/100 ml. Borderline is 130 to 159 mg/100ml, and high risk levels are 160 mg/100 ml or greater. Table 5.5 presents a typical lipid profile.

Dietary treatment is recommended for those with levels of LDL-cholesterol greater than 160 mg/100 ml, or if two other risk factors are present, greater than 130 mg/100 ml. In addition to dietary modifications, drug treatment is recommended if the LDL-cholesterol levels are 190 mg/100 ml or greater with no evidence of coronary heart disease. If there are two

TABLE 5.5

Typical Blood Lipid Profile for an Adult

Lipid	Result	Normal range
Triglycerides (TG)	137 mg/dl	0–210 mg/dl
Cholesterol	163 mg/dl	50–200 mg/dl
HDL	42 mg/dl	30–90 mg/dl
VLDL	27 mg/dl	5–40 mg/dl
LDL	94 mg/dl	50–140 mg/dl
Chol:HDL	3.9 (ratio)	3.7–6.7
LDL:HDL	2.2 (ratio)	

heart disease risk factors already present or evidence of coronary heart disease, then drug therapy concomitant to nutrition modification is the recommended course of treatment when LDL-cholesterol exceeds 160 mg/100 ml.

Older classes of drugs used to treat blood cholesterol, such as bile sequestering agents (i.e., cholestyramine and colestipol) may still be used today. These block the uptake of bile acids by the gut, thereby interfering with the enterohepatic circulation. This forces the liver to replace the lost bile acids through conversion of more hepatic cholesterol into the primary bile acids, thus decreasing the available cholesterol for VLDL synthesis. Also, this effect, in theory at least, would lead to up-regulation of mRNA transcripts for the apoprotein B-100 receptors on the cell membranes. Similarly, the class of drugs that inhibit HMG-CoA reductase (i.e., lovastatin) directly will lower hepatocyte levels of cholesterol and thereby relieve the inhibition of mRNA synthesis for apoprotein B-100. These drugs in particular have been very effective in that blood cholesterol levels may decrease by as much as a third when compared to about a 10% reduction through dietary means. Some early evidence suggests that delayed onset of coronary heart disease is possible with these newer agents.

6

Protein

The name "protein" is derived from the Greek term *proteos*, which means "primary" or "to take place first." Protein was first discovered in the early 19th century, at which time scientists described it as a nitrogen-containing part of food essential to life. While the elemental composition of the other energy nutrients is limited to carbon, oxygen, and hydrogen, protein also contains nitrogen (N) as well as sulfur (S). About one half of the dry weight of a typical human cell is attributed to protein. Some of the most significant roles for proteins are as structural components, contractile filaments, antibodies for immune responses, transporters, neurotransmitters, hormones, and enzymes.

Amino Acids

Proteins are composed of amino acids, many of which also have significant biological functions or are used to make other important molecules such as neurotransmitters and hormones. While approximately 140 types of amino acids are known to exist in nature, a much lower number of amino acids are commonly found as constituents of proteins. Only 20 amino acid are genetically coded, via mRNA. Human proteins also contain modifications of a few of these amino acids (i.e., hydroxylated amino acids); however, the modification takes place after the protein is initially synthesized. Said another way, they are posttranslational modifications of amino acids. Table 6.1 presents the amino acids found in human proteins along with other amino acids found in the human body that are not part of proteins.

A common characteristic of amino acids found in proteins is that they have an asymmetric or alpha (α) carbon, which has attached to it an amino group, a carboxyl group, and a hydrogen atom. The fourth entity attached to the asymmetric carbon is unique from one amino acid to the next (Figure 6.1). This feature has been called the "R" group or "side" group. Glycine is the most simple of these amino acids, as its side group is merely a hydrogen atom.

Amino acids have the potential to present both D and L isomeric forms, with the L form occurring in nature. This is the reverse of carbohydrates, where the D isomer is the type of isomer found naturally. Amino acids are linked together by peptide bonds formed covalently between adjacent OH and amine groups. This is depicted in Figure 6.2.

Amino acids (Figure 6.3) can be classified based on the type of side group they present. The aliphatic amino acids have straight carbon chains, aromatic amino acids have a ring structure, and acidic amino acids and basic amino acids are normally classified separately due to their extreme pH within aqueous solutions. Sulfur-containing amino acids may be recognized as one class (cysteine and methionine), while the imino acid, proline, and its derivative, hydroxyproline, are another class.

TABLE 6.1
Amino Acids Found in the Human Body

Essential Amino Acids Found in Protein	Nonessential Amino Acids Found in Protein[a]	Nonessential Amino Acids Not Found in Protein
Tryptophan	Glycine	Ornithine
Valine	Aspartic acid	Taurine
Threonine	Asparagine	γ-Amino butyric acid
Isoleucine	Proline	
Lysine	Glutamine	
Leucine	Glutamic aid	
Phenylalanine	Arginine	
Methionine	Cysteine	
Histidine	Tyrosine	
	Serine	
	Alanine	

[a] This list can also include posttranslational derivatives of nonessential amino acids such as hydroxyproline, hydroxylysine, and homocysteine.

Human cells are unable to synthesize 8 to 9 amino acids, either at all or in adequate amounts to meet the needs for growth and maintenance. These amino acids, termed dietary *essential amino acids*, are lysine, tryptophan, methionine, valine, phenylalanine, leucine, isoleucine, threonine, and for infants, histidine (Table 6.1). Depending upon conditions and other dietary proteins, methionine and phenylalanine can be converted to cysteine and tyrosine, respectively. However, if the conversion is impaired, the latter amino acids also become dietarily essential as well.

Often the term *limiting* is used in the discussion of the essential amino acid content of various foods. This refers to the fact that one of the essential amino acids present in a food is found in an amount insufficient to support growth or maintenance if it were the sole source of protein. The lack of this amino acid will "limit" the ability of an individual to make protein, regardless of the amount of other amino acids present. All essential amino acids must

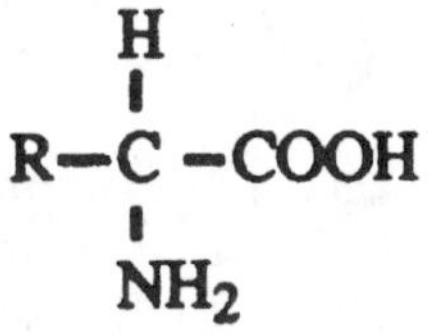

$$\begin{array}{c} H \\ | \\ R{-}C{-}COOH \\ | \\ NH_2 \end{array}$$

FIGURE 6.1
General amino acid structure.

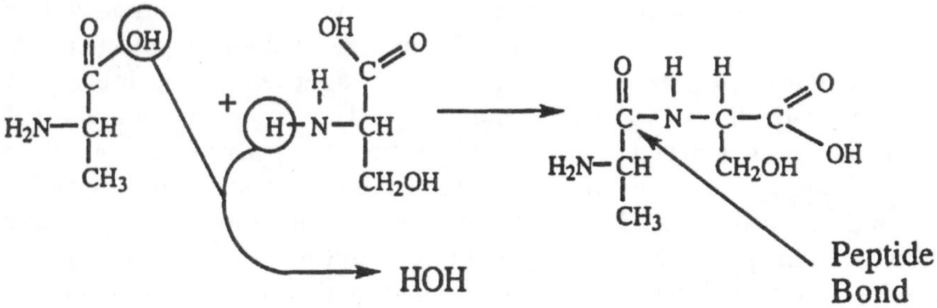

FIGURE 6.2
Formation of a peptide bond between two amino acids.

Name	Abbreviation	Structure
Glutamic Acid	Glu	$HOOC-CH_2-CH_2-CH-COOH$ with NH_2 below the CH
Glutamine	Gln	$H_2N-C(=O)-CH_2-CH_2-CH-COOH$ with NH_2 below the CH
Arginine	Arg	$H_2N-C(=NH)-N(H)-CH_2-CH_2-CH_2-CH-COOH$ with NH_2 below the CH
Lysine	Lys	$CH_2-CH_2-CH_2-CH_2-CH-COOH$ with NH_2 below first CH_2 and NH_2 below the CH
Hydroxylysine	Hyl	$CH_2-CH-CH_2-CH_2-CH-COOH$ with NH_2 and OH below, and NH_2 below the CH
Histidine	His	imidazole ring $-CH_2-CH-COOH$ with NH_2 below the CH
Phenylalanine	Phe	benzene ring $-CH_2-CH-COOH$ with NH_2 below the CH
Tyrosine	Tyr	$HO-$ benzene ring $-CH_2-CH-COOH$ with NH_2 below the CH
Tryptophan	Trp	indole ring $-CH_2-CH-COOH$ with NH_2 below the CH
Proline	Pro	pyrrolidine ring $-COOH$
Hydroxyproline	Hyp	hydroxy-pyrrolidine ring $-COOH$

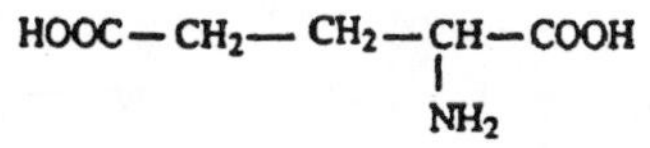

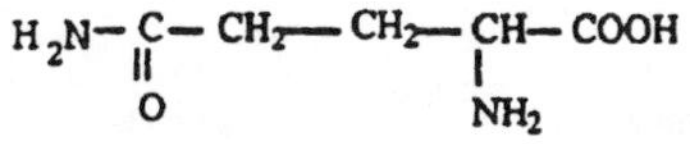

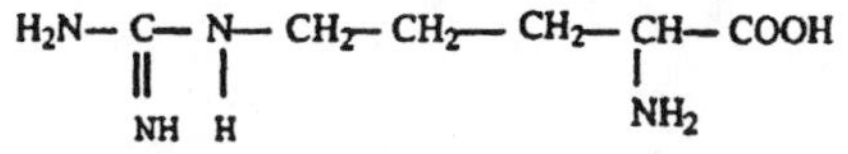

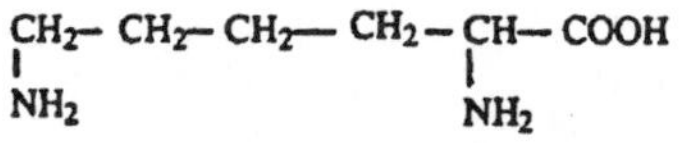

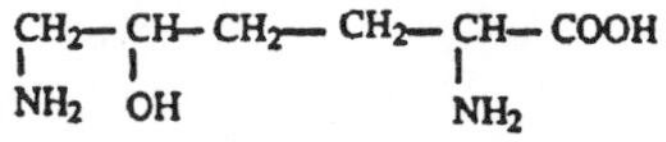

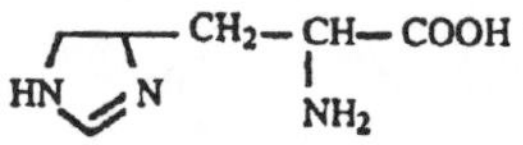

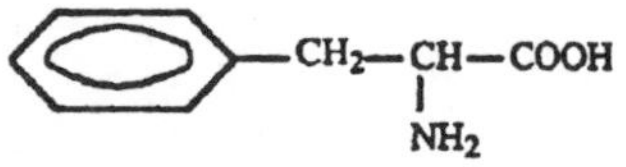

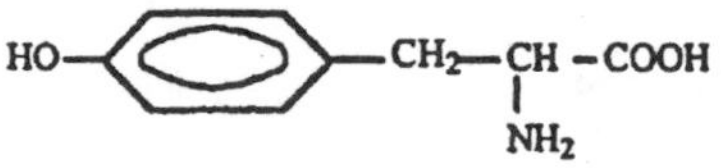

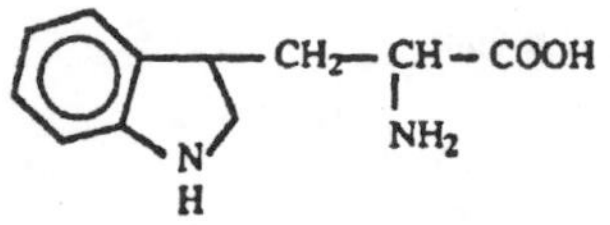

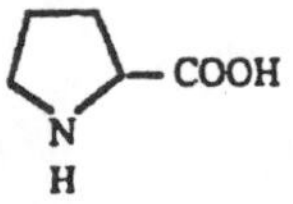

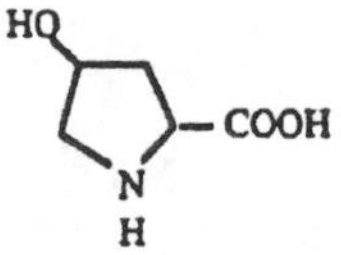

FIGURE 6.3
Amino acids.

(continues)

Name	Abbreviation	Structure
Glycine	Gly	$\begin{array}{c} H \\ | \\ H-C-COOH \\ | \\ NH_2 \end{array}$
Alanine	Ala	$\begin{array}{c} CH_3-CH-COOH \\ | \\ NH_2 \end{array}$
Valine	Val	$\begin{array}{c} CH_3 \\ \backslash \\ CH-CH-COOH \\ H_3C \quad\quad NH_2 \end{array}$
Leucine	Leu	$\begin{array}{c} CH_3 \\ \backslash \\ CH-CH_2-CH-COOH \\ H_3C \quad\quad\quad NH_2 \end{array}$
Isoleucine	Ile	$\begin{array}{c} CH_3 \\ \backslash \\ CH_2 \\ \backslash \\ CH-CH-COOH \\ H_3C \quad NH_2 \end{array}$
Serine	Ser	$\begin{array}{c} CH_2-CH-COOH \\ | \quad\quad | \\ OH \quad NH_2 \end{array}$
Threonine	Thr	$\begin{array}{c} CH_3-CH-CH-COOH \\ | \quad\; | \\ OH \; NH_2 \end{array}$
Cysteine (Cystein)	Cys	$\begin{array}{c} CH_2-CH-COOH \\ | \quad\;\; | \\ SH \quad NH_2 \end{array}$
Methionine	Met	$\begin{array}{c} CH_2-CH_2-CH-COOH \\ | \quad\quad\quad\quad | \\ S-CH_3 \quad\quad NH_2 \end{array}$
Aspartic Acid	Asp	$\begin{array}{c} HOOC-CH_2-CH-COOH \\ | \\ NH_2 \end{array}$
Asparagine	Asn	$\begin{array}{c} H_2N-C-CH_2-CH-COOH \\ \| \quad\quad\quad | \\ O \quad\quad\; NH_2 \end{array}$

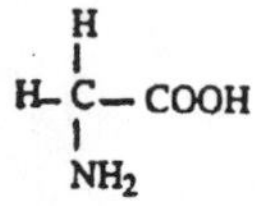

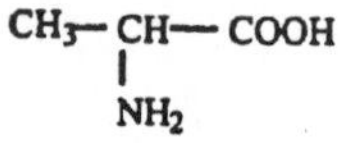

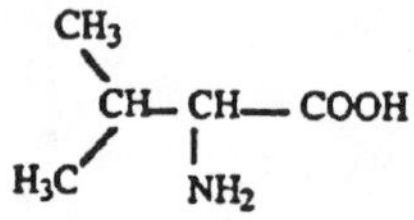

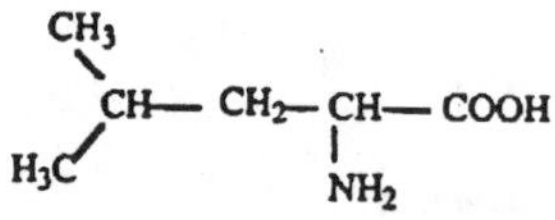

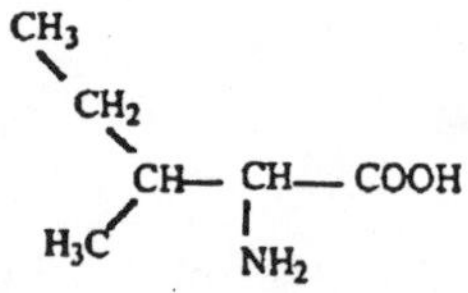

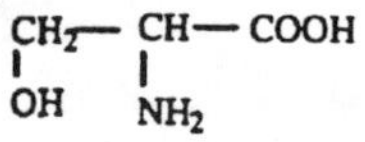

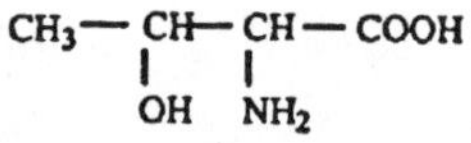

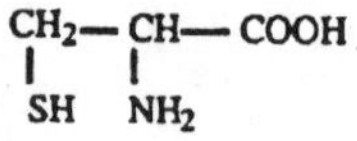

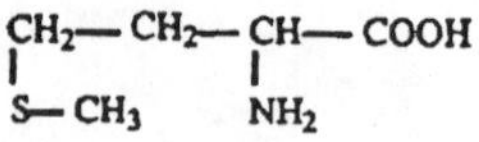

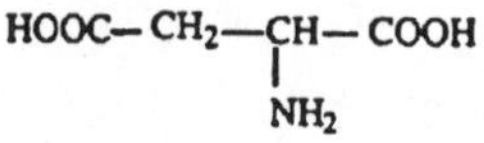

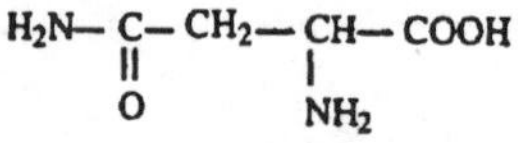

FIGURE 6.3 (continued)
Amino acids.

be present simultaneously, and in appropriate quantity, in order to make protein. If one essential amino acid is not present in the right amount, the whole synthesis process comes to a halt at a level associated with the quantity of the limiting amino acid.

The occurrence of particular amino acids within proteins is neither random nor equally distributed. Alanine is quite common, whereas methionine and tryptophan are not as common. Collagen, the most abundant protein in the human body, being about one fourth of total protein mass, has a disproportionate amount of glycine, proline, and hydroxyproline.

Protein Structures

The sequencing of an amino acid determines its three-dimensional nature. It is really the side chains that impart this character. Some side chains are large, while others are small; some are charged, while others are neutral; and some can form hydrogen and disulfide bonds with other amino acids to stabilize a structure. These characteristics all contribute to the final conformational design of a protein.

The *primary* polypeptide chain, as translated or synthesized, is termed the primary structure. The R groups of adjacent amino acids are located on opposite sides *(trans)* of the straight chain and are without interaction. The secondary structure of a protein is determined by the number and sequence of amino acids. The secondary structure refers to chemical interactions among the amino acids forming the primary structure via hydrogen bonds and disulfide linkages. The hydrogen bonding occurs between the C=O and HN of different amino acids. Spiral, globular, or flat sheet arrangements are common (i.e., α-helix, β-pleated sheet) as depicted in Figure 6.4. The secondary structure is believed to be the lowest energy state for a particular protein in a given environment. The protein α-helix is similar to the α-helix of DNA in that it is right-handed. The protein α-helix contains 3.6 amino acids per turn, with the R groups extended outward. The β-pleated sheet has the peptide sequence folding in a hairpin loop and doubling back, running in an antiparallel manner. R groups alternate between the inside and outside of the backbone and antiparallel chains are linked together by hydrogen bonding.

Tertiary structures of proteins are produced by the coiling of molecules and bonding within molecules, which determines the general shape of proteins, for instance, fibrous and globular. Fibrous proteins, which typically are not soluble in water, are long and tough fibers. Keratin of hair, skin, and nails, collagens and elastins of connective tissue, fibrin of blood, and actin and myosin proteins composing muscle are good examples. Globular proteins, which are relatively compact and fairly soluble in most solvents, are polypeptide chains folded into compact spheres. Examples include most enzymes, protein hormones, and blood proteins. Finally, the quartenary structure of proteins involves two or more polypeptide chains interacting to form functional entities. Insulin, hemoglobin, and immunoglobins are examples.

Links of amino acids can vary tremendously in length. In general, the system below can be applied. Molecular weight, the weight of a molecule obtained by totaling the masses of its constituent atoms, can also be applied in classifying protein subgroups. Oftentimes protein mass is expressed as dalton units. A dalton is an arbitrary unit of mass equal to 1/12 the mass of carbon 12 or 1.657×10^{-24} grams.

dipeptide   = linkage of 2 amino acids

peptides   = linkage of between 3 and 10 amino acids

polypeptide = linkage of more than 10 amino acids and typically less than 100 amino
                   acids

proteins   = very long linkages of amino acids (>100) and/or more than one linkage
                   complexed together (some scientists label amino acid links >50 as
                   proteins)

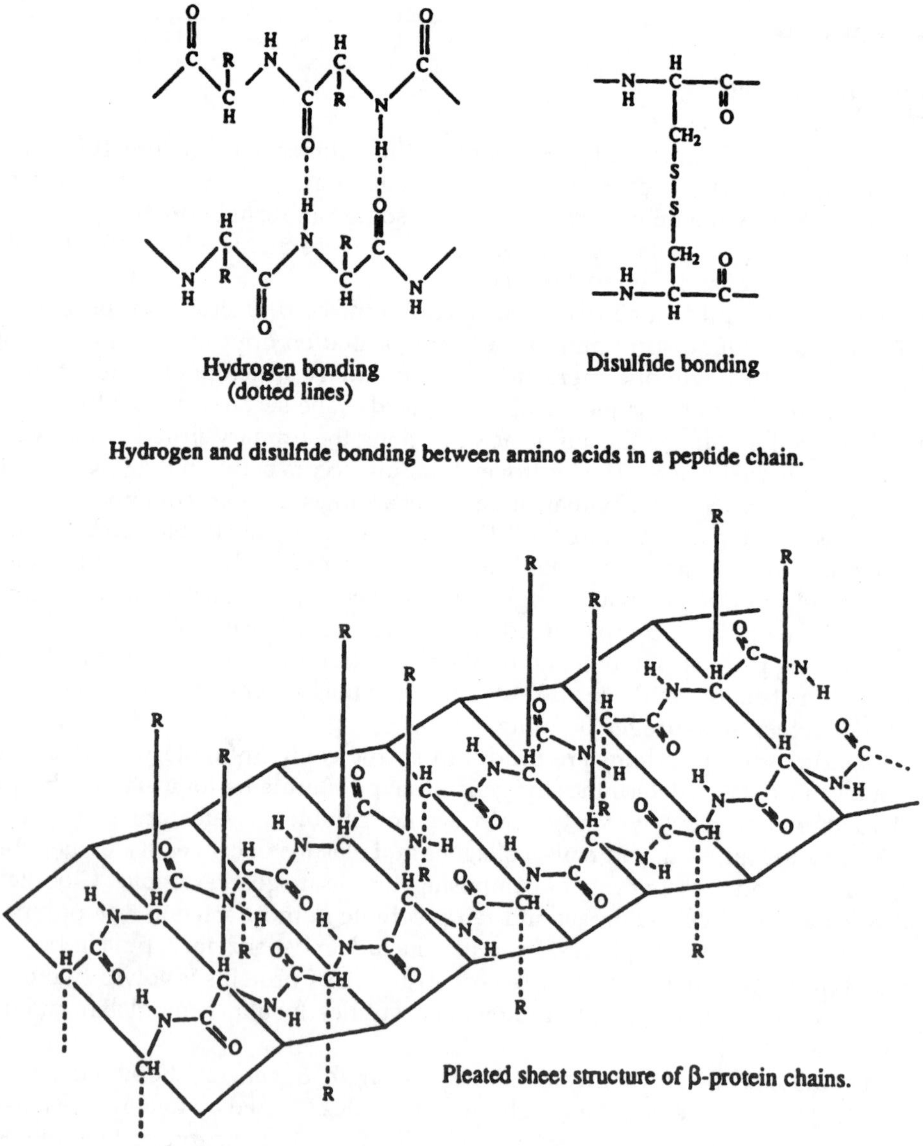

Hydrogen bonding
(dotted lines)

Disulfide bonding

Hydrogen and disulfide bonding between amino acids in a peptide chain.

Pleated sheet structure of β-protein chains.

FIGURE 6.4
Basic protein structures.

Dietary Protein, Digestion, and Absorption

Food Protein

Since protein is vital to life, all organisms will contain protein. However, the content of protein in organisms will vary. In general, foods of animal origin will have a greater protein content than plants and plant-derived foods. This is largely due to the constituent skeletal muscle of animals. The protein content of skeletal muscle or animal flesh is about 22% (Table 6.2). In fact, water-packed tuna derives more than 80% of its energy from protein. It is estimated that more than 65% of the protein that Americans eat is derived from animal sources. In comparison, many African and Asian societies derive only about 20% of their protein from animals.

TABLE 6.2
Approximate Protein Content of Selected Foods

Food	Protein (g)
Beef (3 oz)	30
Pork (3 oz)	42
Cod, poached (32 oz)	21
Oysters (32 oz)	17
Milk (1 c)	8
Cheddar cheese (1 oz)	7
Egg (1 large)	6
Peanut butter (1 tbl)	8
Potato (1)	3
Bread (1 slice)	2
Banana (1 med)	1
Carrots, sliced (2 c)	1
Apple (1)	2
Sugar, oil	0

Protein Digestion and Absorption

Compared to carbohydrate and lipid digestion discussed previously, protein digestion is perhaps a little more complex in that a variety of enzymes and tissues are involved with the breakdown into end products. The regulation of the hormones associated with protein digestion is also more involved then perhaps with carbohydrate and fat digestion.

The stomach is the first major organ involved in protein digestion. The HCl-rich secretion of parietal cells has a pH of 0.8 to 0.9, which, when mixed with other components of gastric juices, allows for a very acidic environment (pH 1.5 to 2.5) during digestion. With regard to protein digestion, the acidity of stomach juices has two primary functions. First, it activates pepsin from its zymogen form as well as creating a favorable pH for its proteolytic activity. Second, the acidity of stomach juice allows for the *denaturing* of proteins. Denaturing is the straightening and uncoiling of proteins, thereby allowing greater access to proteolytic enzymes. HCl may also directly hydrolyze proteins, but the extent is perhaps not significant.

Pepsin is a key enzyme that begins the process of protein hydrolysis after HCl has uncoiled or linearized the proteins to some extent. The mucosal chief cells secrete pepsin in the zymogen form, pepsinogen. HCl stimulates the conversion of pepsinogen to pepsin by the loss of a portion of the NH_2-terminus amino acid sequence. The optimal pH for enzyme activity of pepsin is <3.5. When pH rises above 5.0, the activity of pepsin declines rapidly. Pepsin, as is the case with other digestive proteolytic enzymes, cleaves proteins and peptides at specific peptide bonds. Pepsin will hydrolyze at peptide bonds involving the carboxyl group of the aromatic amino acids such as phenylalanine, tryptophan, and tyrosine. There is also some evidence that it may cleave where leucine and acidic amino acids are found.

Some individuals lack the ability to secrete HCl (achlorhydria) or have decreased secretion (hypochlorhydria). This condition is especially prevalent among the elderly. This results in decreased protein hydrolysis and digestion, which may have clinical consequences and require special dietary measures.

When the partially broken down protein products enter the small intestine, the pancreatic proteolytic enzymes, namely, *trypsin, chymotrypsin*, and *carboxypeptidases A and B*, are the major enzymes that result in further digestion. However, all are secreted from the pancreas in inactive zymogen forms. Trypsinogen, chymotrysinogen, and procarboxypeptidases A and B are the zymogen forms of trypsin, chymotrypsin, and carboxypeptidases A and B, respectively. The mucosal intestinal cells secrete the enzyme *enterokinase*, which will cleave off a hexapeptide from trypsinogen to form active trypsin. Once formed, trypsin can also perform the hexapeptide cleavage of trypsinogen, yielding more trypsin. The activation of trypsin is a critical step in protein digestion as trypsin also converts the other inactive pancreatic enzymes to the active forms. Trypsin acts upon the peptides linkages involving the carboxyl groups of arginine and lysine. It is an endopeptidase since it cleaves proteins and peptides internal to the chain.

Chymotrypsinogen is an endopeptidase and is specific for linkages involving the carboxyl groups of a phenylalanine, tyrosine, and tryptophan. Carboxypeptidase has two forms, an A and a B form. Inactive forms (procarboxypeptidase) reaching the small intestine are also activated by trypsin. Carboxypeptidase A contains zinc and hydrolyzes the carboxyl terminal resides that possess aromatic and aliphatic linkages. The B form acts upon terminal arginine or lysine residues. Both carboxypeptidase forms are considered exopeptidases in that they will cleave off amino acids at the carboxyl end of the polypeptide.

The pancreas also synthesizes and releases a substance known as trypsin inhibitor. This compound prevents the autoactivation of the inactive trypsinogen molecules in secretory vesicles in the pancreas. This prevents autodigestion of the pancreas. However, many times when there is pathology to the pancreatic parenchyma or obstruction of pancreatic exocrine ducts; large quantities of pancreatic secretions are pooled and overwhelm the limited quantity of trypsin inhibitor. Within a few hours, the pancreas sustains autodigestive damage resulting in inflammation or acute pancreatitis.

The final hydrolysis of the peptides produced by pancreatic enzymes will occur at the surface of the microvillus membranes of the intestinal mucosal cells. The *aminopeptidases* will take the peptides and yield individual amino acids and oligopeptides (3 or 4 amino acid fragments). Aminopeptidases are considered exopeptidases. Thus, the net result of luminal digestion in the small intestine is short oligopeptide fragments, dipeptides, and amino acids.

The absorbed form of protein is primarily individual amino acids. However, along with amino acids, dipeptides, small oligopeptides and polypeptides, and possibly intact or nearly intact proteins can be taken into enterocytes. With regard to whole proteins, this event is insignificant in adults, adolescents, and children. However, during infancy, it does occur and has physiological significance. While some absorption may occur between cells, most occurs by enterocyte pinocytosis. This is particularly important for infants, since the fetus does not synthesize antibodies. Gamma globulins in the colostrum may be absorbed by the small intestine of the newborn in order to convey passive immunity from the mother during the neonatal period. This occurs within the first few hours of birth. The subsequent consumption of more mature breast milk proteins eventually limits this activity. Breast milk lactoferrin in infants may also be absorbed by pinocytosis. This protein binds iron in breast milk and is thought to promote iron uptake by the infant.

Absorption-free amino acids occurs, primarily in the ileum of the small intestine. As with monosaccharides, the absorption of amino acids is via an energy dependent carrier mediated mechanism. There are several transport carriers for amino acids. All of these carriers have the following elements in common:

1. Transport is against a concentration gradient
2. Carrier is specific for L-isomers; it will not absorb D-isomers
3. Energy in the form of ATP is required
4. Sodium and vitamin B_6 are required
5. Carboxyl, amino, and alpha-H groups are required groups

Separate amino acid carriers are present in the microvillus membrane. These carriers will transport four groups of amino acids:

1. Neutral
   a. Aromatic amino acids: tyrosine, tryptophan, and phenylalanine
   b. Aliphatic amino acids such as alanine, serine, threonine, valine, leucine, isoleucine, and glycine
   c. Methionine, histidine, glutamine, asparagine, and cysteine.

The common feature among these amino acids is the nonpolar side groups. However, each amino acid will have a different binding affinity to the carrier that follows Michaelis-Menton kinetics similar to those of enzymes. Those amino acids with greater affinities, such as methionine, can inhibit those amino acids with lower affinities, such as threonine.

2. Basic amino acids: specific for lysine, arginine, ornithine, and cystine.
3. Dicarboxylic acids: glutamic and aspartic acids.
4. Amino acids: proline and hydroxyproline. Glycine may also use this carrier in addition to the neutral carrier. Other amino acids such as taurine, D-alanine and γ-aminobutyric acid.

Proline and hydroxyproline can also be absorbed by the neutral carrier system, but may be insignificant due to competitive inhibition with other amino acids. For all of these systems, there is a coupling with sodium for absorption, similar to that previously detailed for glucose and galactose monosaccharide absorption (Figure 6.5). The Na^+/K^+ pump is maintained by an ATPase enzyme, whereby the concentration of Na^+ is greater outside of the mucosal cell. Na^+ binds to the membrane carrier as does the amino acid, and the complex transverses the membrane so that sodium is going down its concentration gradient. The energy requirement is for maintaining the ion gradient.

Dipeptides, tripeptides, and tetrapeptides may be absorbed by humans, and this route of uptake may be more significant than once thought. In fact, the uptake of amino acids via this route may be faster than from equivalent mixtures of free amino acids. Dipeptidases and aminopeptidases have been isolated from the cytosolic fractions of intestinal mucosal

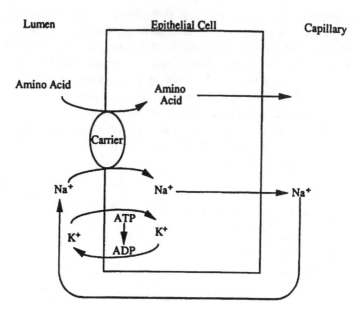

FIGURE 6.5
Active absorption of amino acids in enterocytes.

cells. This suggests that some of the final steps in peptide hydrolysis occur inside the cell, however, only amino acids leave the mucosal cell for entry into the portal blood. Evidence of this comes from two human genetic diseases, (1) Hartnup disease and (2) cystinuria. In Hartnup disease there is a defect in the ability to transport free neutral amino acids. In cystinuria, there is reduced ability to absorb dibasic amino acids and cystine. Despite the inability of individuals to transport certain essential amino acids, the patients afflicted with these diseases show no evidence of protein malnutrition. Dipeptides given to these patients show a disappearance from the lumen, indicating uptake. The uptake of dipeptides occurs mostly in the jejunum and for free amino acids in the ileum. The available data suggest that for dipeptides the neutral, basic, or acidic ones all share the same carrier. The system appears to be sodium dependent, but evidence also suggests that a sodium-independent mechanism may also coexist.

There are tetrapeptidases in the brush border of the microvillus membrane that will hydrolyze tetrapeptides into tripeptides and free amino acids. Tripeptidases are present in both membrane and cytoplasm in equal amounts. Dipeptidases are found commonly in the mucosal cell cytoplasm.

Dietary Protein Quality

Protein quality is different from quantity. Quantity refers to the amounts of nitrogen in the food. Nitrogen comprises approximately 16% of the weight of most amino acids and therefore of proteins in general. Quality refers to the essential amino acid content in a protein compared to the needs of human cells, collectively. If the availability of essential amino acids is not adequate to meet the needs of cells to synthesize proteins, then protein synthesis is limited. The availability of essential amino acids in cellular pools largely reflects the composition and quantity of dietary protein. If the amount of one or more essential amino acids in a food protein is relatively low in comparison to human protein as a whole, then that amino acid(s) is referred to as *limiting*. Food proteins able to provide all essential amino acids in proportions meeting human proteins are called *complete* or *high biological value proteins*. The following definitions of terms may help:

High biological value protein (complete protein): contains all nine essential amino acids in proportion to human protein and will support growth and maintenance. This is normally protein of animal origin.

Low biological value protein (incomplete protein): contains all nine essential amino acids, but not in the proportional amounts to meet the body's need. Plant proteins will often fall into this category. Corn is such an example because it is low in the amino acid lysine.

There are several methods used to assess the relative quality of a protein. Some have advantages over others, and many of these methods are used in the food industry to assess the quality of protein in foods. The measures used to assess protein quality always compare the quality of a particular protein to a *reference protein*, which is also a high quality protein. One such protein that is highly digestible and has an essential amino acid content similar to human protein is egg protein. In fact, egg protein is probably the most "perfect" protein source for humans in that the correct balance of amino acids appears to be present and available. Another commonly used reference protein is the milk-based protein casein.

Biological value (BV) is the amount of nitrogen digested, absorbed, and used by the body but not excreted. Egg protein has a BV of 100 or is 100% efficient. The assessment of BV begins with an analysis of the nitrogen content of food, urine, and feces. A test diet that is protein-free also needs to be included in this method. Urinary nitrogen represents absorbed amino acids that have been deaminated. Fecal nitrogen represents unabsorbed amino acids and nitrogen from sloughed off intestinal cells and nitrogen comprising the enzymes. To determine the endogenous protein excretion and the nitrogen from sloughed off cells and digestive enzymes, a protein-free diet is needed to subtract the difference. The following formula best illustrates this concept:

$$BV = \frac{\text{Dietary N} - (\text{urinary N} - U_0) - (\text{Fecal N} - F_0)}{\text{Dietary N} - (\text{Fecal N} - F_0)} \times 100$$

where:

Dietary N = nitrogen content of the food consumed

Urinary N = nitrogen in the urine while consuming the test protein

U_0 = nitrogen content of the urine when consuming the protein-free diet

Fecal N = nitrogen in the feces while consuming the test protein

F_0 = nitrogen content of the feces when consuming the protein free diet

A protein with a BV of 70 or more is considered capable of supporting growth, assuming caloric value of the diet is adequate. This means that 70% of the nitrogen absorbed is retained. However, one consideration is that this does not take into account differences in digestibility between various proteins. For instance, it is generally known that plant protein sources are less digestible than animal sources, since the cell wall of plant foods may interfere with digestive enzymes binding to the substrates. To correct for this problem, another measure can be applied, *net protein utilization* (NPU). This measure expresses how efficiently protein is used by an organism such as a human. It accounts for both the digestibility of the protein and the BV. The NPU is therefore the BV multiplied by the digestibility:

$$\text{Digestibility} = \frac{\text{Diet N} - (F - F_0)}{\text{Diet N}} \times 100$$

Thus NPU represents the percent of the dietary nitrogen retained while BV represents the percent of the absorbed nitrogen retained. Generally, the NPU is almost always lower than the BV. For instance, the BV of egg is 100% and the NPU is 94%. However, for peanuts, both the BV and NPU are 55%.

Another commonly used measure of protein quality is the *protein efficiency ratio* (PER). This is perhaps the simplest method of determining protein quality; however, it does require some chemical analysis. The basic idea is to calculate the weight gain of a growing animal in relation to its protein intake when energy is ample and protein source is fed at an adequate level. The adequate level for protein when using a laboratory rat, which is the common approach, is 9% protein expressed on an energy basis. Growing rats are usually given the test protein at weaning or 21 days of age and allowed free access to the test diet for a 28 day period. A control group of rats is used that has casein as a control protein source. The expression is therefore as follows:

$$\text{PER} = \frac{\text{weight gain (g)}}{\text{protein intake (g)}}$$

Casein usually will yield a PER value of 2.5. This means that for every gram of protein consumed by the growing rats, a body weight gain of 2.5 g was obtained. Egg protein usually has a PER value of 3.9, while soybeans have a value of 2.3 and peanuts 1.7.

Another commonly used method for assessing protein quality is the *chemical score*, sometimes referred to as the *amino acid score*. This method requires that a particular test and reference protein be analyzed for their essential amino acid content. The expression is:

$$\text{Score} = \frac{\text{mg amino acid in 1 g test protein}}{\text{mg amino acid in reference protein}} \times 100\%$$

The content of each essential amino acid in the test and reference proteins are determined and the smallest score is by definition the score applied to that particular protein, as the amino acid found in the smallest amount is the limiting amino acid. Either egg or milk protein is typically employed as the reference protein. Egg has a score of 100, while when cow's milk is compared to egg, it has a score of 95. Beef has a score of 69, soybeans 47, and corn 49. The correction for the amino acid score for digestability of a given protein will be discussed below.

Roles of Amino Acids and Proteins in Metabolism

All enzymes are proteins and function to catalyze biochemical reactions by lessening the energy requirements for a particular chemical reaction. In general, enzyme names end in -*ase* following the type of reaction they catalyze. For instance, a transferase will facilitate group transfers from one molecule to another (i.e., alanine transferase). Chemical reactions, and the enzymes that facilitate their action, have been placed into six classes, each having numerous subclasses. The six classes of enzymes are *oxidoreductases, transferases, hydrolases, isomerases, lyases,* and *ligases* (Table 6.3).

TABLE 6.3
Classifications of Enzymes and General Function

Enzyme Class	General Function
1. Oxidoreductase	In these reactions one substrate is oxidized while another is reduced
2. Transferases	In these reactions a functional group is transferred between substrates
3. Hydrolases	In these reactions water splits an ester, ether, peptide, glysyl linkage, acid anhydride, carbon–carbon bond, carbon–halide bond, or phosphorus–nitrogen bond
4. Lyases	In these reactions two groups are removed from a substrate, leaving a double bond
5. Isomerases	In these reactions there is an interconversion of isomers—optical, geometric, and positional
6. Ligases	In these reactions a covalent bond is formed, utilizing the hydrolysis of ATP or some other high-energy compound

Proteins are important transportation components of the blood. For example, *hemoglobin* in red blood cells endeavors to transport oxygen. There are about 3×10^{13} red blood cells and about 900 g of hemoglobin in an adult man. Each subunit of hemoglobin contains one heme group with a centralized iron atom that can bind oxygen. Hemoglobin has a molecular weight of approximately 67,000 Da and has four subunits — 2 α chains of 141 amino acids each and 2 β chains of 146 amino acids each. Hemoglobin in the form of $2\alpha2\beta$ is often referred to as hemoglobin A. About 2.5% of hemoglobin is in the form of hemoglobin A_2 in which the 2 β subunits are replaced by 2 δ subunits ($2\alpha,2\delta$), also containing 146 amino acids each. Ten amino acid residues differ in the δ chains in comparison to the β chain. Fetal hemoglobin (hemoglobin F) is also similar to hemoglobin A except that its 2 β subunits are replaced by 2 γ subunits, thus $2\alpha2\gamma$. Here again the β subunits and the γ subunits contain 146 amino acids each; however, this time there is a difference in 37 amino acid residues.

Other important transport proteins include plasma proteins. With the exception of antibodies and γ-globulin and some endothelial secreted proteins, plasma proteins are largely synthesized and secreted by the liver. The total protein content of plasma for an adult is 7.0 to 7.5 g/100 ml. Plasma proteins contain simpler molecules as well as conjugated proteins such as glycoproteins and lipoproteins. *Albumin*, a 610-amino acid single chain protein with a molecular weight of 69,000, is the principal plasma protein. Its concentration is usually 3.5 to 5.0 g/100 ml. Albumin is a principal transporter for substances such as fatty acids, bile acids in the portal circulation, and many other substances, including several minerals. Other transport proteins found in the blood include transferrin, ceruloplasmin, and vitamin D-binding protein (DBP). Protein-containing lipoproteins are major transporters of lipids and lipid-soluble substances (i.e., fat-soluble vitamins).

Clotting factors are synthesized in the liver and released in a zymogen form. These include factors V, VII (proconvertin), VIII (antihemolytic factor), IX (Christmas factor), X (Stuart factor), XI (plasma thromboplastin), XII (Hageman factor), XIII (transaminase), fibrinogen, and prothrombin. The mechanism of clotting incorporates a cascade of events or stages, each serving to amplify the process. The final reaction in the cascade results in the activation of *fibrinogen* to *fibrin*, which forms a cross-linking structure, the structural basis of the clot. Conversely, the liver also secretes *plasminogen*, which, when activated to *plasmin*, serves to dissolve clots.

Muscle contraction is based upon contractile proteins such as myosin, actin, troponin, and tropomyosin. Myosin is a major body protein as well as a major muscle protein, accounting for 55% of muscle mass. It contains three pairs of proteins, one pair of heavy chains and two different pairs of light chains and is about 460,000 Da. The heavy chains alone are about 1800 amino acids long, which are among the longest in the human body. Actin is a smaller protein with a molecular weight of about 45,000. As initially synthesized, actin is a globular protein (G-actin) which can then polymerize with other actin molecules to form a fibrous structure called F-actin (Figure 1.23). Tropomyosin is also a fibrous protein that binds to F-actin and serves to cover myosin binding sites on actin monomers when a muscle is not being stimulated to contract. There are three principal troponin molecules, all of which are in some manner associated with one another, as well as with tropomyosin. The C subunit binds calcium when intracellular calcium levels increase during stimulation. This results in a conformational change in the troponin complex which ultimately results in the uncovering of myosin binding sites on actin by physically moving tropomyosin structures.

Several hormones are protein structures or modified amino acids. Insulin and glucagon, which are pivotal hormones involved in energy nutrient metabolism, are examples. The hypothalamus alone will produce nine hormones of a protein or modified amino acid nature. These include thyrotropin-releasing hormone (TRH), somatostatin, growth hormone releasing hormone (GHRH), prolactin-inhibiting hormone (PIH), prolactin-releasing hormone (PRH), Melanocyte-stimulating hormone (MSH), inhibiting hormone, MSH-releasing hormone, gonadotropin-releasing hormone, and corticotropin-releasing hormone. The anterior pituitary gland produces eight protein-based hormones, including thyroid-stimulating hormone (TSH), growth hormone (GH), prolactin, MSH, luteinizing hormone (LH), follicle-stimulating hormone (FSH), and adrenocorticotropic hormone (ACTH). FSH, LH, and TSH are glycoproteins comprised of two subunits, an α subunit which is identical and a β subunit which differs between the hormones.

Connective tissue protein structures such as collagen and elastin provide strength and elasticity properties to human tissue. As mentioned above, collagen is the most abundant protein in the human body. It is generally an insoluble fibrous protein found in tendons, bones, cartilage, skin, the cornea, and in interstitial spaces. About 30% of its amino acids are glycine, while proline, hydroxyproline, and hydroxyserine contribute about 20%. Collagen as synthesized by fibroblasts is helical in structure, and three collagen helices are twisted together to form a larger left-handed helix called tropocollagen. Multiple tropocollagen helicies are cross-linked together to form a strong collagen fiber. Copper, iron, and vitamin C are all vital in the production of collagen fibers. Elastin is a protein also found in connective tissue and is an especially important component of vascular tissue such as the aorta and other arteries and arterioles. It allows for expansion of a vessel under pressure and recoil as pressure subsides. Elastin is especially rich in lysine and glycine.

A major protein of hair, skin, and nails is α-keratin. It has a secondary protein structure in the form of an α-helix. Like collagen, several keratin helices are twisted together and stabilized by disulfide bonds, to form thicker fibers. Commercially available "permanent wave" solutions disrupt the disulfide bonds.

Protein is also an important factor in water balance. Since proteins cannot diffuse through a semipermeable membrane, they exert osmotic pressure in either the intracellular or extracellular fluid, or across organelle membranes. A normal concentration of protein in the plasma, especially albumin, is fundamental in balancing the water between tissue and the blood. If protein intake is insufficient, a decreased concentration of protein in the plasma results and water deposits into tissues, resulting in *edema*.

Acid–base balance is another function, since proteins act as natural buffers and amino acids can ionize and provide both acidic and basic groups. The carboxyl group helps neutralize excess base and the amine group neutralizes excess acid. The natural buffering capacity of amino acids and some proteins (i.e., carbonic anhydrase) is critical for cellular and extracellular environments and metabolic functions and biochemical reactions.

Additionally, antibodies are composed of protein. It is not unusual to find decreased resistance to infections in areas of the world where protein intake is low or insufficient. Membrane transport carriers (i.e., GLUT4, Na^+/K^+ ATPase) and receptors are also proteins, as are many intracellular binding entities such as metallothionein and ferritin. The visual pigment opsin is a protein found in the retina of the eye.

In addition to being building blocks for proteins, amino acids may be used to construct other molecules, or their carbon skeleton can be used in energy metabolic pathways. From an energy perspective, amino acids may be classified either as *ketogenic* or *glucogenic*. Phenylalanine, tyrosine, leucine, and isoleucine are degraded to acetoacetate and are ketogenic. Other amino acids are degraded to pyruvate, oxaloacetate, α-ketoglurate, succinate, and fumarate, which can be used in gluconeogenesis to produce glucose, and thus are glucogeneic.

Beyond intermediates of energy pathways, certain amino acids are also precursors of critical biochemical compounds. As alluded to already, some amino acids give rise to other amino acids as in the conversion of phenylalanine to tyrosine. Tyrosine itself is a precursor of thyroid hormone (T_3/T_4), dopamine, epinephrine, and norepinephrine. Sulfur-containing amino acids such as taurine give rise to bile compounds. Tryptophan is metabolized to serotonin, a critical neurotransmitter. The most simplest amino acid, glycine, is involved in the formation of the porphyrin ring of hemoglobin as well as creatine. Hydroxyproline and hydroxylysine are important components of collagen. Table 6.4 summarizes the functions of some of these amino acids used to make various substances.

TABLE 6.4
Amino Acid-Derived Substances

Substance	Amino Acids Utilized in the Synthesis
Choline	Serine
Niacin	Tryptophan
Glutathione	Cysteine, glycine, glutamic acid
Serotonin	Tryptophan
Carnitine	Lysine, methionine
Carnosine	Histidine, alanine
Creatine	Arginine, glycine, methionine
Pyrimidines	Asparate, glutamine
Purines	Aspartate, glutamine, glycine
Epinephrine	Tyrosine or phenylalanine
Norepinephrine, dopamine, thyroid hormone	

The amino acid methionine is a principal molecule involved in single-carbon unit transfer mechanisms used in molecular synthesis operations. The enzyme methionine adenosyl transferase catalyzes the ATP-requiring conversion of methionine to *S*-adenosyl methionine (SAM). This enzyme is abundant in the liver, which is the primary site of methionine metabolism. SAM is the principal methyl donor in human cells and is used to create molecules such as carnitine, creatine, epinephrine, and purines. Upon removal of the methyl group from SAM the compound *S*-adenosyl homocysteine is created (SAH), which can be converted to homocysteine (Figure 8.34). In order for methionine to be regenerated from homocysteine, vitamin B_{12}, 5-methyl THF (a folate form), and betaine must be present, with the latter compound donating a single carbon unit. Homocysteine can also be converted to the nonessential amino acids serine and cysteine. Recently, attention has been focused upon the relationship between homocysteinemia and the risk of heart disease. This will be discussed in Chapter 16.

Taurine and ornithine are two amino acids that have fundamental roles in the human body but are not incorporated into protein. Taurine has a fundamental role in retinal operations related to vision, in membrane stability, as a component of bile acids, and possibly as a neurotransmitter. Ornithine is vital in the disposal of nitrogenous waste molecules (ammonia) via the urea cycle, which is discussed below.

Metabolism of Amino Acids

Transamination and Deamination

Amino acids are unique from other energy nutrients in that they contain the element nitrogen. The removal of nitrogen or its transfer is necessary for the utilization of amino acids as an energy source as well as for the creation of nonessential amino acids and other molecules. *Transamination* reactions, involving an aminotransferase enzyme, transfer the amino group to an α-keto acid, while *deamination* reactions, catalyzed by deaminases, remove amine groups to form ammonia.

Aminotransferases bind to the substrate amino acid and pass the amine group to pyridoxal phosphate (PLP), which is a form of vitamin B_6. Pyridoxal phosphate is also bound to the aminotransferase. The amine group is then passed to an acceptor α-keto acid that binds with PLP and the enzyme. Pyruvate and α-ketoglutarate are the two α-keto acids utilized most in transamination reactions and aminotransferase enzymes are specific to an α-keto acid and an amino acid. *Alanine-pyruvate transaminase* and *glutamate α-ketoglutarate transaminase* are present in most human cells and an increase in the cardiac and hepatic isomeric forms present in the plasma is a diagnostic tool for cardiac and hepatic pathology. The glutamate-α-ketoglutarate transaminase is shown in Figure 6.6.

Nitrogen can also be removed from amino acids by deamination. For instance, oxidative deamination of glutamate yields α-ketoglutarate and free ammonia (Figure 6.6). This deamination is catalyzed by glutamate dehydrogenase, an enzyme which uses NAD or NADP as electron acceptors. In peroxisomes, D-amino acids undergo oxidative deamination by amino acid oxidases which use FAD and FMN as electron acceptors.

As discussed in more detail below, amino groups can be removed from amino acid to create free ammonia. Glutaminase, asparaginase, and the amino acid oxidases all produce ammonia; however, glutamate dehydrogenase generates the most ammonia. This hepatic enzyme is pivotal in amino acid disposal via urea synthesis.

1. Transamination

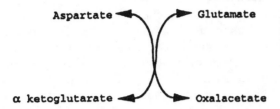

Aspartate can donate its amino group to α ketoglutarate which becomes glutamate while aspartate becomes oxalacetate. The reverse can also occur.

2. Oxidative deamination

$$\text{Glutamate} + \text{NAD(P)}^+ + \text{HOH} \longrightarrow \alpha \text{ ketoglutarate} + \text{NAD(P)H}^{++}$$

$$+ \text{ NH}_3$$

3. Amino acid oxidase

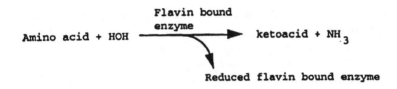

FIGURE 6.6
General reactions involving the transfer or removal of amino groups.

Synthesis of Amino Acids

Discussion of the synthesis of amino acids is limited to nonessential amino acids and posttranslational derivatives of nonessential amino acids (i.e., hydroxyproline). Glutamate provides most of the nitrogen used in the synthesis of nonessential amino acids. As mentioned above, two nonessential amino acids rely upon the presence or appropriate metabolism of essential amino acids for their creation. Tyrosine is synthesized by hydroxylation of the phenylalanine and cysteine is formed with the help of methionine. Many amino acids are derived from intermediates of glycolysis and the Krebs cycle. Serine can be synthesized from the glycolytic intermediate 3-phosphoglycerate. Serine can then serve as a precursor for glycine and cysteine. While the carbon skeleton and nitrogen of cysteine are derived from serine, methionine is needed to supply sulfur. Alanine is produced via the transamination of pyruvate.

The nonessential amino acids derived from Krebs cycle intermediates include aspartate, asparagine, glutamate, glutamine, proline, and arginine. Aspartate is derived from oxaloacetate via transamination, and asparagine can then be synthesized from aspartate by amidation. Glutamate is derived from α-ketoglutarate either by transamination or by the addition of ammonia via glutamate dehydrogenase. Glutamine, proline, and arginine are also produced from glutamate. Glutamine is generated via amidation, while proline and arginine are derived from glutamate semialdehyde, which is the result of the reduction of glutamate. Proline requires the cyclization of glutamate semialdehyde, while the creation of arginine requires glutamate semialdehyde to first be converted to ornithine which is eventually converted to arginine by way of urea cycle reactions.

The amino acid composition of several proteins contains modifications of nonessential amino acids such as hydroxyproline, hydroxylysine, and homocysteine. The modifications occur after the initial protein chain has been synthesized on ribosomes, and thus the modifications are called *posttranslational* events. Hydroxylysine and hydroxyproline occur almost exclusively in collagen. These amino acids are formed by dioxidation reactions, and iron, copper, vitamin C, and α-ketoglutarate are required. 3-Methyl histidine is formed posttranslationally from the amino acid histidine. This amino acid is found almost exclusively in actin protein. While most actin quantatively is found in muscle, some actin is found in other tissue, such as the intestines where actin shafts yield support to microvilli. Some actin is also found in platelets as well. Upon proteolysis, 3-methyl histidine is released from these cells, and it is not reincorporated into new proteins. It diffuses out of cells and is excreted in the urine. Because of the greater relative mass of muscle to other actin-containing tissue, most of the 3-methyl histidine in the urine is attributed to muscle catabolism during fasting, starvation, or prolonged activity.

Degradation of Amino Acids

Once nitrogen is removed from amino acids, the remaining molecule is referred to as the *carbon skeleton*. When carbon skeletons of amino acids are degraded, the major products are pyruvate, acetyl CoA, intermediates of the Krebs cycle, and the ketone body acetoacetate. As alluded to above, amino acids whose carbon skeleton forms pyruvate or intermediates of the Krebs cycle, are deemed glucogenic, as they can be used to form glucose in the liver via gluconeogenesis. Those amino acid skeletons that become acetyl CoA and acetoacetate are deemed ketogenic, as they can form ketone bodies. While most amino acids are either glucogeneic or ketogenic, a few amino acids, namely, tryptophan, phenylalanine, tyosine, and isoleucine, are both.

Those amino acids whose carbon skeletons are used to form pyruvate include serine, glycine, cysteine, hydroxyproline, threonine, tryptophan, and alanine, with the latter forming pyruvate directly via a transamination reaction. Serine dehydratase converts serine to pyruvate by first removing water; then a hydrolysis reaction removes ammonia. Glycine, on the other hand, is first converted to serine and then pyruvate. In the first reaction, a single carbon unit is donated to glycine by N^5, N^{10}-methylene tetrahydrofolate, a folic acid form.

As mentioned above, hydroxyproline which is prominent in collagen, but not found in most other proteins, undergoes a series of reactions that ultimately produce pyruvate and glyoxylate. The nitrogen of hydroxyproline is removed by transamination. Cysteine's carbon skeleton forms pyruvate by one of two mechanisms. In the first, cysteine must first be transaminated to form thiopyruvate and then sulfur is removed to form pyruvate; while in the second, sulfur is first removed and then cysteine dehydratase removes ammonia in a hydrolytic reaction. In either case the removal of sulfur creates H_2SO_4.

The initial reaction in the catabolism of threonine creates glycine and acetaldehyde. Glycine can be converted to pyruvate, as mentioned above, while acetaldehyde is oxidized by FAD to create acetate, which itself is condensed with coenzyme A to yield acetyl CoA. Thus, threonine is both glucogenic and ketogenic, as is tryptophan. Tryptophan catabolism results in the formation of pyruvate and acetoacetate.

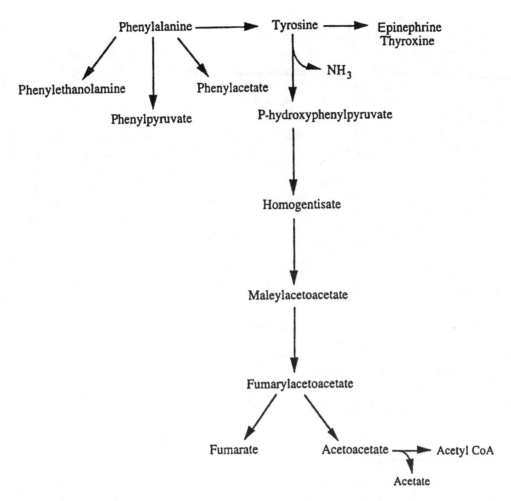

FIGURE 6.7
Catabolism of phenylalanine.

Those amino acids whose carbon skeletons form Krebs cycle intermediates are glutamate, glutamine, proline, arginine, histidine, asparagine, aspartate, threonine, methionine, homocysteine, valine, and isoleucine. Aspartate is converted into oxaloacetate via a transamination reaction involving α-ketoglutarate and forming glutamate in the process. Asparagine's carbon skeleton is also converted to oxaloacetate; however, asparagine must first be deaminated by asparaginase to aspartate.

The carbon skeletons of arginine, histidine, proline, and glutamine can all be converted to α-ketoglutarate. However, they are first converted to glutamate, which, via oxidative deamination, is converted to α-ketoglutarate. Glutamate can also be used in a transamination reaction that forms alanine and α-ketoglutarate.

Parts of methionine, isoleucine, and valine are used to form succinyl CoA. The catabolism of these amino acids first allows for the formation of either propionyl CoA or methylmalonyl CoA, which are oxidized to succinyl CoA in the same reactions that oxidized odd-chain-length fatty acids. The catabolism of methionine first involved the production of *S*-adenosyl methionine which subsequently loses its methyl group, producing *S*-adenosyl homocysteine. Further enzymatic processing results in the cleavage of adenosine and the addition of serine to yield cystathionine. Cystathionine is subsequently cleaved to form cysteine and homoserine. Cysteine is converted to pyruvate as discussed above. Meanwhile oxidative deamination of homoserine yields α-ketobutyrate, which is then decarboxylated and activated by the attachment of coenzyme A to form propionyl CoA. Further carboxylation to methylmalonyl CoA and subsequent molecular rearrangement produces succinyl CoA.

Phenylalanine and tyrosine are converted to fumarate. The first step in phenylalanine breakdown is the formation of tyrosine (Figure 6.7). The first reaction is catalyzed by phenylalanine hydroxylase, and a genetic predisposition resulting in diminished activity of this enzyme results in the increased formation of alternative phenylalanine metabolites (phenylethanolamine, phenylpyruvate, phenylacetate) which can result in poor growth and development especially of the brain. This condition is often called phenyketonuria or PKU. Tyrosine is transaminated by tyrosine transaminase to form *p*-hydroxyphenylpyruvate. The acceptor of the transferred amino group is α-ketoglutarate. A copper-containing enzyme that also requires ascorbate yields homogenizate which is then ultimately metabolized to fumarylacetoacetate, which is split to yield fumarate and acetoacetate.

There are five amino acids that are converted to acetoacetate. These amino acids are lysine, leucine, phenylalanine, tyrosine, and tryptophan. The latter three have been discussed above. Leucine and lysine will be discussed here.

Leucine is the only amino acid that is only ketogenic. This is to say that it does not produce glucogenic intermediates. The product of leucine metabolism is similar to isoleucine and valine, except that leucine yields acetoacetate and acetyl CoA. Lysine, on the other hand, is both ketogenic and glucogenic. While there is some uncertainty about the true final glucogenic product, the breakdown of lysine yields acetoacetate.

Disposal of Amino Acid Nitrogen

Disposal of amino acid-derived nitrogen in the form of ammonia is crucial for the survival of humans. Increased serum levels of ammonia result in a toxicity syndrome, with the brain being a major site of impact. Ammonia is produced either by cellular degradation of amino acids and nucleic acids or by the metabolism of intestinal bacteria. Glutaminase, asparaginase, histidases, serine dehydratase, cysteine dehydratase, and amino acid oxidases all produce ammonia. By far the major source of cellular ammonia comes from glutamate dehydrogenase. This mitochondrial enzyme catalyzes the removal of glutamate nitrogen collected from amino acid transaminase reactions. As urea synthesis occurs within the mitochondria, primarily in the liver and secondarily in the kidneys, the liberated ammonia can be immediately utilized.

Tissues other than the liver and kidneys will not synthesize urea. Therefore, ammonia liberated in cellular reactions can be used to convert glutamate to glutamine. In fact, if a cell starts with α-ketoglutarate, two ammonia molecules can be transported as glutamine. Muscle tissue forms alanine and glutamine in efforts to transport excess nitrogen generated by the degradation of amino acids. Alanine is produced in muscle by the transamination of pyruvate via alanine transaminase. During a fasting state, alanine and glutamine account for as much as 50% of the amino acids released from skeletal muscle into circulation. Alanine circulates to the liver and is transaminated to pyruvate, which serves as a gluconeogenic precursor, while glutamine serves as an energy source for the intestines and a gluconeogenic precursor for the kidneys.

Urea Cycle

The urea cycle consists of five reactions that convert ammonia, CO_2, and the α-amino nitrogen of aspartate into *urea*. Two of the reactions occur within the mitochondria, while the remaining reactions occur in the cytoplasm (Figure 6.8). In the preliminary reaction, carbon dioxide in the mitochondria is phosphorylated, via ATP, and subsequently condensed to ammonia using the energy released by the hydrolysis of another ATP molecule. The enzyme catalyzing the reaction is carbamoyl phosphate synthase and the product is *carbamoyl phosphate*. While still in the mitochondria, carbamoyl phosphate is condensed with ornithine, via ornithine transcarbamoylase, to form *citrulline*. Phosphate is released in the reaction, and citrulline enters the cytosol. Next citrulline condenses with aspartate via arginosuccinate synthase to form *arginosuccinate*, which is subsequently split by a lyase enzyme into fumarate and arginine. The arginase enzyme then hydrolyzes arginine to form ornithine and urea.

There is some disagreement as to the fate of fumarate formed by the splitting of arginosuccinate. It is more probable that fumarate is hydrated in the cytosol to form malate, which is then oxidized to oxaloacetate (OAA) by cytosolic malate dehydrogenase. Finally, oxaloacetate accepts an amino group from glutamate to reform aspartate.

Protein Requirements

The measures discussed above are methods of determining quality of proteins. The amount of protein, or nitrogen, required by a human is another matter. This concept is called *nitrogen balance*. If one is in nitrogen balance, that means that the amount of nitrogen from protein consumed/day is equal to the amounts of protein nitrogen lost per day. $N_{in} = N_{out}$ is nitrogen equilibrium. To measure balance, the losses of nitrogen in urine, feces, and sweat are determined and the sum of these is subtracted from the amount ingested. A positive nitrogen balance occurs when the body is building tissue, so that more nitrogen is retained than is excreted by the body or $N_{in} > N_{out}$. A negative nitrogen balance occurs when the amount of nitrogen lost is greater than the amount of nitrogen retained: $N_{in} < N_{out}$. Tissue proteins are being catabolized in excess of synthesis.

There are several methods available to determine protein or nitrogen requirements in humans. The *factorial method* is used where obligatory nitrogen losses are determined. This refers to the nitrogen loss in urine, feces, sweat, nails, and dermal sources when a protein-free diet is given to test subjects. Adequate energy is provided in the diet in an attempt to prevent endogenous muscle from being used for energy. The grams of N in each of the above routes of loss is assessed daily until the loss levels out. At the point of leveling, this is referred to as the endogenous loss. Fecal nitrogen will be present even on a protein-free diet, since digestive enzymes and sloughed off cells will be present. All of the nitrogen loss sources are then added up for a given individual. Table 6.5 presents the estimated daily nitrogen loss for a 70-kg adult male.

A 70-kg male loses about 54 mg of N/kg body weight per day ± 2 SD. This increases the estimated nitrogen requirement to 70 mg N/kg body weight per day. To convert this to the amount of protein, the factor 6.25 is used, since 16% of the protein by weight is nitrogen (100/16 = 6.25). This converts to 0.45 g of protein per kilogram body weight per day. However, the nitrogen requirement assumes a linear response, which in reality does not exist. As the level of nitrogen in the diet increases toward the balance figure, the efficiency declines. Said another way, the relationship is curvilinear as the nitrogen in the diet

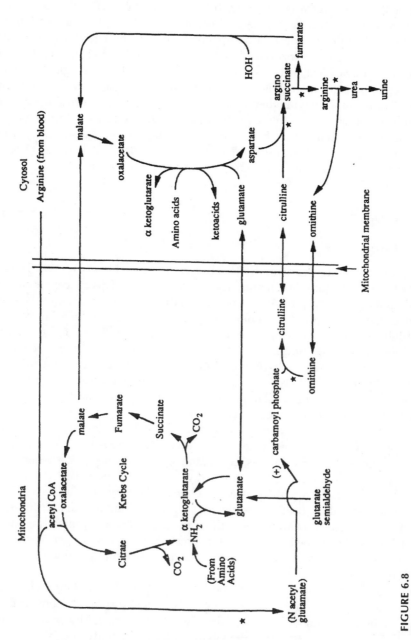

FIGURE 6.8
The urea cycle.

TABLE 6.5
Estimated Daily Loss of Protein by Various Routes

Route	Daily Loss (mg N/kg body weight/day)
Urine	37
Feces	12
Cutaneous	3
Minor routes (nasal secretions, expired breath, seminal fluid)	2

TOTAL = 54 mg.

approaches the requirement level. The efficiency of protein utilization therefore declines. The loss of efficiency is estimated to be at 30%. Therefore, the requirement for dietary protein is increased by this percentage, or from 0.45 to 0.57 g protein per kilogram body weight per day. Here, egg protein is the sole source of nitrogen. If other proteins are used, then the protein requirement must be adjusted upward accordingly. In American and other Western diets, the diet protein quality is about 75% of the quality of egg protein. The requirement for protein when this is taken into account is

$$0.57 \text{ g protein per kg body weight per day} \times \frac{100}{75} = 0.8 \text{ g protein per kg body weight per day}$$

For a 70 kg male, 56 g of protein per day is needed to meet the nitrogen requirement. This is essentially the Recommended Dietary Allowance for males. This assumes the energy levels are adequate, since energy levels may influence protein requirements. When calories are supplied at a level of 45 kcal/kg body weight per day, egg protein has a nitrogen requirement of 0.65 g/kg body weight per day. At higher energy levels of 57 kcal/kg body weight per day, the protein requirement declined to 0.45 g protein per kilogram body weight per day. Also, the 30% decline in efficiency in egg protein as the nitrogen level approaches balance levels may not apply to other protein sources.

Another method used is the *nitrogen balance method*. The minimum amount of dietary protein that is needed to keep the subject in nitrogen equilibrium is the objective. For infants and children, optimal growth and not zero nitrogen balance is the criterion used. The expression for this approach is simple:

$$\text{Balance} = \text{diet intake} - 7(\text{urine N} + \text{fecal N} + \text{skin N}) \times 6.25$$

A positive nitrogen balance is anabolic or represents net deposition, whereas a negative balance is catabolic and represents net loss of nitrogen. A limitation of this method is that at zero balance, it does not reveal whether there have been shifts within organs or body compartments. The loss of nitrogen by one route may be compensated for by decreased loss from another route.

Amino Acid Requirements

How much of an essential amino acid should be consumed is not a simple process to determine. Also, minimum levels of nonessential amino acid nitrogen may be required when determining the minimal intake needed for an essential amino acid. To study the requirement of an amino acid, a partially purified diet in which synthetic amino acids are incorporated must be used. When any one of the essential amino acids is excluded from the diet, subjects will immediately fall into negative nitrogen balance. The missing amino acid is then fed at graded levels until the criteria for adequacy are met. Accepted essential amino acids levels are listed in Table 6.6.

TABLE 6.6
Essential Amino Acid (EAA) Requirements by Age Categories (mg/kg/day)

Amino Acid	Adult EAA	10-12 years	2 years of age
Tryptophan	3.5	4	12.5
Threonine	7	35	37
Isoleucine	10	30	37
Leucine	14	45	73
Lysine	12	60	64
Methionine + Cystine (S-containing)	13	27	27
Phenylalanine + Tyrosine (aromatic)	14	27	69
Valine	10	33	38

It is well known that when an essential amino acid is present in an inadequate amount, protein synthesis ceases. This process is believed to have a molecular basis or control point. More specifically, the initiation complex is most likely affected by the lack on an essential amino acid. A *eukaryotic initiation factor* (eIF) is thought to play a pivotal role. eIF-2 is phosphorylated with GTP to produce an eIF-2-GTP complex. The tRNA for methionine normally forms a complex with eIF-2-GTP. However, when one essential amino acid is missing, the enzyme eIF-2 α-kinase is activated and will phosphorylate the eIF-2-GTP, which blocks the formation of the 43S initiation complex required to initiate protein synthesis.

Organisms have other adaptation mechanisms to deal with low protein intakes and in particular the essential amino acids. In rats and humans, amino acid oxidation is minimalized when individuals are fed a low protein diet. When the dietary protein levels of specific essential amino acids are increased, oxidation will increase only after a level is reached to meet the needs of optimal growth.

The K_m, or Michaelis-Menton constant, of the enzymes responsible for both amino acid oxidation and mRNA synthesis is critical. The K_m value for an enzyme is an index of the affinity of that enzyme for a particular substrate. Basically, the lower the value the greater the affinity, and vice versa. Thus if the K_m is high for a particular enzyme, then a relatively higher concentration of a substrate is needed to have an appreciable effect upon the enzyme activity. K_m values for amino acid oxidative enzymes are high and for mRNA they are low. On a low protein diet, there is reduced amino acid substrate for the enzymes. Since the oxidative enzymes require a higher concentration of amino acids to increase the reaction rate, a low protein diet will decrease the activity of these enzymes, and thus amino acid catabolism is kept to a minimum. However, mRNA synthesis will still proceed since the K_m values are low. Therefore, for a human consuming a low protein diet, protein synthesis will continue. This is to say that humans will direct more of the limited amino acids into protein synthesis.

Some mention of the urea acid cycle enzymes is appropriate in regards to conditions where protein intake is limited. The liver is the site of the urea acid cycle to excrete nitrogenous waste and toxic ammonia compounds. Altering dietary protein intake alters the activity of urea cycle enzymes. For instance, when protein synthesis decreases, so does the activity of the urea acid cycle enzymes. Liver arginosuccinate synthetase, for example, declines in activity when rats are fed a low protein diet. Furthermore, the mRNAs responsible for the coding of urea acid cycle enzymes also decline in a parallel fashion.

The enzymes responsible for nitrogen removal through the urea acid cycle and those enzymes used for tissue amino acid metabolism do not vary in the same fashion in response to a low protein diet with respect to essential vs. nonessential amino acids. As protein intake increases, the activity of enzymes responsible for the catabolism of nonessential amino acids varies in direct response to the dietary protein intake in a linear fashion. However, for essential amino acids, such as branched-chain ketoacid dehydrogenase, this activity is relatively low when protein intake is low and below the requirement. Once the protein level has increased to the requirement level or above, then the enzyme activity increases in a linear fashion. Thus, organisms must have at their disposal unique mechanisms to derive as much gain from the essential amino acids when protein intake is low.

Determination of Protein Intakes by Food Source, Based on Limiting Amino Acids

Knowledge of the amino acid composition of various protein sources facilitates the ability to determine what levels of protein are needed in the diets of humans to meet minimum needs. Protein quality differs substantially in different areas of the world. Protein digestibility and the amino acid score, as discussed previously, are critical in determining protein requirements. Also, the Food and Drug Administration, as part of the Nutrition Labeling Regulation of 1993, required the protein digestability-corrected amino acid scoring method of protein quality evaluation for labeling of food products intended for children over 1 year of age and adults.

To calculate the protein intake for a person of a particular age, the FAO of the World Health Organization developed guidelines, including publishing what is termed "Safe Levels of Protein Intake." These are levels of protein which, when consumed on a daily per kilogram body weight basis will meet the amino acid requirements for an individual of a certain age. Safe levels have been established for the reference proteins milk, egg, meat, and fish by three different age ranges (Table 6.7). The age groups are adult, ages 1 to 6 years, and 6 to 12 years. After age 12, the adult values are used. To apply this information, the protein digestibility also needs to be known. However, rather than analyzing a meal for each protein fraction and determining separate digestibilities, the WHO has simplified the process by using one of two values. If a diet is composed of coarse food items, whole grain

TABLE 6.7

Safe Levels of Reference Protein (mild, egg, meat, and fish) by Age Group

Age	Safe Level of Reference Protein (g/kg/d)
Adults	0.75
Children (preschool; ages 1 to 6 yr)	1.10
Children (school; 6 to 12 yr)	0.99

cereals, and vegetables, then a digestibility of 85% may be a close approximation. If refined cereals are more likely, then a digestibility of 95% is suggested.

A critical piece of information that is needed is the amino acid scores for the essential amino acids of the diet consumed. This allows for the determination of one or more limiting amino acids. Lysine, methionine (+ cysteine), threonine, and tryptophan are the amino acids most limiting in the world's diets. The minimum levels of each of these amino acids has been determined for the three age ranges and the level of the amino acids present in a typical diet as well. From such data, the amino acid scores for these four amino acids can be determined and thus the limiting amino acid(s) determined in each diet. With this information, it is possible to calculate the amount of dietary protein required for either maintenance and/or growth. For example, a preschool child has a reference requirement for lysine of 58 mg/g protein. A rural Tunisian diet provides 33 mg/g protein with respect to lysine. The amino acid score is (33/58) × 100% or 57%. The safe level of protein intake for a preschool aged child is 1.10 g/kg body weight per day. The diet is likely to be coarse, and thus a digestibility of 85% may be assumed. From this information, one may calculate the amount of protein this child should consume from the diet available to meet the minimum amino acid requirement:

1.10 g of protein per kilogram body weight per day × (100%/85%) × (100%/57%)

= 2.27 g of protein per kilogram body weight per day

Thus, 2.27 g of protein per kilogram body weight per day from a rural Tunisian diet needs to be consumed for this child to stay in positive nitrogen balance. Knowing the protein content of various foods, the amount of total quantity of food needed may be determined. While this approach is not likely to be practical on an individual basis, it does give relief agencies, government agencies, and related institutions some guidelines to use in estimating food production needs, imports, and emergency food aid.

Excess Dietary Protein

Is it possible to eat too much protein? In the U.S., the amount of protein consumed is seldom a problem as it can be in other parts of the world. However, there is some concern that Americans may be consuming too much protein. Most studies suggest that Americans as a nation consumed twice the required levels needed. The question must then be posed: can this apply a detrimental influence upon human health? While this area is still debated, some causes for concern have been suggested. These causes include increased renal stress leading to impaired function; bone demineralization; an increased incidence of colon cancer due to the type of bacteria present in a high nitrogen environment; and obesity, particularly in this country where high protein foods are often high in fat. Consuming individual amino acid supplements has also been suggested to have detrimental possibilities. Because of shared amino acid absorption transport systems, increased consumption of individual amino acids with a meal may reduce the absorption of other amino acids, potentially leading to imbalance. Supplements of individual amino acids, unless there is deficiency in a meal, should not be taken in conjunction with protein-rich meals.

Protein Undernutrition

Whether the issue is lack of total protein or poor protein quality, it is well known that *kwashiorkor* is the result. It is often difficult to separate out protein malnutrition from undernourishment of other nutritional factors. *Protein-energy malnutrition* (PEM) is the most prevalent form of undernutrition in the world. Not only is kwashiorkor a problem, but *marasmus* may occur, or a combination of both. Kwashiorkor is a disease resulting from the lack of dietary protein. Marasmus results from a lack of energy or calories (lack of food) and protein. In kwashiorkor, one may consume seemingly adequate energy, but without enough protein. In this disease, the subject becomes "pot-bellied" due to edema, has depigmented hair (red and white), easily pluckable hair, a moon face appearance, facial expressions that resemble agony, skin lesions, fatty liver, decreased antibodies and greater susceptibility to disease, and the victim does have some body fat.

Individuals suffering from marasmus are emaciated. This results from excessive muscle wasting. Also, there is minimal body fat present. Clinically, marasmus is most commonly observed in 6- to 18-month-old children who were not breast-fed or who were weaned onto poor diets. Even when adequate protein is present, their bodies will use it for energy, and thus symptoms close to kwashiorkor may appear in the individual suffering from marasmus. Marasmus victims display excessive crying, mostly due to hunger. Meanwhile, in kwashiorkor, individuals will experience increased pain. These individuals possess a decreased ability to cry due to impaired brain functions.

A protein-malnourished female will often give birth to small and/or premature infants that are underdeveloped neurologically as well as physically. Brain damage in the toddler stage can result even if the undernutrition does not occur until after birth. Undernutrition at practically any point in the life cycle will lessen resistance to illness and infection. Height and head size may be relatively low in a child or infant. A malnourished child shows little curiosity or eagerness to learn. Such children often have difficulty learning in school as they may have a shorter span of attention and possess an inability to concentrate. A malnourished adult is usually less physically active, may work at a slower pace, and often have poor general health. Also, malnourished individuals may suffer nutritionally from more than just a lack of protein and/or energy. They may have vitamin and/or mineral deficiencies superimposed upon lack of the macronutrients. Around half of the 5 billion world population suffers from undernutrition of some type.

INSIGHT: Causes of Global Protein Undernutrition

The causes may be debatable, but certain elements are common in areas where protein undernutrition and simple undernutrition are prevalent. It was once dogma that over population and inadequate food production were the primary cause of undernutrition. While these aspects contribute, there are other factors, such as greed of those in power or in control; unemployment; lack of productive resources, including natural resources; lack of available land, credit, and proper tools; and lack of technology in many areas. Also, there is a problem with the developed nations transferring their technology to those who could benefit from it. With debt and trade imbalance, cost of oil means more is spent to buy the commodity than a nation may get for a crop, etc. Cultural traditions make things worse many times. Women will often do heavy physical labor even when pregnant to help support the family. They will feed their husbands and older children first as well. Often the wife/mother will eat last, or many times an infant already weaned will get what is leftover.

Catastrophes and weather-related issues such as droughts may influence food supply. War and civil unrest are man's own creation of misery on earth. Declining ecology for agriculture production such as in the sub-Sahara region is an example. Many nations do not have adequate food reserves to get by in case of an emergency. There may be lack of economic incentives to farmers, who may not own their own land. Disease and parasites are a large factor and one that often may be ignored. When considering undernutrition, one must also look at the disease states of those afflicted. Many of them have parasites or infections (malaria, cholera, dysentery, etc.) which will increase nutritional requirement even more.

The U.S. is not without its own undernutrition problems. However, much of the problem is not likely to be related to protein issues. Undernutrition in the U.S. often traditionally has been restricted to economically poor African-Americans, southern Americans, immigrant workers, unemployed minorities and some of the elderly; however, it is now extending into other parts of the population. These include such diverse groups as youngsters, of whom 500,000 are believed to be malnourished. A group termed the "new poor," who are displaced farm families, blue collar laid-off workers, and the change of our economy to a more service economy has left those with manufacturing skills unable to compete. The elderly are at risk, and the incidence is likely to increase, given the aging population. Problems with lack of health insurance programs, rising costs of living, and inflation are problems that contribute. Unfortunately, one does not have to venture far from home to see the growing ranks of the homeless who are also often malnourished. Estimates of the homeless in the U.S. range from 3 to 5 million, which are staggering figures. More than half of the homeless are single mothers. Many of the homeless were once in mental institutions. Low-income women, many of whom are single with children, have undernutrition problems. Ethnic minorities, such as African-Americans and Hispanics are known to have a greater prevalence of malnutrition. The unifying factor, given this list, may best be described in terms of a lack of income with which to buy the nutrient-dense foods.

7

Water

For at least three reasons, an argument can be made that water is the most essential nutrient to humans. First, for an adult about 2 to 3 kg of water is needed daily to balance losses. This amount is substantially greater than requirements for all other essential nutrients. For example, the average daily need for water for an adult is about 40 to 50 times greater than protein needs and about 5000 times greater than need for vitamin C. Second, signs of water deficiency or *dehydration* would be apparent within the first day, while a complete lack of water influx may result in death in as few as 3 to 4 days. Therefore, a deficiency of water leads to the development of deficiency signs at a rate greater than other nutrients. And third, due to the fact that water is the medium of intracellular and extracellular fluids, dehydration or its opposite, overhydration, can not occur without affecting the metabolism of all other nutrients.

Properties of Water

The chemical and physical properties of water, such as its ability to function as a general solvent and its high specific heat, make it a well-suited medium for the human body. Water differs from the other macronutrients in that it is an inorganic molecule consisting of two atoms of hydrogen bonded to one atom of oxygen. The bonding nature is covalent; however the sharing of electrons is far from equal. Oxygen, having 8 protons within its nucleus vs. hydrogen's lone proton, is able to generate a greater electrical pulling force upon the shared electrons (Figure 7.1). This results in a partially positive charge associated with the hydrogen atoms and a partially negative charge associated with the oxygen atom. It is this arrangement that allows for the cohesiveness between water molecules. The hydrogen atoms of one water molecule are electrically attracted to the oxygen atom of nearby water molecules (Figure 7.2). In fact, in a solution containing pure water, individual water molecules can interact with up to four other water molecules in somewhat of a tetrahedral arrangement. This results in the formation of a water lattice. The association between water molecules decreases as temperature increases, or as its phase goes from solid to vapor. Water is solid below 0°C and vaporizes above 100°C. Water also has a relatively low thermal conductivity and, as mentioned above, a relatively high specific heat.

It is the dipolar nature of water molecules that allows for the solubility of many substances. In general, substances having ionic character, such as sodium chloride (Figure 7.3), or polar molecules possessing the ability to hydrogen bond (i.e., alcohols, ketones, and sugars) will demonstrate water solubility. However, larger molecules such as proteins will form colloidal suspension solutions consisting of particles between 1 to 100 nm. Furthermore, water provides a medium for the formation of emulsions. For example, homogenized milk contains an emulsion of fat globules, protein, and other solutes in aggregates with diameters ranging between 1 to 100 μm.

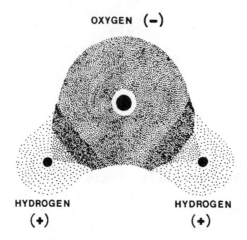

FIGURE 7.1
Water molecule with a partial negative charge associated with oxygen and partial positive charge associated with the hydrogen atoms.

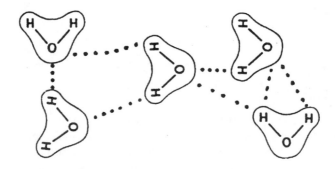

FIGURE 7.2
Hydrogen bonding between adjacent water molecules.

Distribution of Water in the Human Body

The human body is about 60% water by mass. Because adipose tissue is relatively void of water, while skeletal muscle is approximately 73% water, it is the skeletal muscle/fat ratio that is the primary factor in determining body water mass. As men typically have a greater skeletal muscle/fat ratio, they tend to have higher percentages of body water. Water is compartmentalized into the extracellular and intracellular fluids. About 55 to 60% of total body water in an adult is intracellular with the remainder being extracellular. The extracellular compartment is composed of interstitial (between cells) fluid, including the lymph and the fluid within connective tissue, the plasma; fluids within the intestinal tract lumen and joints; and the cerebral spinal fluid (Table 7.1). Collectively, the plasma and the interstitial fluid account for about 27% of the total body water mass. Blood plasma is about 90% water and 10% dissolved and suspended substances such as proteins, electrolytes, urea, and lipoproteins. The daily secretion of water-based intestinal juices is about 6 to 7 liters

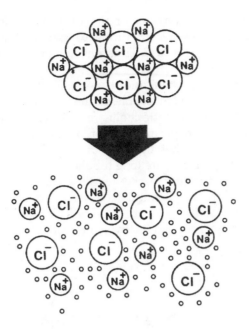

FIGURE 7.3
Ionization of sodium chloride into water (∘).

TABLE 7.1
Distribution of Body Water

Compartment	Approx % of Total Body Water[a]
Plasma	7
Interstitial fluid (including lymph)	20
Cartilage and connective tissue	8
Contents of lumen of GI tract	1
Cerebral spinal fluid	1
Bile	1
Intracellular fluid	60

[a] Approximate % of total body water in 70-kg man (42 l total).

for a typical adult. This includes saliva (1000 ml), gastric secretions (1500 ml), pancreatic secretions (1000 ml), bile (1000 ml), along with secretions from the small intestine (2000 ml) and large intestines (200 ml).

Sweat Water

Water provides the basis for *sweat*, which is a primary mechanism for removing excessive body heat. The core temperature of the human body on average is 37°C (98.6°F). In order for this temperature to remain constant, excessive heat generated through metabolic operations of deep organs or exercising muscle must be dissipated by either conduction, radiation, convection, or evaporation. Evaporation of sweat occurs continuously through-out the day and is particularly augmented during exercise. The evaporation of 1 g of water from the skin surface dissipates 0.58 kcal. Thus, one liter of water evaporation can remove about 580 kcal of heat.

Sweating is largely controlled autonomically and is initiated by stimulating the hypo-thalamus-preoptic area of the brain. Sweat glands are located in skin tissue throughout the body and are innervated by sympathetic cholinergic fibers. Sweat gland activity may also be stimulated by circulating epinephrine and norepinephrine. This becomes particularly important during exercise bouts when the circulating level of these chemicals increase.

Sweat glands, shown in Figure 7.4, are long tubular structures consisting of a deep sub-dermal coiled portion and a duct that reaches to skin surface. The deep coiled portion con-sists of epithelial cells which, when stimulated, secrete a primary sweat solution that is very similar to plasma in its sodium (142 mEq/l) and chloride (104 mEq/l) content. How-ever, the primary secretion will contain relatively little of the other plasma solutes, includ-ing proteins.

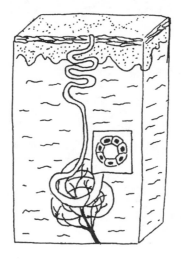

FIGURE 7.4
A sweat gland with underlying sympathetic innervation. Inset of absorptive cells along the tubule of a sweat gland.

As the primary solution flows through the duct it is modified in solute concentration. If the rate of sweating is slow, resulting in a slow rate of flow through the tubule, almost all of the sodium and chloride will be reabsorbed as well as a large portion of the water. Water reabsorption is primarily attributed to the osmotic gradient developed by the reabsorption of sodium and chloride. The reabsorption of water leads to the concentration of the other components of sweat, such as lactic acid, urea, and potassium.

As sweat rate is increased, the transit time through the duct is decreased and so is the reabsorption of sodium, chloride, and water as well. When sweat release is strongly stim-ulated and copious amounts of primary secretion flow through the duct, only about half of the sodium and chloride along with minimal amounts of water are reabsorbed. This results in a final concentration of sodium and chloride of about half of plasma levels.

Urinary Water

Water also provides the basis of urine, which serves as the primary route of excretion of metabolic waste and regulation of the composition of the extracellular fluid. Each human kidney contains about 1,000,000 nephrons, as described in Chapter 1. Collectively, they generate approximately 1 to 2 liters of urine daily. Urine is a composite of water, electrolytes, urea, creatinine, and trace amounts of glucose, amino acids, and proteins.

At rest the kidneys receive approximately 20% of the left ventricular cardiac output or about 1 l/min. In nephrons, water and plasma solutes having a size smaller than about 3 to 7 nm in diameter are filtered into Bowman's capsule under a glomerular capillary pressure which is about 3 times greater than capillaries of other tissue. On a daily basis, about 180 liters of renal filtrate or *ultrafiltrate* is produced. At this point ultrafiltrate has many compositional similarities to plasma. However, it will lack plasma proteins and lipoproteins as well as platelets and blood cells. As ultrafiltrate flows through the tubule system its composition changes and its volume greatly decreases. In fact, reabsorptive operations reduce the filtered fluid volume by about 99%, or from 180 l to about 1 to 2 l.

The first aspect of the renal tubule system, the *proximal convoluted tubule* (PCT), is designed for massive reabsorptive operations. The epithelial cells lining the tubule are endowed with microvilli, which are heavily studded with transport proteins and channels. PCT epithelial cells also have a rich complement of mitochondria, which provide ATP for the extensive active transport operations associated with reabsorption. Glucose and amino acids are completely reabsorbed in the PCT along with much of the electrolytes and water.

Water reabsorption along the length of the nephron tubule system occurs entirely by osmotic diffusion. Water largely moves through relatively loose tight junctions between PCT epithelial cells to reenter the extracellular fluid. This allows a lot of osmotic water reabsorption to occur concomitant to the large reabsorption of ultrafiltrate solutes in the PCT. However, the tight junctions in the ensuing *loop of Henle* and *distal tubule* are more tight and therefore less permeable to water. Thus, water reabsorption in the later aspects of the tubule system takes place mostly by moving through epithelial cells instead of between them. The reabsorption of filtered water attributable to the varying segments of the tubule system is as follows: PCT, 65%; loop of Henle, 15%; and the distal tubule and collecting ducts about 10% each.

The descending thin loop of Henle begins relatively permeable to water; however, the ascending portion is relatively impermeable to water. The distal tubule is also water impermeable. The thick loop of Henle participates in active transport of about three quarters of the remaining sodium and chloride in the tubular fluid to the extracellular fluid. As water is relatively impermeable in this segment, urine becomes diluted. As the tubular fluid moves into the first segment of the distal tubule, more sodium and chloride are removed by active transport operations. This further dilutes urinary fluid, with the exception of urea which too is impermeable in the latter segments of the tubule system. In the later aspect of the distal tubule and the cortical collecting duct, sodium removal is regulated by aldosterone while water reabsorption is regulated by *antidiuretic hormone* (ADH).

ADH is the hormone that dictates the excretion of either dilute or concentrated urine based upon the osmolality of the extracellular fluid. ADH or vasopressin is a peptide consisting of nine amino acids that is secreted by the posterior pituitary gland. The presence of even minute quantities of ADH in the plasma results in marked diuresis or decreased water excretion by the kidneys. If ADH is not present in the plasma, the distal tubule and the collecting duct remain relatively impermeable to water. Thus, the urine would contain a significant amount of water and be very dilute. Contrarily, the presence of ADH evokes structural changes in the epithelial cell plasma membranes in the distal tubule and collecting duct. These changes produce channels which allow water to flow osmotically from the tubule lumen into the epithelial cells.

The release of ADH from the posterior pituitary gland is regulated by specialized neurons called osmoreceptors in the hypothalamus. For example, if a concentrated electrolyte solution is injected into hypothalmic vasculature, ADH neurons in the supraoptic and paraventricular nuclei carry impulses to the posterior pituitary, evoking the release of ADH. Contrarily, injection of a dilute electrolyte solution into an artery serving the hypothalamus ultimately results in an inhibition of ADH release. Normally functioning kidneys can adjust the concentration of urine osmolality from 40 to 1400 mosmol/l, depending on the water status of the human body. The highest solute concentration of urine is limited by the minimum urinary water necessary to excrete nitrogenous waste (principally urea), sulfates, phosphates, and other electrolytes. As mentioned, the maximal concentration is about 1400 mosmol/l for adults and 700 mosmol/l for infants.

Water Balance

No other nutrient experiences as much flux (in/out) on a daily basis as water. Daily water loss from the human body for a nonexercising adult is about 4% of their body mass. This loss must be balanced by water ingestion or infusion to avoid the development of deficiency. The percentage of body water lost daily is approximately 15% of total body weight for infants. Furthermore, unlike all other essential nutrients, water does not have an appreciable storage in the human body. For instance, a reduction in extracellular water content is not buffered by a mobilization of water from some inert storage site. In reality, increased osmolality of the extracellular fluid evokes an osmotic pull on intracellular water. Continuation of extracellular water loss will dehydrate cells. Thus, even slight inadequacy of water supply can result in alterations of physiological function.

Water loss from the human body occurs primarily by the following routes: sweat, excretion of urine and feces, and exhalation of air humidified by the lungs. Generally about 1400 ml of water is lost daily as urine. This quantity will increase relative to water ingestion and decrease relative to increased losses by other means. Urinary water loss is strongly influenced by ADH as discussed above, allowing for urine to be very concentrated or very dilute. However, in order to remove potentially deleterious nitrogenous waste molecules such as urea, obligatory water loss is about 400 to 600 ml/d.

About 200 ml of water is lost daily within feces, while about 600 ml of water is lost in both mild sweating and exhalation of humidified air. Because mild daily sweating or perspiration and the exhalation of air humidified by the lungs generally goes unnoticed they, and other minor water-loss mechanisms such as lacrimal secretions of the eyes, are often referred to as *insensible* losses. Mild sweating is often separated from activity-induced sweat, which has a higher mineral content and is visually obvious. The amount of water loss by mild sweating is related to body surface area. On average this process allows a continual removal of excessive body heat totally about 250 to 400 kcal/d.

Sweating becomes a significant route of water loss during athletic training or competition or for individuals in warmer climates. Furthermore, over a span of a few weeks a person can acclimate to increase the sweat rate from about 700 to 2000 ml/h. The increased production of sweat is attributable to increased capabilities of sweat glands. In addition, the sweat produced will be much more dilute than in an unacclimated individual.

Cumulative water output must be balanced by water made available to the body in order to prevent dehydration. Water is made available primarily by oral ingestion. Approximately two thirds enters as pure water or other water-based fluids, while the remaining third is consumed as part of food or produced metabolically. Several foods are excellent sources of water due to their high water content. For instance, many fruits and vegetables are 85 to 95% water by mass (Table 7.2).

TABLE 7.2
Water Content of Various Foods[a]

Food	Approx Water (%)
Tomato	95
Lettuce	95
Cabbage	92
Beer	90
Orange	87
Apple juice	87
Milk	87
Potato	78
Banana	75
Chicken	70
Bread, white	35
Jam	28
Honey	20
Butter	16
Rice	12
Shortening	0

[a] Approximate % of total weight.

The metabolic generation of water accounts for about 200 to 300 ml of water daily. The complete oxidation of fuel substrates results in the production of water. For instance, the oxidation of 1 mole of glucose generates 6 moles of water.

$$C_6H_{12}O_6 + 6\,O_2 \longrightarrow 6\,CO_2 + 6\,H_2O$$

Water requirements are based upon replenishing water lost by the processes named above. It is often difficult to accurately estimate water losses as approximately half is lost by insensible routes (mild sweating and humidification of breath). General recommendations for water consumption for adults is 1 ml/kcal (1.5 ml/kcal for infants and children) of energy expenditure under average environmental conditions. Recommendations can be increased to 1.5 ml/kcal to cover variations in activity level, sweating, and renal solute load. Water requirements are augmented during pregnancy and lactation. The expanded extracellular fluid space, the needs of the fetus, and the amniotic fluid increase water requirements by about 30 ml/d. Human breast milk is about 87% water. Since the average milk secretion is 750 ml/d for the first 6 months, the increased water need would approximate 600 to 700 ml/d.

The perceived need for water is commonly called *thirst*. Thirst is controlled by the hypothalamus. There is a direct correlation between plasma osmolality and the intensity of thirst. This also means that an individual must be slightly dehydrated prior to the initiation of thirst. Reductions in extracellular fluid volume also evoke thirst, independent of plasma osmolality. For example, a hemorrhage and subsequent reduction in extracellular fluid volume will result in thirst without changes in plasma osmolality. The effect of a reduced extracellular fluid volume upon thirst is mediated in part by the renin–angiotensin mechanism. Renin secretion is increased by hypovolumenia and subsequently results in an increase in angiotensin II. Angiotensin II acts on a specialized region in the diencephalon to stimulate neural activity associated with thirst.

Water Deficiency (Dehydration) and Intoxification

In extreme situations, failure to ingest or infuse water can result in death within several days. Mild or early dehydration can result in significant alterations in physiological operation. Perhaps those most affected by early dehydration would be training or competing athletes. A loss of water approximating 2% of body weight as water can result in significant reduction in athletic ability. If dehydration continues, allowing a loss of approximately 5% in body weight as water, cramping and heat exhaustion can result. Furthermore, a reduction in body water approximating 7 to 10% of body weight as water can result in hallucinations and the development of heat stroke. Coma, shock, and death may soon follow.

Factors that might expedite the development of critical dehydration include severe protracted diarrhea and/or sodium deficiency. Severe dehydration causes a shift in fluid from intracellular and interstitial fluids to the vascular compartment. Eventually, though, the vascular volume is reduced to a critical level and results in the reduction in venous return to the heart and ultimately a diminished cardiac output and reduced blood pressure. Tissue perfusion is reduced and organs such as the brain starve for oxygen and nutrients. Furthermore, dehydration reduces the ability to remove excessive heat in sweat, leaving an individual prone to hyperthermia and heat stroke.

Excessive water is eliminated as urine, a process regulated primarily by antidiuretic hormone (ADH) and influenced by the urinary excretion of other substances. For most individuals without renal or endocrine considerations, this poses minimal threat unless voluntary ingestion or infusion is extreme.

8

Vitamins

It is legend that the term *vitamine* was coined in the early 1900s when a biochemist named Casimir Funk described a vital amine (nitrogen)-containing component of food. Subsequently newly discovered food-derived substances purported to be vital to human operation were also called vitamines. However as scientists observed that many of these substances did not contain nitrogen, the "e" was dropped from "vitamine," converting it to the more familiar term *vitamin*.

In order for a substance to be recognized as a vitamin it must be organic and be an essential player in at least one necessary chemical reaction or process in the human body. Also, a vitamin cannot be made in the human body, either at all, or in sufficient quantities to meet individual needs. Later discussion will include two vitamins, niacin and vitamin D, that can be made in the human body and two others, vitamin K and biotin, that can be made by bacteria inhabiting the large intestine. Vitamins are noncaloric substances and are required in relatively small amounts — micrograms to milligram quantities. The basis for the recommendations for vitamin intake in the U.S., the RDAs, was discussed in more detail in Chapter 2.

Water Solubility

As water is the principal component of the human body, which includes the blood (transport), and it is the basis of digestive juices (absorption) and the urine (primary metabolic excretion route), the vitamins are broadly classified based upon their water solubility (Table 8.1). Many general statements can be made about the water-soluble and fat-soluble vitamins with regard to digestion and absorption, transport from the intestines, plasma circulatory mechanisms, storage, and the timing to onset of deficiency and toxicity. The fat-soluble vitamins will be discussed first.

TABLE 8.1
Vitamins

Water-Soluble Vitamins	Fat-Soluble Vitamins
Vitamin C	Vitamin A
Thiamin	Vitamin D
Riboflavin	Vitamin E
Vitamin B_6	Vitamin K
Vitamin B_{12}	
Folate	
Biotin	
Niacin	
Pantothenic acid	

Fat-Soluble Vitamins

The fat-soluble vitamins are very dependent upon the processes of normal lipid digestion and absorption, such as the presence of bile and the incorporation into chylomicrons in the intestinal mucosa. Any situation whereby there is decreased bile production and/or delivery to the small intestine would greatly decrease fat-soluble vitamin digestion and absorption. Fat-soluble vitamins are less likely to be removed by urinary excretion as they are typically transported aboard lipoproteins or in association with a transport protein or complex. In general, it requires relatively longer periods of time to bring about deficiency. The most outstanding exception is vitamin K.

Vitamin A

First identified in 1914 and its structure elucidated in 1930, vitamin A or *preformed vitamin A* (provitamin A) has three primary forms. Retinol is an alcohol, retinal is an aldehyde form, and retinoic acid (acid form) is derived from retinal. Vitamin A consists of a ring structure attached to a hydrocarbon tail that terminates with a variable chemical group, either a alcohol, aldehyde, or acid. The nature of the double bonds in the hydrocarbon tail can vary between *cis* and *trans* configurations. For instance retinol, which is regarded as the vitamin A parent compound is *all-trans* retinol. The form of vitamin A vital to vision is 11-*cis* retinal, while 13-*cis* retinoic acid is used to treat cystic acne.

Previtamin A refers to cartotenoid structures which include the carotenes and xanthophylls. Carotenes and xanthophylls differ slightly in that true carotenes are purely hydrocarbon molecules (i.e., lyopene, α-carotene, β-carotene, γ-carotene), the xanthophylls (i.e., lutein, capsanthin, cryptoxanthin, zeaxanthin, astaxanthin) contain oxygen in the form of a hydroxyl, methoxyl, carboxyl, keto, and epoxy groups. Carotenoids have the potential to be converted into retinol within human cells. The most obvious cartenoid in foods is β-carotene; however, other forms such as α-carotene and γ-carotene are nutritionally significant as well. The structures of vitamin A compounds as well as various carotenoids are presented in Figures 8.1 and 8.2.

α-Carotene and β-carotene differ in the location of a double bond in a ring, while one of what would be a ring of γ-carotene rings is actually open (Figure 8.2). These differences will influence the carotene's efficiency of conversion to vitamin A. There are hundreds of carotenoids found in nature; however, only about 50 or so demonstrate the ability to be converted to vitamin A. Of these carotenoids, only a half dozen or so are found in the diet in appreciable amounts. For instance, β-carotene is perhaps the most potent in its ability to be converted to vitamin A, while α-cartotene, γ-carotene, and cryptoxanthin have about 40 to 60% of the potency of β-carotene. Conversely, other carotenoids such as xanthophyll, zeaxanthin, and lycopene have virtually no vitamin A potency.

Dietary Sources of Vitamin A and Carotenoids

All-trans retinols are generally found in foods esterified to fatty acids. Retinyl palmitate is among the most abundant forms. Retinyl esters are found only in certain animal products such as liver, fish liver oils, egg yolks, milk, and butter. Vitamin A-fortified milk and milk products are among the major contributors of vitamin A in certain countries. Vitamin A in the previtamin A-carotenoid form is found in plant sources, mainly in orange and dark green vegetables and some fruits such as squash, carrots, spinach, broccoli, papaya, sweet

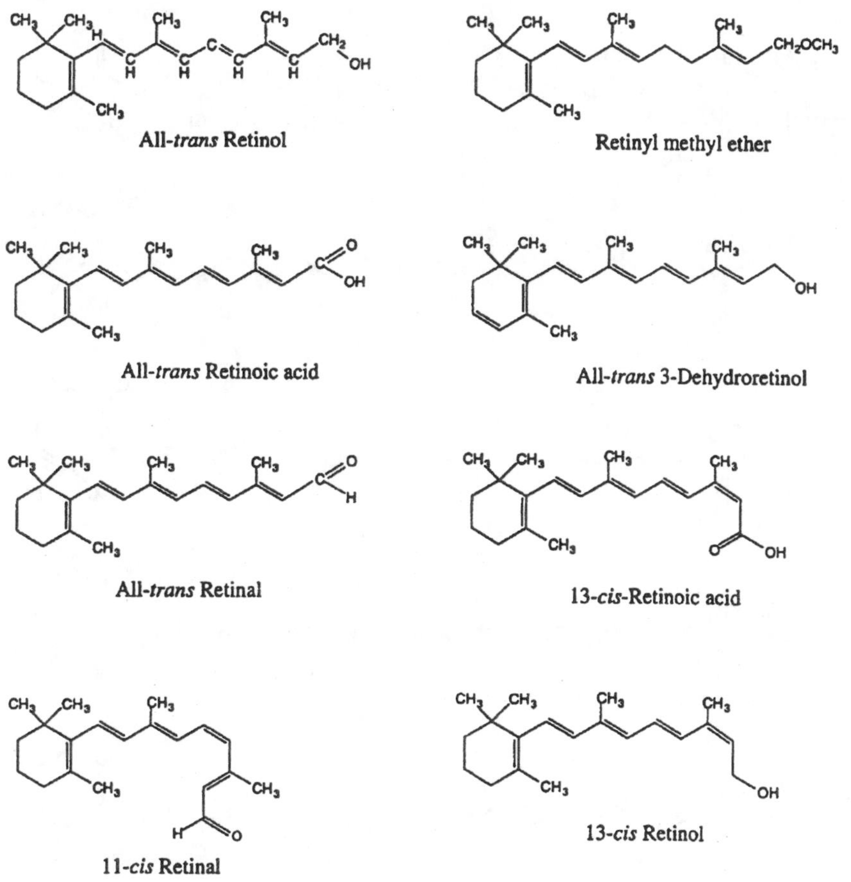

FIGURE 8.1
Structures of vitamin A compounds.

potatoes, pumpkin, cantalope, and apricots. Food sources of vitamin A are presented in Table 8.2.

Digestion and Absorption of Vitamin A and Carotenoids

Retinyl esters and carotenoids complexed with proteins must be liberated prior to absorption. This is accomplished mainly by pepsin and proteases in the small intestine. Removal of fatty acids of retinyl esters is accomplished by pancreatic lipase, and cholesterol esterase as well as other intestinal esterases rather than having a specific esterase. Free carotenoids and retinols integrate into micelles and most likely traverse the enterocyte plasma membrane by passive diffusion. As much as 70 to 90% of the retinol is absorbed. Meanwhile, the efficiency of carotenoid absorption will vary tremendously and probably decreases as carotenoid concentration increases in the intestinal lumen. For example, the absorption of β-carotene may be 20 to 50%, while the absorption of other carotenoids may be as low as 3 to 10%. The intake of carotenoids in America is typically around 1 to 3 mg/d, while in other countries, wherein the inhabitants eat more fruits and vegetables, this amount is increased. Dietary fat is important for the digestion and absorption of both *pre* and *pro* vitamin A forms; however, the presence of bile salts may be even more critical for carotenoids.

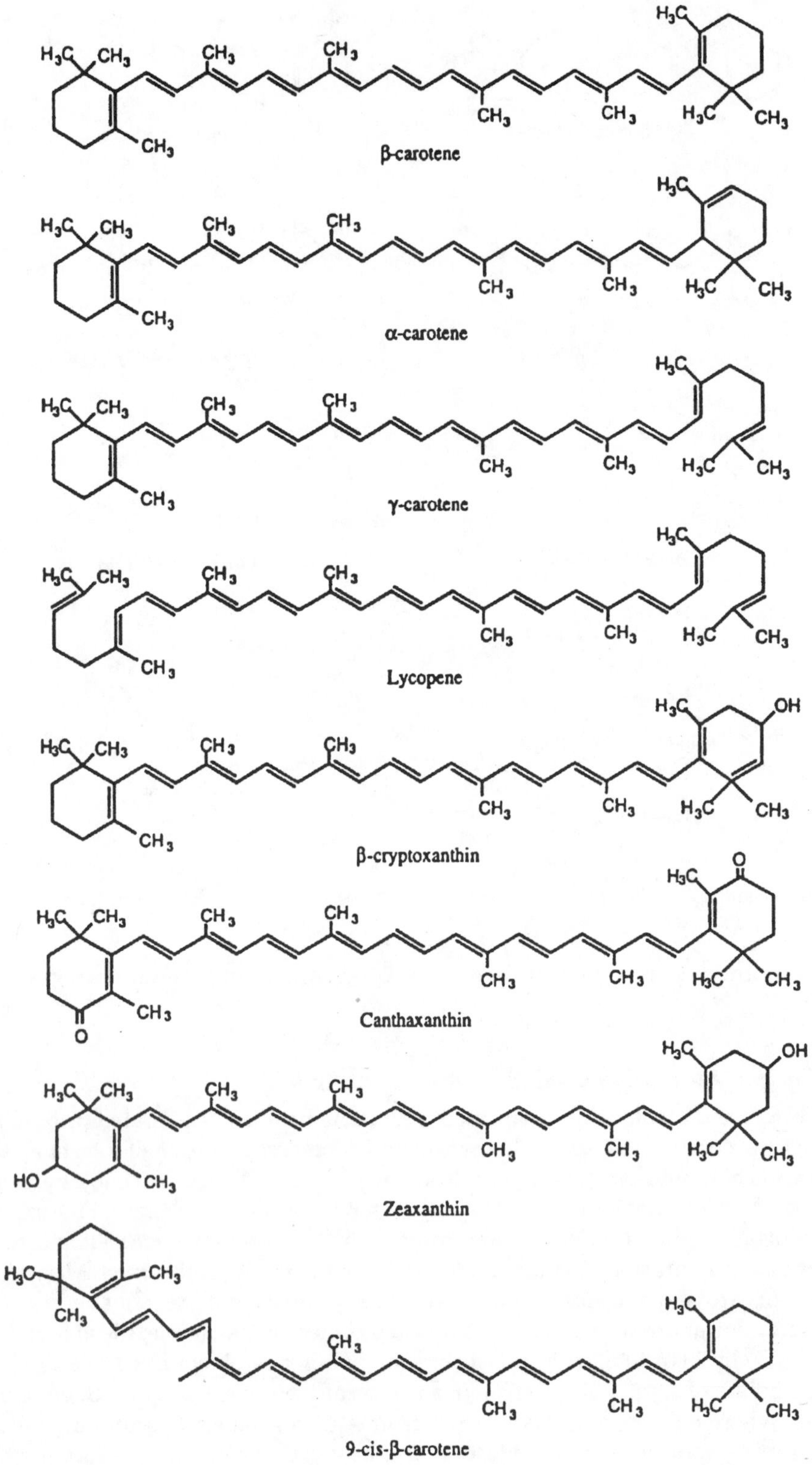

FIGURE 8.2
Structures of carotenoids having vitamin A activity.

TABLE 8.2
Vitamin A Content of Selected Foods

Food	Vitamin A (RE)
Vegetables	
Pumpkin, canned (2 c)	2,712
Sweet potato, canned (2 c)	1,935
Carrots, raw (2 c)	1,913
Spinach, cooked (2 c)	739
Broccoli, cooked (2 c)	109
Winter squash (2 c)	53
Green peppers (2 c)	40
Fruits	
Cantaloupe (3 whole)	430
Apricots, canned (2 c)	662
Nectarine (1)	101
Watermelon (1 c)	59
Peaches, canned (2 c)	188
Papaya (2 c)	78
Meats	
Liver (3 oz)	9,124
Salmon (3 oz)	53
Tuna (3 oz)	14
Eggs	
Egg (1)	95
Milk and milk products	
Milk, skim (1 c)	149
Milk, 2% (1 c)	139
Cheese, American (1 oz)	82
Cheese, Swiss (1 oz)	65
Fats	
Margarine, fortified (1 tsp)	46
Butter (1 tsp)	38

[a] RE = Retinol equivalents.

Within the enterocyte some of the β-carotene (*all-trans*) and other carotenoids can be converted to retinol by cleavage at the central double bond by *β-carotene 15,15′-dioxygenase*. In the case of β-carotene, enzymatic cleavage yields two molecules of retinal. The conversion of carotenoids to vitamin A depends on the activity of this enzyme which itself is dependent upon the structure of the carotenoid, as well as the efficiency of the enzymatic cleavage. The retinal that is formed can be converted to retinol by *retinaldehyde reductase*. This reaction requires NADH for its reducing equivalents. Futhermore, the central acting enzyme can also convert 9-*cis* β-carotene to a mixture of 9-*cis* and *all-trans* retinals.

Retinal formed in enterocytes can also associate with a protein called *cellular retinoid binding protein (CRBP)* type II and be reduced to retinol and then esterified to a long-chain fatty acid. Phosphatidylcholine (lecithin) is the primary provider of fatty acids while acyl CoA is the secondary provider.

Retinyl esters, retinol, and carotenoids (carotenes and xanthophylls) are packaged into chylomicrons, which are released from enterocytes and enter the lymphatic circulation. Because the long-chain fatty acids esterified to retinol are derived primarily from lecithin, the fatty acid composition of lymph retinyl esters is independent of the fatty acid composition of the associated meal. Retinyl palmitate usually accounts for about 50% of the retinyl esters, while retinyl stearate contributes about 20 to 30% and retinyl oleate and retinyl linoleate make relatively smaller contributions. Vitamin A and carotenoids are taken up primarily by hepatocytes as components of chylomicron remnants.

Plasma Transport

In the liver, vitamin A, as *all-trans* retinol, complexes with *retinol-binding protein (RBP)* forming, which circulates in the plasma. The synthesis of RBP by hepatocytes is regulated by vitamin A status. The normal serum retinol concentration is 45 to 65 mg/100 ml for adults. Other vitamin A forms such as retinoic acid, β-glucoronide, retinyl ester, and retinoyl β-glucuronide are also transported in the plasma, but in a much lower amount. The carotenoids circulate as components of lipoproteins with the principal ones being α-carotene, β-carotene, lycopene, cryptoxanthin lutein, and zeaxanthin. The carotenes appear to associate more with LDL, while the xanthophylls are found in both LDL and HDL. While the concentration and relative concentrations of different carotenoids varies with dietary intake, β-carotene typically represents 15 to 30% of plasma carotenoids.

Storage of Vitamin A and Cell Binding Proteins

Vitamin A is stored very well with greater than 90% being found in the liver and distributed between two liver cell types. Liver parenchyma cells (hepatocytes) contain mostly retinyl esters derived from chylomicron remnants. In addition, these cells also synthesize RBP. *Stellate* cells, which comprise 5 to 15% of total liver cells, are distinct from parenchyma cells, in that they are relatively small nonphagocytic fat-storing cells. As much as 80% of a healthy adult's vitamin A may be stored in lipid globules within these cells. Stellate cells are found associated with other tissue and can also store vitamin A, but to a much smaller extent than in the liver.

Carotenoids can be irreversibly converted to retinal. Retinal itself can be reversibly reduced to retinol or converted to a Schiff base of retinal (Figure 8.3). The conversion of retinal to retinol occurs in many tissues. Retinol can be reversibly converted to retinyl phosphate (minor pathway), retinyl esters, and retinyl β-glucuronide, as well as irreversibly to retinoic acid. Retinoic acid can be irreversibly converted to retinoyl coenzyme A (minor pathway) and retinoyl β-glucuronide or be irreversibly converted to inactive structures such as 5,6 epoxyretinoic acid, 4-hydroxy retinoic acid, 4-oxoretinoic acid, or other metabolites. In addition, vitamin A structures can undergo isomerization reactions to convert *trans* to *cis* configurations and vice versa.

Within cells, retinol, retinoic acid and retinal associate with CRBPs. As mentioned above, retinal binds with CRBP type II in enterocytes, where it is converted to retinol. Retinol in many other cells binds to CRBP, while in the interphotoreceptor space of the eye it binds to

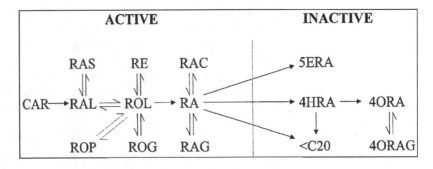

FIGURE 8.3

Metabolism of vitamin A: retinol (ROL); retinal (RAL); carotenoid (CAR); retinoic acid (RA); Schiff base of retinal (RAS); retinyl ester (RE); retinyl phosphate (ROP); retinoyl β-glucuronide (RAG); retinoyl coenzyme A (RAC); 4-hydroxy retinoic acid (4HRA); 4-oxo retinoic acid (4ORA); 4-oxo retinoyl β-glucuronide (4ORAG); oxidized metabolites <20C (<20C). (Adapted from Olson, J.A., Vitamin A, in *Present Knowledge in Nutrition*, 7th ed. © 1996 International Life Sciences Institute, Washington, D.C. With permission.)

interphotoreceptor (interstitial)-binding protein (IRBP). Retinal in the eye associates with *cellular retinal-binding protein (CRALBP)* and retinoic acid in several tissues binds to *cellular retinoic acid binding protein (CRABP)*. CRABP type II is present in many tissues of newborns.

Functions of Vitamin A and Carotenoids

The most recognizable function of vitamin A is its involvement with the eye and normal vision. After *holo*-RBP binds with specific receptors on retinal pigment epithelial cells of the eye, retinol enters the cells and is isomerized to 11-*cis* retinol. 11-*cis* Retinol is transported by IRBP to rod outer segments where it undergoes oxidative conversion to 11-*cis* retinal, which then associates with a specific lysine residue in the membrane protein *opsin*, forming *rhodopsin*, as depicted in Figure 8.4. When exposed to light, the 11-*cis* retinal component of rhodopsin isomerizes, causing a series of conformational changes in the protein. An intermediate form of changing rhodopsin, called metarhodopsin, interacts with the G-protein transducin. Guanosine diphosphate (GDP) is subsequently replaced on transducin with guanosine triphosphate (GTP), which activates phosphodiesterase which then hydrolyzes cGMP to GMP.

As cGMP is involved in maintaining rod sodium channels in an open position, the decrease in rod cell cGMP concentration results in a reduction in sodium flux through the channel, which allows for hyperpolarization of the membrane potential and the generation of an action potential. Neural impulses are then transmitted to the optic center of the brain. In the process of interacting with transducin, metarhodopsin is split to *all-trans* retinal and opsin, which can then form another complex with available 11-*cis* retinal.

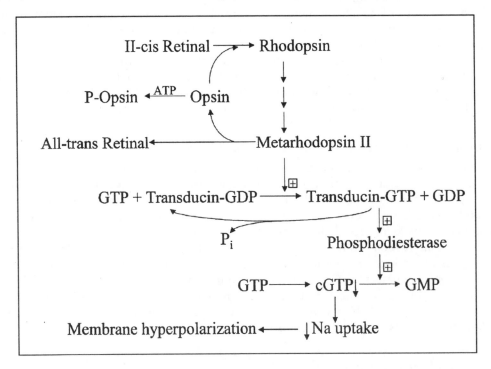

FIGURE 8.4

Involvement of vitamin A, as 11-*cis* retinal, in vision. Retinol (ROL); retinal (RAL); carotenoid (CAR); retinoic acid (RA); Schiff base of retinal (RAS); retinoyl coenzyme A (RAC); 4-hydroxy retinoic acid (4HRA); 4-oxo retinoic acid (4ORA); 4-oxo retinoyl β-glucuronide (4ORAG); oxidized metabolites <20C (<20C). (Adapted from Olson, J.A., Vitamin A, in *Present Knowledge in Nutrition*, 7th ed. © 1996 International Life Sciences Institute, Washington, D.C. With permission.)

Perhaps the second most-recognized function of vitamin A is its involvement in cell differentiation. There are two sets of nuclear retinoic acid receptors (RXR and RAR), both with subgroups designated α, β, γ. RXR specifically binds 9-*cis* retinoic acid, while RAR binds either 9-*cis* retinoic acid or *all-trans* retinoic acid. After binding vitamin A, both RAR and RXR form *dimer* complexes. The term dimer refers to an event whereby two molecular complexes specifically interact and proceed to have a purposeful function. RAR complexes with RXR, while RXR can also complex with either vitamin D receptor (VDR) or triiodothronine (T_3) receptor (TR). Typically these dimeric interactions lead to activation of specific gene expression. However, if RAR dimerizes with *jun* (a nuclear transcription factor), the result can be inhibitory upon gene expression. Typically *jun* complexes with *fos*, another transcription factor, and the result is stimulatory with regard to cell proliferation.

Retinoic acid may also form retinoylated proteins which approximate the size of nuclear receptors. Scientists speculate that this may also influence cell proliferative activities as well. In addition, retinoic acid may be involved in the expression of *hox* genes which appear to be involved in the sequential development of embyonic tissue.

Vitamin A may also be involved in the synthesis of certain glycoproteins which are key components of the plasma membrane. Glycoproteins are important for cell communication, cell recognition, cell aggregation, and cell adhesion properties. Interestingly, here the impact of vitamin A may not be at the nuclear level. It is speculated that retinyl phosphate is converted to retinyl phosphomannose, which in turn can transfer mannose to an accepting glycoprotein. This is another possible mechanism for the involvement of vitamin A in cell proliferation and differentiation.

Other functions of vitamin A include reproduction processes, bone development and maintenance, and immune system function. The mechanisms for vitamin A involvement in these operations still remain vague at present.

Carotenoids appear to function as antioxidants as they possess the ability to squelch free radical substances. For example, β-carotene and lycopene are able to interact with singlet oxygen radicals while β-carotene can also squelch peroxyl radicals. The ability of carotenoids to squelch free radicals is attributed to their double bond system.

Nutrient Relationships for Vitamin A and Carotenoids

Vitamin A appears to have significant relationships with vitamins E and K, protein, and the minerals zinc and iron. Vitamin E appears to be necessary for the cleavage of β-carotene to retinal, while a greater consumption of vitamin E (>10× RDA) may reduce β-carotene absorption and/or conversion to retinol in enterocytes. Meanwhile, excessive intake of vitamin A seems to interfere with vitamin K absorption.

Protein malnutrition can result in a reduced synthesis of RBPs. Meanwhile, a zinc deficiency can also reduce RBP production as well as reduce the mobilization of retinyl esters from storage in hepatocytes. On the other hand, vitamin A also seems to be involved in iron metabolism, since a deficiency results in a microcytic anemia characteristic of iron deficiency. It is unclear whether vitamin A is influencing iron metabolism, storage, or key differentiation steps in red blood cell formation.

Excretion of Vitamin A and Carotenoids

Oxidized products of vitamin A are conjugated to glucuronide and excreted as a component of bile. This accounts for about 70% of vitamin A losses. Carotenoid metabolites are also added to bile for excretion. The remaining 30% of vitamin A metabolites are voided in the urine.

Recommended Levels of Vitamin A Intake

The 1989 RDA stated that vitamin A recommended levels were 800 µg Retinol Equivalents (RE) for an adult woman and 1000 µg or 1 mg RE for an adult man. In light of significant impact of vitamin A upon developing embryonic and fetal tissue, recommendations for a woman are not increased during pregnancy. However, the RDA is elevated during lactation. The recommendations are listed as RE with respect to the conversion of carotenoids to vitamin A. Here 1 RE is defined as 1 µg of retinol or 6 µg of β-carotene.

Deficiency

Vitamin A deficiency is perhaps the leading cause of nonaccidental blindness in children worldwide. It has been estimated that as many as one half million school-aged children go blind each year due to vitamin A deficiency. Common signs of deficiency include night blindness and xerophthalmia. Bitot's spots on the eyes of young children are used as a diagnostic indicator. Bitot's spots appear as foamy, whitish accumulations in the conjuntiva of the eye.

Toxicity

At doses approximating ten times the RDA (~10 g/d), signs of hypervitaminosis including decreased appetite, dry, itchy, flaky skin, headache, hair loss, bone and muscle pain, ataxia, nausea, vomiting, dry mouth, and eye irritation and conjunctivitis may develop. Reabsorption of a fetus, abortion, and the development of birth defects are the most serious side effects of hypervitaminosis. At higher intakes, yet not enough to cause physical deformities, learning disabilities in progeny have been observed. Serum retinol levels may be augmented fourfold (>200 µg/100 ml) as more and more retinol is incorporated into lipoproteins. The delivery of retinol to peripheral tissue in lipoproteins, and not as a RBP complex, has been suggested to be a factor in the development of toxicity.

11-*cis* Retinoic acid (isotretinoin, accutane) is the vitamin A form used to treat severe cystic acne. Accutane is taken orally, typically at dosages between 0.5 to 1.0 mg/kg/d with a maximum of 2 mg/kg/d. The dosage is split and taken twice daily with food for 15 to 20 weeks with 2-month intermissions between 20-week treatments. The side effects are similar to those mentioned above and clinical signs include proteinuria, hematuria, hyperuricemia, hypertriglyceridemia, and hyperglycemia. Because of the high risk of physical abnormalities associated with vitamin A toxicity, women of child-bearing years utilizing accutane should ensure proper contraception. Conversely, there does not appear to be significant concern of carotenoid toxicity.

Vitamin D

Although long known for its fundamental role in calcium and phosphorus metabolism, vitamin D is now recognized to be involved in numerous aspects of human physiology. Vitamin D has also been regarded as a having questionable vitamin status for two reasons. First, vitamin D can be synthesized in the human body in adequate quantity, provided exposure to sunlight and associated organ (skin, liver, and kidney) function; and second, it functions more as a hormone, as its activity is dependent upon vitamin D first interacting with a receptor.

The chemical structures for vitamin D were determined in the 1930s. Vitamin D_2 (ergocalciferol) was produced via ultraviolet irradiation of ergosterol. Vitamin D_3 (cholecalciferol)

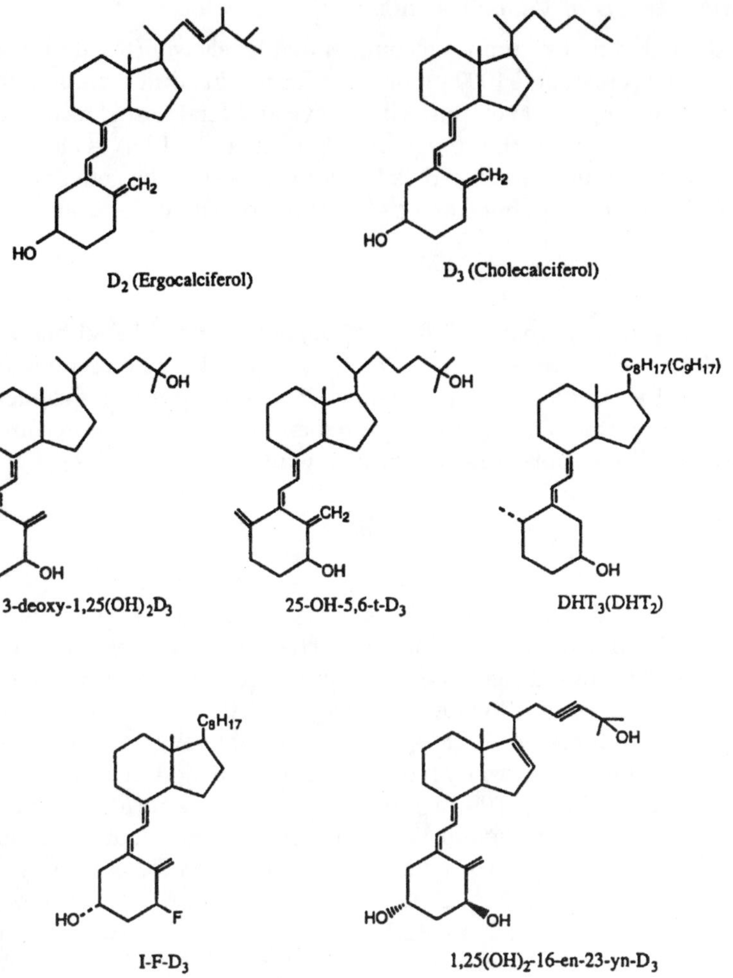

FIGURE 8.5
Compounds with varying vitamin D activity.

was produced by irradiating 7-dehydrocholesterol. Figure 8.5 shows the molecular structures of these vitamin D-related molecules. While 7-dehydrocholesterol and ergosterol carry the 4-ring structure that is characteristic of a steroid, vitamin D_2 and D_3 are actually secosteroids as one of their rings is broken. Both of these structures will be referred to as vitamin D.

Sources

In humans, as in most higher mammals, vitamin D_3 is created photochemically as ultraviolet light converts a precursor sterol 7-dehydrocholesterol to cholecalciferol. This reaction takes place as sebaceous oil glands secrete 7-dehydrocholesterol onto the skin surface. Cholecalciferol can then be reabsorbed to varying depths within the skin. Double bonds present at the 5th and 7th carbons in the B-ring structure are necessary for this conversion, which in essence opens the B-ring. As long as humans receive adequate exposure to sunlight, it is questionable as to whether dietary vitamin D is needed. However, because adequate exposure to sunlight is not possible in some geographic regions and seasons and in conjunction with recommendations to reduce exposure to sunlight to decrease the risk of skin cancer, dietary vitamin D is still deemed essential.

Dietary vitamin D is derived mostly from foods of animal origin. Eggs, liver, fatty fish, and butter are the best natural sources. The fortification of milk has greatly improved its vitamin D content, augmenting it from approximately 0.03 to 0.13 to 1.0 µg/100 g. Therefore, fortified milk and dairy products made from fortified milk are also among the better sources of vitamin D and certainly the major contributors to the human diet. Margarine has also been fortified to contain approximately 11.0 µg/100 g. A listing of foods and their vitamin D content is presented in Table 8.3.

TABLE 8.3
Vitamin D Content of Selected Foods

Food	Vitamin D (µg)
Milk	
Milk, all (1 c)	2.5
Fish and seafood	
Salmon (3 oz)	4.9
Tuna (3 oz)	3.4
Shrimp (3 oz)	3.2
Meats	
Beef liver (3 oz)	0.3
Eggs	
Egg (1)	0.7

Absorption and Transport of Vitamin D

Vitamin D becomes incorporated into micelles in the small intestine and enters mucosal enterocytes by passive diffusion. Approximately half of vitamin D is absorbed along the length of the small intestine, with the majority absorbed in the more distal aspects. Once within enterocytes, vitamin D is incorporated into chylomicrons which reach the systemic circulation via the lymphatic circulation. Some of the vitamin D is actually transferred from plasma chylomicrons to circulating vitamin D binding protein (DBP). Vitamin D carried aboard chylomicrons will be taken into hepatocytes as chylomicron remnants are removed. Meanwhile, the vitamin D transported by DBP can be delivered to extrahepatic tissue such as skeletal muscle and adipocytes. DBP also picks up cholecalciferol created in the skin. About 40% of circulating vitamin D is transported by chylomicrons and the remaining 60% is transported by DBP.

Metabolism

Vitamin D is in effect a prohomone. Its activity requires first its interaction with a *vitamin D receptor (VDR)*. Furthermore, the efficiency of binding to VDR is tremendously increased after two hydroxylations to its molecular form. Upon reaching the liver, either by chylomicron remnant removal or by transport by DBP, vitamin D is hydroxylated at carbon 25 by *25-hydroxylase*. Existing active vitamin D status is fundamental in the efficiency of this enzyme, in that, when vitamin D status is low, the efficiency increases. Vitamin D is converted to *25-hydroxycholecalciferol* or more simply $25\text{-}(OH)D_3$.

The enzyme *1α-hydroxylase (1α-OHase)* catalyzes the conversion of 25-(OH)D$_3$ to 1,25-(OH)$_2$D$_3$, the most potent metabolite of vitamin D. This enzyme is found in renal cells lining the proximal tubule. The activity of the enzyme is enhanced by PTH and insulin-like growth factor-I (IGF-I) and inhibited by calcium and phosphorus. 1α-OHase is part of the enzyme systems associated with cytochrome P$_{450}$. The general metabolism of vitamin D is presented in Figure 8.6 and the structural differences between vitamin D and 1,25-(OH)$_2$D$_3$ are presented in Figure 8.7.

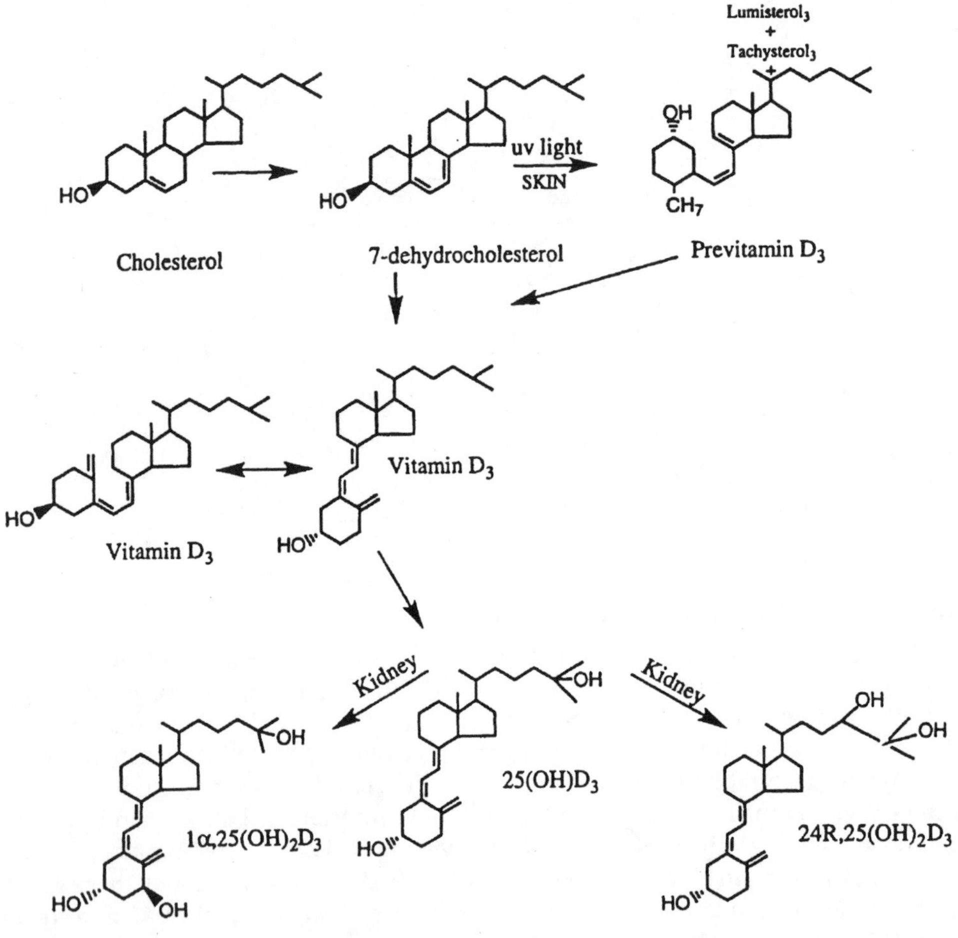

FIGURE 8.6
Synthesis of 1,2-dihydroxycholecalciferol, using cholesterol as the initial substrate.

Vitamin D Receptor and Functions

The vitamin D receptor (VDR) is a member of the superfamily of nuclear receptors that regulate gene expression. VDR was first cloned in the 1980s. The gene for VDR is located on chromosome 12 and it has characteristics similar to other nuclear receptor genes, both in structure of heteronuclear RNA and posttranscriptional processing. VDR is expressed in bone, intestines, and kidneys as well as in stomach, heart, brain, and other tissue.

The VDR exerts its influence once associated with a specific ligand, namely, 1,25-(OH)$_2$D$_3$. The VDR/1,25-(OH)$_2$D$_3$ complex controls specific gene expression by first

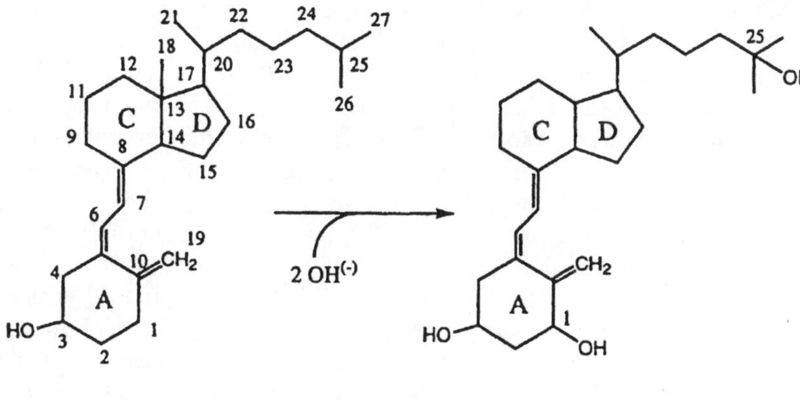

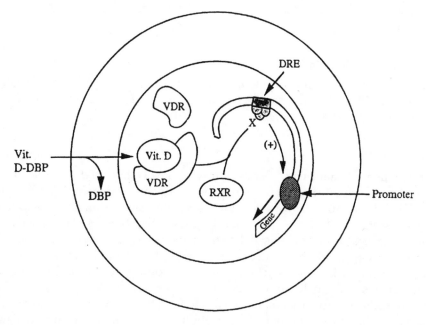

FIGURE 8.7
Chemical structure of vitamin D and 1,25-dihydroxycholecalciferol. Note the addition of the hydroxyl groups at carbons 1 and 25 in the active metabolite.

associating with vitamin A/retinoid X receptor (RXR) to form a dimer and then interacting with specific vitamin D responsive elements (VDREs) in target genes (Figure 8.8). VDREs are short sequences of DNA and are found in DNA regions associated with 1,25-$(OH)_2D_3$-activated genes such as osteocalcin, osteponin (expressed in osteoblasts), β_3 integrin (found in osteoclasts and macrophages), 24-OHase and calbindin-D (kidney).

FIGURE 8.8
Schematic representation of the interaction of vitamin D to VDR and subsequent genetic activity. The 1,25-$(OH)_2D_3$/VDR complex first forms a dimer with a vitamin A receptor (RXR) and then interacts with vitamin D-responsive elements.

Active vitamin D, via VDR association, affects calcium and phosphate homeostasis. Hypocalcemia results in the secretion of PTH, which increases 1α-OHase activity in the kidneys. In turn, this will increase the quantity of $1,25\text{-}(OH)_2D_3$. Vitamin D stimulates calcium and phosphate absorption from the gut, bone calcium and phosphate resorption, and renal calcium and phosphate reabsorption. The net effect of these activities is to increase circulatory levels of calcium. In the intestines, $VDR/1,25\text{-}(OH)_2D_3$ induces the expression of key proteins involved in calcium and phosphorus absorption. Calbindin and intracellular membrane calcium-binding protein (IMCBP), both calcium-binding proteins in the intestinal mucosa are synthesized in response to $VDR/1,25\text{-}(OH)_2D_3$. $VDR/1,25\text{-}(OH)_2D_3$ is believed to also increase the activity of brush border alkaline phosphatase, which increases the availability of phosphorus for absorption by cleaving phosphate ester bonds with other molecules. In addition, $VDR/1,25\text{-}(OH)_2D_3$ may modulate the quantity of brush border phosphate carriers. In bone tissue, $VDR/1,25\text{-}(OH)_2D_3$ is probably involved in the differentiation of stem cells into osteoclasts which mediate bone resorption and the mobilization of calcium and phosphate into the blood.

$VDR/1,25\text{-}(OH)_2D_3$ may regulate the differentiation of hair follicles. VDR "knockout" mice develop alopecia. The alopecia persists even after mice are provided a "rescue diet" consisting of relatively high amounts of lactose, calcium, and phosphate that correct PTH levels and normalize bone mineralization. Also, $VDR/1,25\text{-}(OH)_2D_3$, is likely to be involved in the differentiation of skin epidermal cells.

The $VDR/1,25\text{-}(OH)_2D_3$ complex plays a pivotal role in feedback regulation of the level of $1,25\text{-}(OH)_2D_3$ produced by renal tubular cells. Thus, $VDR/1,25\text{-}(OH)_2D_3$ is involved in the turnover of one of its own constituents. The 24-OHase enzyme is markedly enhanced by $1,25\text{-}(OH)_2D_3$ in a VDR-dependent manner. This occurs in both renal tissue and all vitamin D target tissue. Both $1,25\text{-}(OH)_2D_3$ and $25\text{-}(OH)D_3$ serve as substrates for 24-OHase. In the past it was believed that 24-hydroxylated D-metabolites were not functional; however, it may be that they are involved in some aspect of bone metabolism and/or bone formation via an uncharacterized receptor.

Recommended Levels of Intake

The RDA for vitamin D for infants over 6 months of age, children, and adolescents is $10\ \mu g$ daily. During adulthood, which is not associated with rapid growth, the vitamin D recommendations are reduced to $5\ \mu g$ daily.

Deficiency

In children, vitamin D deficiency results in a syndrome called *rickets* in which the associated characteristics result from a failure of growing bone to mineralize. As the epiphyseal cartilage of bone continues to grow, it is not properly replaced with matrix and hydroxyapatite. This results in a "bowing" of longer weight-bearing bones such as the femur, tibia, and fibula of the legs, dysformations of the knee region, and curvature of the spine. Vitamin D deficiency during adulthood reduces calcium and phosphate absorption. As bone turnover occurs, the matrix is preserved; however, bone progressively losses its mineralization. Loss of mineral resulting in decreased bone density is referred to as *osteomalacia*. Vitamin D deficiency, despite poor dietary intake, can be avoided by adequate exposure to sunlight.

People with lighter skin color require only about 10 to 15 minutes of summer sun exposure to make adequate amounts of vitamin D; while the necessary exposure time for people with darker skin color seems to increase relative to the degree of skin color. Also, the ability to make vitamin D appears to be stronger in youth and decreases relative to age.

Vitamin E

Like many other vitamins, vitamin E is not necessarily a single molecule, but a class of related molecules possessing similar activity. There are eight or so vitamin E molecules which can be subdivided into two major classes, *tocopherols* (α, β, γ, δ) and *tocotrienols* (α, β, γ, δ). Structurally the tocotrienols have unsaturated phytyl side chains, while tocopherol side chains are saturated. Meanwhile, the α, β, δ, and γ forms of tocopherols and tocotrienols are based upon the number and position of methyl groups attached to chromanol ring (Figure 8.9). The structures of α-tocopherol and α-tocotrienol are presented in Figure 8.10. All-rac α-tocopheryl acetate is used in the fortification of food.

Food Sources

The best sources of vitamin E include plant oils such as cottonseed, corn, sunflower, safflower, soybean and palm oils, and oil-derived products such as margarine, shortenings,

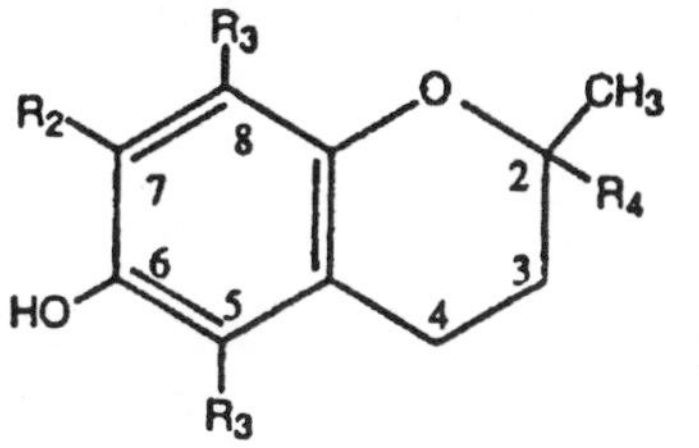

$R_1 R_2 R_3 = CH_3$ or H

$$R_4 = CH_2(CH_2CH_2\overset{\overset{\displaystyle CH_3}{|}}{C}HCH2)_3H \ \text{(Tocols)}$$

or

$$CH_2(CH_2CH = \overset{\overset{\displaystyle CH_3}{|}}{C}- CH_2)_3H \ \text{(Tocotrienols)}$$

α-Tocol or Tocotrienol have $R_1, R_2, R_3 = CH_3$

β-Tocol or Tocotrienol have $R_1, R_3 = CH_3$; $R = H$

γ-Tocol or Tocotrienol have $R_2, R_3 = CH_3$; $R_1 = H$

δ-Tocol or Tocotrienol have $R_3 = CH_3$; $R_1 R_2 = H$

ϵ-Tocol or Tocotrienol have $R_1 = CH_3$; $R_2, R_3 = H$

ζ-Tocol or Tocotrienol have $R_1, R_2 = CH_3$; $R_3 = H$

η-Tocol or Tocotrienol have $R_2 = CH_3$; $R_1, R_3 = H$

FIGURE 8.9
Structures of naturally occurring compounds having vitamin E activity.

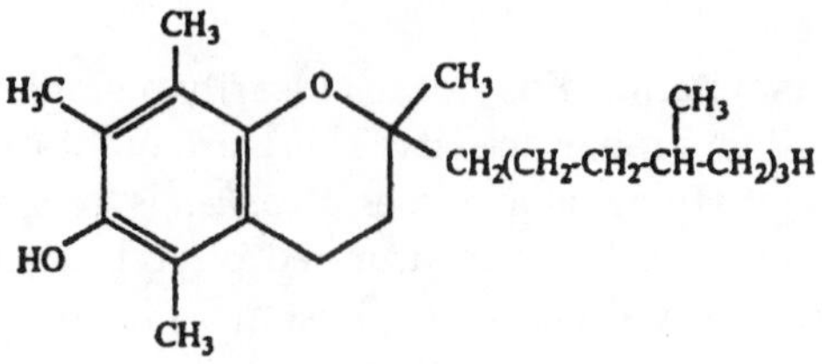

α-Tocopherol (5, 7, 8 Trimethyltocol)

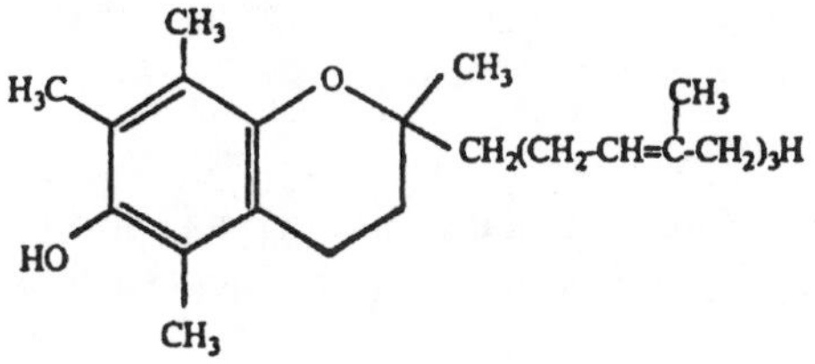

α-Tocotrienol (5, 7, 8 Trimethyltrienol)

FIGURE 8.10
Basic structures of vitamin E.

and mayonnaise. Wheat germ and its oil and nuts are also rich sources. Some fruits and vegetables, such as peaches and asparagus, are fair sources, while meats and fish contain appreciable amounts (Table 8.4). The tocopherols are more widely distributed in nature than the tocotrienols and therefore will be more nutritionally significant. α-Tocopherol is the most prevalent form as well as the most potent. For this reason, the RDA for vitamin E is given in α-tocopherol equivalents (α-TE), where 1 α-TE unit has the activity of 1 mg of α-tocopherol. The average adult intake of vitamin E approximates the RDA, which is 8 to 10 mg α-TE daily.

Absorption and Transport

The absorption efficiency of vitamin E is about 20 to 50%. However, as the dosage increases, the efficiency of absorption decreases. For example, at doses approximating 200 mg or higher, the efficiency of absorption falls to 10% and less. With respect to its lipid nature, vitamin E must first be solubilized into micelles within the lumen of the small intestine. Esterases produced by the pancreas and intestinal mucosa will digest vitamin E esters. Free vitamin E then appears to penetrate enterocytes via passive diffusion and is then incorporated into chylomicrons for export into the lymphatic circulation. Once chylomicrons reach the systemic circulation their triglyceride is progressively translocated into peripheral tissue by lipoprotein lipase; some vitamin E can enter the tissue as well. Furthermore, some vitamin E can translocate into circulating HDL. However, the majority of absorbed vitamin E remains in chylomicron remnants and is released in hepatocytes as remnants are removed and catabolized.

In liver cells, vitamin E binds to a cytosolic protein called *hepatic tocopherol transfer protein (HTTP)*, which preferentially interacts with the α-tocopherol. HTTP releases vitamin E into VLDL under construction in the endoplasmic reticulum or Golgi apparatus. Intuitively then, the predominant form of vitamin E in the plasma will be α-tocopherol. α-Tocopherol can remain in VLDL during lipolytic transformation to LDL and then circulate within LDL.

TABLE 8.4
Vitamin E Content of Selected Foods

Food	Vitamin E Content (mg α-TE)
Oils	
Oils (1 tbl)	1.7
Margarine (1 tbl)	1.8
Nuts and seeds	
Sunflower seeds (1 c)	70
Almonds (1 c)	20
Peanuts (1 c)	10
Cashews (1 c)	1.0
Vegetables	
Sweet potato (1 c)	0.5
Collard greens (1 c)	1.6
Asparagus (2 c)	5.4
Spinach, raw (1 c)	0.6
Grains	
Wheat germ (1 tbl)	—
Bread, whole wheat (1 slice)	0.3
Bread, white (1 slice)	—
Seafood	
Crab (3 oz)	0.9
Shrimp (3 oz)	0.7
Fish (3 oz)	1.6

Some vitamin E can also translocate into HDL. Typically, the plasma content of α-tocopherol is 5-20 µg/ml in adults. It is lower in children and infants, especially in preterm infants.

Storage and Excretion

While vitamin E is found in tissue throughout the body, such as the adrenals, heart, lungs, and brain, perhaps the most significant sites of storage are the liver, adipose tissue, skeletal muscle, and lipoproteins. The liver represents a more transient site of storage as turnover or rate of release is very rapid. Therefore, the hepatic vitamin E concentration does not increase significantly under normal conditions. This is largely attributed to the delivery of vitamin E to VLDL construction sites by HTTP. Adipose tissue, on the other hand, accumulates vitamin E slowly and the rate of turnover is also very slow. Vitamin E is found largely within the lipid droplet compartment of adipocytes or associated with membranes. While the concentration of vitamin E remains somewhat constant in most other tissue, concentration in adipose tissue increases linearly with dietary intake. Also, because of its large contribution to human mass, skeletal muscle is considered a significant store of vitamin E. Last, lipoproteins are the principal transport vehicle for vitamin E in the blood. During a fasting state, most of the α-tocopherol in males can be found in LDL and in HDL in women.

Vitamin E is excreted from the body by several mechanisms. First, the major route of α-tocopherol excretion is as a component of bile and subsequent incorporation into feces. Fecal vitamin E is also derived from enterocyte-secreted vitamin E and sloughed off enterocytes. Some vitamin E may be excreted from the body as a component of skin secretions and dermal exfoliation. Also, two metabolites of α-tocopherol have been identified in the urine. α-Tocopheronic acid and α-tocopheronolactone can both be conjugated to glucuronic acid and excreted in the urine (Figure 8.11). While these metabolites are typically present to a

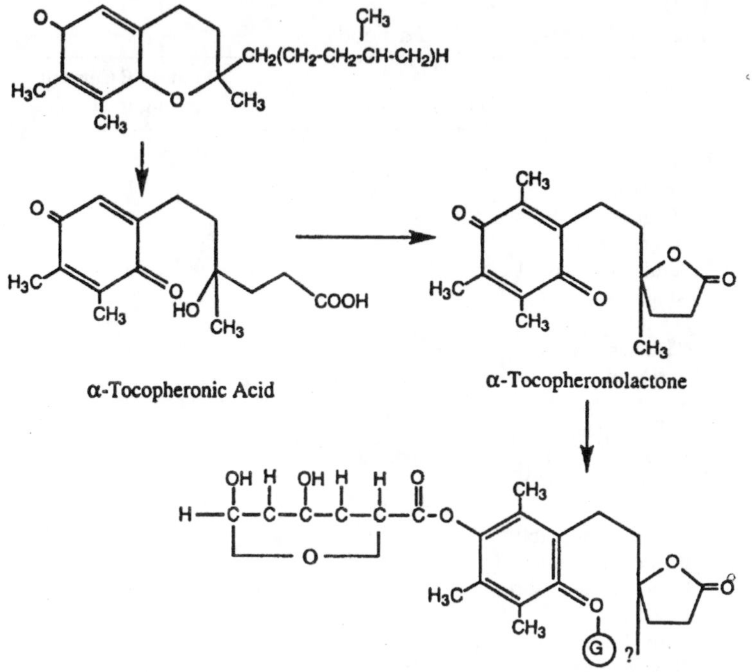

FIGURE 8.11
Excretory pathway for the tocopherols.

minimal degree, their concentration in the urine rises proportionately to increased vitamin E intake.

Function of Vitamin E

Without question, the predominant function of vitamin E is that of an antioxidant necessary for the maintenance of cellular membrane integrity. Vitamin E prevents the oxidation (peroxidation) of the unsaturated fatty acid component of membrane phospholipids. Furthermore, there are differences in the concentration of unsaturated fatty acids between the plasma membrane and membranes of the various organelles as well as between the same membranes in different tissue. For instance, the membranes of the mitocondria and endoplasmic reticulum contain a higher concentration of unsaturated fatty acids and are therefore at greater risk of free radical peroxidation. Membranes of tissue with a relatively higher risk of lipid peroxidation include lungs, brain, and red blood cells, due to a higher degree of unsaturation of fatty acids, metabolism, and oxygen presence.

Free radicals are either taken into the human body or created within cells. They are atoms or molecules with one or more unpaired electrons. This renders them unbalanced and highly reactive. Many free radicals are oxygen related, such as the *superoxide radical* (O_2^-), *peroxy radical* (O_2^{2-}), *hydroxyl radical* ($OH^\bullet$), and *peroxide* (H_2O_2). Within cells, free radicals can be generated by the reduction of oxygen, such as occurs in the endoplasmic reticulum, via the cytochrome P_{450} system, and mitochondria, via the electron transport chain. In the process of interacting with a free radical, tocopherol molecules are oxidized to form a tocopheroxyl radical, which can then be re-reduced to tocopherol by vitamin C, glutathione, and maybe ubiquinone.

Recommended Levels of Intake

The U.S. RDA for vitamin E is 10 mg of α-tocopherol equivalents for adult males and 8 mg of α-tocopherol equivalents for adult females. Pregnancy and lactation increase the recommendations to 10 and 12 mg, respectively, while the recommendation for infants is 3 mg and children 7 to 10 years of age is 7 mg.

As there is disparity in bioactivity between the different molecular forms of vitamin E, with α-tocopherol being the most potent, food vitamin E is listed in α-tocopherol equivalents (α-TE). β-tocopherol has only about 25 to 50% of the bioactivity of α-tocopherol while γ-tocopherol only has about 10 to 30%, and α-tocotrienol about 25 to 30% the bioactivity. Therefore, the α-TE units associated with a food is based on the amount of α-tocopherol, as well as the potential vitamin E activity contributions made by the other forms.

Deficiency

Because of the general availability of vitamin E in popular foods, deficiency related to inadequate intake is rare. However, conditions resulting in maldigestion of lipids, such as cystic fibrosis, celiac disease (nontropical sprue), and hepatic and biliary insufficiencies, can result in a compromised vitamin E status. Also, situations in which enterocyte lipoprotein production is impaired, such as *abetalipoproteinemia*, can also compromise vitamin E status.

The onset to deficiency signs and symptoms is very long in adults who, prior to the development of a maldigestion or malabsorption situation, had normal vitamin E stores. It may take a year or so before plasma vitamin E levels fall to critical levels associated with deficiency signs. Furthermore, it may take as long as a decade before neurological signs of deficiency appear. In infants and children experiencing hepatic or biliary insufficiencies the onset to deficiency is much more rapid as their stores have not been fully developed.

Manifestations of a vitamin E deficiency are assumed to have their origins in the degeneration of cellular membranes. The destruction of red blood cell membranes can result in hemolytic anemia. Degeneration of neuronal and muscular membranes may result in cerebellar ataxia and muscular weakness. Retinal degeneration has also been reported.

Toxicity

Relative to the fat-soluble vitamins discussed above, vitamin E is relatively nontoxic. In fact, vitamin E is recognized as one of the least toxic of all the vitamins. Intakes as high as 500 to 800 mg of α-TE for several months to years have not resulted in significant effects. However, gram doses may result in fatigue, muscle weakness, and gastrointestinal distress. Infants, especially preterm infants may be more sensitive to relatively higher doses of vitamin E.

While toxic effects of supplementing vitamin E are not a large concern, it should be understood that it may impact the absorption and function of other fat-soluble vitamins. For instance, gram doses of vitamin E appear to hinder vitamin K absorption. Furthermore, gram doses of vitamin E may impede the involvement of vitamin K in blood clotting while also increasing the effect of oral coumarin anticoagulent drugs. The involvement of vitamin D in bone mineralization may be altered by excessive vitamin E intake, while the absorption of β-carotene as well as its conversion to vitamin A may be hindered as well.

Vitamin K

First recognized in the 1930s, vitamin K is a group of naturally occurring or synthetically created 2-methyl-1,4-naphthoquinones with a hydrophobic substitution at the number 3 position of the structure (Figure 8.12). The form of vitamin K naturally occurring in green plants is *phylloquinone*, which has a phytyl group at the number 3 position. Bacteria produce a number of forms of vitamin K called *menaquinones*, which have an unsaturated multiprenyl group at the number 3 position. The most common menaquinones have 6 to 10 isoprenoid groups which are abbreviated MK6 to MK10. *Menadione* is the synthetic version of vitamin K, which is primarily used in animal feeds.

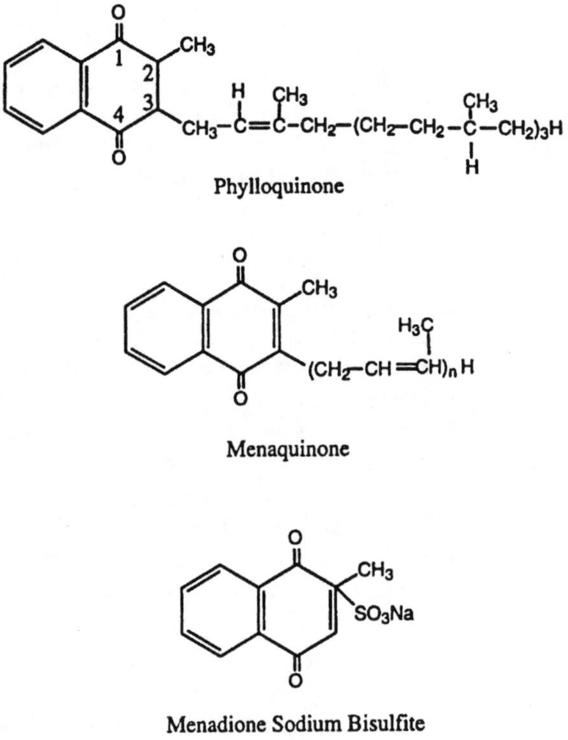

Phylloquinone

Menaquinone

Menadione Sodium Bisulfite

FIGURE 8.12
Structures of vitamin K.

Sources

In the human diet, vitamin K is largely provided by plant foods; however the vitamin K content of many foods has yet to be determined. Good sources appear to be spinach, broccoli, brussels sprouts, cabbage, lettuce, and kale, while some vitamin K is provided by cereals, meats, nuts, legumes, dairy products, and fruits. Vitamin K may also be derived from bacteria in the human colon, primarily anaerobes such as *Escherichia coli* and *Bacillus fragilis*.

Absorption and Transport

It appears that phylloquinone is taken into enterocytes in the small intestine via an active, saturable process. This primarily takes place in the duodenum and jejunum, with the latter being the primary site of absorption. Conversely, menaquinones and menadione seem to cross the wall of the intestine via passive diffusion, which occurs mostly in the distal small intestine and the colon. This allows the menaquinones synthesized by bacteria in the colon to be absorbed, although the extent to which this occurs is still unclear. The absorption of vitamin K in the small intestine is positively influenced by the presence of pancreatic and biliary seretions, especially bile acids.

Vitamin K entering mucosal cells is incorporated into chylomicrons which enter the lymphatic circulation and, in turn, the systemic circulation. As chylomicron remnants are removed from circulation, vitamin K enters hepatocytes. Once in the liver, vitamin K can be metabolized and then incorporated into VLDL for export. The plasma concentration of phylloquinone is about 0.14 to 1.17 ng/ml. The duration of diet-derived vitamin K in the liver is not very long, and thus, the liver is not considered a significant site of storage for this vitamin. Typically, the vitamin K content of the liver is less than 20 to 25 ng/g of liver tissue. However, it should be recognized that hepatic turnover of menaquinones is much slower than phylloquinones, allowing for a large concentration difference (tenfold or more) in the liver.

Functions

The fact that vitamin K is essential for proper clotting of the blood in response to a hemorrhage has been known for at least 60 years. For the several decades that followed, it was assumed that the assistance in blood clotting might be the only physiological role of vitamin K. However, in the last few decades, newer roles of vitamin K have emerged. Vitamin K influences physiological processes, such as blood clotting, by posttranslation carboxylation of glutamic acid residues, to form γ-carboxyglutamic acid, in key proteins.

The coagulation of blood requires a series of "activation" reactions involving clotting factors synthesized in the blood. This is depicted in Figure 8.13. The final reaction in the series is proteolytic activation of fibrinogen to fibrin, which forms the structural basis of an insoluble fibrous network at the site of a hemorrhage. The enzyme that catalyzes this reaction is thrombin, which itself circulates as an inactive enzyme (zymogen) called prothrombin or clotting factor II. Four clotting factors, including prothrombin, are dependent upon vitamin K for normal function.

Factor X is vitamin K dependent and is the factor responsible for activating prothrombin to thrombin. Factor X is activated by one of two means. First, it can become functional via a series of activation reactions beginning with factor XII and involving factors XI and IX, the latter of which is also vitamin D dependent. The initial reaction occurs as the inactive form of factor XII interacts with exposed collagen fibers at the site of a hemorrhage. Collagen fibers would normally not be exposed to the blood as they are part of the interstitial connective tissue (i.e., basal laminae) of endothelial cells and local tissue. However rupture of the endothelial lining would expose the underlying connective tissue. This series of events leading to activation of prothrombin is called the *intrinsic pathway*.

The second mechanism leading to the activation of prothrombin tissue is called the *extrinsic pathway*. Here clotting factor VII, one of the vitamin D-dependent proteins, is activated by a tissue factor called *thromboplastin*. Activated factor VII then activates factor X, which activates prothrombin. As both the intrinsic and extrinsic pathways involve clotting factors are dependent upon vitamin K posttranslational modification, the proper coagulation of blood is sensitive to vitamin K status. Anticoagulant drugs, such as coumarin and warfarin, inhibit the action of vitamin K.

In addition to the clotting factors discussed above, four other proteins (C, M, S, and Z) involved in the regulation of blood clotting appear to be vitamin K dependent as well.

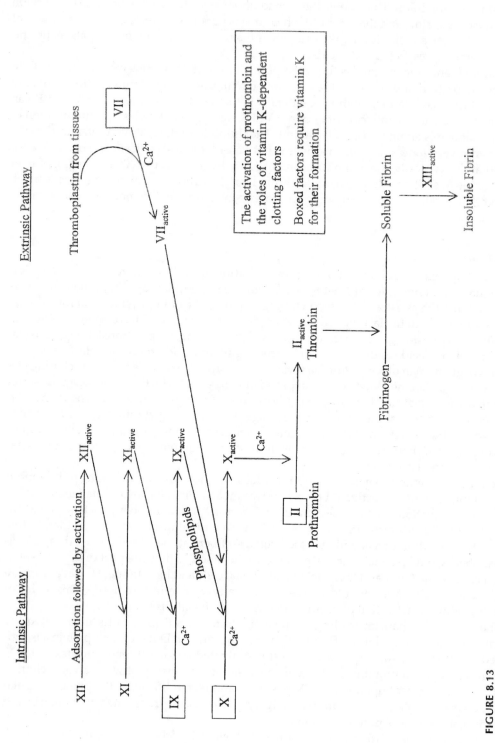

FIGURE 8.13

Cascade of events leading to the activation of insoluble fibrin which provides the structural foundation for a blood clot.

Protein C is a protease that appears to inhibit coagulation, while protein S appears to promote the breakdown of the fibrin network and thus the clot. Meanwhile protein M may be involved in the conversion of thrombin from prothrombin.

Other vitamin K-dependent proteins have been identified in tissues such as bone and kidneys. In bone, two proteins, called bone Gla protein (BGP or osteocalcin) and matrix Gla protein (MGP), are modified posttranslationally by carboxylation reaction of specific glutamic acid residues involving vitamin K. "Gla" makes reference to glutamic acid, and carboxylated glutamic acid residues are able to bind calcium. Osteocalcin, which is expressed under the influence of vitamin D, is produced in osteoblasts in bone and the dentine of teeth. MGP is associated with the matrix of bone, dentine, and cartilage. The specific roles of these proteins are still being investigated.

In addition, another protein has been identified in the renal cortex which, too, is dependent upon posttranslational modification involving vitamin K. Here again, the modification is carboxylation of specific glutamic acid residues. This protein is referred to as kidney Gla protein (KGP) and its physiological significance is also under investigation.

Recommended Levels of Intake

Vitamin K was added to the list of nutrients having an RDA in 1989. For infants less than 6 months of age and greater than 6 months of age, 5 µg and 10 µg are recommended, respectively. Children range between 10 to 30 µg, while adolescents and adults range between 45 to 80 µg. Pregnancy and lactation do not increase the vitamin K recommendation above the highest level for women (65 µg).

Deficiency and Toxicity

Unlike other fat-soluble vitamins, vitamin K is not stored very well in human tissue and appreciable amounts are lost in the urine and feces daily. This presents a theoretical opportunity for a rapid onset to deficiency. However, vitamin K is relatively abundant in the diet and respectable amounts are also absorbed from intestinal bacterial synthesis, thereby making vitamin K deficiency uncommon in adults. The typical American adult may actually eat 5 to 6 times the RDA.

Opportunities for vitamin K deficiency do arise in infancy. There does not seem to be an appreciable transfer of vitamin K from the mother to the fetus. Therefore, newborns are born with very limited stores. Also, a newborn's digestive tract is sterile and will not develop a mature bacterial population for months. Additionally, maternal breast milk is not a good source of vitamin K. All of these factors place infants at greater risk for developing a vitamin K deficiency, which can lead to poor blood clotting and hemorrhage, among other considerations. With these concerns in mind, pediatricians will routinely treat newborns with vitamin K.

One other situation may raise concern regarding the development of a vitamin K deficiency. Those individuals utilizing antibiotics for long periods of time are at a greater risk for vitamin K deficiency. Certain antibiotics can remove vitamin K-producing bacteria from the colon, results in a greater risk of deficiency, especially if individuals are consuming a low vitamin K diet and/or experiencing problems with lipid digestion. But the combination of these factors is indeed rare. Conversely, vitamin K is relatively nontoxic in natural forms; however, there have been situations of toxicity from chronic use of excessive vitamin K in the synthetic menadione form.

Water-Soluble Vitamins

The water-soluble vitamins contain many more compounds as compared to the fat-soluble vitamins. Typically, when one refers to the water-soluble vitamins, the so-called "B vitamins" and vitamin C are included. While the fat-soluble vitamins are not directly involved in energy metabolism, one characteristic of most water-soluble vitamins is a direct involvement in such operations. Their involvement is largely in the form of coenzymatic activity associated with metabolic pathways for carbohydrates, protein (amino acids), fat, and ethanol. Notable exceptions are vitamins C and B_{12} and folic acid. While these three water-soluble vitamins are not coenzymes in energy pathways, they are indeed coenzymes for other key operations. Therefore, coenzyme function is the most salient characteristic of this class of vitamins.

While much has been said pertaining to the potential of toxicity for the fat-soluble vitamins, due to their longer storage time in tissue, water-soluble vitamins, are also toxic in large quantities, although in excesses far greater than that observed for the fat-soluble vitamins.

Vitamin C (Ascorbic Acid)

Vitamin C has long been a controversial and popular vitamin among scientists and the general public. Deficiency of vitamin C or *ascorbate* results in one of the most famous nutrition-related diseases throughout time, *scurvy*. Scurvy prevailed until the mid 18th century, and was the scourge of sailors who were at sea for extended time periods. It was not unusual to observe fleets of ships return with 90% of the crew dead and/or incapacitated with scurvy. In 1754, the British navy hired the physician, James Lind, to investigate the disease. He became aware that the disease was not of microbial origin, but one that was associated with the diet. Eventually he determined that the juice from one sour lime would protect individuals from the disease. As a result of his findings, the British navy, via the suggestion of Captain James Cook, required ships to carry one citrus fruit for each man per day for the estimated time of the voyage. The practice of sucking the juice of limes by British sailors by legend said to have resulted in the nickname, "Limeys." It was not until 1933 that the Hungarian scientist, Albert Szyent-Gyorgyi, isolated the active principle from his native Hungarian green peppers. Following the isolation of ascorbate, he and Haworth, a carbohydrate chemist, worked out its structure. Szyent-Gyorgyi received the Nobel Prize in 1936 for his work on vitamin C.

Ascorbate is a derivative of glucose. Through a series of reactions shown in Figure 8.14, glucose is converted to glucuronate, then l-gulonolactone, where the latter compound is oxidized via l-gulonolactone oxidase to yield ascorbate. Unfortunately, humans are unable to carry out the reaction because they lack this enzyme. The guinea pig, primates, bats, and some fish (catfish) are unable to synthesize ascorbate. On the other hand, many animals, such as rats and chickens, are able to synthesize vitamin C.

A biochemically useful property of vitamin C is that it can both donate and accept hydrogen readily. The reduced form of vitamin C is termed *dehydroascorbic acid* (Figure 8.15). Glutathione facilitates the production of the reduced form. Both forms of the vitamin are equally active, and this interconversion makes it a good antioxidant. This property also makes vitamin C useful for food protection, especially in canned foods.

The vitamin has several centers of asymmetry. Both D and L isomer forms exist, but it is the L form that is active in humans. In contrast, the reverse is true in regard to glucose,

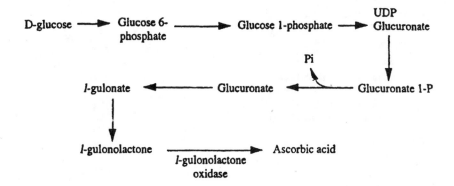

FIGURE 8.14
Biosynthesis of ascorbic acid.

where the D form is the active form. If ascorbate is oxidized, it will form diketogulonic acid, which is inactive. These are also substitutions that may occur on carbon atoms of the molecular structure. The methoxyl group on carbon 6 may be substituted by a methyl group. Also, a 7-carbon structure may exist where an additional CH_2OH group may be added. In both situations, both of these forms are still active.

Vitamin C is heat labile, readily dissolves in water, and is destroyed by alkali solutions, but is stabilized by acid solutions. Oxidation, as suggested above, will destroy the vitamin, whereas reduction stabilizes it. Vitamin C will absorb light, whereupon it is destroyed. Contact with iron and copper will readily oxidize ascorbate and destroy its activity.

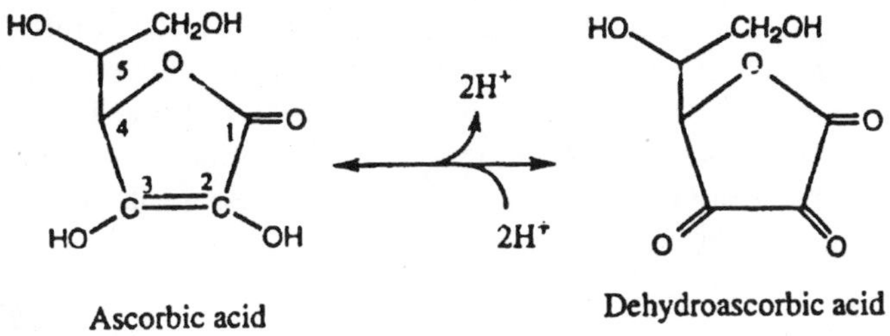

FIGURE 8.15
Chemical structures of ascorbic acid and dehydroascorbic acid.

Food Sources

Vitamin C is available in many fruits and vegetables, with excellent sources being cantaloupe, kiwi, mango, honeydew melon, citrus fruits, papaya, strawberries, watermelon, asparagus, broccoli, brussels sprouts, cabbage, cauliflower, green and red peppers, and plantains. Vitamin C is susceptible to breakdown during certain cooking, processing, and storage procedures (i.e., heat or cooking in neutral or basic medium). For instance, potatoes can lose almost half of their vitamin C by boiling; and spinach can endure nearly an entire loss of its vitamin C if it is stored for 2 to 3 days at room temperature. Therefore, for practical purposes, citrus fruits and other vitamin C-containing fruits usually are better dietary sources of vitamin C, as they are generally eaten fresh and raw. Table 8.5 presents a listing of the vitamin C content in select foods.

TABLE 8.5
Vitamin C Content of Selected Foods

Food	Vitamin C (mg)
Fruits	
Orange juice, fresh (1 c)	124
Kiwi (1)	75
Grapefruit juice, fresh (1 c)	94
Cranberry juice cocktail (1 c)	90
Orange (1)	70
Strawberries, fresh (1 c)	84
Cantaloupe (3)	63
Grapefruit (1)	51
Raspberries, fresh (1 c)	31
Watermelon (1 c)	15
Vegetables	
Green peppers (2 c)	95
Cauliflower, raw (2 c)	142
Broccoli (2 c)	164
Brussels sprouts (2 c)	65
Collard greens (2 c)	48
Cauliflower, cooked (2 c)	112
Potato (1)	29
Tomato (1)	23

Absorption

The efficiency of vitamin C absorption appears to be high, and is primarily a sodium-dependent and gradient-coupled carrier mechanism in the small intestine. On the contrary, the oxidized form of vitamin C, dehydroascorbate, demonstrates a relatively low uptake and is probably absorbed via a passive mechanism. At an intake level up to 180 mg/d, about 80% of the vitamin C is absorbed. Above that level, saturable levels are achieved and much of the additional absorption is due to passive absorption. It is estimated that at doses approaching 5 g only about one fourth is absorbed. However, this can still lead to significant levels of absorption, since 25% of 5 g is 1.25 g.

Functions

Vitamin C is a cofactor in several important enzymatic reactions. It is an activator of a hydroxylase enzyme involved with collagen synthesis. As mentioned in Chapter 6, collagen is the most abundant protein in the human body and is found in tendons, bones, cartilage, skin, the cornea, and in interstitial spaces. About 30% of its amino acids are glycine, while proline, hydroxyproline, and hydroxylysine contribute about 20%. Collagen, as synthesized by fibroblasts, is helical in structure, and three collagen helixes are twisted together to form a larger left-handed helix called *tropocollagen*. Multiple tropocollagen helicies are cross-linked together to form a strong collagen fiber. Hydroxylation of the proline, produces hydroxyproline in collagen chains allowing for cross-linking via prolylhydroxylase. This is significant in that every third amino acid in collagen is proline. The hydroxylation of lysine allows for more extensive collagen associations in the extracellular space. Prolyl and lysyl hydroxlases both require iron as a cofactor, and vitamin C functions as a reductant maintaining iron in a reduced state.

Vitamin C is well known for aiding in the absorption of iron by promoting the ferrous (Fe^{2+}) iron state. Iron in this oxidation state is better absorbed than when in the ferric (Fe^{3+}) state. While this may be extremely important in iron-deficient individuals, it is still not clear at this time whether excessive vitamin C consumption increases the risk of iron overload. However, preliminary research indicates that it may not be a concern, as vitamin C consumption of 1 to 2 g daily does not appear to increase iron status indicators such as ferritin.

Vitamin C is probably necessary for two reactions in the formation of carnitine. (The synthesis of carnitine is discussed in greater detail in Chapter 14.) The reactions involving vitamin C are hydroxylations and are very similar to those discussed for collagen synthesis. The two enzymes, *trimethyllysine hydroxylase* and *4-butyrobetaine hydroxlase*, require iron as a cofactor, and vitamin C is the preferred reductant. Carninitine is needed to transport longer chain fatty acids across the mitochondrial inner membrane so that they can engage in β-oxidation.

The hydroxylation reaction that converts the amino acid phenylalanine to tyrosine is catalyzed by *phenylalanine hydroxylase*, an iron-containing enzyme found in the liver and kidneys. A substrate for this reaction is tetrahydrobiopterin, which is converted to dihydrobiopterin. Vitamin C is needed to regenerate tetrahydropterin from dihydrobiopterin. Vitamin C participates in another key reaction in the metabolism of tyrosine catalyzed by the copper-dependent enzyme *p-hydroxyphenylpyruvate*. Further still, the *dopamine β-hydroxylase* reaction produces norepinephrine from dopamine, which was derived from tyrosine, and requires ascorbate to reduce copper at its active site. The adrenal glands are the primary site of this reaction, and this tissue has the highest concentration of vitamin C in comparison to other tissues or organs. Vitamin C appears to be needed to allow for a release of some of the adrenal hormones into the circulation. Vitamin C may therefore play a role in stress reactions.

Vitamin C is also known for its antioxidant capacity. As an antioxidant it seems to be very efficient in reducing superoxide (O_2^-) and hydroxyl radicals ($OH^\cdot$) as well as hydrogen peroxide (H_2O_2). Also, recent investigative efforts have revealed that vitamin C promotes the reduced form of vitamin E, which itself can help protect LDLs from oxidation. Therefore, in this manner vitamin C may indirectly decrease the development of atherosclerotic lesions.

Recommended Levels of Intake

Currently, the RDA for adults is set at 60 mg; however, the actual requirement is probably much lower than the recommended amounts. During pregnancy, the RDA is 70 mg and for the first 6 months of lactation it is 95 mg, and declines slightly to 90 mg in the second 6 months of lactation. Interestingly, smokers present lower serum levels of vitamin C than nonsmokers, as the metabolism of vitamin C is greatly enhanced. Thus, it takes about twice the amount of dietary vitamin C to achieve similar serum levels to non-smokers.

Deficiency

A deficiency of vitamin C is known to result in several symptoms, the most significant of which is the syndrome, scurvy. This disease is characterized by abnormal bone growth, joint pains, bleeding gums, and tiny petechial hemorrhages beneath the skin. While normal blood clotting is hindered, the capillaries become very weak, because the underlying connective tissue is compromised due to impaired collagen synthesis. An abrasion to the surface of the skin may result in many petechial hemorrhages in individuals with scurvy. Hemorrhaging will occur around hair follicles, in the jaw, gum–tooth area, muscles, bones, the gastrointestinal tract, and kidneys. Teeth may become loose and fall out in severe cases. Susceptibility to infections due to the wound exposure is a possibility. Edema occurs, due to a shift in osmotic pressure resulting from the loss of blood proteins during episodes of hemorrhaging. Infants develop a scorbutic rosary where the rib cage exhibits swollen joints. In milder cases, rheumatic-like pain is frequent. Other signs and symptoms of mild deficiency include yellowish complexion, listlessness, and some psychic disturbances (in both mild and severe deficiencies) as a result of imbalances in neurotransmitters. As little as 10 mg of vitamin C may be enough to prevent signs of scurvy. The adult RDA of 60 mg allows higher serum levels and will prevent the development signs of scurvy for at least 1 month if vitamin C was removed from the diet. Scurvy is not a problem in the U.S. today, although individuals afflicted with poverty or alcoholics may show some of the symptoms.

Toxicity

Vitamin C is one of the most popular nutritional supplements. It has been purported to be a prophylactic or treatment for the common cold as well as for cancer. Vitamin C supplementation, in quantities approaching gram-doses, has been advocated by several scientists, including Nobel Prize winners. However, most of the scientific community does not support such aggressive suggestions.

Vitamin C toxicity can produce *rebound scurvy*. In children and adults, as well as during fetal life, humans developed an enzymatic mechanism to destroy excessive vitamin C. Therefore, supplementation by individuals or pregnant women results in higher levels of these enzymes in their tissue, including fetal tissue. Thus, an infant is at higher risk of vitamin C deficiency if it consumes only breast milk, which is a marginal vitamin C source at best. Also, children and adults supplementing with larger doses of vitamin C can also develop rebound scurvy once the supplement is removed. It is recommended that an individual should taper their reduction in vitamin C supplementation.

Chronic excessive vitamin C ingestion can lead to inaccurate readings on blood glucose tests (due to pancreatic β cell damage), intestinal bleeding and other anomalies of the digestive tract, adrenal failure, reduced fertility and bone growth, suppression of mitosis, hemolytic reactions, and kidney stone formation. Calcium oxalate crystals are the most prominent component of kidney stones. Oxalates are a primary metabolite of vitamin C and are voided in the urine.

Asians and individuals of African or Middle-Eastern descent appear more sensitive to vitamin C toxicity. Hemolytic anemia is common among these groups who supplement well above normal doses of vitamin C. It is generally recommended that supplementation of 100 to 300 mg/d is sufficient, and up to 1 g/d is safe. Above that there may be increased risk associated with supplementing.

Thiamin (Vitamin B$_1$)

Thiamin was first recognized as essential in 1896 by Eijkman, a Dutch physician who traveled to the Dutch East Indies to help prisoners. He altered their food supply by removing brown rice and providing polished rice. The prisoners became sick, as did pigeons who normally fed from the rice. Some of the pigeons that had access to the hulls did not suffer or were found to be recovering from the disease. Eijkman shifted the diets of the prisoners back to the brown rice and noticed a great improvement in the reversal of symptoms. He discovered that there was a water-soluble material left behind by the polishing of rice. Later, Duneth and Jansen, who worked in Eijkman's laboratory, isolated and crystallized the active factor. Then, in 1912, Casmir Funk determined that the active factor was amide (nitrogen-containing structure) and referred to it as a vital amine or *vitamine*, as discussed at the onset of this chapter. Williams, at the University of Texas in 1936, discovered the structure and synthesized the vitamin.

Thiamin is comprised of two chemical components: a *pyrimidine* group and a *thiazole* ring (Figure 8.16). A methylene group bridges the two groups together. The molecule may be split at this methylene group with sodium bisulfite or the enzyme *thiaminase*, the latter of which is found in fish or the bracken fern. At one time, mink breeders fed raw fish to the animals, and the minks died, as a result of a thiamin deficiency due to the thiaminase activity. The methyl group at the 2 position of thiamin may be replaced with an ethyl or propyl group, but this results in a less active vitamin. Replacement with a butyl group actually results in antithiamin activity.

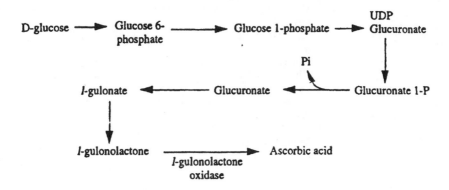

FIGURE 8.16
The structure of thiamin.

If the amino group at position 6 can be replaced by an OH group, the resulting compound is referred to as oxythiamine, which has antivitamin activity. Oxythiamine exacerbates thiamin deficiency symptoms related to nervous tissue. If the sulfur group at position 1 is replaced by an ethylene group, the compound is referred to as pyrithiamine, which is also an antivitamin and accentuates the fluid imbalance associated with thiamin deficiency. It should be pointed out that these derivatives are laboratory synthesized and do not occur in nature. Other compounds may interact with thiamin to cause it to become inactive, such as potassium phosphate, copper and iron salts.

Dietary Sources

Good sources are pork (probably the best), whole grains, enriched or fortified cereals, liver, poultry, fish eggs, potatoes, legumes, nuts, dark green vegetables, brewer's yeast and wheat germ (Table 8.6). All of the thiamin available in plant sources is in the form of thiamin. On the contrary, almost all of the thiamin in animal sources is phosphorylated, with 80% being *thiamin pyrophosphate (TPP)* (Figure 8.17) and the remainder being *thiamin monophosphate (TMP)* and *thiamin triphosphate (TPPP)*. As mentioned above, certain foods, such as raw fish, contain thiaminases, which inactivate thiamin. Cooking (heat) inactivates thiaminases. Other antithiamin factors include tannic and caffeic acids. These substances are heat-stable and are found in foods such as coffee, tea, betel nuts, brussels sprouts, and blueberries.

TABLE 8.6
Thiamin Content of Selected Foods

Food	Thiamin (mg)
Meats	
Pork roast (3 oz)	0.8
Beef (3 oz)	0.4
Ham (3 oz)	0.4
Liver (3 oz)	0.2
Nuts and seeds	
Sunflower seeds (1 c)	0.82
Peanuts (1 c)	0.64
Almonds (1 c)	0.18
Grains	
Bran flakes (1 c)	0.6
Macaroni (2 c)	0.1
Rice (2 c)	0.1
Bread (1 slice)	0.1
Vegetables	
Peas (1 c)	0.4
Lima beans (1 c)	0.4
Corn (1 c)	0.1
Broccoli (1 c)	0.1
Potato (1)	0.1
Fruits	
Orange juice (1 c)	0.2
Orange (1)	0.1
Avocado (2)	0.2

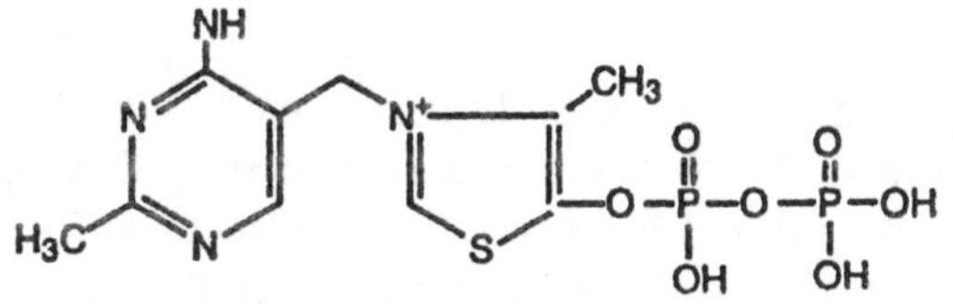

Thiamin pyrophosphate (TPP)

FIGURE 8.17
The structure of thiamin pyrophosphate.

Digestion, Absorption, and Transport

Thiamin phosphates must be digested by intestinal phosphatases to yield free thiamin. Absorption of thiamin is high and takes place rapidly primarily in the jejunum and secondarily in the duodenum and ileum. The uptake actively occurs against a concentration gradient, with metabolic inhibitors reducing the uptake. For instance, *in vivo* and *in vitro* findings have revealed that inhibitors of Na^+/K^+-ATPase and a lack of sodium could inhibit thiamin uptake. Passive absorption does occur and may be significant when luminal thiamin content is high. Intake levels greater than 5 mg daily will result in an increase in passive diffusion. Alcohol reduces thiamin absorption. However, it does not appear that mucosal uptake is inhibited, but more likely that the transfer of thiamin to the serosal side is inhibited via an inhibition of Na^+/K^+-ATPase.

Thiamin can be phosphorylated within mucosal enterocytes to form TMP. Thiamin is transported across the basilateral membrane via an active, sodium-dependent mechanism. Thiamin is transported in the plasma, primarily as TMP and secondarily as thiamin, within red blood cells and, to a lesser degree, other blood cells. It appears that only TMP and thiamin are able to cross cellular plasma membranes, therefore explaining the relative lack of the other polyphosphorylated forms of thiamin in the blood.

Metabolism and Functions

An adult body may contain approximately 30 mg of thiamin. While about one half of body thiamin can be found in skeletal muscle, other tissues of higher thiamin concentration include those with high metabolic expenditure, such as the heart, liver, brain, and kidneys. Thiamin is necessary for biochemical reactions involving the metabolism and release of energy from carbohydrates. Thiamin is largely active as TPP which is formed in tissue by the reaction series presented in Figure 8.18. Basically, this form of thiamin is needed for oxidative decarboxylation of α-keto acids (pyruvate and α-ketoglutarate) and 2-keto sugars via a transketolase reaction, in which an aldehyde group is removed from the molecule.

The pyruvate dehydrogenase enzyme complex is necessary for the conversion of pyruvate to acetyl CoA. This reaction occurs within the mitochondrial matrix and the acetyl CoA created is then available to condense with oxaloacetate (OAA) to form citrate, the first molecule of TCA or the Krebs cycle. TPP is a critical component, along with lipoic acid, Mg^{2+}, NAD^+, and coenzyme A. Thiamin, as TPP, is also necessary for a key reaction of the

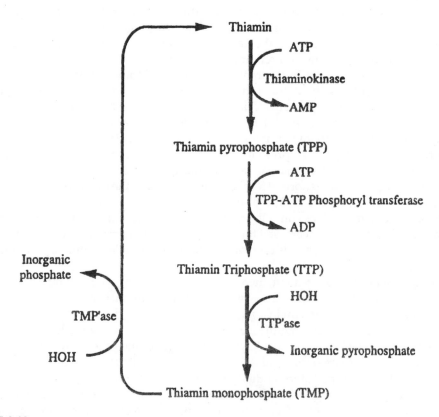

FIGURE 8.18
The synthesis of thiamin pyrophosphate via the phosphorylation of thiamin.

Krebs cycle whereby α-ketoglutarate is converted to succinyl CoA. The necessary components of the α-ketoglutarate dehydrogenase enzyme complex, which catalyzes this reaction, are the same as for pyruvate dehydrogenase. In both of these thiamin-dependent reactions, NADH is produced which delivers electrons to the electron transport chain for ATP generation.

Thiamin, as TPP, also functions at an important step in the cytosolic *hexose monophosphate shunt* or *pentose phosphate pathway*. Here TPP functions as a coenzyme for a transketolase reaction. The metabolic significance of the pentose phosphate pathway is the generation of NADPH for synthetic operations and ribose for nucleic acid synthesis. Thiamin also appears to be important in the membrane conduction of nervous tissue, although its involvement is purely speculative at this time.

Recommended Levels for Intake

Recommendations for thiamin intake are in milligram quantities. For infants, 0.3 and 0.4 mg are recommended for infants less than 6 months and more than 6 months of age, respectively. For children, the recommended level is 0.7 to 1.0 mg, and for adolescent and adult males the recommendation ranges between 1.2 to 1.5 mg, while for adolescent and adult females it ranges between 1.0 to 1.1 mg. During pregnancy the recommendation increases to 1.5 mg and is further increased to 1.6 mg during lactation.

Deficiency

Severe thiamin deficiency produces mental confusion and muscular cramps which are characteristic of the disease syndrome called *beriberi*. The polishing of rice, which is a staple food for many countries, has led to the development of *beriberi*. Polishing removes the thiamin in the rice hulls. The general refining (polishing, milling, refining) of grains, leaving only the endosperm, results in the removal of most of the thiamin. For instance, the endosperm only contains about 3% of the thiamin in a kernel of wheat. The remainder of thiamin is split between the germ (64%) and the bran layers (33%). Because of this, the U.S. government passed the *Enrichment Act*, which made it mandatory for food manufacturers to resupply thiamin and other vitamins and minerals to products which used refined cereal products (i.e., flours). Figure 4.7 presents the compartments of a typical cereal grain.

One characteristic of *beriberi* may be cardiac enlargement. It has been observed that the size of the heart can return to normal if thiamin is returned to the diet in adequate amounts. In thiamin deficiency, there is inefficient utilization of carbohydrate which can also lead to CNS-related problems such as convulsions, head retractions, and spasms. Muscular anomalies can also occur, such as decreased tonus, improper peristalsis, and constipation. Anorexia is also a deficiency sign, as it is for many of the water-soluble vitamins, particularly the B vitamins.

In addition to cardiac enlargement, there appears to be a change in heart rate; however, this seems to vary among species. In humans, tachycardia is common; in rats bradycardia results. Fluid imbalances are also frequent in *beriberi*. In humans, the cachexia produced occurs with a marked loss of body fluids. An individual in this state appears as a walking skeleton, and this is referred frequently as the "dry" type of *beriberi*. On the other hand, edema or fluid accumulation in tissue can occur, and the individual presents a bloated appearance. When this occurs in thiamin-deficient individuals it is referred to as "wet" *beriberi*.

Milder signs of thiamin deficiency can be observed, including fatigue, irregular heart beat, a burning sensation in the feet, muscle cramps and a loss of "tickle" in the fingers. A simple test used to diagnose thiamin deficiency is to have an individual sit on a table.

Under normal conditions, the feet should be parallel to the floor. In deficiency, the foot points to the floor in what is referred to as "foot drop syndrome."

Thiamin Toxicity

Thiamin ingestion in amounts exceeding 125 mg/kg body weight can cause physiological problems. Edema, nervousness, sweating, tachycardia, tremors, an increased incidence of sores caused by the herpes virus, increased allergic reactions, fatty liver, and hypotension may occur. In rats, sterility has even been reported.

Riboflavin (Vitamin B_2)

Riboflavin was discovered shortly after the discovery of thiamin. It is synthesized in all plants and microorganisms, but not by higher organisms. This substance is fundamentally important in energy metabolism and occurs in foods and in the human body as either riboflavin or as *flavin mononucleotide (FMN)* or *flavin adenine dinucleotide (FAD)* bound to protein complexes (Figure 8.19 and 8.20). Other names given to riboflavin include vitamin B_2, vitamin G, lactoflavin, hepatoflavin, and ovoflavin. In 1917, riboflavin was shown to be a growth factor in yeast and it was also revealed that this substance was relatively heat stable, yet broken down to inactive structures with exposure to light (Figure 8.21). In solution, riboflavin produces a greenish-yellowish color which is readily obvious in urine. In 1935, the structure and synthesis of riboflavin had been achieved. The name "riboflavin" is derived from ribose, a component of this vitamin, and *flavus* which is Latin for yellow.

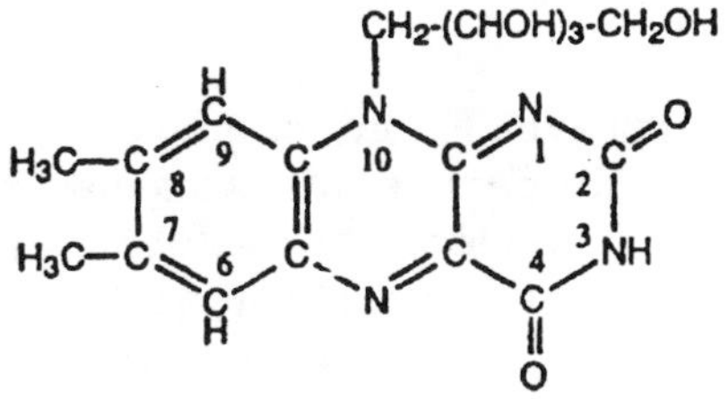

FIGURE 8.19
The structure of riboflavin.

Dietary Sources

Riboflavin is found in many foods, especially milk and dairy products (i.e., yogurt, cottage cheese), leafy green vegetables, beef liver, beef, and other meats. (Table 8.7) About one half of the riboflavin provided in the American diet comes by way of milk and milk products. Meats are also a primary supplier of dietary riboflavin. As mentioned above, riboflavin appears to be more stable in heat, certainly more so than vitamin C and thiamin. However, significant riboflavin losses in foods are experienced when exposed to light. For instance, milk will lose about one third of its riboflavin activity when exposed to sunlight for about 1 h. Fortunately, most milk producers no longer package their product in clear containers such as glass bottles. This helps milk retain most of its riboflavin. Sun-drying and cooking foods in an open pot can lead to significant riboflavin losses as well. Also, like other water-soluble vitamins, riboflavin can be "washed away" during boiling and thawing (thaw drip). And, like for so many other vitamins and minerals, the refining or milling of cereal

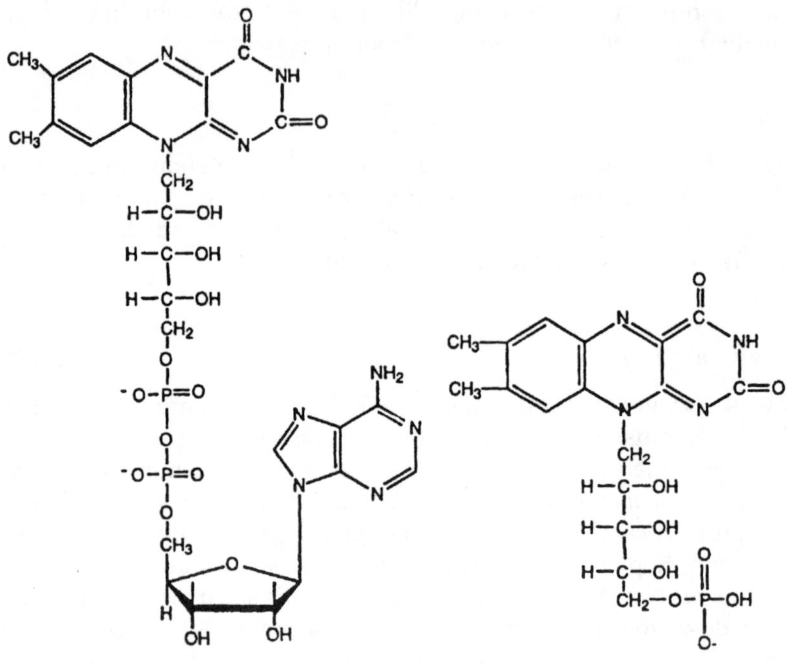

FIGURE 8.20
Structures of the coenzyme forms of riboflavin. FAD is flavin adenine dinucleotide and FMN is flavin mononucleotide.

grains removes most of the riboflavin. For instance, a kernal of wheat only has about 32% of the riboflavin within the endosperm, while the remaining riboflavin is distributed throughout the germ (26%) and bran layers (42%). Riboflavin is added to foods utilizing refined cereal grain products as per the Enrichment Act.

Absorption and Transport

The coenzyme forms FAD and FMN represent most of the riboflavin in the diet. In the small intestine, these coenzymes are acted upon by pyrophosphatases and phosphatases in the upper portion of the small intestine. The free riboflavin is absorbed by a saturable transport system that is rapid and proportional to dose before reaching a plateau at approximately 25 mg/d. Apparently the presence of bile salts facilitates the uptake of thiamin, and there is evidence that suggests that this uptake is also a sodium-dependent process. Once riboflavin is absorbed by the mucosal cells, it can be rephosphorylated to FMN. Riboflavin can dissolve into the plasma, while about one half is bound to proteins, primarily albumin and secondarily globulins, fibrinogen, and other proteins. FMN is mostly found in the plasma bound to proteins, again primarily albumin.

Metabolism and Roles

Tissues having a greater riboflavin concentration include the heart, liver, and kidneys. While the concentration of riboflavin in the brain is not as great as in the tissues just

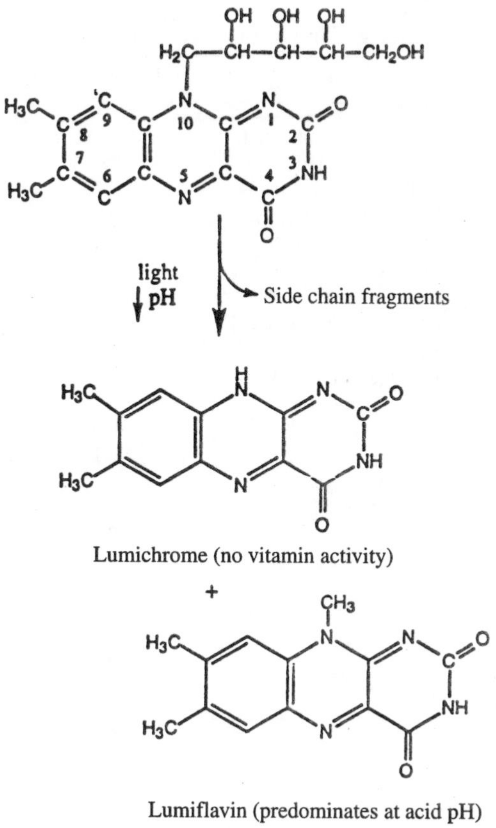

FIGURE 8.21
Degradation of riboflavin by light and acidic conditions.

mentioned, the brain does seem more resistant to changes in riboflavin status elsewhere in the human body. This suggests some form of regulation. It is estimated that the reserve of riboflavin in an adult is equivalent to the metabolic demands for 2 to 6 weeks. Riboflavin is voided primarily in the urine.

In cells of all tissue, riboflavin can be interconverted to FMN and FAD as depicted in Figure 8.22. In the coenzyme forms (FAD and FMN), riboflavin facilitates the release of energy from carbohydrates, fat, and protein through both the Krebs cycle and mitochondrial electron transport as well as other electron transfer mechanism. Both compounds serve their basic roles in accepting electrons (and H^+) in biochemical reactions (Figure 8.23).

FMN is a cofactor for enzymes such as NADH dehydrogenase, which transfers electrons from NADH to ubiquinone of the electron transport chain and L-amino acid oxidase and lactate dehydrogenase (interconversion of pyruvate and lactic acid). FAD is a coenzyme for enzymes such as cytochrome reductase, succinate dehydrogenase (Krebs cycle reaction), acyl CoA dehydrogenase (β-oxidation of fatty acid), D-amino acid oxidase (degradation of D-amino acids), xanthine oxidase (oxidation of hypoxanthine and xanthine to uric acid), and monoamine oxidase (degradation of amine structures such as tyramine).

TABLE 8.7
Riboflavin Content of Selected Foods

Food	Riboflavin (mg)
Milk and milk products	
Milk, whole (1 c)	0.4
Milk, 2% (1 c)	0.4
Yogurt, low fat (1 c)	0.5
Milk, skim (1 c)	0.4
Yogurt (1 c)	0.5
Cheese, American (1 oz)	0.1
Cheese, cheddar (1 oz)	0.1
Meats	
Liver (3 oz)	0.2
Pork chop (3 oz)	0.3
Beef (3 oz)	0.3
Tuna (3 oz)	0.1
Vegetables	
Collard greens (2 c)	0.3
Broccoli (2 c)	0.2
Spinach, cooked (2 c)	0.1
Eggs	
Egg (1)	0.2
Grains	
Macaroni (2 c)	0.1
Bread (1 slice)	0.8

Recommended Levels of Intake

The most recent RDAs for riboflavin range from 1.2 to 1.8 mg for adolescents and adults. During pregnancy, 1.8 mg is recommended. For lactation, the RDA is 1.8 mg for the first 6 months, but decreases to 1.7 mg in the second 6 months. The requirements for riboflavin, like those of thiamin, are again best described on an energy basis, or more specifically, on a 1000-kcal intake basis.

Deficiency and Toxicity

A decrease in energy release is the most obvious result of riboflavin deficiency, due to its critical role in the Krebs cycle and breakdown of fatty acids. The nervous system is typically the first region to develop problems, due to the reliance upon carbohydrate as an energy source. *Photophobia* or fear of light can occur. There is increased vascularity around the eyeball, allowing for the appearance of "bloodshot" eyes. A riboflavin-deficient individual exhibits signs of discoordination. Overt signs of deficiency also include cracked skin around the mouth (*cheilosis*), inflamed lips, and sore, inflamed tongue (*glossitis*) which develops a glossy appearance. The skin can over secrete a waxy material (*sebacea*) resulting in seborrheic dermatitis, and anorexia is common. The enrichment of foods has made riboflavin deficiency rare in the U.S.; however, it is still prominent in countries where milled grain is a major portion of the dietary intake.

On the other hand, there does not appear to be great concern regarding riboflavin toxicity. Much of the excessive riboflavin present in the human body is rapidly voided in the urine. Unlike the urinary loss of most other substances, riboflavin removal is visually obvious as urine turns a bright yellow. This effect is noticeable even with smaller doses of riboflavin. Gastrointestinal discomfort has been noted when intake levels exceed 1000 mg/d.

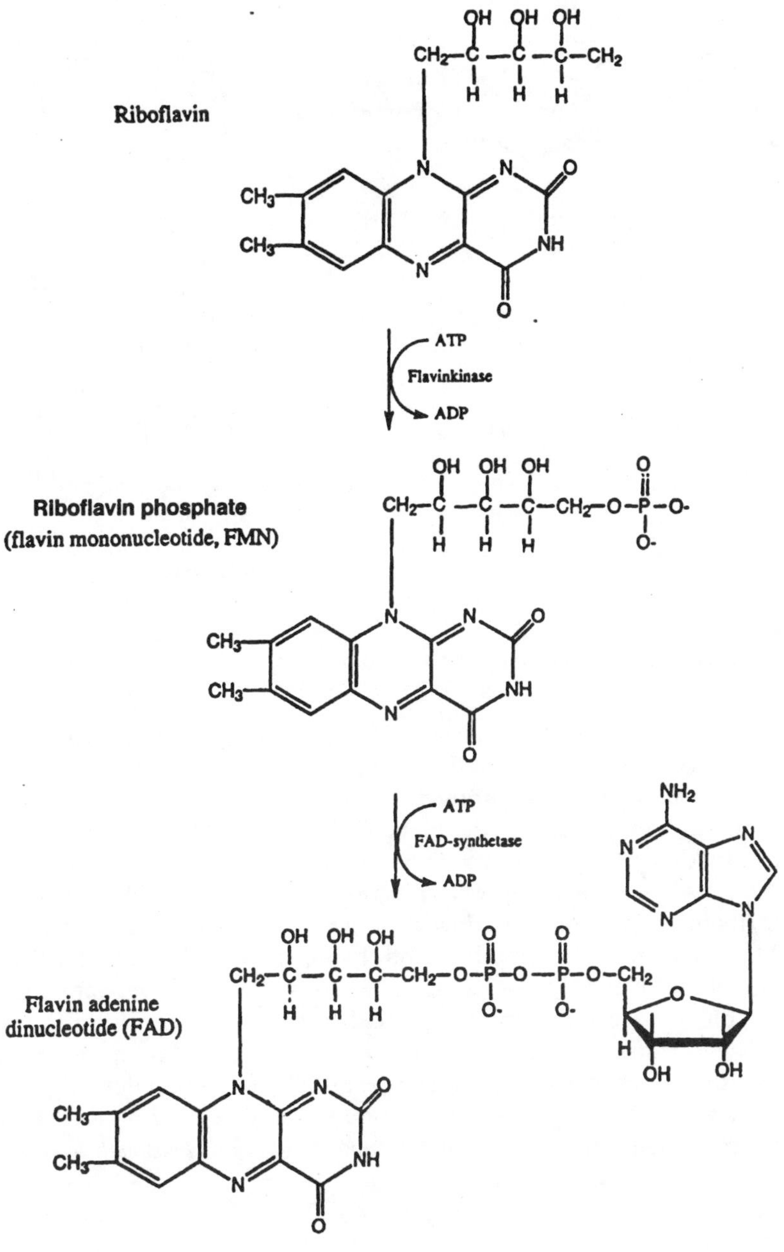

FIGURE 8.22
Synthesis of FAD and FMN.

Niacin (Vitamin B$_3$)

Niacin has an rather interesting history and has been known since 1864. Niacin deficiency leads to *pellagra* and in rural areas of the southeastern United States had significant outbreaks of this disease from that time until about 1935. The chemical structure of niacin was known and the disease pellagra was known, but the association of the two was not made until later. In fact, pellagra was thought to be an infectious disease. In the mid-1920s the

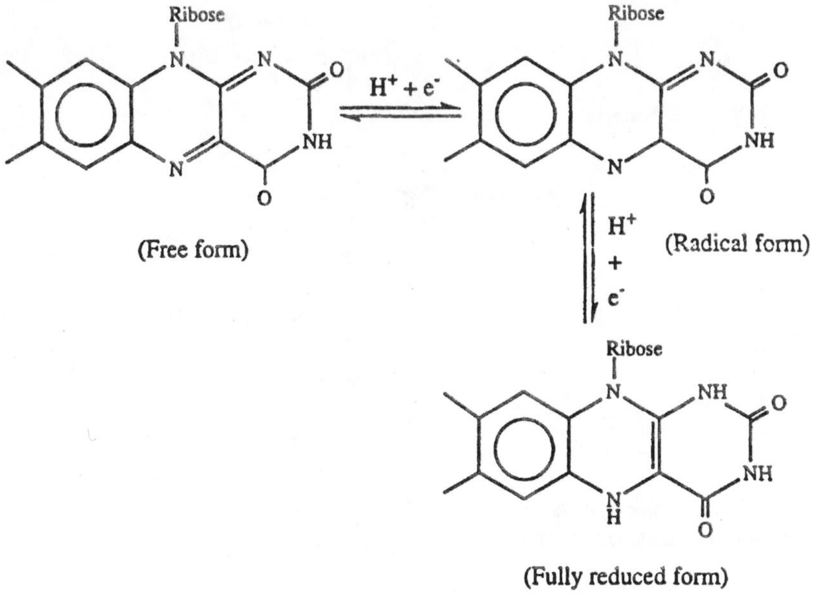

(Free form)

H⁺ + e⁻

Ribose

(Radical form)

H^+
+
e^-

(Fully reduced form)

FIGURE 8.23
Mechanism of action of the riboflavin portion of the coenzyme form of riboflavin.

U.S. Public Health Service sent a physician, Joseph Goldberger, to rural areas of the Southeast to deal with what was thought at the time to be an infectious disease. He noticed that the rural poor consumed a monotonous diet of fatback, molasses, and grits (white corn). These food items are completely devoid of niacin. He realized that if he changed the diet of the afflicted individuals, there appeared to be less severe symptomology. When the fatback, molasses, and grits were combined with milk, meat, or fresh vegetables, either alone or in combination, there was a great resolution in the symptoms . He became convinced that pellagra could be cured by dietary intervention. Later, in the 1930s, Conrad Elveghem was able to show that niacin cured "black tongue" in dogs, the canine version of pellagra.

Niacin is typically present as nicotinic acid (niacin) or nicotinamide, as shown in Figure 8.24. The pyrimidine ring with a carboxyl group at carbon number 3 is nicotinic acid. Similarly, the presence of an amine group at this same carbon defines the structure as *nicotinamide. Niacin* is active in the human body in two coenzyme forms: *nicotinamide adenine dinucleotide (NAD)* and *nicotinamide adenine dinucleotide phosphate, (NADP).* Both are involved in electron transfer operations.

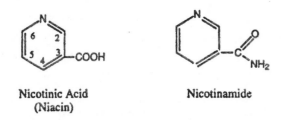

Nicotinic Acid
(Niacin)

Nicotinamide

FIGURE 8.24
Chemical structures of niacin (nicotinic acid) and nicotinamide.

Sources

Nicotinic acid and nicotinamide are found well distributed throughout most foods. Brewer's yeast, most fish, pork, beef, poultry, mushrooms, and potatoes offer a higher niacin content (Table 8.8). Plant foods contain nicotinic acid, while animal foods will contain nicotinamide, as well as the coenzyme forms NAD, and NADP. Niacin forms in foods appear relatively stable in most forms of cooking and storage, while some losses may be experienced when boiling foods, as the vitamin leaches out of a food, and during the thaw–drip.

TABLE 8.8
Niacin Content of Selected Foods

Food	Niacin (NE)[a]
Meats and seafood	
Liver (3 oz)	14.0
Tuna (3 oz)	10.3
Turkey (3 oz)	9.5
Chicken (3 oz)	7.9
Salmon (3 oz)	6.9
Veal (3 oz)	5.2
Beef, round steak (3 oz)	5.1
Pork (3 oz)	4.5
Haddock (3 oz)	4.3
Scallops (3 oz)	1.1
Nuts and seeds	
Peanuts (1 oz)	4.9
Vegetables	
Asparagus (1 c)	1.0
Grains	
Wheat germ (1 oz)	1.5
Rice, brown (2 c)	5.9
Noodles, enriched (2 c)	0.2
Rice, white, enriched (2 c)	2.9
Bread, enriched (1 slice)	0.9
Milk and milk products	
Milk (1 c)	0.2
Cheese, cottage (1 c)	0.1

[a] 1 NE = 1 mg niacin and 60 mg tryptophan.

Nicotinic acid can also be formed in human cells. The starting molecule is the essential amino acid tryptophan, depicted in Figure 8.25. It is estimated that only about 3% of tryptophan is utilized in this manner. This process is considered inefficient for niacin production as it requires approximately 60 mg of tryptophan to create 1 mg of niacin. This is largely due to the potential to irreversibly create intermediate molecules such as kynurenic acid and xanthuremic acid. The process of niacin formation is also influenced by the levels of tryptophan and niacin ingested, protein and energy intake and vitamin B_6 (involved in four reactions), and riboflavin nutriture.

Digestion and Absorption

Niacin in its coenzyme forms must be digested to nicotinamide. This is accomplished by *glycohydrolase* in the small intestine. While some absorption of nicotinic acid and nicotinamide can occur in the stomach, most absorption takes place in the small intestine. Nicotinamide and nicotinic acid appear to be taken up by mucosal enterocytes via a

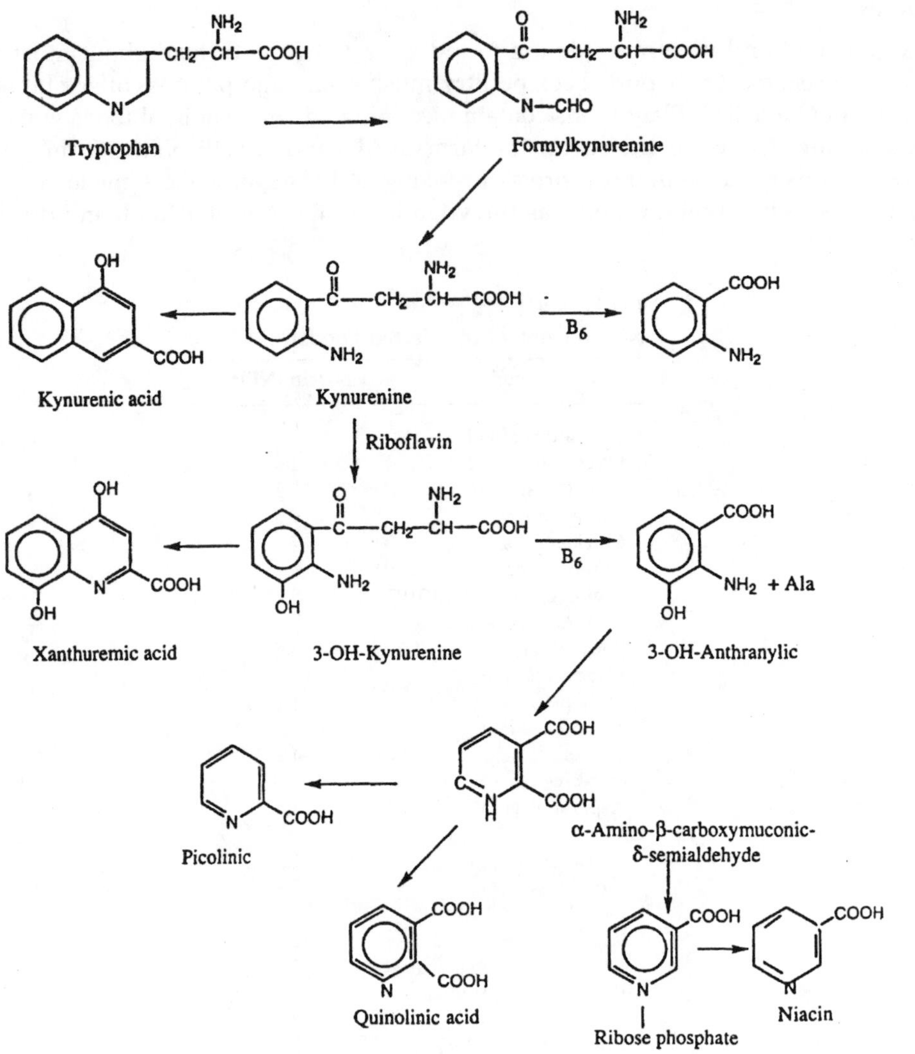

FIGURE 8.25
Biosynthesis of niacin from tryptophan.

sodium-dependent and saturable, facilitated diffusion carrier mechanism at lower luminal concentrations. As the luminal concentration increases, more niacinamide and nicotinic acid are absorbed by simple passive diffusion.

Metabolism and Functions

Nicotinic acid and niacinamide are both found in the plasma freely dissolved or bound to proteins (15 to 30%). In all human cells, nicotinamide is converted to NAD. Nicotinic acid can also be converted to NAD; however this seems to occur mostly in the liver. NAD can be phosphorylated to form NADP. NAD and NADP are involved in more than 200 enzymatic reactions, most of which are dehydrogenase reactions, and many are reversible. While most of the functions associated with NAD and NADP is attributable to their redox potential, more nonredox roles are becoming known.

With regard to carbohydrate utilization for ATP synthesis, NAD (NAD$^+$) is reduced in one reaction of glycolysis, the conversion of pyruvate to acetyl CoA in the mitochondria, and three reactions of the Krebs cycle (Figures 11.4 and 11.10). One NADH is created for each "turn" of β-oxidation of fatty acids, and the acetyl CoA created in this process can condense with oxaloacetate to form citrate (Figure 11.13). Two NADH are generated per ethanol molecule metabolized by alcohol dehydrogenase (Figure 11.16). The NADH generated by these reactions can be transferred to the electron transport chain for ATP generation. Beyond energy metabolism, NAD is involved in vitamin B$_6$ metabolism, as pyridoxal is converted to pyridoxic acid, a primary excretory metabolite. Beyond redox operations, NAD probably serves as a donor of ADP-ribose for posttranslational modification of proteins associated with chromosomes (i.e., histone and nonhistone proteins). Also, NAD is speculated to be a possible component of glucose tolerance factor (GTF).

NADP differs from NAD in that while most of the NADH generated is used to transfer electrons to the electron transport chain, most of the NADPH is used in synthetic processes. NADP is reduced to NADPH in 2 oxidative reactions of the pentose phosphate pathway (Figure 11.9). As mentioned previously, the pentose phosphate pathway is a means of generating NADPH for fatty acid synthesis. NADP is also reduced to NADPH by cytosolic malic enzyme, and this NADPH can be used for fatty acid synthesis as well. NADPH is also needed for cholesterol synthesis. In the rate-limiting reaction involving HMG-CoA reductase, 2 NADPH are used (Figure 5.11). NADPH is also used in steroid hormone synthesis and the synthesis of deoxynucleotides for DNA. NADPH may also be used by cells to help reduce dehydroascorbic acid to ascorbic acid.

Recommended Levels for Intake

Recommended intakes of niacin are expressed as niacin equivalents or milligram (mg) NE. Sixty milligrams of tryptophan is equal to 1 mg of niacin, and this factor is taken into consideration when determining the RDA. The range of intakes recommended for infants is 5 to 6 mg NE. For adolescents and adults, the recommendations range from 13 to 19 mg NE, and for those individuals who are more than 51 years of age, to 13 to 15 mg NE. During pregnancy and lactation, 17 mg NE and 20 mg NE are recommended, respectively.

Deficiency

As mentioned above, niacin deficiency can result in a syndrome called pellagra. Severe pellagra is characterized by the 4 Ds: dermatitis, diarrhea, dementia, and death. Gastrointestinal disturbances are common, including glossitis, stomatitis, abdominal discomfort, and severe diarrhea. The skin tends to become affected in areas exposed to light and in contact with heat. Lesions on the skin also develop, with loss of cells and desquamation. Dementia can occur, characterized by disorientation and confusion. A manic type of behavior may also be observed. The use of *isoniazid*, an antituberculosis drug and an antivitamin, can produce niacin deficiency symptoms relatively quickly, especially if the diet is previously marginal in niacin. An encephalopathy syndrome develops. Uncontrollable sucking reflexes, stupor, delirium, and agitated depression are common mental symptoms. Many victims of pellagra ended up in mental institutions because the dementia is irreversible.

Pharmacological Use and Toxicity

Nicotinic acid (niacin) is often prescribed in gram doses as a drug to lower blood cholesterol, LDL-cholesterol, and triglyceride levels in individuals with hypercholesterolemia and hypertriglyceridemia. Usually the dosage required varies depending on activity, age and sex of the individual. It is believed that nicotinic acid decreases mobilization of fatty acids from adipocytes, thereby decreasing circulation and uptake by the liver and incorporation into VLDL.

Large doses of niacin in the above form may produce toxic side effects such as heart abnormalities, GI problems, abnormal blood tests, hot flashes, skin irritations, liver damage, elevated blood glucose and peptic ulcers.

Vitamin B$_6$

Szent-Gyorgyi in 1935 demonstrated that dermatitis in rats was due to a new B complex factor. In 1939, Harris and Folks synthesized Vitamin B$_6$. A few years later, compounds were identified that had similar properties to the synthesized vitamin. In 1945, pyridoxal phosphate was discovered as an active coenzyme.

Vitamin B$_6$ appears in the body in six chemical forms. These forms are *pyridoxamine* (the amine form), *pyridoxal* (the aldehyde form), *pyridoxine*, or *pyridoxol* (the alcohol form), all of which have a 5′ phosphate derivative (Figure 8.26). Chemically, pyridoxine is stable to light and heat in acid solutions, but not at neutral or alkaline pH. Pyridoxal is probably the least stable.

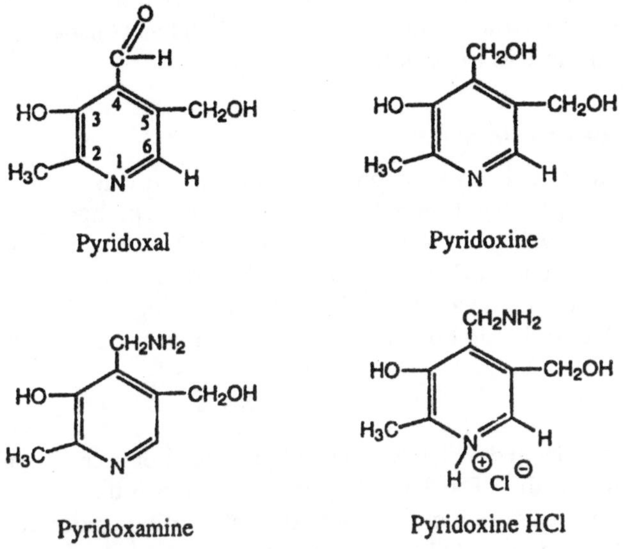

Pyridoxal

Pyridoxine

Pyridoxamine

Pyridoxine HCl

FIGURE 8.26
Structures of naturally occurring vitamin B$_6$. Pyridoxine hydrochloride is the commercially available form.

Food Sources

All six forms of vitamin B$_6$ are found in foods. Pyridoxine is mostly found in plant foods with better sources being bananas, navy beans, and walnuts (Table 8.9). Pyridoxal and pyridoxamine and their 5′-phosphorylated derivatives are almost exclusively found in animal products with better sources being meats, fish, and poultry. Vitamin B$_6$ is fairly stable in cooking processes; however, some losses are experienced with prolonged exposure to heat, light, or alkaline conditions as alluded to above. Also, the milling or refining of cereal grains removes vitamin B$_6$. For instance, the endosperm of a kernel of wheat contains only 6% of the pyridoxine, while the remainder is located in the germ (21%) and bran layers (73%).

TABLE 8.9
Vitamin B$_6$ Content of Selected Foods

Food	Vitamin B$_6$ (mg)
Meat and seafood	
Liver (3 oz)	0.8
Salmon (3 oz)	0.7
Chicken (3 oz)	0.4
Ham (3 oz)	0.4
Hamburger (3 oz)	0.4
Veal (3 oz)	0.4
Pork (3 oz)	0.3
Beef (3 oz)	0.2
Eggs	
Egg (1)	0.3
Legumes	
Split peas (2 c)	0.3
Beans, cooked (2 c)	0.2
Fruits	
Banana (1)	0.6
Avocado (2)	0.9
Watermelon (1 c)	0.2
Vegetables	
Brussels sprouts (2 c)	0.5
Potato (1)	0.7
Sweet potato (2 c)	0.2
Carrots (2 c)	0.3
Peas (2 c)	0.3

Absorption

Pyridoxal phosphate in the gut will react with an intraluminal intestinal alkaline phosphatase or other phosphatases to remove the phosphate group. Absorption of the three nonphosphorylated forms of vitamin B$_6$ then takes place by diffusion primarily in the jejunum. If the luminal concentration of the phosphorylated forms is high, then some will be absorbed as well. Vitamin B$_6$ absorption is relatively efficient and ranges roughly between 70 to 85% at physiological doses. However, the efficiency of absorption will decrease as the intake increases. Within enterocytes, some of the pyridoxine can be phosphorylated to pyridoxine phosphate via pyruvate kinase. Also, pyridoxal can be converted to PLP via the kinase. In essence, this is a method of trapping the vitamin within the mucosal cell and preventing movement back into the lumen.

Metabolism and Function

About 60% of the circulating vitamin B$_6$ is in the form of PLP and is transported either within cells such as erythrocytes or is bound to albumin. Circulating pyridoxal is also found in red blood cells as well as bound to albumin. Some pyridoxamine is also found in the blood. The liver is a primary organ involved in the metabolism of vitamin B$_6$. *4-Pyridoxic acid* and *pyridoxal lactone* are metabolites of PLP produced by tissue and are excreted in the urine (Figure 8.27). The former compound represents as much as one half of vitamin B$_6$ found in the urine. There are also two antivitamin B$_6$ compounds, desoxypyridoxamine and a methyl ester of pyridoxamine. They are thought to be produced by bacterial synthesis of the vitamin in the gut, but the general consensus is that they are insignificant to overall human vitamin B$_6$ status.

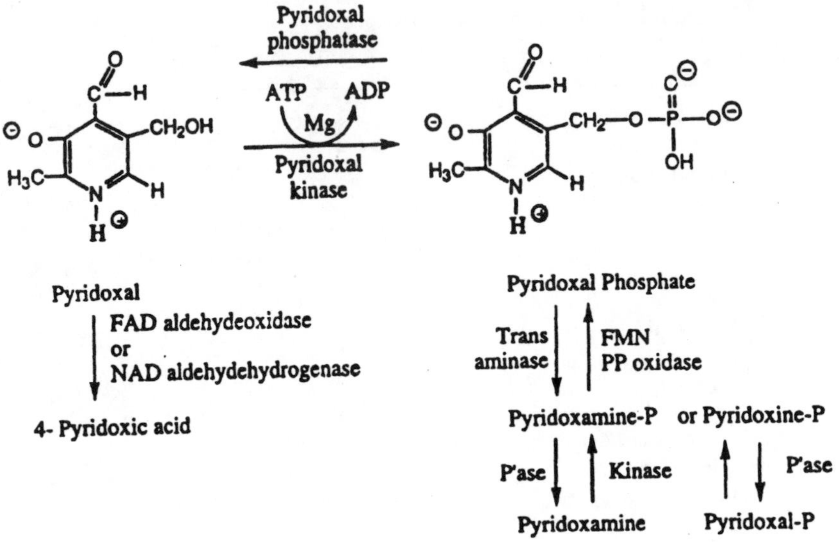

FIGURE 8.27
Phosphorylation of pyridoxal.

The functions of PLP are numerous, as it is involved in several metabolic pathways. The main function of PLP is to convert one type of amino acid to another type by transferring the amino group of one amino acid to a carbon skeleton in a Schiff base mechanism. This is called "transamination" (Figures 6.6 and 8.28). Transamination reactions reversibly pass an amino group from a donor amino acid to an α-keto acid such as pyruvate and α-ketoglutarate. For instance, alanine amino transferase (ALT) passes the amino group from alanine to an α-keto acid to form pyruvate and an α-amino acid. More likely than not, α-ketoglutarate accepts the amino group to form glutamic acid (glutamate). In another reaction, aspartate amino transferase (AST) catalyzes the transfer of an amino group from aspartate to an α-keto acid to form an α-amino acid and oxaloacetate. ALT is sometimes referred to as alanine-pyruvate transaminase.

During fasting and starvation or prolonged aerobic exercise, muscle cell α-ketoglutarate receives an amino group from branch-chain amino acids (leucine, isoleucine, valine) and aspartate to form glutamate. Subsequently the amino group of glutamate can be transferred to pyruvate to form alanine, via alanine amino transferase. Alanine can then be released from skeletal muscle and circulate to the liver for conversion back to pyruvate and gluconeogenesis. PLP is also critical for the deamination of certain amino acids via deaminase enzymes. As discussed earlier in this text, transamination and deaminase reactions are important for several reasons. First, they may allow the generation of carbon skeletons of amino acids for energy and other metabolic pathways. Also, transamination reactions allow for the creation of certain nonessential amino acids. PLP is also involved in decarboxylation reactions as well as in transulfhydration and desulfhydration reactions. For instance, the formation of γ-aminobutyric acid (GABA) from glutamate as well as the synthesis of serotonin from 5-hydroxytryptophan require PLP (Figure 8.29). PLP is pivotal in the formation of several other neurotransmitters, such as histamine, dopamine and norepinephrine. PLP is involved in the creation of the nonessential amino acid cysteine from methionine, the conversion of tryptophan to niacin, and the breakdown of glycogen as it may positively influence glycogen phosphorylase activity.

PLP is important to the production of aminolevulinic acid, which is necessary in heme production. Here, succinyl CoA condenses with glycine to form an intermediate molecule

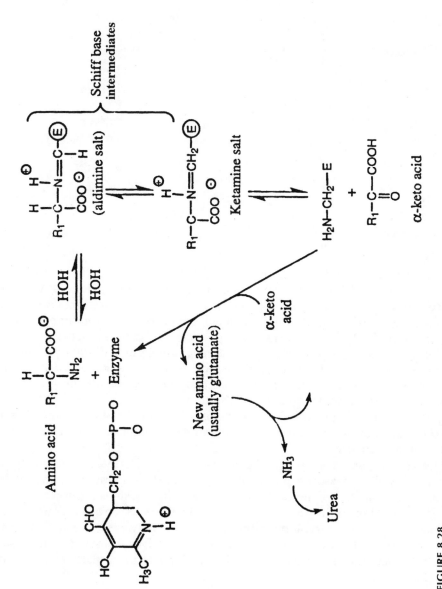

FIGURE 8.28
Schiff base mechanism for pyridoxal phosphate. R_1 represents an amino acid, encircled E is an apoenzyme.

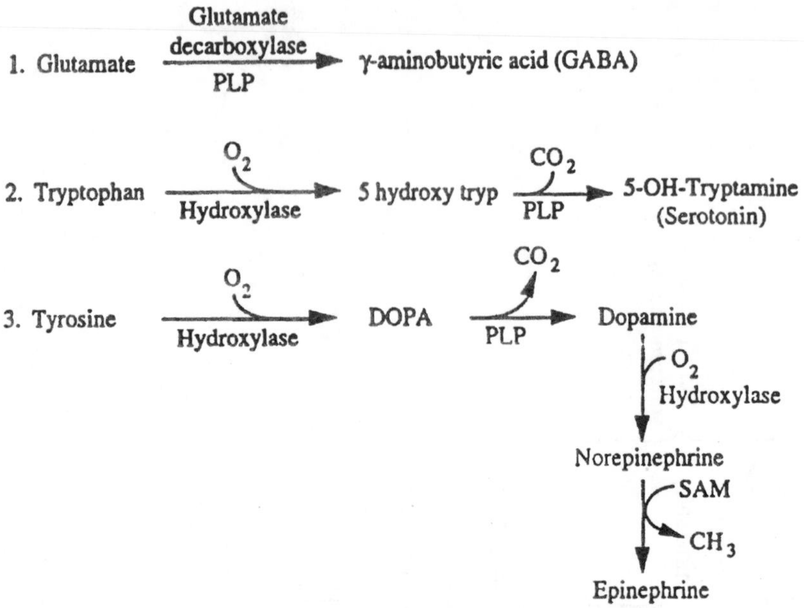

FIGURE 8.29
Formation of key neurotransmitters involving vitamin B_6.

which is subsequently decarboxylated by ALA synthetase (involving PLP), forming ami-nolevulinic acid (Figure 8.30). This compound is in turn dehydrated to form protoporphy-rin and heme. PLP also appears to be required for the incorporation of iron into the heme molecule. The importance of vitamin B_6 in hemoglobin formation is very important, as is demonstrated during a deficient state as hypochromic microcytic anemia occurs.

Interestingly, vitamin B_6 is probably involved in sphingolipid and other phospholipid synthetic processes. Research involving rodents, which began in the 1930s, demonstrated that a vitamin B_6 deficiency resulted in decreased body fat, decreased liver lipids, and an impairment in lysosomal lipid degradation. The conversion of the omega-3 polyunsatu-rated fatty acid linoleic acid to arachidonic acid is also dependent on PLP. Vitamin B_6 status also influences the immune system, as deficient animals demonstrated a hindered cell-mediated immune response.

Several tests can be performed to evaluate vitamin B_6 status. The most direct and perhaps most commonly applied measure is plasma PLP. However, it is important to note that other nutrition physiological factors, such as increased protein intake, smoking, and age can also influence PLP levels. In addition to plasma PLP, vitamin B_6 status can be evaluated by mea-suring urinary metabolites of tryptophan and methionine pathways as well as erythrocyte transaminase activity. However, the use of oral contraceptives is known to increase the activity of these transaminases, but decrease vitamin B_6 pools, particularly in the blood.

Recommended Levels of Intake

The 1989 RDA for vitamin B_6 ranges from 1.4 to 2.0 mg for adolescents and adults. During pregnancy an additional 0.2 mg is recommended, totaling 2.2 mg, and for lactation, an additional 0.1 mg, is recommended, to total 2.1 mg.

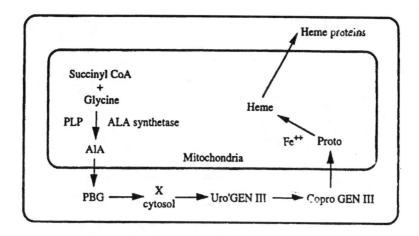

Abbreviations used:
ALA — aminolevulnic acid
PBG — porphobilinogen
Uro GEN III — uroporphyrinogen III
Copro GEN III — coproporphyrinogen III
Proto — protoporphyrin IX
X — intermediates
Enzymes catalyzing heme biosynthesis are omitted,
  except ALA synthetase

FIGURE 8.30
Role of pyridoxal phosphate in heme biosynthesis.

Deficiency and Toxicity

Cases of vitamin B_6 deficiency, while rare, have been reported. Infants fed formula, whereby vitamin B_6 was accidentally destroyed by the high-heat treatment process of autoclaving, developed vitamin B_6 deficiency. Individuals being treated for tuberculosis are at increased risk of vitamin B_6 deficiency, as isoniazid drugs commonly prescribed are antagonists to vitamin B_6. Other drugs such as penicillamine, corticosteroids, and anticonvulsants can also inhibit vitamin B_6 activity. The production of acetaldehyde formed by alcohol (ethanol) metabolism may in turn destroy some vitamin B_6-associated structures.

Vitamin B_6 deficiency affects the CNS and can cause convulsions, particularly in infants and children, as well as other behavioral abnormalities. Depressive symptoms and peripheral neuritis are often observed. Poor growth, decreased antibody formation, and some vague symptoms such as weakness, irritability, and insomnia have also been reported. A dermatitis with lesions around the mouth, eyes, and nose is common. Niacin levels may also be depleted or lowered, which may confound the deficiency signs. Some inborn errors of metabolism have an impact on vitamin B_6 metabolism. For instance, in cystathionurea, where cystathione lyase is deficient, supplementation with vitamin B_6 may be used to help treat the disease. The immune response in humans may be compromised by poor vitamin B_6 status increasing the risk of infection and illness.

At one time, vitamin B_6 was advocated by health food stores as a treatment for premenstrual syndrome (PMS). Some woman who were taking 2 g/d developed toxic symptoms, such as pins and needles in the feet, caused by irreversible nerve damage. Numbness of the

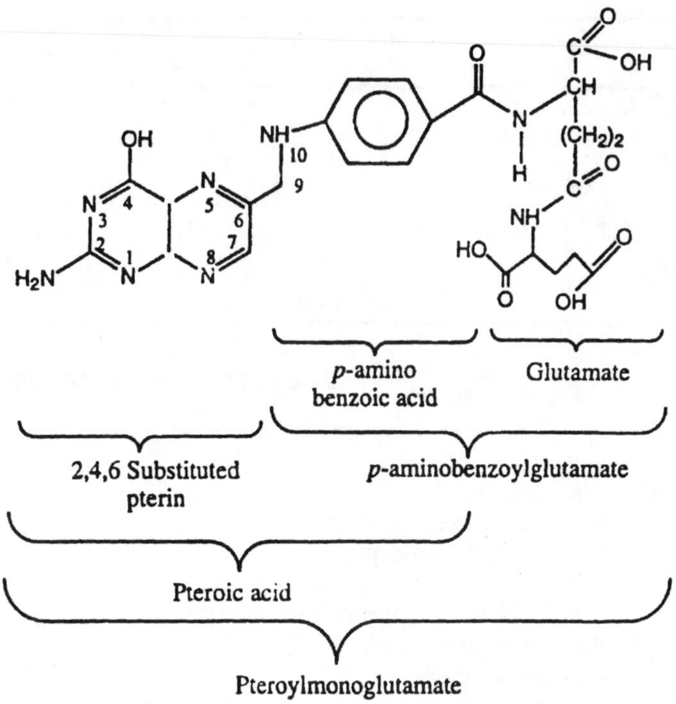

FIGURE 8.31
Structure of folic acid.

mouth can also occur. With regard to pregnancy, a drug once used for morning sickness, called Bendectin, a derivative of vitamin B_6, was commonly prescribed. This drug was banned by the FDA because of evidence that women who consumed it had a higher incidence of stillbirths, birth defects, and sudden infant death syndrome.

Folic Acid (Folate)

In 1930, folic acid was first termed "Wills factor." For a while it was confused with vitamin B_{12}, since a deficiency in both led to a similar type of anemia. In 1938, the term "vitamin M" was given to the folate in food, as it was recognized as an essential growth factor in monkeys. In 1939, folate was also called "factor U," and by 1940 the term "*Lactobascillus caessei* growth factor" was coined.

The structure of folic acid is best described as a complex of individual compounds as depicted in Figure 8.31. A *pterin* nucleus is bound to *paraaminobenzoic acid (PABA)* to form *pteroic acid*. Glutamic acid is linked to the PABA portion of pteroic acid, forming folate or pteroylmonoglutamatic acid or pteroylmonoglutamate. While all three components of folate can be synthesized by humans, there is a lack of the conjugase enzyme that condenses these components to form folate. Therefore, folate remains dietary essential.

Dietary Sources

Folate is available in a wide variety of foods derived from both animal and plant sources (Table 8.10). Better sources include vegetables such as asparagus, mushrooms, brussels sprouts, broccoli and turnip greens, legumes such as lima beans and peas, nuts, some fruits

TABLE 8.10

Folate Content of Selected Foods

Food	Folate (μg)
Vegetables	
Asparagus (1 c)	265
Brussels sprouts (1 c)	95
Black-eyed peas (1 c)	360
Spinach, cooked (1 c)	130
Lettuce, Romaine (1 c)	15
Lima beans (1 c)	110
Peas (1 c)	360
Sweet potato (1 c)	22
Broccoli (1 c)	160
Fruits	
Cantaloupe (1)	35
Orange juice (1 c)	75
Orange (1)	40
Grains	
Oatmeal (1 c)	50
Wild rice (1 c)	20
Wheat germ (1 T)	20

such as citrus and their juices, organ meats, and whole grain products. The name folate is derived from *folium* with respect to some of the better providers of this vitamin to the diet. Nonorgan meats are not a good source of folate. Furthermore, the limited availability of folate in meats is drastically reduced during cooking, as folate is generally unstable in heat. This also means that foods consumed raw will retain more of their folate content. It is estimated that as much as 50 to 80% of the folate in foods may be lost during processing and preparation.

Absorption

As naturally found in foods, folate may have as many as nine or more glutamate residues attached to PABA. However, only the monoglutamate form is found in human plasma. Thus, polyglutamates must be digested to the absorbable monoglutamate form. This process is performed by intestinal *conjugases* or *γ-glutamylcarboxypeptidases*, which are primarily active in the jejunum. These enzymes are both soluble and membrane-bound proteins. Most of the folate absorbed is believed to occur via a sodium-dependent, saturable, carrier-mediated mechanism on the brush border. A reduction in folate absorption caused by cyanide uncoupling of oxidative phosphorylization has made it clear that folate absorption is an energy-requiring process. However, when the luminal concentration of folate increases, passive absorption increases as well. Passive absorption may account for 20 to 30% of folate absorption, even at physiological doses. While bioavailability will vary between food sources, the net absorption of folate is approximately 50%. The bioavailability of cooked lima beans may be 95 to 96% or as low as 25% in romaine lettuce.

As at least one of the conjugases is zinc dependent, zinc deficiency can decrease folate absorption. Excessive alcohol consumption as well as drugs such as sulfinpyazone, phenylbutazone, ethacrynic acid, and furosemide (Lasix) will also decrease folate absorption by inhibiting digestion or competing for absorptive mechanisms. Once inside the mucosal enterocyte, folic acid may be reduced successively to *dehydrofolate* and then *tetrahydrofolate* (*THF*) and then methylated primarily at the N^5 position to form N^5-*methyl THF*.

Metabolism and Functions

Folate may be transported in portal and systemic blood, either freely dissolved or bound to blood proteins. While some of the folate is bound to albumin, it has a relatively low affinity for folate. Folate circulates as a monoglutamate. Folate-binding proteins (FBPs) have also been identified within blood cells, as well as in the plasma, and they have a higher binding affinity. Folate is taken into cells in a carrier-mediated fashion, which may require energy. Those human cells that turnover will have higher folate content. These include red blood cells, hepatocytes, and epithelial cells.

Within cells, the folate molecular structure can be metabolized in three ways. First, glutamic acid residues can be added to form polyglutamate forms of folic acid. This probably serves to "trap" folate within a cell. Second, folate is reduced on the pterin nucleus, at N^5 and N^8, and at C^6 and C^7, giving rise to tetrahydrofolate as depicted in Figure 8.32. (As stated above, tetrahydrofolate is abbreviated as THF or it is often abbreviated as H_4-folate or other ways.) $NADPH_2$ is required for the reduction as catalyzed by dihydrofolate reductase. Once in the THF form, which is sometimes referred to as the "active" form, the structure can accept single carbon moieties (Figure 8.33).

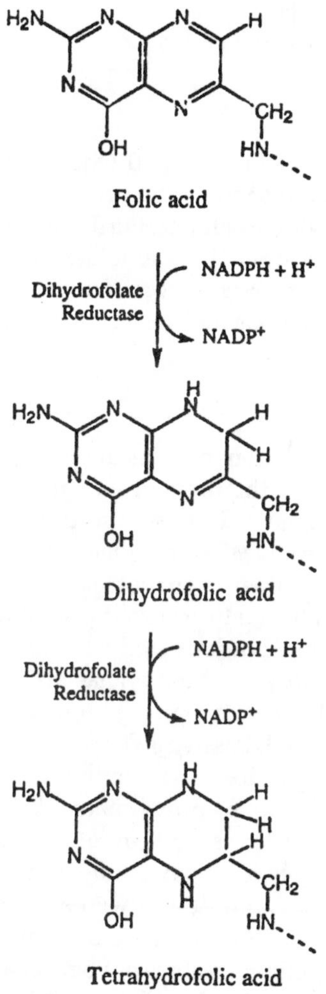

Folic acid

Dihydrofolate Reductase

$-$ NADPH + H$^+$

$\rightarrow$ NADP$^+$

Dihydrofolic acid

Dihydrofolate Reductase

$-$ NADPH + H$^+$

$\rightarrow$ NADP$^+$

Tetrahydrofolic acid

FIGURE 8.32
Activation of folic acid.

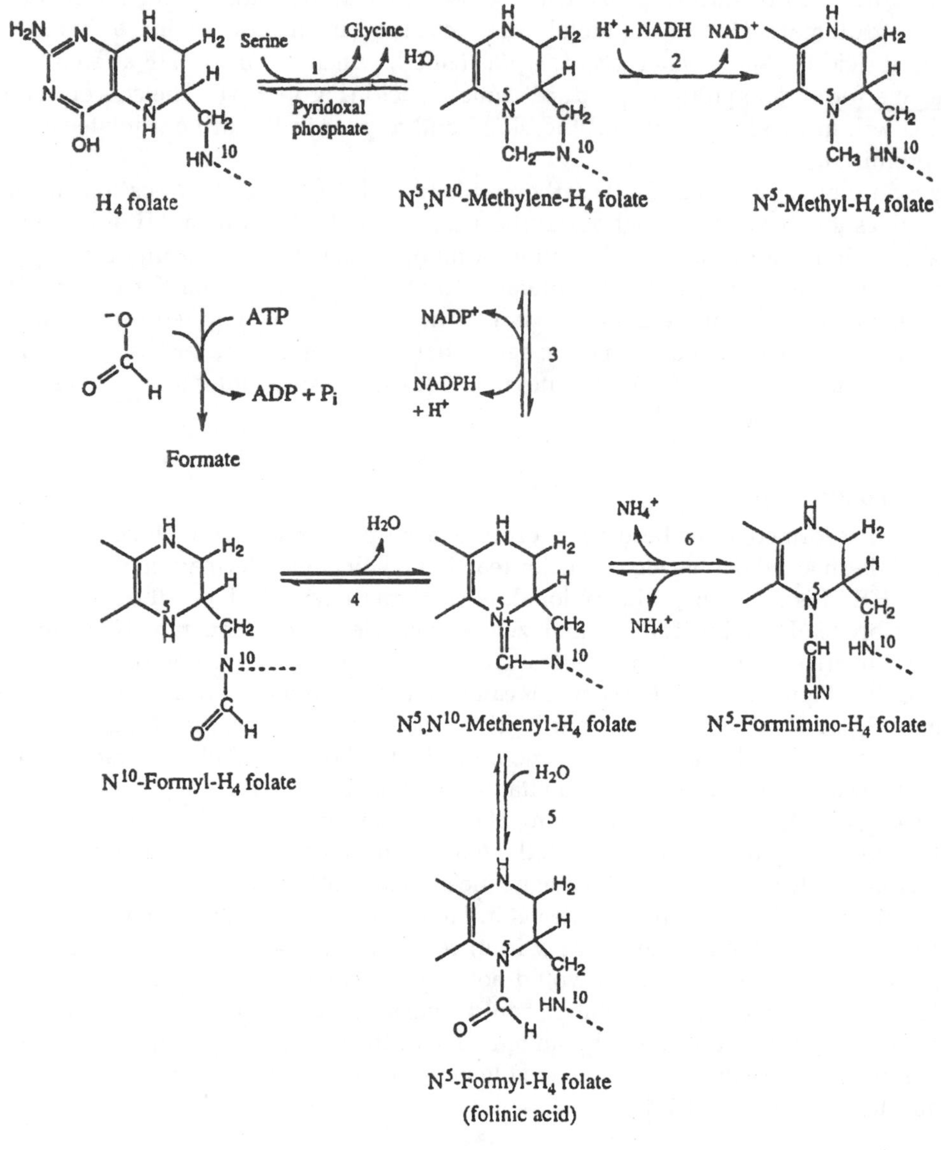

FIGURE 8.33
The interconversion of one-carbon moities attached to THF.

Carbon moieties or units can attach at the N^5 or N^{10} position or form a bridge between these positions. The carbon units are in the form of a methyl group as in N^5 *methyl THF*, an aldehyde group as in N^{10} *formyl-THF*, an imino group as in N^5 *formimino THF*, a methylene bridge as in N^5,N^{10} *methylene THF*, and a methylidyne bridge as in N^5,N^{10} *methylidyne/ methenyl THF*.

Once carbon moieties are attached to THF, then folate can become involved in a variety of synthetic and other metabolic processes. For instance, the single carbon unit from folate is used to make the amino acid methionine from homocysteine and serine from glycine as well as to synthesize nucleic acid precursor molecules (i.e., dTMP and purines). This is depicted in Figure 8.34. Because of this function and the need for replicating cells to copy their DNA prior to cell division, folate is recognized as one of the most important vitamins with regard to tissue turnover. Folate is also necessary in the complete catabolism of histidine to glutamate. One of the metabolites involved in the conversion of histidine to glutamic acid is *N-formiminoglutamic acid (FIGLU)*, which requires THF as a cofactor to remove a formimino group to produce glutamic acid (Figure 8.34). The concentration of FIGLU will increase in tissue and the blood and appear in the urine if folate stores are compromised.

Beyond the acquisition of single carbon units to THF, there are other possible molecular derivatives that have physiological significance. An aldehyde group at N^5 or N^{10} is possible as is an imino group at the N^5 position. Aminopterin, which has an amino group at N^4, is an antineoplastic drug and has antifolate activity. Other antivitamin forms are possible and are useful as chemotherapeutic agents, since folic acid is required for cell division. Methotrexate is one chemotherapeutic agent that inhibits folate metabolism as it hinders dihydrofolate reductase activity. The net result of methotrexate inhibition is a decrease in the conversion of folate to THF.

Methyl-Folate Trap

Once THF is formed, it can become involved in a couple of reactions in which a single-carbon unit is attached. However, the major reaction results in the formation of N^5,N^{10} methylene THF. This reaction is bidirectional. N^5,N^{10} methylene THF can then be converted irreversibly to N^5 methyl THF as catalyzed by methylene-THF reductase. N^5 methyl THF can be converted back to THF via the transfer of the methyl group to homocysteine to form methionine (Figure 8.34). This reaction is catalyzed by methionine synthase which requires vitamin B_{12} as a coenzyme. If vitamin B_{12} is deficient within a cell, then folate can become trapped as N^5 methyl folate. As more and more THF follows the pathway just described, a cell will become void of THF. Thus, a vitamin B_{12} deficiency can create a conditional folate deficiency, thereby explaining why many of the manifestations associated with deficiencies in these vitamins are the same. In fact, the macrocytic anemia that results from the conditional folate deficiency is used as a diagnostic indicator of a vitamin B_{12} deficiency.

If folate is provided by dietary means in larger doses, as with supplements, it would decrease the need for THF recycling within cells, via the vitamin B_{12}-required reaction. Therefore, the macrocytic anemia would not result and a vitamin B_{12} deficiency could go undetected. As folate supplementation could "mask" a vitamin B_{12} deficiency, folate levels in supplemental form are federally limited. One of the manifestations of a protracted and severe vitamin B_{12} deficiency is irreversible neurological alterations and the most critical manifestation would be death.

Recommended Levels for Folate Intake

Today, it is debated whether the current RDA for folate should be increased, given recent information regarding folate as it relates to spina bifida, still births, and even heart disease implications later on in life. The 1989 RDA for folate ranges from 150 to 200 µg for adolescents and adults. During pregnancy, the RDA is 400 µg, and declines to 280 µg during the first 6 months of lactation, and is then reduced slightly to 260 µg in the second 6 months of lactation. Whether the RDA during pregnancy should be increased further, especially during pregnancy, is still being debated.

Folate Deficiency and Toxicity

Deficiency will lead to a *megaloblastic macrocytic anemia*, as just mentioned. Here, red blood cells are large and immature and their numbers are reduced. This results in reduced

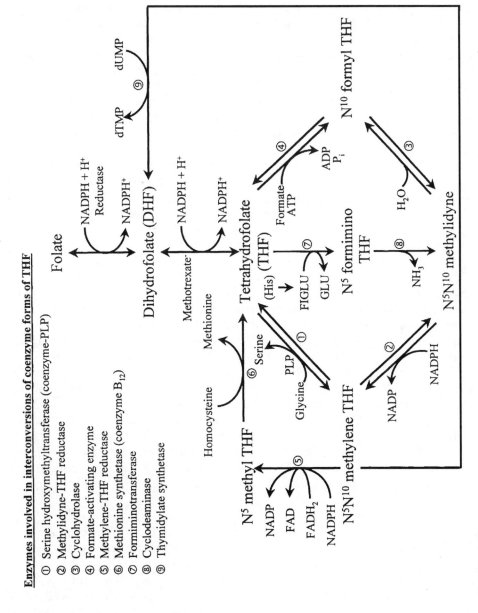

FIGURE 8.34
Metabolism of folic acid forms. From Grof, J.L. et al., *Advanced Nutrition and Human Metabolism*, West Publishing, NY, 1995.)

oxygen-carrying capacity of the blood. Pathological changes to the digestive tract mucosa also result from a folate deficiency. Mucosal villi shorten and the digestive tract wall thins. Much of this is due to a reduced ability of the mucosal lining to replace enterocytes being sloughed off into the lumen of the intestinal tract. Leukopenia, or decreased white blood cell count, is another sign of folate deficiency.

As folate is fundamentally important in rapidly dividing cells, good folate status is paramount during pregnancy, and the requirement increases accordingly. Individuals at greater risk of folate deficiency include those with chronically poor folate intake, women who have experienced multiple births, those enduring malabsorption situations (i.e., celiac disease), leukemia, Hodgkin's disease, cancer, burns, and even alcoholics. Cancer increases folate requirements due to the high reproductive rate of cancerous tissue.

Psychosis and mental deterioration are associated with folate deficiency. In pregnancy, neural tube defects have also been associated with elevated plasma homocysteine levels and low levels of folate. In a multinational study spanning nearly a decade, the recurrence risk of neural tube defect was reduced by 72% with periconceptual (4 weeks before and 8 weeks after conception) folate supplementation of 4 µg daily.

Folate supplements greater than 400 µg daily is considered a pharmacological dosage. While intakes of 15,000 µg resulted in insomnia, malaise, irritability, gastrointestinal problems, and decreased zinc status, other reports of folate supplementation stated that there were no significant effects in taking 10,000 µg for months to years. However, as mentioned above, folate supplementation potentially can mask a vitamin B_{12} deficiency.

Vitamin B_{12}

Vitamin B_{12} was the last of the water-soluble vitamins to be isolated and have its structure identified. This is partly due to this vitamin's relatively small requirement in comparison to other water-soluble vitamins. However, as far back as 1822, cases of anemia were described that were at that time believed to be due to a disorder of the gastrointestinal tract. As this particular type of anemia was associated with a potentially fatal prognosis, it became known as *pernicious anemia*, whereby "pernicious" meant "to lead to death." In 1860, Flint suggested that many of the individuals with this particular type of anemia exhibited degeneration of the stomach, and the glandular structures of the stomach appeared abnormal. In 1929, Castle demonstrated that normal gastric secretions contained a peptide that he called *intrinsic factor (IF)*. Furthermore, it was hypothesized that this IF combined with an extrinsic factor, and the combination of the two factors alleviated pernicious anemia. In 1948, Rickes, Smith, and Packer isolated vitamin B_{12} and in that same year, Beck demonstrated that vitamin B_{12} was the extrinsic factor or anti-pernicious anemia factor.

Vitamin B_{12} is composed of four pyrrole rings forming a porphyrin structure, as shown in Figure 8.35. This central part of the compound is called a corrin ring. The central core of the molecule contains cobalt, and thus the chemical name for this vitamin became known as cobalamin. There are a number of related compounds that have cobalamin-like activity. One compound is cyanocobalamin, where a cyanide (CN) group is present and attached to the cobalt atom and exists above the ring complex. The CN group must be removed before the molecule can be used as an active vitamin. Other substances can be attached to cobalt instead of cyanide, also existing above the ring structure, for instance, OH (hydroxocobalamin), CH_3 (methylcobalamin), H_2O (hydrocobalamin), NO_2 (nitrocobalamin), and 5′ deoxydenosyl (5′ deoxyadenosylcobalamin) as well as others. Below the ring a heterocyclic nitrogen side-chain may be present or nothing may be attached. Often a 5,6-dimethylbenzimidazole moiety is present as part of the attachment below the ring. Cobalt is in the Co^{3+}

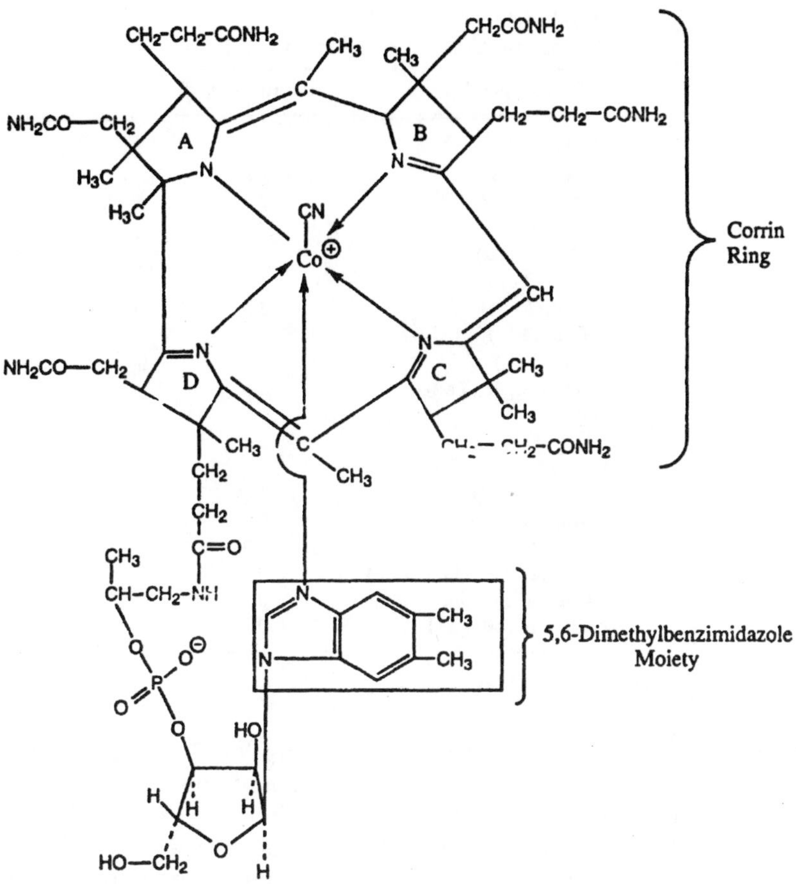

FIGURE 8.35
The vitamin B_{12} form, cyanocobalamin.

oxidation state and may form 6 bonds, 4 with the pyrrole nitrogen atoms, 1 with a attachment structure below the ring and one of the substances mentioned previously (i.e., CN, CH_3) in structures above the ring. Vitamin B_{12} is a rather stable compound. Subjecting it to extreme heat such as 100 to 120°C does not destroy the vitamin; however, intense ultraviolet light and visible light will result in significant destruction. Vitamin B_{12} is water soluble, especially in acid type solutions; however, acids will reduce its activity. The presence of other metals such as iron and copper, strong oxidizing elements, can also destroy the vitamin. It is insoluble in chloroform and other fat solvents. Vitamin B_{12} is synthesized by microorganisms and it also may be synthesized in a laboratory, although the latter is a difficult procedure.

Food Sources, Digestion, and Absorption

Vitamin B_{12} is only available from animal sources. However, animals derive their vitamin B_{12} from microbes inhabiting their digestive tract. The best sources of vitamin B_{12} are meats, fish, poultry, shellfish, eggs, milk, and milk products (Table 8.11). The vitamin B_{12} content in these foods is modest, however, compatible with human needs.

In order for vitamin B_{12} to be absorbed it must bind to IF, which is produced by the parietal cells of the stomach mucosa. IF is a glycoprotein with a molecular weight of approximately 50,000. This protein essentially protects vitamin B_{12} from degradation as it moves

TABLE 8.11
Vitamin B_{12} Content of Selected Foods

Food	Vitamin B_{12} (µg)
Meats	
Liver (3 oz)	6.8
Trout (3 oz)	3.6
Beef (3 oz)	2.2
Clams (3 oz)	2.0
Crab (3 oz)	1.8
Lamb (3 oz)	1.8
Tuna (3 oz)	1.8
Veal (3 oz)	1.7
Hamburger (3 oz)	1.5
Eggs	
Egg (1)	0.6
Milk and milk products	
Milk, skim (1 c)	1.0
Milk, whole (1 c)	0.9
Yogurt (1 c)	0.8
Cheese, American (1 oz)	0.2
Cheese, cheddar (1 oz)	0.2
Cheese, cottage (1 c)	0.5

through the intestinal tract to the ileum, the site of absorption. While the large intestine can also absorb some vitamin B_{12}, the mechanism is generally undefined. This absorption is more significant for bacterial synthesized B_{12}.

Vitamin B_{12} in foods is generally bound to proteins. Cooking of food will release some of the vitamin, and pepsin in stomach juice will free the remaining protein-bound vitamin B_{12}. The free vitamin then attaches to *R-proteins* which are present in the saliva and gastric juices. Vitamin B_{12} has a greater affinity for R-proteins than for IF. However, as R-proteins undergo subsequent digestion by proteases, vitamin B_{12} is released to IF to create a B_{12}-IF complex. Next, the B_{12}-IF complex will bind to specific receptors on the brush border and cross the intestinal mucosa, where B_{12} is released from IF and transferred to *transcobalamin II*. For the B_{12}-IF complex to attach to the receptor site, ionic calcium and a pH greater than 6.0 are needed. Vitamin B_{12} is transported into the mucosal enterocytes against a concentration gradient, so it is an active process and saturable as well. With pharmacological doses of vitamin B_{12}, an increasing percentage of absorption is attributable to passive diffusion. At lower levels of ingestion (i.e., 0.1 µg) absorption is approximately 80% efficient; however, as the dosage increases the percentage of absorption decreases.

Vitamin B_{12} is released on the serosal side to the portal blood supply most likely by pinocytosis. Transcobalamin II is the major plasma transport protein for this vitamin. *Transcobalamin I* is another protein that can transport vitamin B_{12} in the plasma, and it is also involved in vitamin B_{12} storage in the liver. Transcobalamin II is the major form in which the vitamin is delivered to the tissues. Methylcobalamin is the primary vitamin B_{12} form found in the blood, accounting for as much as 80%, while 5′ deoxyadenosylcobalamin makes up most of the remaining vitamin B_{12} in the blood.

Metabolism and Function

Vitamin B_{12} is somewhat unique compared with the other water-soluble vitamins in that it has significant storage and retention. The liver possess the greatest concentration of vitamin B_{12} and the total content of the liver may be 1.5 µg. Other tissue, such as the brain, kidneys, bone, spleen, and muscle also present relatively higher concentrations than other tissue. In the liver, the major form of the vitamin is 5'-deoxyadenosylcobalamin, which, as mentioned above, contrasts with the blood, in which the major form is methylcobalamin. In hepatocytes, vitamin B_{12} is added to bile, which flows to the small intestine. As mentioned above, vitamin B_{12} complexes with IF and is subsequently reabsorbed in the ileum and returns to the liver in the portal blood. Therefore, vitamin B_{12} experiences enterohepatic circulation. The vitamin B_{12} which is not absorbed from biliary secretions is excreted in the feces, thus making bile the primary means of ridding excessive vitamin B_{12}. About 40 µg enters biliary secretions daily; however, almost all is reabsorbed. Some urinary losses occur as well, and a typical urinary loss may be 0.025 µg/d.

Vitamin B_{12} appears to be involved in perhaps as few as three chemical reactions. One of the reactions involved is the conversion of homocysteine to methionine (Figure 8.34). Here, methylcobalamin is the coenzyme form and N^5 methyl THF is the methyl source. In this reaction, homocysteine methyltransferase (methionine synthetase) binds to vitamin B_{12} and N^5 methyl THF transfers the methyl moiety to cobalt of vitamin B_{12}. At this point, the methyl group, now bound to vitamin B_{12}, will be transferred to homocysteine to produce methionine. As mentioned in the discussion of folate, if there is a lack of vitamin B_{12}, an accumulation of N^5 methyl THF occurs. This is known as the "methyl folate trap." This creates a lack of reduced folate or THF, which is needed for nucleic acid metabolism. Such a block is responsible for the megaloblastic anemia characteristic of both vitamin B_{12} and folate deficiency.

Another reaction in which vitamin B_{12} plays a critical role is the conversion of L-methylmalonyl-CoA to succinyl CoA (Figure 8.36). Methylmalonyl CoA is produced from the catabolism of propionyl CoA, which itself is produced from the β-oxidation of odd-chain length fatty acids as well as the amino acids methionine, threonine, and isoleucine. This reaction is an isomerization reaction and requires the enzyme L-methylmalonyl CoA mutase along with the coenzyme 5'-deoxyadenosylcobalamin. In vitamin B_{12} deficiency, methylmalonyl CoA and methylmalonic acid accumulate in the blood. The latter compound is formed when methylmalonyl CoA is split. As neural tissue utilizes propionic acid, this may explain the peripheral neuritis that accompanies vitamin B_{12} deficiency.

In another chemcial reaction utilizing vitamin B_{12} as a coenzyme, L-leucine is isomerized to β-leucine, and vice versa. β-Leucine is created by intestinal bacteria and can be converted to L-leucine in a limited manner. Oppositely, L-leucine can be converted to β-leucine, which can undergo subsequent transamination. The latter mechanism requires PLP and is believed to be an alternative means of leucine catabolism.

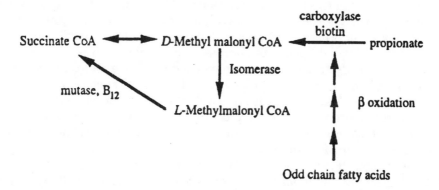

FIGURE 8.36
Overall reaction sequence in the conversion of propionate to succinate. Note the involvement of biotin and vitamin B_{12} as coenzymes.

Recommended Levels of Intake

The 1989 RDA for vitamin B_{12} is 2.0 µg for both adults and adolescents. For pregnancy, the RDA is 2.2 µg and increases to 2.6 µg during lactation. As mentioned above, the recommendations for vitamin B_{12} are small relative to other water-soluble vitamins. For instance, the next lowest recommendation for a water-soluble vitamin is folate, which is still 100× greater than vitamin B_{12} for adult males.

Deficiency

Individuals with limited amounts of vitamin B_{12} in their diets or who have a lack of intrinsic factor can develop pernicious anemia. The whole body turnover of vitamin B_{12} in an otherwise healthy adult is only about 0.1% daily. Therefore, it could take many months to years to develop a deficiency in an adult who previously was a well-nourished person. However, the limited development of vitamin B_{12} stores in infants in conjunction to being weaned to a vegetarian-based diet would be a greater risk. Also, individuals with gastric anomalies such as gastric by-pass and stapling or excessive pathology to the gastric mucosa would be at increased risk as well. These individuals would have a decreased ability to reabsorb the biliary vitamin B_{12}, due to a reduced presence of IF and R-proteins. In fact, as much as 95% of the vitamin B_{12} deficiencies in America are explained by malabsorption, not dietary intake. This disease is characterized by abnormally large immature red blood cells or macrocytic megaloblastic anemia. Accompanying symptoms include weakness, indigestion, abdominal pain, constipation altering with diarrhea, sore and glossy tongue, and damaged nerve fibers, via demyelination and degeneration. An individual can also exhibit a psychosis. These red blood cells are identical to those developed in a folate deficiency, leading to some confusion regarding treatment. As mentioned above, treating the individual with folate supplements may reverse the anemia, while the vitamin B_{12} deficiency worsens.

Biotin

Bateman in 1916 observed that feeding raw egg white resulted in toxic symptoms such as dermatitis in animals. Boas in 1927 further demonstrated that feeding particular food items could prevent this dermatitis In 1936, Koel and Tonnis isolated biotin from liver and at that same time proposed its structure. It was not until 1942 that the definite structure of biotin was proven by Vdu Vigneaud. At times, biotin was referred to as vitamin H.

Biotin is composed of two rings and a carbon chain that ends with a carboxyl group, as shown in Figure 8.37. Its scientific name is *cis*-hexahydro-2-oxo-1*H*-thieno-(3,4-d) imidazole-4-pentanoic acid. It has two rings, one that contains sulfur at the number 1 position. Biotin is stable in heat and light, both ultraviolet and visable, as well as in air when in its dry state. It is relatively soluble in both ethanol and water, with a relatively greater solubility in the former medium. When biotin is dissolved in an aqueous or solution environment, its properties change and it is susceptible to destruction by ultraviolet light or oxidation in either strong acid or alkali conditions. Humans are unable to synthesize biotin; however microorganisms in the gut will, and use cysteine as the source of sulfur. This allows gut microbial synthesis as a source of biotin to humans. There are as many as eight isomeric forms of biotin, but what is termed the D-biotin form has the greatest vitamin activity in humans. Biotinol and biocytin are two derivatives that have some biotin activity.

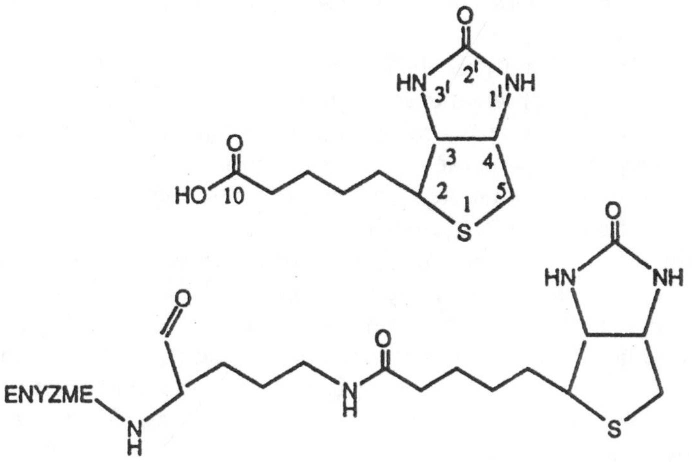

FIGURE 8.37
Biotin.

Biotin

Biotin in foods is fairly widespread, as it is found in every living cell. Better sources include organ meats, egg yolks, brewer's yeast, legumes, nuts, soy flour and soybeans, whole grains, and certain ocean fish. While egg yolks are a concentrated source of biotin, egg whites contain a protein called *avidin*, which has an extremely high affinity for biotin and substantially decreases its availability for absorption. Avidin is not stable in heat and is inactivated by cooking. In addition to food, biotin is produced by microbes in the human colon. Some of the biotin is believed to be absorbed.

Digestion and Absorption

In food, biotin is found either free or bound to proteins. The protein-bound form can be liberated via proteases yielding free biotin forms, predominantly biotin and secondarily biocytin. An intestinal enzyme, which also appears to be in the blood, can cleave the lysine portion bound to biocytin, to release biotin. Biotin is absorbed by facilitative diffusion, mostly in the jejunum of the small intestine. The presence of avidin, as provided by rough eggs (whites) would significantly decrease biotin absorption efficiency; however, cooking denatures the avidin and eliminates this potential problem.

Metabolism and Function

Biotin is transported primarily as free biotin and bound to plasma proteins such as albumin, α- and β-globulins, and a biotin-binding protein. It is excreted largely by urinary filtration as biotin and to a minor degree, biotin metabolites such as bisnorbiotin, biotin sulfone, and biotin sulfoxide. Biotin appears to be stored, at least to a minor degree, in muscle, brain, and the liver.

Biotin is critical, as it is needed to metabolize carbohydrates, fatty acids, and the amino acid leucine. The carboxylase enzymes that require biotin as a coenzyme are *acetyl CoA carboxylase*, *β-methylcrotonyl CoA carboxylase*, *pyruvate carboxylase*, and *propionyl CoA carboxylase*. Essentially, these enzymes attach to biotin as does carbon dioxide, where the carbon dioxide (via HCO_3^-) is added to a substrate. Biotin is activated in cells to biotinyl

5′-adenylate before it becomes involved in these complex processes. The activation process requires ATP and magnesium.

Acetyl CoA carboxylase catalyzes the addition of carbon dioxide to acetyl CoA to form malonyl CoA in the cytosol of cells such as hepatocytes and adipocytes. This energy-requiring reaction is the first step in fatty acid synthesis. Propinyl carboxylase catalyzes another biotin-dependent reaction. Here, the addition of carbon dioxide to propionyl CoA, again via HCO_3^-, results in D-methylmalonyl CoA, which subsequently is converted to succinyl CoA and enters the Krebs cycle (Figure 8.36).

In a third biotin-dependent reaction, pyruvate carboxylase converts pyruvate in the mitochondria to oxaloacetate. Depending upon the metabolic state of the cell, oxaloacetate can be utilized for gluconeogenesis or condense with acetyl CoA to form citrate, the first molecule of the Krebs cycle. The last carboxylase reaction is involved in the catabolism of leucine. Here β-methylcrotonyl CoA carboxylase catalyzes the conversion of β-methylcrotonyl CoA to β-methylglutaconyl CoA, which is subsequently split to acetoacetate and acetyl CoA. There may be other not well-defined reaction pathways where biotin has a role, including deamination of some amino acids, tryptophan metabolism, purine synthesis, oxidative phosphorylation, and synthesis of tRNA.

Recommended Levels for Intake

At this time there is not a RDA for biotin, but there is an estimated daily safe and adequate intake (ESADDI). For adolescents and adults, the range is from 100 to 200 µg. Meanwhile, the recommendation for infants is 35 µg/d for the first 6 months and 50 µg for the second 6 months. Recommendations for children between 1 to 10 years of age range between 65 to 120 µg.

Deficiency and Toxicity

Biotin deficiency does not occur naturally, except if the intake is marginal and there is a chronic consumption of raw egg whites. Most of the cases of known biotin deficiency are the result of individuals with an inborn error of metabolism when there is insufficient biotinase activity to free the lysine from the biotin. In documented animal studies, as in cases of human biotin deficiency, a dermatitis is the most striking deficiency symptom. The skin presents patches of dried out tissue and a scaly nature. In these areas, the loss of the cells results in a grayish hue.

Biotin deficiency results in a loss of epithelial cells, and the tongue papillae are compromised as is the mucosal lining of the gastrointestinal tract. Anorexia and nausea have also been documented. Alopecia, growth retardation, auditory and visual loss, metabolic acidosis, and elevated blood ammonia levels are other symptoms. On the contrary, biotin toxicity has yet to be documented.

Pantothenic Acid

Pantothenic acid first gained notice around 1931 when a pellagra-like dermatitis was described by Ringrose. In 1933, Williams gave the name "pantothenic acid" to a compound that was a growth factor for yeast. In 1939 the compound was identified as an antidermatitis factor in chicks. Then, in 1940, Williams synthesized pantothenic acid, followed by the

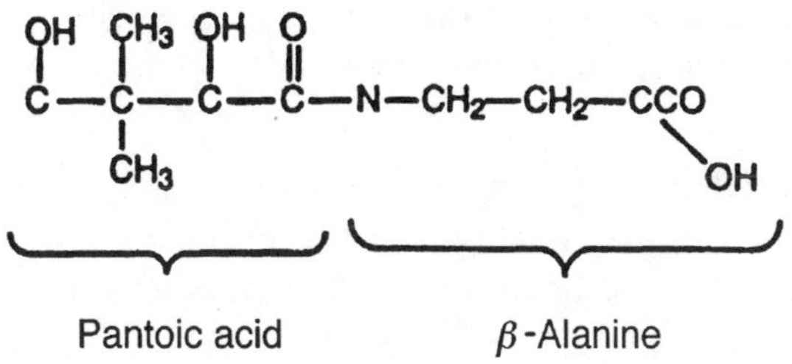

FIGURE 8.38
Pantothenic acid.

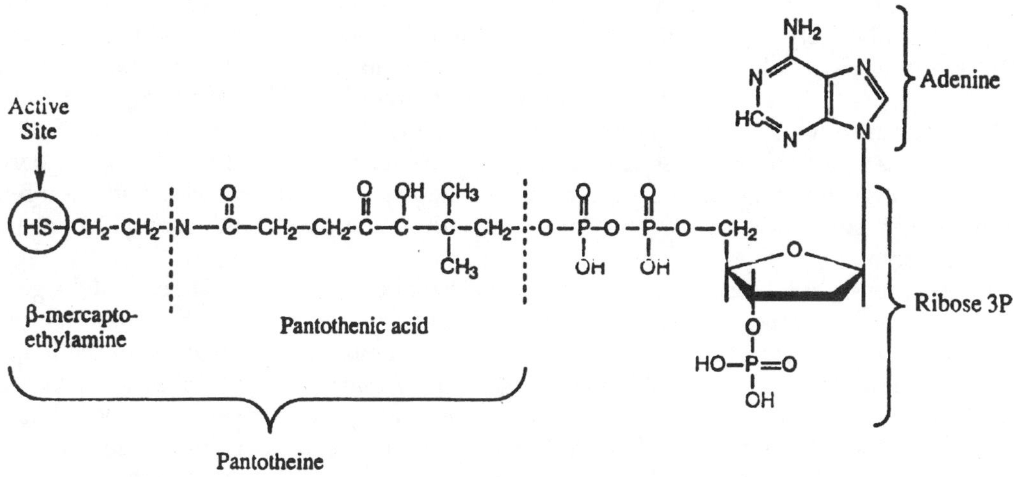

FIGURE 8.39
Coenzyme A.

characterization of coenzyme A as being the active form of pantothenic acid by Kaplan and Lipmann in 1948.

While pantothenic acid is active as a structural component of coenzyme A (Figures 8.38 and 8.39), pantothenic acid itself is composed of two principal parts: *β-alanine* and *pantoic acid*. Its scientific name is dihydroxy-β,β-dimethylbutyryl-β-alanine. Pantothenic acid is stable in air and light when in the dry state. It is soluble in both water and acetic acid. At neutral pH in solution, it is stable, but it is readily destroyed by heat and alkali or acid pH. It may also decompose when heated.

Food Sources

Pantothenic acid is widespread in foods, from both animal and plant sources. In fact, its name is derived from the Greek word *pantos* which means "from every side" or "from everywhere." Richer sources include certain organ meats, egg yolk, meats, fish, whole grain cereals, legumes, mushrooms, broccoli, avocados, and royal jelly from bees.

Digestion and Absorption

Almost all (85%) of the pantothenic acid in foods is provided as part of coenzyme A. During digestion, pantothenic acid is liberated, first to pantotheine which is then converted to pantothenic acid. Absorption, occurring principally in the jejunum, is mostly of a passive nature and the efficiency of absorption is approximately 50% with physiological doses and decreases as the dosage increases. Pantothenol and salts of pantothenate (i.e., calcium pantothenate) are typically used in supplements.

Metabolism and Function

Absorbed pantothenic acid is transported in the portal vein. In the plasma, pantothenic acid is found largely in the form of coenzyme A in RBC. Free coenzyme A is also found in RBCs, as well as dissolved in the plasma, but to a lesser extent. Pantothenic acid excretion is mainly by renal filtration and typical urinary pantothenic acid levels are 1 to 4 μg daily. The mechanism for uptake of pantothenic acid by various tissue differs between active and passive processes. For instance, in the liver and cardiac and skeletal muscle, panthenic acid is transported into cells in a sodium-dependent, active process. On the other hand, in the central nervous system as well as in adipose and renal tissue, uptake appears to be passive.

Once in cells, pantothenic acid is largely used to make coenzyme A. Because of the general involvement of coenzyme A in energy metabolism, its concentration is higher in more metabolically active tissue such as the heart, liver, kidneys, adrenal gland, and the brain. Coenzyme construction is shown in Figure 8.40. Briefly, pantothenic acid is phophorylated to 4′ phosphopantothenate in an ATP-requiring step catalyzed by the enzyme pantothenate kinase. Then, cysteine is attached to 4′–phosphopantothenate to form 4′–phosphopantothenyl cysteine in another ATP-requiring reaction. The addition of cysteine provides coenzyme A with a fairly exposed sulfur region. Subsequently CO_2 is removed from 4′–phosphopantothenyl cysteine producing 4′–phosphopantotheine, which in turn is converted to dephosphocoenzyme A and then to coenzyme A in two ATP-requiring reactions. The first of the last two reactions utilizes ATP as a source of AMP. AMP is added to the molecule and the last step involves phosphorylation of a hydroxyl group of dephosphocoenzyme A.

Coenzyme A, and thus pantothenic acid, is fundamentally involved in the metabolism of the energy providing nutrients: carbohydrates, protein, fat, as well as alcohol (ethanol). Coenzyme A bonds to the carboxylic acid portion of molecules as its sulfur forms a *thio-ester* covalent link. This is said to "activate" the molecules, thereby allowing them to proceed in subsequent reactions of energy pathways. One of the most common molecules that coezyme A activates is acetic acid (acetyl CoA), which is the product of fatty acid and certain amino acid oxidations as well as the product of pyruvate and ethanol oxidation. Propionic acid is also activated by coenzyme A to form propionyl CoA. Propionic acid is either found in foods such as fish or derived from the oxidation of odd-chain fatty acids and certain amino acids (methionine, leucine, isoleucine), and methylmalonic acid (methylmalonyl CoA) formed as an intermediate in the conversion of propionyl CoA to succinyl CoA. Succinic acid is also activated to succinyl CoA, which is a Krebs cycle intermediate, as well as other key intermediate acids.

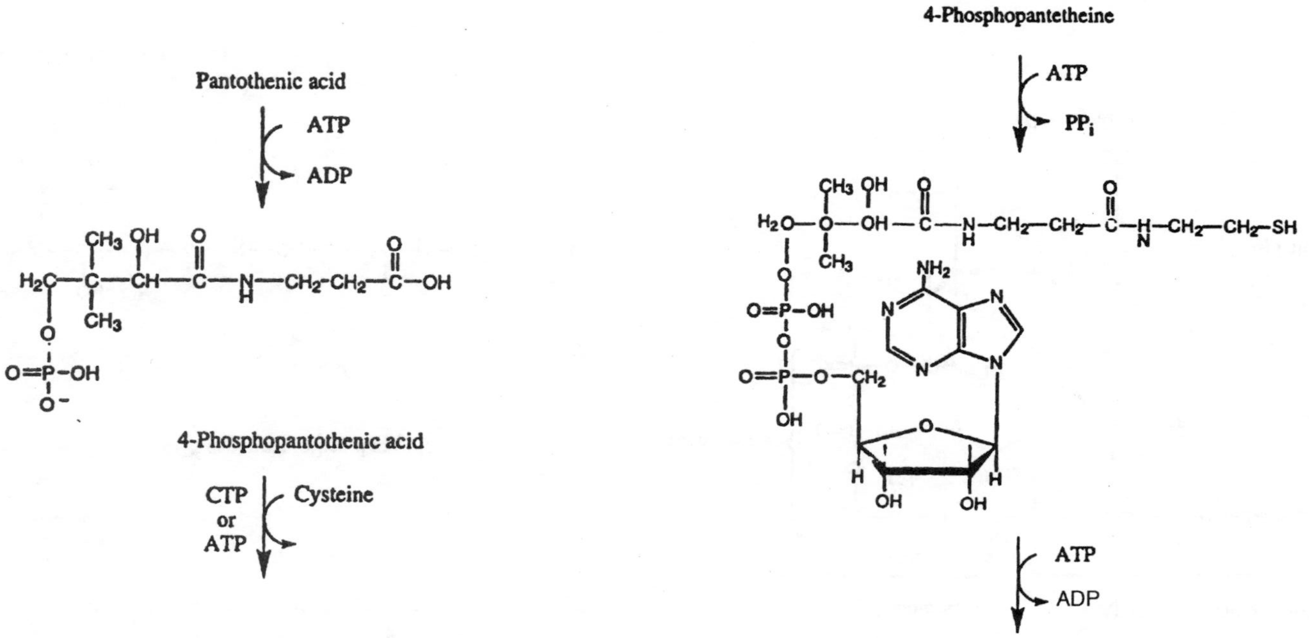

FIGURE 8.40
Mechanism for the formation of coenzyme A, using pantothenic acid as a building block.

(continues)

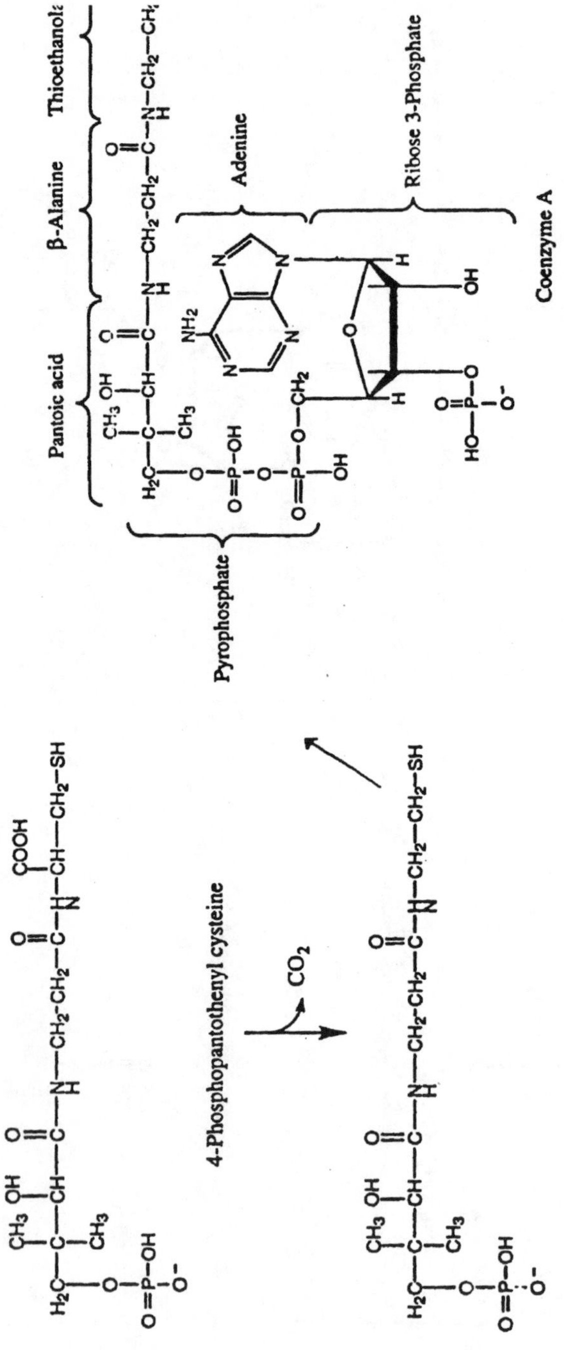

FIGURE 8.40 (continued)

As mentioned numerous times in this text, acetyl CoA can condense with oxaloacetate to form citrate, the first molecule of the Krebs cycle. Acetyl CoA can also be used to make ketone bodies in the liver, as well as being the building block for fatty acid and cholesterol synthesis. Furthermore, when fatty acids are to become involved in processes such as β-oxidation or attachment in phospholipids they must first be activated by binding of coenzyme A.

A second function of pantothenic acid is to serve as a component of *acyl carrier protein* (ACP) whose structure is shown in Figure 8.41. ACP is a component of the large fatty acid synthase (FAS) discussed in Chapter 5. ACP, as a component of FAS, binds to nascent fatty acids during the synthetic process. Other functions of pantothenic acid are somewhat more vague. As coenzyme A, pantothenic acid may be involved in the posttranslational acetylation of key cellular proteins such as histones and cytoskeletal proteins, thereby increasing their stability against proteases such as ubiquitin.

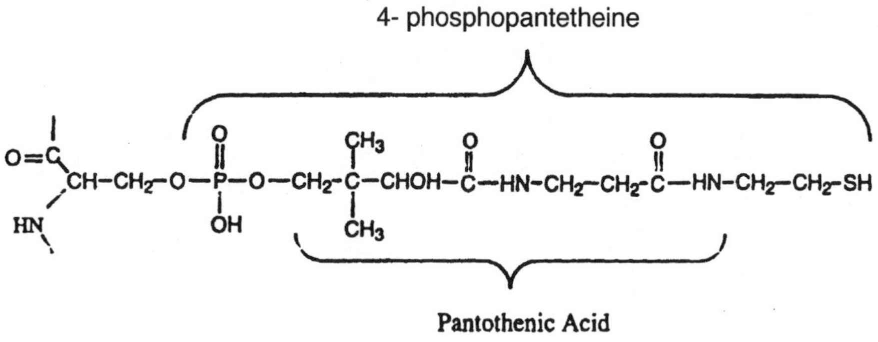

4- phosphopantetheine

Pantothenic Acid

FIGURE 8.41
Acyl carrier protein (ACP).

Recommended Levels of Intake

Currently there is not a RDA for pantothenic acid. An estimated and safe adequate intake is 4 to 7µg for adults. For infants, 2 µg and 3 µg are recommended in the first 6 months and after the first 6 months, respectively. Children and adolescent recommendations are 3 to 4 µg.

Deficiency and Toxicity

Deficiency of pantothenic acid is rare and takes several weeks to develop. In experimental studies, a pantothenic acid deficiency can be produced by feeding L-isomers of pantothenic acid. Other antagonist of pantothenic acid include methylpantothenic acid, pantoyl-amino-ethanothiol, and pantoyl taurine. Symptoms of a pantothenic acid deficiency include "burning feet syndrome," which is a feeling of tingling and tenderness in the feet. Other symptoms include headache, fatigue, impaired motor function, muscle cramps, disturbances of the digestive tract, and vomiting. However, more extreme manifestations can result, such as ulcerations, cardiac tachycardia, hypotension, reduced eosinophil output, hypochromic anemia, and hypoglycemia. Pantothenic acid, however, is not stored well in the human body and urinary levels reflect dietary intake. There have been no reports of pantothenic acid toxicity at present.

Suggested Readings

Berdanier, C.D., *Advanced Nutrition: Micronutrients*, CRC Press, Boca Raton, FL, 1995.

Combs, G.F., *The Vitamins*, Academic Press, San Diego, CA, 1992.

Present Knowledge in Nutrition, Ziegler E.E. and Filer, L.J., Eds., ILSI Press, Washington, D.C., 1996.

Groff, J.L., Gropper, S.S., and Hunt, S.M., *Advanced Nutrition and Human Metabolism*, West Publishing, New York, N.Y., 1995.

9

Major Minerals

In comparison to the macronutrients discussed in the preceding chapters, the requirement of minerals and their contribution to total body weight is relatively small. For instance, while some 20 to 25 minerals are known to have human physiological significance, collectively they constitute less than 5 to 6% of total human mass. On the other hand, water, protein, fat, and carbohydrates make up the majority of the remaining human mass.

Minerals are typically divided into two general categories: major minerals and trace minerals (Table 9.1). Minerals whose estimated average daily dietary need is 100 mg or more and represent more than 0.01% of total human mass are considered *major* minerals. This is to say that, for a 70-kg individual, a particular major mineral would contribute at least 7 g to their total body mass. However, many nutritionists prefer to classify the minerals based solely upon dietary need. The major minerals include calcium (Ca), phosphorus (P), sodium (Na), potassium (K), chloride (Cl), and magnesium (Mg). Sulfur (S) is often included in this category because of its contribution to human mass; however, its dietary need remains questionable. Only the major minerals will be discussed in detail in this chapter. The remaining minerals, deemed minor or trace minerals, will be discussed in the next chapter.

TABLE 9.1
Minerals of the Human Body

Major Minerals	Trace Minerals
Calcium	Iron
Phosphorus	Copper
Sulfur	Selenium
Potassium	Manganese
Sodium	Iodine
Chloride	Fluoride
Magnesium	Vanadium
	Cadmium[a]
	Tin[a]
	Chromium
	Boron
	Zinc
	Molybdenum
	Nickel
	Arsenic
	Cobalt[a]
	Silicon[a]
	Lithium[a]

[a] Dietary essentiality questionable despite presence in body.

Calcium

Calcium is a divalent cation (Ca^{2+}) and is the most abundant mineral in the human body. It accounts for roughly 40% of total mineral mass and about 1.5% of total body mass. Approximately 99% of the calcium within the human body is located within bone and teeth where it provides more of a structural service. The remaining 1% of body calcium is found within intracellular and extracellular fluids. This calcium plays more functional roles. Calcium nutrition has become a concern for many individuals because of the heightened incidence of osteoporosis as human life expectancy continues to increase. Also, calcium has become a consideration for many individuals as more is becoming known about its potential involvement in cancer prevention and hypertension.

Dietary Sources

Dairy products tend to be the greatest contributors of calcium to the human diet. As much as 55% of calcium in the American diet is derived from dairy products. For instance, a glass of milk will supply about 300 mg of calcium. Beyond dairy products, good sources of calcium include sardines, oysters, clams, tofu, molasses, almonds, calcium-fortified foods, and dark green leafy vegetables such as broccoli, kale, collards, mustard, and turnip greens (Table 9.2). Other vegetables such as spinach, rhubarb, chard, and beet greens contain respectable amounts of calcium. However, *oxalates* and *phytate* found in these foods can bind to calcium in the digestive tract and decrease its absorption. For example, as little as 5% of the calcium in spinach is actually absorbed.

Calcium-containing complexes rank among the most popular individual nutrient supplements. For the most part, these supplements are used with hopes to increase bone density and or to perhaps minimize the rate of bone calcium loss. Amino acid chelates of calcium, calcium carbonate, calcium acetate, calcium citrate, as well as calcium gluconates, phosphates, lactates, and oyster shells are the most common forms of calcium supplements.

TABLE 9.2
Calcium Content of Selected Foods

Food Source	Calcium (mg)
Milk and milk products	
Yogurt, low fat (1 c)	448
Milk, skim (1 c)	301
Cheese, Swiss (1 oz)	272
Cheese, cheddar (1 oz)	204
Ice cream (1 c)	180
Ice milk (1 c)	180
Custard (2 c)	150
Cottage cheese (2 c)	70
Vegetables	
Collard greens (2 c)	110
Spinach (2 c)	90
Broccoli (2 c)	70
Legumes and products	
Tofu (2 c)	155
Dried beans (2 c)	50
Lima beans (2 c)	40

Here the associated molecule is merely ionically complexed to calcium. About 36 to 42% of the calcium in calcium carbonate is absorbed. This is perhaps the most widely used calcium supplemental form. The calcium in calcium citrate, calcium acetate, calcium lactate, and calcium gluconate is absorbed at about 24 to 36%. Recently, calcium citrate malate (CCM) has been utilized by some food manufacturers (i.e., manufacturers of orange juice), as researchers have reported very efficient absorption. Calcium supplements should be taken with a snack or meal, and it is not advised to take single large doses since calcium supplements will be better absorbed when distributed throughout the day.

Absorption

Calcium, either derived from foods or supplements, is in the form of insoluble salts. Therefore, in order for calcium to be absorbed it must be liberated to its ionized form. However, calcium in its ionized form may also form chelates with certain dietary factors such as other minerals and fiber-associated substances. These ionic chelations can potentially decrease calcium absorption, especially in more neutral pH environments such as the small intestine.

Several factors that may decrease the absorption of calcium include: (1)presence of oxalate, phytate, and fibers in foods; (2) rapid movement of food through the intestine as with higher fiber intake; (3) very high fat diet or decreased fat digestion; (4) excess vitamin A intake; (5) excessive dietary phosphorus and magenesium. A calcium:phosphorus ratio of 1:1 to 3:1 is considered optimal. Magnesium, is also a divalent cation and it is believed that magnesium can compete with calcium for absorptive mechanisms. Interestingly, decreased physical activity may also be associated with decreased calcium absorption efficiency. Table 9.3 lists many of the factors that influence calcium absorption.

TABLE 9.3
Factors Influencing Calcium Absorption

↑ Calcium Absorption	↓ Calcium Absorption
↑ Vitamin D and PTH[a]	↓ Vitamin D and PTH[a]
lactose during same meal	phytate, fiber, and
↑ Need (growth, pregnancy,	oxalates during same meal
lactation)	↓ Need

[a] PTH = parathyroid hormone.

Phytate (inositol hexaphosphate) is found in fibrous plant sources such as legumes, nuts, and cereals. A molar ratio greater than 0.2 of phytate:calcium has been suggested to increase the risk of calcium deficiency. Oxalate can also bind ionized calcium in the digestive tract and decrease its absorption. Oxalate is found in various vegetables (i.e., spinach, eggplants, beets, celery, greens, okra), fruits (i.e., berries), nuts (i.e., peanuts and pecans) and beverages (tea, Ovaltine, cocoa). High fat diets, or decreased fat digestion, may decrease calcium absorption by allowing for the formation of calcium soaps. These soaps are ionically formed between the acid portion of a fatty acid and calcium.

Contrarily, calcium absorption is enhanced by several factors. These factors include: (1) healthy vitamin D status; (2) acid conditions in the digestive tract (prevents precipitations); (3) presence of lactose in the digestive tract; (4) lack of stress; (5) distribution of calcium intake throughout the day rather than at one time; and (6) increased physiological need (i.e., growth, pregnancy, lactation, decreased calcium status). The effect of a more acidic pH in the digestive tract is most likely related to a reduction in the formation of calcium chelations.

Lactose can also facilitate the absorption of calcium. The constituent monosaccharides of lactose may be more responsible for the positive influence upon calcium absorption. This effect is probably more significant in infants than for adults. Also, while some fermentable fibers such as pectin can bind calcium in the digestive tract, microbes in the colon may liberate some of the calcium and thereby allow for some calcium absorption in the large intestine. It has been suggested that as much as 4% of dietary calcium is absorbed in the colon. Normal bile acid presence may assist in calcium absorption by promoting proper fat digestion and decreasing the formation of calcium–fatty acid soaps.

The absorption of calcium occurs along the length of the small intestine. There appear to be two transport processes responsible for the absorption of calcium. The first process is a saturable, active mechanism which involves a calcium-binding protein (CBP) or *calbindin*. Calbindin is located along the small intestine, but is more abundant in the duodenum and proximal jejunum. In the upper portion of the small intestine, the efficiency of calcium absorption is greater, but since the chyme stays in contact with the remainder of the small intestine for a greater period of time, the total amount absorbed is greater in the distal portion of the small intestine. The absorption of calcium occurs in a three-step process. First, calcium is transferred through the microvillus membrane. Next, calcium is transported or escorted through the cell to decrease its interaction with intracellular molecules. Last, calcium exits from the cell across the basolateral membrane into the extracellular fluid and subsequently into the blood. Vitamin D (1,25-$(OH)_2D_3$) regulates all three steps. Vitamin D enters intestinal mucosa cells and binds to a receptor. The vitamin D-receptor complex translocates to the nucleus and binds to promoter regions to stimulate the transcription of CBP as well as an intracellular membrane calcium binding protein (IMCBP). These proteins bind to the calcium that enters the mucosal cells. This may keep the free calcium levels minimized, thereby decreasing any potential interference with other intracellular metabolic processes. Organelles, such as the mitochondria and Golgi apparatus, may also bind calcium and facilitate its absorption by assisting in the movement of calcium towards the basolateral membrane. In any event, the calcium bound to these proteins or organelles are released into the extracellular fluid. Release into the extracellular fluid requires ATP and a vitamin D-regulated Ca^{2+}/Mg^{2+} ATPase. Sodium may also be exchanged for calcium during membrane transport.

Aging appears to decrease the efficiency of calcium absorption. As explained in Chapter 8, vitamin D-regulated absorption of calcium becomes impaired as less 1,25-$(OH)_2 D_3$ is made in response to parathyroid hormone (PTH). Reduction in estrogen in menopausal and postmenopausal women is also associated with a reduced vitamin D-mediated calcium absorption.

The second mechanism for calcium absorption also occurs throughout the small intestine and appears to be a nonsaturable paracellular process. Here calcium moves between enterocytes instead of moving through them. This route of calcium absorption becomes more significant as calcium intake increases. Also, it should be mentioned that larger intakes of calcium appear to hinder iron absorption.

Blood Calcium Levels and Regulation

The total amount of calcium in the blood is 8.8 to 10.8 mg/100 ml. Calcium is found in the blood mainly bound to protein (~40%) or independent (~50%). Albumin is the primary transport protein. The remaining 10% of circulating calcium is complexed with sulfate, phosphate, or citrate.

Blood calcium is very tightly regulated by several endocrine factors. Contrary to public belief, dietary calcium levels do not significantly influence blood calcium levels. Alterations in blood calcium levels occur as a result of endocrine balance. As blood calcium levels fluctuate towards the lower end of the normal range, parathyroid hormone (PTH) levels in the blood increase. Parathyroid hormone supports the reestablishment of normal serum calcium levels by: (1) increasing calcium absorption from the intestine; (2) mobilizing calcium from bone via stimulating osteoclasts; and, (3) reducing kidney excretion of calcium and increasing tubular reabsorption. Vitamin D will also help regulate the level of calcium in the blood by interacting with the function of PTH. Vitamin D will stimulate the production of CBP and IMCBP the small intestine mucosa, as discussed above, thereby facilitating calcium absorption. Contrarily, calcitonin is secreted by the thyroid glands when blood calcium levels increase. Calcitonin will increase calcium deposition into bones, thereby removing it from the blood. This effect, along with a decreased influence of PTH and vitamin D, will result in a lowering of the level of serum calcium.

Physiological Role

As alluded to above, calcium has both structural and functional significance. As most body calcium is found as part of mineral complexes in hard tissue such as bone and teeth, this has become its most recognizable role. However, calcium is involved in several functional aspects of human physiology such as nerve impulse transmission, regulation of muscle contraction, maintenance of acid–base (pH) balance, regulation of biochemical reactions, and blood coagulation. In fact, from an immediate homeostatic regulation perspective, this limited quantity of calcium is actually much more important.

Calcium is part of structurally important components of bones and teeth. Bone and teeth are about two thirds mineral by weight, with the remainder being mostly water and protein, and small amounts of lipid and other organic substances. Two complexes containing mostly calcium and phosphate provide hardness and rigidity to these tissues. These complexes are calcium phosphate ($Ca_3(PO_4)_2$) and hydroxyapatite ($Ca_{10}(PO_4)_6OH_2$). These mineral complexes also serve as a storage for calcium and phosphorus. It is this portion of bone that is depleted during bone demineralization diseases such as osteomalacia and osteoporosis. The finer structural aspects of bone and calcium's involvement will be reviewed in Chapter 19.

Calcium is also associated with proteins in bone, cartilage, and dentine as ionic calcium binds with proteins such as bone Gla protein (BGP or *osteocalcin*) and matrix Gla protein (MGP). Both of these proteins are believed to promote mobilization of bone calcium. This notion that is supported by reports that their expression is stimulated by $1,25\text{-}(OH)_2 D_3$.

Beyond bone, the remaining 1% of calcium in our body is found distributed in the blood and other tissue such as muscle, nerves, and glands. As mentioned above, it is this portion of body calcium that is crucial to human function and survival on a millisecond-to-millisecond, second-to-second, minute-to-minute basis. The level of ionized calcium in the intracellular fluid is about 1/10,000 of that extracellular levels. The concentration of calcium in the intracellular fluid is maintained at 100 nmol/l. Maintaining such low intracellular levels of calcium prevents activational events, as described below, as well as precipitation with phosphates and other anions. While cytosolic calcium levels are indeed at their nadir, calcium is sequestered within organelles such as mitochondria, nucleus, and the endoplasmic reticulum (sarcoplasmic reticulum in muscle tissue). Low intracellular fluid calcium levels are maintained by Ca^{2+} pumps located on the plasma or organelle membranes.

Calcium is involved in the function of excitable cells, namely, muscle fibers and neurons. Calcium, via so called slow calcium–sodium channels in the SA node of the heart, initiate the electrical signal or action potential that stimulates cardiac muscle to contract. Furthermore, the influx of calcium, via voltage-gated membrane channels on the plasma membrane and sarcoplasmic reticulum, initates cardiac muscle contraction. In skeletal muscle, an increase in the intracellular calcium concentration evokes fiber contraction as well. Calcium binds with troponin C, which evokes a conformational change in this protein which ultimately uncovers binding sites on actin. This allows myosin to form crossbridges and perform a *power stroke* which results in sarcomere shortening and fiber contraction. After the stimulus for contraction is removed, calcium is pumped back into the sarcoplasmic reticulum and across the plasma membrane to reestablish the extremely low intracellular fluid ionized calcium concentration. The sarcoplasmic reticulum contains a calcium binding protein called *calsequestrin* which allows for a 10,000-fold greater calcium concentration during an unstimulated state.

Smooth muscle contraction differs somewhat from skeletal and cardiac muscle. First, smooth muscle contains relatively fewer voltage-gated sodium channels and many more voltage-gated calcium channels. Therefore calcium, not sodium, is responsible for the initiation and propagation of the action potential. Second, the source of calcium to initiate contraction is derived primarily from the extracellular fluid as the sarcoplamic reticulum system is not developed in smooth muscle. Thus, whereas most of the calcium influx in stimulated skeletal muscle is derived from the sarcoplasmic reticulum, nearly all of the calcium influx in smooth muscle is across the plasma membrane. Last, smooth muscle does not contain troponin. Therefore, calcium has the capability to evoke smooth muscle contraction by a mechanism that is unique from other muscle tissue.

While the intitiation and propagation of neuron action potentials is largely attributed to other ions, namely, sodium and potassium, the release of neurotrasmitter at the synaptic junction is reliant upon calcium. As an action potential reaches a nerve terminal, voltage-gated calcium channels open and calcium enters the intracellular fluid. It is believed that the increase in intracellular calcium allows for neurotransmitter-containing vesicles to migrate to and fuse with the plasma membrane. Neurotransmitters are thereby released into the synaptic gap.

Calcium functions as a second messenger. The binding of certain hormones to plasma membrane receptors results in the opening of calcium channels and an increase in the intracellular calcium concentration (Figure 1.30). Calcium is then able to bind with calmodulin, a protein with four calcium binding sites. The binding of calcium to calmodulin evokes a conformational change in the protein structure. The presence of calmodulin/calcium complexes results in several intracellular events, including the regulation of the activity of key enzymes. For example, myosin light-chain kinase, which is involved in smooth muscle cell contraction, is dependent upon calmodulin. Also, phosphorylase kinase is calmodulin dependent. Phosphorylase kinase activates phosphorylase, which is a key enzyme involved in glycogen degradation.

Calcium is pivotal for blood clotting as it is necessary for the conversion of factors VII, IX, and X to their active forms, as well as the conversion of prothrombin to thrombin during the clotting cascade. Last, calcium appears to be involved in sperm motility and enzyme release upon penetration of the granulosa cell mass surrounding an ovum.

Recommended Levels for Intake

The RDA quantities for calcium are the highest among the nonenergy providing nutrients, with the exception of another mineral, phosphorus. The recommendations for water are also higher than for calcium; however, specific RDA quantities have not been designated for water. For adolescents, 11 to 24 years of age, the RDA for calcium is 1200 mg. This is higher than the 1980 level for 19 to 24-year-old adults, which was 800 mg. The RDA above 24 years of age is 800 mg, and for pregnant and lactating women the RDA is 1200 mg. On a per weight basis, children have a higher requirement. Some organizations, like the World Health Organization (WHO), suggest lower calcium intakes of 400 to 500 mg/d for adults.

The RDA set for calcium take into consideration daily losses of calcium by way of urine, skin, and feces along with an absorption rate of about 20 to 40% in adults and up to 75% in children and during pregnancy. The average calcium intake for American men appears to meet the RDA level for all ages except for those over 55 years. Contrarily, the calcium intake for American women is recognized as below the RDA for all age groups. Some nutritionists attribute the lower intake for women to weight-loss dieting and the substitution of milk with diet soft drinks.

Deficiency

A deficiency of calcium, whether from decreased provision or absorption or increased excretion, can result in numerous disease situations, especially pertaining to bone. If the deficiency occurs during growing years, poor bone mineralization will occur. Bones become soft and pliable due to a lack of mineralization. This can result in a bowing of the legs similar to *rickets*.

In adults, two forms of bone disease may develop related to calcium. *Osteomalacia* is a demineralization of bone, primarily peripheral bones, due to loss of calcium and phosphorus crystals rendering the remaining bone soft. This bone disease can result from a diet that is chronically poor in calcium or poor vitamin D status. *Osteoporosis* which affects mostly older women is characterized by loss in the total amount of bone. Osteoporosis has a multiple etiology, not just less calcium over a lifetime, but decreased estrogen and lack of exercise. The bones affected in osteoporosis are more likely to be central bones such as the hip and spine. Osteoporosis reviewed in greater detail in Chapter 19.

Other situations such as excessive calcium loss in our urine or a vitamin D deficiency may also result in a reduction in blood calcium. Whatever the case may be, it will affect the calcium concentration found in tissue such as nerve, muscle, and glands. Low blood calcium levels are associated with irritability of nervous tissue, including the CNS, and skeletal muscle cramping.

Toxicity

Today, it is not uncommon to find people ingesting very large supplemental amounts of calcium. Sometimes, their intake can climb above ten times their RDA. Although the efficiency of calcium absorption decreases as its dietary content increases and with optimal physiological status, passive paracellular absorption can still lead to increased absorption. Also, other factors, such as gram doses of vitamin C and increased vitamin D ingestion or hyperparathyroidism may increase calcium status. While fairly uncommon, excessive body calcium, over time, can lead to increased calcium deposition in tissue such as muscle (including our heart), blood vessels, and lungs. This will affect the activity of these tissues by making them more rigid. Renal filtration is the primary route of calcium excretion and increased calcium in the ultrafiltrate may render an individual more prone to calcium containing renal stones (i.e., calcium oxalates).

Phosphorus

Phosphorus is the sixth most abundant element (by weight) in the human body and second most abundant mineral behind calcium — and, like calcium, most of the phosphorus (~85%) in the human body is found in bone. Whether one is addressing the phosphorus in food or in the body, this mineral is almost exclusively in the form of *phosphate* (PO_4).

Dietary Sources

Food sources with a higher content of phosphorus include meat, poultry, eggs, fish, milk and milk products, cereals, legumes, grains, and chocolate (Table 9.4). Many soft drinks contain phosphorus in the form of *phosphoric acid*. Coffee and teas also provide some phosphorus. Phosphorus occurs in foods in both an inorganic form and as a component of organic molecules such as phospholipids, phosphoproteins, and phosphorylated sugars. The type of food determines the relative amount of either inorganic or organic sources. For instance, most phosphorus in meats and more than half of the phosphorus in milk is complexed in organic molecules. As much as 80% of the phosphorus in grains (i.e., wheat, oats, corn, rice) is part of phytate (inositol hexaphosphate). Phytate is composed of the carbohydrate inositol with up to six phosphate groups esterified to the carbon atoms in the ring. Phytate is the plant storage form of phosphorus.

Digestion and Absorption

Most phosphorus is absorbed in its inorganic form. Therefore phosphate, as part of organic molecules, must be liberated by digestive enzymes. A notable exception is the phosphate from phytate, which has very limited absorption due to a lack of the *phytase* enzymes in humans. However, yeast preparations used in the production of breads contain phytase. This phytase can liberate as much as one half of the phosphate available from the grain's phytate.

A meal containing a considerable quantity of magnesium and/or calcium can decrease phosphorus absorption. Magnesium and phosphates may form chelates in the intestinal lumen, thereby decreasing the absorption efficiency for both substances. By contrast, a meal low in magnesium will enhance phosphate absorption. Also, aluminum-containing substances ingested with a meal can decrease phosphate absorption. For instance, 3 g of *aluminum hydroxide* can reduce phosphorus absorption by one half. Aluminum hydroxide and magnesium hydroxide are common ingredients in antacids.

Phosphorus absorption is believed to take place throughout the small intestine. The efficiency of absorption is about 50 to 70% with a typical intake and as high as 90% when phosphorus intake is low. The efficiency of absorption is not impaired by physiological phosphorus status; thus hyperphosphatemia is possible with higher intakes over time.

The absorption of phosphorus probably involves two mechanisms: first, an active, saturable, carrier-mediated process, and second, a diffusion system that demonstrates a linear nature. Vitamin D stimulates the absorption of phosphorus via the active transport mechanism.

TABLE 9.4

Phosphorus Content of Selected Foods

Food	Phosphorus (mg)
Milk and milk products	
Yogurt (1 c)	233
Milk (1 c)	228
Cheese, American (1 oz)	211
Meat and alternatives	
Pork (3 oz)	105
Hamburger (3 oz)	97
Tuna (3 oz)	139
Lobster (3 oz)	152
Chicken (3 oz)	118
Nuts and seeds	
Sunflower seeds (1 c)	1015
Peanuts (1 c)	549
Peanut butter (1 tbl)	59
Grains	
Bran flakes (1 c)	227
Bread, whole wheat (1 slice)	64
Noodles, cooked (2 c)	76
Rice, cooked (1 c)	68
Bread, white (1 slice)	—
Vegetables	
Potato (1)	128
Corn (2 c)	261
Peas (2 c)	228
Broccoli (2 c)	116
Other	
Milk chocolate (1 oz)	61
Cola (12 oz)	45
Diet cola (12 oz)	41

Serum Phosphorus Levels

About 70% of the phosphorus in the blood circulates as part of phospholipids, primarily in lipoproteins, cells, and platelets. The remaining 30% is largely dissolved inorganic phosphates (HPO_4^{2-} and $H_2PO_4^-$) and to a lesser degree phosphate is bound to proteins or complexed to calcium or magnesium. The range for inorganic phosphate in adult blood is approximately 2.5 to 4.5 mg/100 ml. As a large portion of dietary phosphorus is absorbed, proper renal excretion is paramount. As much as two thirds of dietary phosphorus is excreted in the urine.

Physiological Roles

Phosphorus, as phosphate, has numerous functions in the human body. First, it is a component of high-energy molecules, such as ATP, GTP, and creatine phosphate (Figures 9.1 and 13.2). The enzymatic cleavage of phosphate bonds in these molecules liberates significant quantities of energy that drive many cellular reactions and operations. This includes

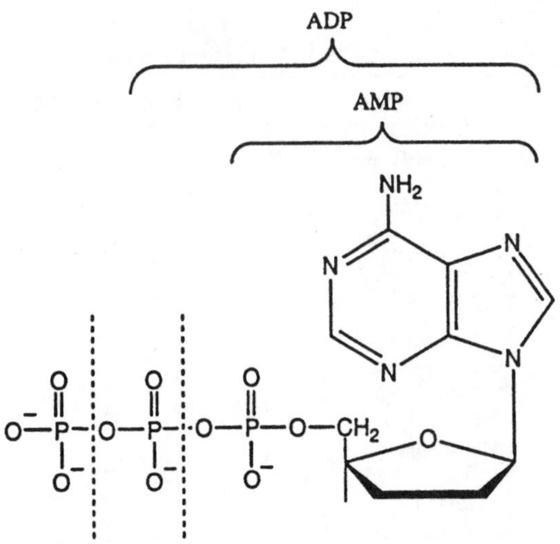

FIGURE 9.1
ATP molecule displaying phosphate groups connected by ester bonds.

the absorption of many nutrients, muscle cell contraction, and maintenance of ionic concentrations across plasma membranes.

Phosphate, as a component of phospholipids (Figure 1.3), provides structure to cellular membranes, while phosphate found in bone and teeth is a component of hydroxyapatite and calcium phosphate crystals. Phosphate is also an important component of nucleic acids. In fact, bases are linked together in a nucleic acid polymer by phophodiester bonds (Figure 1.8). Last, phosphate is involved in regulating the pH of the extracellular fluid. Phosphates in the ultrafiltrate, largely as sodium phosphates, can react with secreted hydrogen ions and keep them from being reabsorbed.

$$Na_2HPO_4 + H^+ \longrightarrow NaH_2PO_4 + Na^+$$

Recommended Levels of Intake

The RDA for phosphorus is the same as for calcium in efforts to maintain a proper calcium:phosphorus balance in the diet. Many nutritionists recommend that the calcium:phosphorus ratio should not fall below 1:2. The recommended intake for phosphorus parallels calcium recommendations at 800 to 1200 mg daily for adults.

Deficiency and Toxicity

As most foods contain phosphorus, a deficiency is somewhat rare under normal circumstances. Toxicity is also rare, perhaps with the exception of infants who receive a high-phosphorus-containing formula. However, most commercially available infant formulas are not a threat in regard to their phosphorus content.

Magnesium

Like calcium, magnesium is a divalent cation. Typically an adult body will contain 20 to 28 g of magnesium. More than half and up to two thirds of this mineral is associated with bone tissue. On a mass basis, magnesium is the 12th most abundant element in the human body, contributing about 1% of human mass. It is the fourth most abundant cation in the human body; however, it is the second most abundant intracellular cation next to potassium. Magnesium is the third largest element in the human diet, following calcium and phosphorus.

Dietary Sources

Magnesium is found in a variety of foods, with better sources including whole grain cereals, nuts, legumes, spices, seafood, coffee, tea, and cocoa (Table 9.5). Chlorophyll contains magnesium. Therefore, plant components rich in chlorophyll, such as green leaves, will be a source of magnesium. Certain processing techniques, such as the refining of grains and polishing of rice, may result in significant losses of magnesium. Also, some magnesium can dissolve into cooking water during boiling, resulting in some losses there as well.

TABLE 9.5
Magnesium Content of Selected Foods

Food	Magnesium (mg)
Legumes	
Lentils, cooked (1 c)	72
Split peas, cooked (1 c)	71
Tofu (1 c)	256
Nuts	
Peanuts (1 c)	184
Cashews (1 c)	332
Almonds (1 c)	477
Grains	
Bran buds (1 c)	243
Rice, wild, cooked (1 c)	52
Wheat germ (2 tbl)	45
Vegetables	
Bean sprouts (1 c)	22
Black-eyed peas (1 c)	91
Spinach, cooked (1 c)	157
Lima beans (1 c)	81
Milk and milk products	
Milk (1 c)	33
Cheese, cheddar (1 oz)	8
Cheese, American (1 oz)	6
Meats	
Chicken (3 oz)	15
Beef (3 oz)	18
Pork (3 oz)	10

Absorption

The absorption of magnesium occurs along the length of the small intestine, as well as to a limited degree in the colon. However, if small intestinal absorption of magnesium is impaired, the absorption in the colon can play a major role in maintaining magnesium balance in the body. Also, absorption in the ileum may be a saturable process, whereas absorption in the more proximal small intestine is not.

Magnesium absorption from our digestive tract is fair (25 to 60%), while certain factors can certainly influence this efficiency. For example, a low body magnesium status results in a higher percentage of absorption. Vitamin D also appears to increase magnesium absorption to a limited, yet significant degree. Contrarily, a high magnesium diet, excessive dietary calcium, phosphate, phytate, and excessive fatty acids will decrease the efficiency of magnesium absorption. The unabsorbed fatty acids can form magnesium–fatty acid soaps in a manner similar to the formation of calcium–fatty acid soaps. As mentioned above, calcium and magnesium may compete for similar absorptive mechanisms.

Tissue Content and Excretion

An adult contains about 0.5 g of magnesium per kilogram of fat-free body weight. About 60% of the magnesium in humans is located in bones, while the remaining portion is found in the extracellular fluid (~1%) and in soft tissue (~39%). About 50 to 55% of plasma magnesium is dissolved as an independent ion. Alternately, about 32% of circulating magnesium is bound to plasma proteins, such as albumin, and the remaining magnesium is complexed to negatively charged substances such as citrate, phosphate, or other anions.

Magnesium is excreted from within the body primarily through urinary loss. Circulating magnesium becomes part of the ultrafiltrate, with the exception of that associated with plasma proteins. As much as 95 to 97% of the magnesium in the ultrafiltrate is reabsorbed. However, as circulating levels of magnesium increase so will renal excretion.

Physiological Roles

Bone magnesium should be separated into (1) the magnesium associated with the crystal lattice which may have been laid down during development; and (2) magnesium associated with the surface of bone which represents a magnesium pool. Most of the nonbone magnesium is in soft tissue, especially skeletal muscle. In these tissues it is ionically associated with membrane phospholipids, proteins, nucleic acids, and ATP.

Magnesium forms an electrical union with the negatively charged oxygen atoms of the phosphate tail of ATP. This interaction appears to add stability to the molecule and assist ATP-dependent reactions, especially kinase reactions that transfer an ATP phosphate group to another molecule.

Magnesium is believed to be necessary or at least important in over 300 enzyme-catalyzed reactions. Therefore, magnesium is a key factor for most metabolic pathways. For instance, hexokinase, glucokinase, and phosphofructokinase (PFK), key reactions in glycolysis are dependent upon magnesium (Figure 9.2). Other magnesium-dependent enzymes include mevalonate kinase, phosphomevalonate kinase, and squalene synthetase, which are involved in cholesterol synthesis. Creatine kinase, which synthesizes creatine-phosphate, and acyl CoA synthetase, a key ezyme in β-oxidation, are also magnesium dependent, as are alkaline phosphatase and pyrophosphatase. Some general operations that

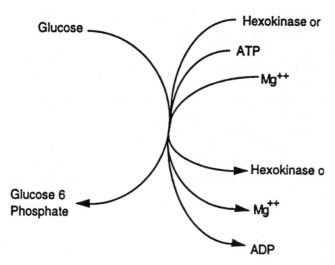

FIGURE 9.2
Magnesium involvement in hexokinase activity.

require magnesium include: amino acid activation, DNA replication and RNA transcription, nucleic acid synthesis, protein synthesis, and cAMP formation from adenylate cyclase.

Magnesium is vital for the proper activity and metabolism of other nutrients. For instance, magnesium is needed for PTH secretion as well as its hormonal affects upon bone, the kidney and intestines. Magnesium is also necessary for the hydroxylation of vitamin D (cholecalciferol) in hepatocytes. This reaction is the preliminary step in converting vitamin D to its most active form.

Calcium and magnesium are antagonists in many biochemical reactions. Increasing the magnesium content of the blood produces anesthesia. Generalized depression of blood pressure and the respiratory system can also occur as blood magnesium levels increase. An intravenous dose of magnesium can be fatal.

Recommended Levels for Intake

The RDA for magnesium is 40 and 60 mg for infants during their first 6 months and their second 6 months of life, respectively. Magnesium recommendations are systematically raised during childhood from 80 mg for those 1 to 3 years of age, and then 120 and 170 mg for children between the ages of 4 to 6 and 7 to 10, respectively. During adolescence and adulthood, recommendations for males will vary between 270 to 400 mg and for nonpregnant females between 280 to 300 mg. Pregnancy increases recommendations to 320 mg, while 355 and 340 mg of magnesium are recommended for lactating women during the first 6 months and the second 6 months, respectively.

Deficiency and Toxicity

While magnesium is found in a variety of foods and deficiency is somewhat rare, excessive vomiting, diarrhea, alcohol abuse, renal and endocrine disease, and protein malnutrition may lead to deficient status. Excess use of diuretics may result in deficiency of magnesium as well as other nutrients. Subtle reductions in blood magnesium content can effect the release of PTH and its activity. Furthermore, a magnesium deficiency can alter the ability of protein pumps to maintain optimal sodium and potassium concentration differences across cell membranes. This largely reflects magnesium's ability to stabilize ATP, which is the power source for pumping ions across cell membranes. Thus, the proper function of excitable and other cells is jeopardized during magnesium deficiency. Muscle tetany and impaired CNS function are deficiency symptoms.

Like a couple other minerals, toxicity induced by a high dietary intake of magnesium can be thwarted by appropriately functioning kidneys. However, magnesium in excess may pose physiological problems in that it may enhance the excretion of calcium, phosphorus, and potassium. A chronic excess of magnesium has been suggested to result in renal damage or renal insufficiency.

Sodium, Chloride, and Potassium

Sodium, potassium, and chloride (chlorine) can be discussed in tandem as their metabolic and biochemical functions are so interrelated. Furthermore, the heavy utilization of *sodium chloride* (table salt) as a flavorant and food preservative allows for many foods to be significant providers of both sodium and chloride.

Sodium is the primary cation found in the extracellular fluid, while potassium is the primary intracellular cation. The chloride anion is usually associated with sodium and therefore is more concentrated in the extracellular fluid. These elements are heavily involved in the proper maintenance of water balance across cellular membranes as well as establishing the electrical potential across plasma membranes. Often these elements are referred to as *electrolytes* because of their ability, as well as other ions, to conduct an electrical charge when dissolved in water.

Dietary Sources

The typical American diet includes about 3 to 7 g of sodium daily; however the natural sodium content of most foods is very low. As much as 50 to 75% of the sodium in the American diet is actually added to foods by food manufacturers for taste or preservation. Another 15% is added by individuals during cooking and by "salting" foods at the table. The sodium occurring naturally in foods such as eggs, milk, meats, and vegetables may only account for about 10 to 15% of the total sodium intake by Americans. Last, drinking water may contribute to sodium intake along with certain medicines, mouthwash, and tooth pastes (sodium fluoride). Foods with the greatest contribution of sodium to the American diet include luncheon meats, snack chips, french fries, hot dogs, cheeses, soups, and gravies. Table 9.6 provides a listing of select foods and their sodium content. Food labels in the U.S. require manufacturers to list the sodium content of a food on a per serving basis. Furthermore, any claims made by the manufacturer regarding the sodium content must follow the criteria listed in Table 9.7.

Like sodium, the natural chloride content of most foods is very low. However, some fruits and vegetables do contain respectable amounts of chloride. Sodium chloride (NaCl) provides nearly all of the chloride in the diet. NaCl is approximately 60% chloride and 40% sodium, by weight. Thus, a food containing 1 g of sodium chloride would contain approximately 400 mg of sodium and 600 mg of chloride.

TABLE 9.6
Sodium Content of Selected Foods

Food	Sodium (mg)
Meat and alternatives	
Corned beef (3 oz)	964
Ham (3 oz)	1120
Fish, canned (3 oz)	458
Sausage (3 oz)	784
Hot dog (1)	585
Bologna (1 oz)	278
Milk and milk products	
Cream soup (1 c)	1060
Cottage cheese (1 c)	918
Cheese, American (1 oz)	405
Cheese, parmesan (1 oz)	454
Milk, skim (1 c)	125
Milk, whole (1 c)	120
Grains	
Bran flakes (1 c)	306
Corn flakes (1 c)	300
Bagel (1)	379
English muffin (1)	264
Bread, white (1 slice)	130
Bread, whole wheat (1 slice)	148
Crackers, Saltines (4 sq)	156
Other	
Salt (1 tsp)	2325
Pickle, dill (1)	833
Broth, chicken (1 c)	776
Ravioli, canned (1 c)	930
Broth, beef (1 c)	782
Gravy (1 c)	1535
Italian dressing (2 tbl)	231
Pretzels, thin (5)	255
Olives, green (5)	468
Pizza, cheese (1 slice)	490
Soy sauce (1 tsp)	343
Bacon (3 slices)	382
French dressing (2 tbl)	427
Potato chips (10)	119
Catsup (1 tbl)	182

TABLE 9.7
Labeling Guidelines for Sodium Claims

Label Claim	Actual Content
Sodium free	Must contain < 5 mg sodium per serving
Very low sodium	Must contain ≤ 35 mg sodium per serving
Low sodium	Must contain ≤ 145 mg sodium per serving
Reduced sodium	75% Reduction in sodium content
Unsalted	No salt added to recipe
No added salt	No salt added to recipe

Unlike sodium and chloride, potassium is not routinely added to foods. Potassium is naturally found in most foods in the diet. Rich sources of potassium are typically fresh foods, without processing, as some losses of potassium can occur. Fresh fruits and vegetables rank among the best potassium sources. Tomatoes, carrots, potatoes, beans, peaches, pears, squash, oranges, and bananas are all notable for their high potassium content (Table 9.8). Along with fruits and vegetables, milk, meats, whole grains, coffee, and tea are also among the most significant contributors to our daily potassium intake. Many athletes refer to bananas as "potassium sticks" with respect to their potassium content, although their potassium content is not necessarily outstanding compared to many other fruits or vegetables.

TABLE 9.8
Potassium Content of Selected Foods

Food	Potassium (mg)
Vegetables	
Potato (1)	510
Squash, winter (1 c)	896
Tomato (1)	273
Celery (1 stalk)	115
Carrots (1)	233
Broccoli (1 c)	286
Fruit	
Avocado (1)	1204
Orange juice (1 c)	473
Banana (1)	467
Raisins (1 c)	1089
Prunes (4)	250
Watermelon (1 c)	176
Milk and milk products	
Yogurt (1 c)	380
Milk, skim (1 c)	407
Meats	
Fish (3 oz)	293
Hamburger (3 oz)	137
Lamb (3 oz)	287
Pork (3 oz)	197
Chicken (3 oz)	147
Grains	
Bran buds (1 c)	817
Bran flakes (1 c)	105
Raisin Bran (1 c)	349
Wheat flakes (1 c)	379

Absorption

The absorption efficiency of sodium, potssium, and chloride rank among the highest of the nutrients. For instance, as much as 90 to 95% of these minerals is absorbed, as less than 10% of dietary sodium, potassium, or chloride appears in the feces. Thus, renal excretion becomes the primary route of regulating physiological levels of these minerals.

Sodium appears to be absorbed by three primary mechanisms: (1) Na^+/glucose cotransport system occurring along the length of the small intestine; (2) Na^+/Cl^- cotransport system occurring throughout the small intestine and in the proximal colon; and (3) an electrogenic Na^+ transport mechanism occurring in the colon. Sodium is also involved in the transport of certain amino acids, dipeptides, tripeptides, and some of the water-soluble vitamins across the apical membrane of enterocytes in a mechanism similar to the Na^+/glucose transporter.

Unlike sodium, the mechanisms for potassium absorption are not entirely clear. Absorption does appear to take place along the length of the intestines, with perhaps the colon being a major site of absorption. Some research has suggested that potassium enters enterocytes via a K^+/H^+ antiport, ATPase pump. Potassium may also diffuse across the apical membrane via channels. Potassium also appears to diffuse across the basolateral membrane into the extracellular fluid via potassium channels. Extracellular potassium is necessary for the movement of sodium across the basolateral membrane as well, as it is utilized in a Na^+/K^+ ATPase antiport system.

Chloride is absorbed along the length of the small intestine, and its absorption is often associated with sodium absorption, in efforts to maintain electrical neutrality. With the exception of the Na^+/Cl^- cotransport mentioned above, most chloride absorption occurs in a paracellular manner as chloride appears to be able to navigate to tight junctions between enterocytes.

Tissue, Urinary, and Sweat Content

Humans have approximately 1.8 g sodium per kilogram of fat-free body weight. For example, an average 70-kg adult male body would contain about 83 to 97 g of sodium. The serum concentration averages in the range of 300 to 355 mg of sodium per 100 ml. About 30 to 35% of total body sodium is located in bone associated with the surface of mineral crystals. This probably serves as a reservoir of blood sodium to avoid potential *hyponatremia*. The remainder of body sodium is found primarily dissolved within extracellular fluid, and sodium accounts for greater than 90% of the blood cation content. Meanwhile, about 88% of chloride is found in the extracellular fluid, while the remainder is located intracellularly. Chloride's negative charge serves to neutralize the positive charge of sodium. As discussed in Chapter 7, the sodium and chloride content of sweat increases with the rate of sweating. Unlike sodium and chloride, about 97 to 98% of body potassium is located within intracellular fluid. It is the predominate intracellular cation. About 2.6 g of potassium per kilogram fat-free body weight can be expected. The concentration of potassium in serum is 14 to 22 mg/100 ml.

The regulation of these elements in the body is primarily accomplished by the adrenalcorticoids: *deoxycorticosterone*, *aldosterone*, and the pituitary octapeptide *antidiuretic hormone* (ADH or vasopressin) and oxytocin. These hormones all act upon the kidney tubules to increase sodium retention. The kidney filters sodium out and the element is reabsorbed by the proximal tubule. The distal tubules are also active in secreting potassium as promoted by these hormones.

Physiological Functions

Sodium, potassium, and chloride are the primary electrolytes in human fluids. Other important electrolytes include HCO_3^- (bicarbonate), magnesium, calcium, sulfate (SO_4^{2-}), and phosphates (PO_4^{2-}). All are dispersed throughout the extracellular and intracellular fluids and their concentrations are listed in Table 9.9. While all electrolytes contribute at least to some degree in the establishment of the electrical potential across plasma membranes, in general, sodium, potassium, and chloride contribute the most. While an electrical potential exists across the plasma membrane of essentially all cells, without doubt it is most important in the so called *excitable cells* (muscle cells and neurons). In excitable cells, ion flux through gated channels allows for rapid and transient changes in the membrane potential. This, of course, is the action potential, the hallmark of excitable cells. During nerve transmission and muscle contraction, sodium diffuses intracellularly, while potassium diffuses extracellularly, serving as the basis of the action potential. The cell will quickly reestablish the concentration gradients after an impulse or contraction has occurred utilizing a Na^+/K^+ ATPase pump.

TABLE 9.9
Electrolyte Composition in Extracellular and Intracellular Fluid

Ion	Extracellular Fluid	Intracellular Fluid
Sodium (Na^+)	142 mEq/l	10 mEq/l
Potassium (K^+)	4 mEq/l	140 mEq/l
Chloride (Cl^-)	103 mEq/l	4 mEq/l
Calcium (Ca^{2+})	2.4 mEq/l	0.0001 mEq/l
Magnesium (Mg^{2+})	1.2 mEq/l	58 mEq/l
Bicarbonate (HCO_3^-)	28 mEq/l	10 mEq/l
Phosphates (PO_4^{2-})	4 mEq/l	75 mEq/l
Sulfates (SO_4^{2-})	1 mEq/l	2 mEq/l

Chloride, is a component of hydrochoric acid, which is responsible for the acidic nature of the stomach. Hydrochloric acid is secreted by parietal cells in oxyntic glands of the stomach mucosa. Chloride is also secreted along the digestive tract as a means of maintaining electrical neutrality. Chloride may be the only ion actively secreted by the digestive tract mucosa.

In red blood cells, the cellular waste product, CO_2, will react with water in the presence of carbonic anhydrase to produce HCO_3^-. When the HCO_3^- content increases in the cell, it will diffuse out of the cell. Chloride will be brought into the cell in order to maintain electrical neutrality. The transport of chloride and HCO_3^- occurs simultaneously, via a transmembrane transport protein. This process allows for more carbon dioxide to circulate to the lungs. In the lungs, the reverse occurs. Since the reversible carbonic anhydrase catalyzes an equilibrium reaction, more and more bicarbonate is converted to CO_2 and water. The equilibrium reaction proceeds in this direction in the lungs as CO_2 diffuses into the alveloi and is expired. These reactions are collectively referred to as the *chloride shift*.

Recommended Levels of Intake

In contrast to a typical sodium intake of several grams per day, the adult dietary requirement may be as low as 100 to 500 mg of sodium daily. The minimum requirement for chloride for an adult is about 700 to 750 mg/d. As with sodium, the average American dietary intake of chloride is in tremendous excess of requirements. For example, Americans tend to eat about six times the estimated requirement. Again, the major provider of sodium and chloride is NaCl used as a food manufacturing or consumer additive. The average consumption of NaCl for Americans is 10 to 15 g/d. Adult requirements of potassium are approximately 2000 mg daily, a quantity that is easily obtained by a diet accommodating a variety of foods.

Deficiency, Toxicity, and Health Concerns

As noted above, with regard to the extremely efficient absorption of sodium, potassium, and chloride, renal excretion becomes the primary mechanism of body content regulation. Provided there is normal renal filtration and urinary excretion, the removal of these ions can easily occur. The sodium:potassium ratio in the human diet is believed to have changed for many cultures in comparison to the postulated *paleolithic diet*. The sodium:potassium ratio has been estimated at about 0.1–1 for paleolithic humans and between 1.5–2:1 for many developed societies today. Many researchers have suggested that this seeming life-long reversal of the sodium:potassium ratio has impacted humans from a pathophysiological perspective.

There is some evidence to suggest that diets high in sodium increase the renal excretion of calcium. Contrarily, diets rich in potassium seem to decrease the excretion of calcium. This may be significant with regard to life-long diets and the risk of osteoporosis, as will be discussed in Chapter 19. Also, the excess consumption of sodium, or the reversed sodium:potassium ratio, has been implicated as a possible risk factor in the development of hypertension or high blood pressure. There is some evidence to suggest that potassium can lower blood pressure in some individuals and therefore has potential therapeutic value.

Excessive loss of sodium by the body will normally result in a concomitant loss of water from the extracellular compartments. This can lead to a shock-like syndrome as blood volume falls and perfusion of tissue becomes insufficient and veins collapse. Loss of sodium as part of sweat followed by replacement of water only may lead to water intoxication as the sodium concentration in the extracellular fluids becomes further depressed. Symptoms such as loss of appetite, weakness, mental apathy, and uncontrolled muscle twitching are common. Death can results if the condition is severe.

Although our dietary potassium intake is by and large adequate to meet our needs, there are situations that can place us at risk for potassium deficiency. Persistent use of laxatives can result in a lowering of body potassium level by decreasing the amount absorbed from our digestive tract. In addition, chronic use of certain diuretics used to control blood pressure may result in increased urinary loss of potassium. Physicians will routinely monitor the potassium levels of patients following either of these prescribed protocols. Also, frequent vomiting after a meal, either involuntarily or voluntarily, will ultimately reduce potassium absorption.

Renal disease may result in excess excretion of potassium. Diarrhea and vomiting over a period of a few days can lead to a potassium loss that results in muscle weakness, complete paralysis, and failure of the GI tract musculature. Tachycardia and hypotension may also be experienced.

Sulfur

Sulfur is not really an essential nutrient, but rather a vital component of essential nutrients, such as the amino acid methionine, and vitamins biotin and thiamin. Therefore, the physiological significance of sulfur is really a reflection of the metabolism of these substances rather than that of an independent nutrient. Sulfur is also part of several food additives.

Suggested Readings

Berdanier, C.D., *Advanced Nutrition: Micronutrients*, CRC Press, Boca Raton, FL, 1995.
Present Knowledge in Nutrition, Ziegler, E.E. and Filer, L.J., Eds., ILSI Press, Washington, D.C., 1996.
Groff, J.L., Gropper, S.S., and Hunt, S.M., *Advanced Nutrition and Human Metabolism*, West Publishing, New York, N.Y., 1995.

10

Minor Minerals

Minor minerals or trace elements are present in the human body as less than 0.01% of total mass. Furthermore, current recommendations for the intake of each of the minor minerals is less than 100 mg daily. Minor minerals may act as cofactors in human tissues and/or are part of various compounds. Presently, there is a growing body of evidence suggesting that certain minor minerals function at the genetic level. Even though they are present in relatively small amounts, certain minor minerals can be fatal if omitted from the diet or even lethal when taken in excess of needs. Deficiencies of trace elements may result from either lack in the diet and/or malabsorption over a period of time. Furthermore, the amount of a minor mineral in plant or animal source can vary, based upon the soil and water content of the area in which the plant was grown or an animal grazed.

Oftentimes trace minerals are called trace elements or trace metals. It is important to recognize that while all the trace minerals important to human nutrition are indeed elements, they are not all metals. For instance, selenium is not a metal and neither are halogens — fluorine and iodine. By contrast, manganese, iron, copper, molydenum, vanadium, zinc, and nickel are indeed metals. Metals are generally solid and tend to have shiny surfaces. Furthermore, they can be pounded into sheets and drawn into wires. They are also very good conductors of electricity. On the contrary, nonmetals are typically lackluster and are poor conductors of electricity in their elemental form. Nonmetals exist as gases, liquids, and solids. Also, with some exceptions, metals tend to have 1, 2, and 3 valence electrons, while nonmetals tend to have 4, 5, 6, 7, or 8 valence electrons.

Iron

Despite a broad range of oxidation states in nature, iron occurs in the human body, as well as in food, in either the ferrous (Fe^{2+}) or ferric (Fe^{3+}) state. As a minor mineral, iron is the most recognizable by the general population. As far as all minerals are concerned, iron is among the top three most recognizable minerals, along with calcium and sodium. From a disease perspective, iron deficiency is second only to obesity as the most prevalent nutritional problem in the U.S. today, and world-wide iron deficiency affects millions of individuals. While much of the attention regarding iron imbalance has focused upon iron deficiency, recently more attention has been afforded to iron overload.

Diet Sources of Iron

The iron content of the Western diet has been estimated at about 7 mg of iron per 1000 kcal. Iron is present in both animal and plant foods in the form of either *heme* iron or *nonheme* iron. Animal foods contain both heme and nonheme iron, while plants and plant-derived

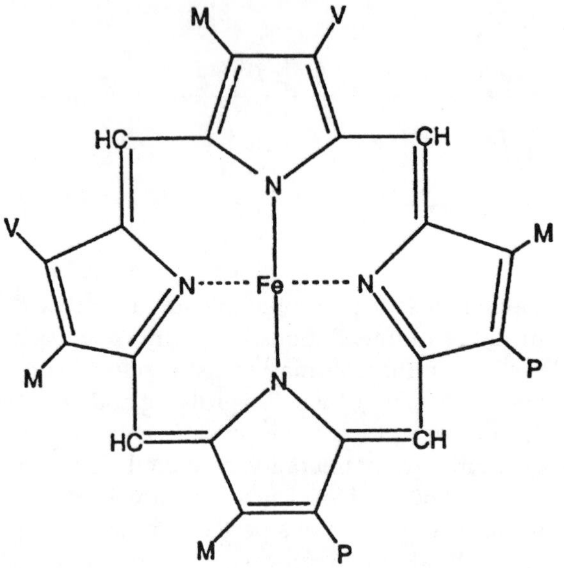

FIGURE 10.1
The structure of heme, showing the centralized atom of iron.

products contain only nonheme iron. About 50 to 60% of the iron in meat, fish, and poultry is in the form of heme. Heme iron is complexed in heme structures such as myoglobin and cytochromes (Figure 10.1). Nonheme iron is found in foods such as cereal grains, legumes, milk, and dairy products. The iron content of select foods is presented in Table 10.1. Cooking in iron pots without enamel increases the iron content of food.

Nonheme iron is less efficiently absorbed (2 to 20%) in comparison to heme iron (25 to 35%). Since the absorption efficiency of both forms of iron are relatively low, it seems likely that the iron content of human body is primarily regulated at the point of absorption. This concept is reinforced by the fact that the efficiency of iron absorption increases significantly during times of greater iron need, such as when our iron stores are low, or during periods of growth, menstruation, and pregnancy. Beyond iron status and need, many factors within the digestive tract appear to affect iron absorption (Table 10.2). This is the primary reason why the ranges of absorption for both forms of dietary iron are so broad.

Iron as part of heme structures requires two stages of digestion. First, heme must be liberated from associated protein structures. This occurs in the stomach and small intestine via the activity of proteases in digestive secretions. Heme, endowed with iron, then crosses the luminal membrane of small intestinal enterocytes intact. Once inside the cell, iron is liberated from the protoporphyrin ring by the action of *heme oxygenase*.

Nonheme iron includes the iron complexed into iron-storage proteins, *ferritin* and *hemosiderin*, and iron-containing enzymes and salts. Nonheme iron is released from food components by digestive secretions. If the iron is associated with a protein, proteases and hydrochloric acid will be necessary for its liberation. Hydrochloric acid will also assist in maintaining the stability of ionic iron by inhibiting its precipitation to anionic entities. Other acids, such as lactic acid, citric acid, and tartaric acid also seem to enhance iron absorption, probably by also stabilizing ionic iron.

Ionic iron appears to be more efficiently absorbed in the ferrous state vs. the ferric state. Two mechanisms for the movement of ionic iron into enterocytes have been suggested: first, a facilitative transport system mediated by a glycoprotein with a molecular weight of

TABLE 10.1

Iron Content of Selected Foods

Food	Iron (mg)
Meat and Alternatives	
Liver (3 oz)	5.3
Round steak (3 oz)	2.5
Hamburger, lean (3 oz)	2.3
Baked beans (2 c)	10
Pork (3 oz)	0.9
White beans (2 c)	33
Soybeans (2 c)	2.9
Fish (3 oz)	0.3
Chicken (3 oz)	0.9
Fruits	
Prune juice (2 c)	6.0
Apricots, dried (2 c)	12.5
Prunes (5 medium)	0.8
Raisins (1 c)	3.0
Plums (3 medium)	0.2
Grains	
Breakfast cereal (1 c) (iron-fortified)	4–18
Oatmeal, fortified (2 c)	13
Bagel (1)	2.5
English muffin (1)	1.4
Bread, rye (1 slice)	1.0
Bread, whole wheat (1 slice)	0.9
Bread, white (1 slice)	0.7
Vegetables	
Spinach (1 c)	1.7
Lima beans (1 c)	3.6
Peas, black-eyed (1 c)	4.3
Peas (1 c)	2.2
Asparagus (1 c)	1.2

160,000, and second, integrin involved movement of iron through the plasma membrane to a protein with a molecular weight of 56,000 in the intracellular compartment. Gastric and intestine luminal factors such as gastric acid, ascorbic acid, and components of meat, fish, and poultry appear to increase the efficiency of nonheme iron absorption. Once inside the enterocyte, iron derived from either diet form may be retained by cellular ferritin or transferred across the basolateral membrane to plasma *transferrin* for systemic distribution.

TABLE 10.2

Factors Influencing Iron Absorption

↑ Iron Absorption	↓ Iron Absorption
Vitamin C	Phytate
Gastric acidity	Oxalates
Meat, fish, poultry	Tannins (in tea)
Increased need:	Decreased need
Pregnancy	Use of antacids
Menstruation	
Growth	

As alluded to above, iron absorption is directly related to physiological need. Absorption may be regulated systemically by the level of plasma transferrin receptors and the rate of erythropoiesis. Furthermore, some evidence also exists for local regulatory factors in mucosal tissue as well. Iron is transported in the plasma to various tissue bound to the glycoprotein transferrin (79,550 M_r). Transferrin can accommodate two atoms of iron; however, only about 30% of the iron-binding sites are occupied with iron under normal conditions.

Vitamin C intake plays a significant role in iron absorption. Quite simply, as vitamin C intake increases in conjunction with the iron-containing source, iron absorption is enhanced. It is likely that vitamin C promotes the formation and stabilization of the ferrous iron, which as mentioned above, is much better absorbed than the ferric form. Living at a high altitude appears to create a greater need for iron. Therefore, a greater iron absorption is needed to synthesize more red blood cells under the control of erythropoietin.

As mentioned above, the presence of meat, fish, and/or poultry (MFP), enhance iron absorption. In fact, 75 units of MFP factor can enhance the absorption of nonheme iron from 2 to 3% to about 7 to 8%. Here, 1 unit is equal to 1.3 g of raw or 1 g of cooked meat, fish, or poultry. Similarly 75 units of ascorbic acid, where 1 unit is equal to 1 mg of vitamin C, can also enhance nonheme tremendously.

There are several factors that will decrease iron absorption. A high phytic acid intake will facilitate decreased absorption. Polyphenolic substances such as mannins in tea; oxalates in spinach, chard, berries, chocolate, teas, and other foods; phytates in whole grains; and the preservative EDTA all can decrease iron absorption by chelation. Interestingly, supplemental doses of calcium may also decrease iron absorption. Supplemental calcium at 600 mg taken in conjunction with 18 mg of either a ferrous or ferric iron salt decreased iron absorption by about 50 to 60%. Beyond supplements, the calcium in milk has also been suggested to reduce iron absorption. These findings suggest that an iron supplement may be most beneficial when taken in the absence of a significant source of calcium. Zinc may also compete with ferrous iron for absorption, via a common transporter, and thus decrease its absorption.

Metabolism and Function

An adult will have about 2 to 5 g of iron distributed throughout his/her body, depending upon diet, gender, size, and menstrual status. Iron is engaged in operations in all human cells and is distributed among metabolic, structural, and transport compartments. About two thirds of the iron in the human body is found within red blood cells as part of oxygen-binding pigment hemoglobin which transports oxygen to the tissues. Each hemoglobin molecule can carry four atoms of iron, and a healthy red blood cell (RBC) can contain 250 million molecules of hemoglobin. Thus, each RBC can carry one billion oxygen molecules. Muscle myoglobin accounts for 10%, and heme and nonheme enzymes account for 2 to 4% of body iron. Ferritin is the primary iron storage protein and is found in many tissues, especially the liver, bone marrow, intestine, and spleen. Augmented synthesis of ferritin occurs in these tissue as they are sites of iron absorption, storage, or RBC catabolism. Ferritin is synthesized as apoferritin, a large protein with 24 subunits and a molecular weight of 440,000. Apoferritin has a 3-dimensional design believed to be similar to a cornucopia or hollow horn. When apoferritin is associated with iron, it is called ferritin, and each ferritin structure can store as much as 4300 atoms of iron. Iron (ferrous) is oxidized by ferroxidase enzyme regions in the porous ferritin shell and the resultant ferric oxyhydroxide (FeOOH) is stored. Ferritin molecules are constantly being synthesized and catabolized. This allows for a contolled intracellular iron pool. Ferritin found in the serum is used as a sensitive indicator of tissue iron status whereby 1 µg of ferritin per liter of serum approximates 10 mg of tissue iron stores. Typically, the ferritin content of adult serum is ≥ 12 µg/l for a woman and ≥ 15 µg/l for a man.

Beyond ferritin, the other iron storage protein is hemosiderin. Hemosiderin is believed to be a breakdown product of ferritin. The ferritin:hemosiderin ratio in the liver is believed to reflect iron storage as the ratio increases with decreasing cellular iron content and vice versa. This reflects an increase in hemosiderin as cellular iron levels increase, not a reduction in ferritin content.

Transferrin is the primary iron transporter in the blood. It is produced in the liver and appears to have two binding sites for minerals such as iron, copper, and zinc. Transferrin has the greatest affinity for ferric iron. After ferric iron, transferrin has the next highest affinity for chromium, followed in descending order by copper, manganese, cadmium, zinc, and last, nickel. Tissue (i.e., liver, spleen, and bone marrow) ferrous iron must be oxidized to ferric iron via ceruloplasmin, the copper transport protein. Therefore, copper deficiency can cause anemia by decreasing circulating iron levels and delivery to sites of erythropoiesis in bone.

Cellular iron levels may control the intracellular levels of both ferritin and *transferrin receptor proteins* at the molecular level. The control is mediated via iron's ability to change the relative stability of the mRNA. This occurs by way of an interaction/noninteraction with a protein known as *iron responsive element-binding protein* (IREP) that affects the synthesis of ferritin and transferrin receptor protein. If iron in the cell is limited or decreased, the level of the transferrin receptor protein increases and that of ferritin decreases. If the IREP is not associated with iron, the protein will bind to the 5′ end of the mRNA for ferritin and block its translation. At the same time, the IREP without iron will also bind to the 3′ end of the mRNA for the transferrin receptor protein and enhance its stability to prevent degradation. This will allow for a greater synthesis of the receptor protein and consequently a greater iron uptake by cells. Conversely, when intracellular iron is high, iron will bind to the IREP, thereby preventing it from binding to mRNA for either protein. Collectively, the iron that is transported as transferrin and stored in the form of ferritin and hemosiderin make up the remaining 20 to 30% of body iron. Iron bound to transferrin makes up a very small portion (3 to 4 mg) of this compartment.

Myoglobin is a transitional oxygen storage protein in muscle, particularly slow-twitch muscle fibers and cardiac muscle cells. *Cytochromes* also contain iron and are components of the electron transport chain in mitochondria and other redux systems, such as the cytochrome P_{450} system in the endoplasmic reticulum, which is involved in the oxidation of organic compounds including alcohol and metabolism of drugs and carcinogens. The iron in myoglobin and cytochromes is found within the heme component. Iron is part of other complexes associated with the electron transport system, namely, NADH dehydrogenase, succinate dehydrogenase, and ubiquinone-cytochrome c reductase. Here iron is present, but not as a component of heme.

Outside of electron transport systems, iron is a component of a couple of heme-containing enzymes, namely, certain *peroxidases, myeloperoxidase,* and *catalase.* Peroxidases are found in leukocytes, platelets, and other tissues involving eicosanoid metabolism. They catalyze the reduction of hydrogen peroxide (H_2O_2) to 2 H_2O in a reaction that proceeds as follows:

$$H_2O_2 + XH_2 \xrightarrow{\text{peroxidase}} 2\,H_2O + X$$

Here X represents several substances that are willing to act as electron acceptors, namely, ascorbate, quinones, and cytochrome c. It is important to note that not all peroxidases contain iron. For instance, glutathionine peroxidase contains selenium at its prosthetic site. Myeloperoxidase, on the other hand, does contain iron at its prosthetic site and is found in relatively large amounts in neutrophil granules. Here, H_2O_2 is used to form a *hypohalous acid*. A hypohalous acid contains a halide element such as Cl^-, Br^- or I^-; however, because of its relative abundance, the hypohalous acid formed is hypochlorous acid (HOCl). Hypochlorous acid is the active ingredient in household bleach and is a powerful oxidant and antimicrobial agent. In humans, hypochlorous acid can react with primary and secondary amines in neutrophils and form chloroamines which are also oxidants, only less potent. These are released at sites of trauma that allow microbial infection. Last, catalase is an antioxidant that converts H_2O_2 to molecular oxygen and water in the following reaction:

$$2H_2O_2 \xrightarrow{\text{catalase}} 2H_2O + O_2$$

Recommended Levels of Intake

The RDA for adult females of childbearing years is 15 mg/d; for males it is 10 mg/d, except for 12 mg/d during ages 12 to 18 years. The RDA drops to 10 mg/d for females greater than 50 years of age. During pregnancy, a total of 30 mg of iron per day is recommended, and a decreases to 15 mg/d during lactation. In light of menstrual losses, the RDA for women is higher than for men. Iron is the only nutrient whereby female recommendations exceed those for men.

Deficiency

When iron stores, which are estimated at about 300 mg in adults, become exhausted, an individual is said to be iron deficient. About 20% of American females have minimal iron stores and are iron deficient, compared to 3% for men. Infants, children, adolescents, and pregnant or menstruating females have a high percent of iron deficiency.

Inadequate iron intake and/or excessive loss will result in a reduction of blood hemoglobin levels. The anemia that results is referred to as a *hypochromic microcytic anemia*, where the RBCs are small and pale in color. Iron deficiency anemia is defined when hemoglobin levels fall well below normal to a level less than 7 g/100 ml of blood; this is referred to as *anemia*. Figure 10.2 presents the involvement of iron, as well as other nutrients in the production of red blood cells. Normal hemoglobin levels for men and women ≥ 14 and 12 g/100 ml of blood, respectively. Borderline anemia exists when blood hemoglobin levels are lower than normal, yet still greater than 7 g/100 ml of blood. When hemoglobin levels are reduced, there is a reduction in the oxygen-carrying ability of the blood. Ultimately, less oxygen delivery to cells can result in lethargy and early fatigue when active. Beyond oxygen transport in the blood, iron deficiency decreases the ability of cells to make ATP by aerobic mechanisms. Furthermore, the activity of all other iron-containing enzymes will likely be reduced as well.

Toxicity (Overload)

Iron toxicity has been reported in both humans and animals. HLA-linked hemochromatosis appears to be one of the most common inborn errors in metabolism among Caucasians of

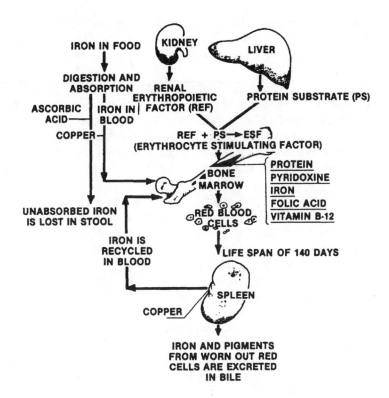

NUTRIENTS NEEDED FOR ERYTHROPOIESIS

I. **MINERALS**

Iron: Core of hemoglobin molecule
Copper: Part of enzyme ferroxidase which converts
        iron to ferric form for release from tissues
        into blood

II. **VITAMINS**

Ascorbic acid: Reduces iron to ferrous form for
        absorption
Pyridoxine: Cofactor in synthesis of hemoglobin
Folic acid and Vitamin B-12: Control division,
        growth, and maturation of red cells

III. **PROTEIN**

Raw material for hemoglobin and red cells

FIGURE 10.2
The nutrients pivotal to erythropoeisis.

European descent. The hemochromatosis locus is linked to the HLA region on the short arm of chromosome 6 and is an autosomal recessive trait. The prevalence of this genetic abnormality may be as high as 12 in 1000 individuals of European descent and is characterized by excessive iron absorption, elevated plasma iron concentration and transferrin saturation, and high iron content in liver parenchyma cells. On the other hand, macrophage iron content is relatively low.

Congenital transferrinemia is an extremely rare disorder characterized by a nearly complete lack of transferrin. This disorder is probably an autosomal recessive anomaly and is accompanied by hypochromic anemia and iron overload involving the liver, heart, and pancreas and an almost complete lack of iron in bone marrow. This disorder, along with a mouse model of hypotransferrin is very suggestive that plasma transferrin is not necessary for the transport of absorbed iron.

More isolated examples of human genetic disposition for iron overload have also been described. One third of the members of a large Melanesian family have been reported to have developed iron overload. Although many characteristics are similar to HLA-linked hemochromatosis, the mode of inheritance appears to be autosomal dominant transmission. Another instance of inherited iron overload heredity was reported in two siblings in a Yemenite Jewish family. This inherited trait is also believed not to be HLA-linked hemochromatosis.

Iron overload has been reported in at least 15 sub-Saharan African countries. The overload is the result of drinking locally brewed beer with a high iron content. The histological alterations to the liver are distinct from alcohol-related insult, and iron accumulates in both hepatic parenchyma cells and macrophages. Necropsy evaluation estimated the incidence of iron overload-induced liver cirrhosis to be greater than 10% in these geographic regions. Further investigation suggested that there is likely an underlying genetic factor concomitant with a high dietary iron consumption.

The forms of inherited anemia, homozygous 8-thalassemia, 8-thalassemia/hemoglobin E, and hemoglobin H disease, all result in ineffectual erythropoiesis in bone marrow. Although the mechanisms are unclear, the ineffective erythropoiesis ultimately leads to augmented iron absorption. The treatment of these diseases involves multiple blood transfusions, which contributes even more iron to these individuals. Initially the overloading of iron results in deposits in the liver; however, with time, iron accumulates in other organs such as the heart and pancreas.

Other forms of anemia associated with ineffective erythropoiesis can increase iron absorption and potentially lead to overload. These anemias include congenital dyserythropoietic anemias, a number of sideroblastic anemias, and many anemias associated with poor iron incorporation into hemoglobin.

Iron overload may also be induced clinically by frequent blood transfusions in patients with aplastic anemia, pure red cell anemia, Blackfan-Diamond syndrome, myelodysplasia, and sickle cell disease. The iron is derived primarily from erythrocyte hemoglobin and excessive iron initially accumulates in macrophages and then liver parenchyma.

Neonatal iron overload has been described as being associated with certain perinatal metabolic disorders such as hypermethionemia and severe fatal liver disease. Animal models have been developed to study iron overload and its related pathology. Rats fed a diet enriched with 2 to 3% elemental (carbonyl) iron over a period of 2 to 4 months develop hepatic nonheme iron concentrations 50 to 100 times normal. Excessive iron deposition in cardiac and pancreatic tissue is modest, and nonhepatic organ toxicity is not evident.

The exact mechanism of toxicity from iron overload is not completely established. However, many investigators agree that the pathological alterations associated with iron overload are probably the result of increased free radical activity initiated by excessive iron. Under normal situations, iron is almost entirely found bound to proteins. However, unbound iron in the reduced ferrous form is believed to contribute to free radical activity by participating in the Fenton reaction, which results in the production of the highly reactive hydroxyl radical (OH·).

$$Fe^{2+} + H_2O_2 \longrightarrow Fe^{3+} \ OH^- + OH·$$

Many investigators have reported the products of lipid peroxidation in various tissues, including liver, plasma, kidney, spleen, muscle, and skin. Increased iron absorption results in hepatic iron overload, which ultimately leads to organelle dysfunction and injury, lipocyte collagen synthesis leading to fibrosis, and possibly alterations in hepatic DNA initiating tumor formation.

Although iron deposition during overload deposits in many tissues such as the heart, lung, kidney, and brain, the liver has received the most investigative attention, most likely because of its prominent involvement in iron storage and also because cirrhosis is recognized as one the most common causes of death with genetic-based hemochromatosis in humans. Rats fed a diet enriched with 2 to 3% carbonyl for 2 to 4 months develop hepatic iron concentrations of 3000 to 6000 µg iron per gram liver. The iron preferentially deposits in periportal hepatocytes, similar to early HLA-linked hemochromatosis and African iron overload. The iron overloaded rats present direct evidence of mitochondrial and microsomal lipid peroxidation along with an increase in the low-molecular-weight pool of catalytically active iron. Further, at hepatic iron concentration at which lipid peroxidation is observed, specific mitochondrial membrane associated activities such as oxidative metabolism and calcium sequestering are decreased. Similarly, microsomal membranes demonstrate decreased cytochrome concentrations, enzyme activities, and calcium sequestration.

Iron overload results in excessive accumulation of iron in hepatocellular lysosomes and appears to increase their fragility. This increase in fragility results in the release of hydrolytic enzymes into the cytosol of hepatocytes, initiating cellular damage. Myers et al. reported that experimental iron-overloaded rat hepatocytes presented lysosomes that were more fragile, enlarged and misshaped. These membranes also demonstrated decreased fluidity, and increased lipid peroxidation as determined by malondialdehyde content.

At liver iron concentrations similar to those observed in HLA-linked hemochromatosis (3000 to 6000 µg of iron per gram liver), experimental iron-overloaded rat mitochondria show increased lipid peroxidation as demonstrated *in vivo* by the presence of conjugated dienes in phospholipid extracts. These investigative efforts also resulted in the determination of a hepatic iron concentration threshold for the presence of lipid peroxidation in mitochondria (1000 to 1500 µg of iron per gram liver) and microsomes (3000 µg of iron per gram liver). It has also been reported that mitochondrial malondialdehyde content is also increased several-fold in experimentally iron-overloaded rats and that this increase in malondialdehyde is likely due to not only increased lipid peroxidation but also an impairment in malondialdehyde metabolism as well. Furthermore, at modest increases in hepatic liver iron concentration, there was a significant impediment of mitochondrial electron transport as exemplified by a 70% reduction in cytochrome c oxidase activity and a 48% decrease in cellular oxygen consumption.

Iron overload also results in hepatic fibrosis. The mechanisms of fibrogenesis in this condition are poorly understood as efforts with experimentally iron-overloaded rats, and baboons have failed to demonstrate a consistent relationship with prolyl hydrolase activity. Morphological investigation of experimental iron overload revealed that hepatic fibrosis was recognized at 8 months, and by 1 year periportal fibrosis was pronounced and concomitant to the identification of cirrhosis in some animals. Investigators have identified that the hepatic levels of type I procollagen mRNA is augmented and that nonparenchymal cells are predominantly involved, most likely activated lipocytes.

Iron overload is also associated with a greater incidence of cancer. Humans with HLA-linked hemochromatosis are about 200 times greater risk of hepatocellular carcinoma. Experimental iron overload rats have presented evidence of an increase in DNA strand breaks with a liver iron concentration of 3130 µg per gram tissue, but not at lower liver iron concentrations (~600 µg/g). Further, a synergistic carcinogenic effect was reported with the combination of iron in conjunction with polychlorinated biphenyls.

Recent concern has been over the reported association of serum ferritin levels with increased myocardial infarction. In a study of over 1900 Finnish males from 40 to 64 years of age, serum ferritin levels greater than 200 µg/l had a 2.2 times greater risk of myocardial infarct compared to males with lower levels. This was after adjustment for other known risk factors, such as cigarette smoking, higher systolic blood pressure, lipoprotein choles-terol levels, etc. In fact, those males with a serum LDL-cholesterol level greater than 193 mg/100 ml had even a greater risk, with the added high serum ferritin levels. Speculation as to the mechanism apparently may be related to the role of iron in free radical generation as reviewed above. Oxidation of LDL-cholesterol is known to result in greater cholesterol uptake by macrophages, which is a key mechanism in foam cell production and subse-quent plaque formation.

Zinc

The major metabolic function of zinc in the human body is as a cofactor for more than 200 enzymes impacting probably every general function in the human body. This makes zinc one of the most ubiquitous micronutrients. Special attention was focused upon zinc after it was determined that zinc works directly at the level of gene expression. Zinc is commonly found as a divalent cation (Zn^{2+}).

Dietary Sources

As zinc is mostly associated with proteins and nucleic acids in organisms, good protein sources are also better zinc sources. For example, some of the best zinc sources in the diet include herring, oysters, clams, poultry, meats, eggs, and legumes (Table 10.3). While whole cereal grains are also a better source of zinc, because the refining or milling process removes most of this mineral. Fruits are also relatively poor sources.

Absorption

Zinc in the intestinal lumina is not only derived from dietary sources but from biliary and pancreatic digestive secretions as well. Zinc associated with proteins and nucleic acids is liberated from these structures via digestive secretions. While the exact mechanisms of zinc absorption are not completely resolved, it does appear to occur along the length of the small intestine, with the jejunum being responsible for most of the absorption. Several fac-tors influence the efficiency of zinc absorption which contribute to its relatively wide range of absorption (12 to 60%). As with several of the transition elements, the absorption of zinc increases as its physiological status decreases, and vice versa. Also, there are several dietary factors that can influence zinc absorption. For instance, zinc availability from soy and wheat may be improved by the addition of casein, cysteine, or histidine, to which zinc binds to preferentially. This is an example of a beneficial chelation. On the other hand, phytate present in grains and legumes can bind zinc and decrease its absorption. However, phytate seems to only have a negative effect in the presence of increased intraluminal cal-cium. Zinc absorption is also decreased by substances such as oxalic acid, found in teas, chocolate, berries, and spinach, and polyphenols, such as tannins present in tea. High dietary fiber intake also may decrease zinc absorption.

TABLE 10.3
Zinc Content of Various Foods

Food	Zinc (mg)
Meat and alternatives	
Liver (3 oz)	4.6
Beef (3 oz)	4.7
Crab (1 c)	4.7
Lamb (3 oz)	4.2
Pork (3 oz)	2.8
Chicken (3 oz)	0.9
Grains	
Wheat germ (2 tbl)	—
Oatmeal, cooked (1 c)	1.7
Bran flakes (1 c)	5.0
Rice, brown (1 c)	1.3
Rice, white (1 c)	0.8
Legumes	
Dried beans, cooked (2 c)	—
Split peas, cooked (2 c)	2.0
Nuts and seeds	
Pecans (1 c)	6.5
Cashews (1 c)	6.2
Sunflower seeds (1 c)	7.3
Peanut butter (2 tbl)	0.5
Milk and milk products	
Cheese, cheddar (1 oz)	0.9
Milk, whole (1 c)	0.9
Cheese, American (1 oz)	0.9

Zinc and iron may also compete for absorption since a iron:zinc intake of 2:1 or higher will substantially reduce zinc absorption in humans. Zinc is more bioavailable as amino acid chelates (zinc–alanine, zinc–glycine) and as zinc gluconate. However, zinc appears to be less available as zinc sulfate and zinc carbonate. Zinc absorption appears to be somewhat positively influenced by the presence of meat. A pancreatic substance such as citrate or picolinic acid may enhance the absorption of zinc. At physiological levels of intestinal zinc, the predominant mechanism of absorption appears to be a carrier-mediated system that may or may not require energy. Zinc is absorbed against a concentration gradient, which is certainly suggestive of an active transport mechanism. Interestingly, metabolic inhibitors do not appear to influence zinc uptake, nor does zinc uptake display saturation kinetics. Therefore, zinc absorption is still somewhat enigmatic. At higher dietary intakes, some paracellular absorption is thought to contribute to the overall absorption in a relative manner.

When zinc enters the mucosal cell, it is destined to one of following fates: (1) it may move back out into the intestinal lumen; (2) it may perform functions within the mucosal cell; (3) it can move into the blood; and/or (4) it may bind to the small molecular weight protein, *thionein*, forming *metallothionein*. High intramucosal zinc levels induce the transcription of mRNA for thionein, a protein with a molecular weight of 6000 to 8000. This compound has a high number of sulfhydryl groups capable of generally chelating divalent cations. The sequestering of minerals to thionein allows for its more popular name, "metallothionein." The excessive zinc, bound to thionein, can then be excreted as mucosal cells are sloughed off. Zinc entering the human body requires a zinc binding ligand called *cysteine-rich protein (CRIP)*, which will transfer zinc primarily to albumin or to other proteins such as transferrin, α-2 macroglobulin, and immunoglobin G (IgG) in the portal blood (Figure 10.3).

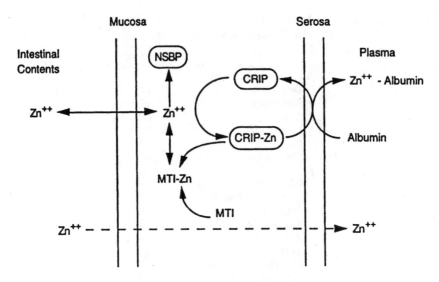

FIGURE 10.3
Intestinal zinc absorption. Passive diffusion is displayed in the lower part of the diagram, while mediated transport is presented in the upper part of the diagram.

One potential consequence of excessive zinc ingestion and the resultant increased synthesis thionein is a sequestering of copper and its subsequent loss in sloughed off cells. Thionein has a greater affinity for copper than zinc, and it has become known that ingesting as little as 18.5 mg of zinc for a couple of weeks significantly decreases copper absorption.

Metabolism and Function

Zinc is found in every human cell, and the average content of the body ranges from 1.5 to 2.5 g, depending upon physical size. Tissues demonstrating a higher concentration of zinc include bone, liver, muscle, kidneys, and the skin. A basic aspect, and perhaps equally as well a fundamental problem, is the issue that zinc is a cofactor for more than 200 enzymes, many of which deal with various aspects of protein synthesis or hormone function of some type. While physiological consequences relating to an absolute or marginal dietary zinc consumption often relate to the effect zinc has upon these enzymes, zinc excess may not have a direct influence upon these target enzymes, and in fact some of the associated physiological consequences may be related to resulting imbalances of other nutrients. This is well documented in the previous section on copper and zinc antagonism. Excess diet zinc may lead to a copper deficiency, which has much different symptoms. Therefore, it becomes a challenge to separate out the direct effects of zinc toxicity from the indirect or secondary effects that it may have at perturbing an imbalance of another essential element.

While zinc is found in all tissue, most of this mineral is actually located in the skeletal muscle (~60%) and bone (~30%). The skin, liver, brain, kidneys, and the heart also have higher concentrations of zinc; however, these concentrations are still small relative to bone and skeletal muscle. Liver zinc content in a newborn infant is greater than an adult man. For instance, 25% of the zinc in newborns is found in the liver. More zinc is probably found in the bones of newborns as compared with adults.

Zinc is primarily found within cells, as its concentration in extracellular fluids is relatively low. It is believed that there is a zinc-selective transport system that allows for the uptake of zinc into tissue. It is possible that zinc carriers, or at least one zinc carrier, is positively influenced by amino acid metabolism within that tissue. Hormonal balance may influence the zinc distribution between extracellular and intracellular fluids. Insulin, glucagon, and glucocorticoids appear to influence liver zinc levels. Glucocorticoids are known to stimulate zinc uptake in hepatic cultured cells. Glucagon may also stimulate zinc uptake by liver cells.

Zinc largely functions as a necessary component of various enzymes. In fact, the number of enzymes whose optimal function relies upon zinc is probably greater than the total number of enzymes that rely on all of the other minor minerals combined. In general, zinc is involved with enzymes that effect pH regulation; ethanol (alcohol) metabolism; bone mineralization; protein digestion; heme manufacturing; antioxidation; immunity; and protein and nucleic acid metabolism. Table 10.4 provides a listing of several zinc-dependent enzymes and their function.

TABLE 10.4
Zinc-Dependent Enzymes and Function

Enzyme	General Function
Alcohol dehydrogenase	Oxidation of ethanol in the cytosol, primarily in hepatocytes
Lactate dehydrogenase	Reversible oxidation/reduction interconversion of pyruvate and lactic acid
Alkaline phosphatase	Primarily involved in mineralization of bone matrix
Angiotensin-converting enzyme	Converts angiotensin I to angiotensin II
Carbonic anhydrase	Interconverts CO_2 and H_2O to carbonic acid to assist in the regulation of CO_2 content of blood as well as pH
Pyruvate dehydrogenase	Converts pyruvate to acetyl CoA within mitochondria
DNA and RNA polymerases	DNA replication and transcription
Superoxide dismutase (SOD)	Cytosolic antioxidant
Aspartate transcarbamylase	Pyrimidine synthesis
Carboxypeptidases A & B	Protein digestion
Phosphodiesterase	Cleaves phosphodiester bonds (i.e., nucleic acids)
Fructose 1,6-bisphosphatase	Gluconeogenesis
Leukotriene hydrolase	Eicosanoid metabolism
Elastase	Digestion of connective tissue elastin
Reverse transcriptase	DNA replication
Gustin	Taste acuity

Zinc also functions directly at the genetic level where it is associated with specialized proteins to form *zinc finger proteins*. Here, zinc binds to histidine and cysteine amino acids in proteins that are known to bind to DNA in the cell nucleus (Figure 10.4). These proteins are referred to as "transcription factors" and control gene expression or repression primarily through targeting promoter regions of genes.

There are two known genetic disorders of zinc metabolism: (1) the decreased ability of zinc to be absorbed by the small intestine can lead to *acrodermatitis enteropathica* — zinc supplementation is the course of treatment; and the familial disorder *hyperzincaemia* results in elevated serum zinc levels, but apparently does not produce any toxicity. Interestingly, zinc overdoses that result in a similar plasma zinc level have been known to be fatal.

Zinc excretion from the human body occurs by several routes. Zinc is primarily lost from the body via fecal excretion. Fecal zinc represents unabsorbed dietary zinc and zinc secreted into the digestive tract via digestion juices (i.e., zinc-containing enzymes, biliary fluids). Also, sloughed off mucosal enterocytes containing metallothionein zinc contribute significantly to fecal zinc content. Exfoliation of skin and sweating allow for about 1 mg of

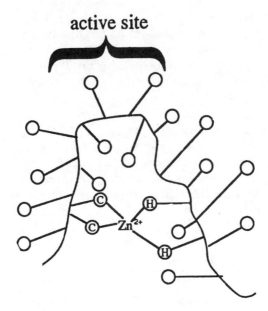

FIGURE 10.4
Zinc binding to cysteine (C) and histidine (H) residues of an enzyme. This serves to stabilize the structure and appropriately expose the catalytic site.

zinc loss daily. Urinary zinc is typically less than 600 µg daily, thus representing a minor route of excretion. Also, a relatively small amount of zinc occurs from the loss of body hair (0.1 to 0.2 mg zinc per gram).

Recommended Levels of Intake

Zinc requirements are influenced by age, gender, health status, condition (pregnancy, lactation), physical activity, and other dietary components. Males have a higher zinc requirement than females after 12 years of age, primarily because of the increased muscle mass. For males greater than 12 years of age and elderly males, 15 mg/d of zinc is recommended as compared to 12 mg/d for females. During pregnancy, the RDA is increased to 15 mg/d. This recommendation is followed by a further increase to 19 mg/d during the first 6 months of lactation and a subsequent reduction to 16 mg/d for the second 6 months of lactation.

Deficiency

Zinc deficiency is characterized by dwarfism, poor sexual performance, deformed bones, poor wound healing, abnormal hair and nails, loss of taste (hypoguesia), gastrointestinal disturbances, poor chylomicron formation, CNS anomalies, and impaired folate and vitamin A absorption. The incidence of zinc deficiency has been commonly observed among Middle Eastern children, especially males, and also in the Hispanic population of Denver, CO. In the Middle East, unleavened bread is frequently consumed, which is high in phytate. Yeast contains phytase which can digest some of the phytate. However, the recipe for the dough of unleavened bread does not include yeast. The high fiber content of their diets and low meat intake also contributes to the problem.

Toxicity

Acute human zinc toxicity rarely occurs. Much of the current knowledge regarding zinc toxicity comes from animal studies and through supplementation with mineral preparations. Animals provided a high diet zinc generally present dysphagia. This could be the result of a reduction in palatibility. Growth rate and even weight loss occur, attributable to decreased food intake. Also, zinc toxicity has been reported to result in rough hair, achromotrichia, emphysema, diarrhea, arthritis-like symptoms, aborted fetuses, stillbirths, etc. A microcytic anemia develops; however, this may be partly explained by a decreased uptake of either copper and/or iron. Also, hemolytic anemia is not uncommon, and renal fibrosis, fatty liver, and liver necrosis have been reported by some scientists. Hypercholesterolemia sometimes occurs with excess zinc, which again may be at least partially explained by a secondary copper deficiency. Excess zinc normally would produce symptoms that mimic deficiencies of copper, iron, manganese and/or calcium. When either one or more of these elements are increased in the diet, the signs of zinc toxicity appear markedly reduced.

Iodine

The role of iodine in humans and animal nutrition has been recognized for a long time. At one time, deficiency of iodine was widespread globally, including the U.S. Today it is still rather problematic in certain areas of the world, such as parts of Africa where an estimated 200 million people are affected (Figure 10.5). Deficiency of iodine results in hypertrophy of the thyroid gland, termed *goiter*. Historically, goiter was documented in the records of the early Greeks. The ancient Greeks used burnt sponges to treat goiter, but this information was lost for a long period of time. It was not until 1850 that the French physician Chatin measured the iodine content of water and various foods of France and noted that the iodine content of the soil correlated with the incidence of goiter. This was published, but forgotten as well. By the early part of the 20th century, iodine became known as a treatment for goiter.

Iodine, as an element, is a halogen. As with other halogens, iodine tends to accept an electron and exist in nature as a negatively charge ion. Therefore, the anion name "iodide" is used interchangeably with "iodine," as are "fluoride" and "fluorine," "chloride" and "chlorine," and "bromide" and "bromine." "Iodide" will be used in this text, as it is the natural state for this element.

Dietary Sources of Iodide

There is a large variability of iodide in food, and intake typically ranges between 100 to 200 µg/d in the U.S. Table 10.5 provides a listing of the iodide content of selected foods. The iodide content of a plant is mostly related to the soil content in which the plant was grown and/or the iodide content of any fertilizers used to cultivate the soil. Furthermore, the iodide content in drinking water usually reflects the iodide content of the rocks and soils through which the water originally flowed or is maintained. The animal content of iodide depends on the plants they consumed or the feed they were provided; for carnivores, it depends upon the plant consumption of their prey. Animal iodide content is also influenced by the content in their water source.

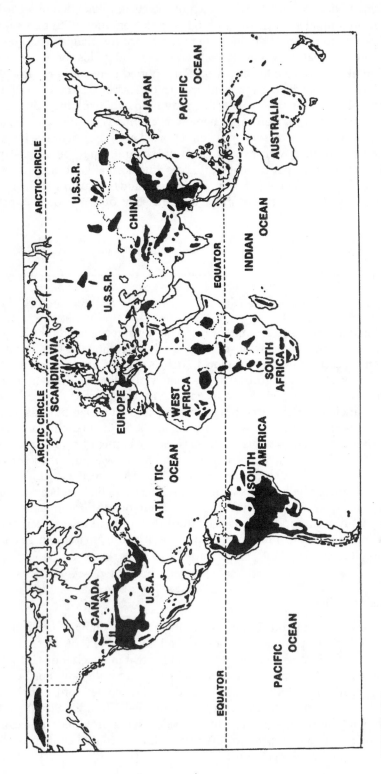

FIGURE 10.5
Goiter areas of the world.

TABLE 10.5

Iodide Content of Selected Foods

Food	Iodide (μg)
Salt, iodized (1 t)	400
Haddock (3 oz)	104–145
Cottage cheese (2 c)	26–71
Shrimp (3 oz)	21–37
Egg (1)	18–26
Cheese, cheddar (1 oz)	5–23
Ground beef (3 oz)	8

Seafood (shrimp, oysters, ocean fish, mollusks) is typically a better source of iodide than fresh-water fish. Dairy foods may be a fair source of iodide. Again, the iodide content of cow's milk reflects either the iodide content of the cow's feed and/or the soil content of the grazing region. Iodide deficiency is for the most part eradicated from many regions of the world, including the U.S., where iodide is added to salt (iodized salt). Iodized salt contains one part sodium iodide for every 1000 parts sodium chloride.

Today, there is a developing concern about the overconsumption of iodine in countries that utilize iodized salt. For instance, in the U.S. excessive use of iodized salt in food manufacturing, preparation, and seasoning results in the ingestion of iodide well in excess of recommendations.

Absorption of Iodide

Along with dietary iodide, some iodide enters the small intestine via biliary secretions. The amount of iodide in biliary secretions is influenced by iodide status. The absorption of iodine occurs efficiently along the length of the intestinal tract including the stomach. This results in nearly complete absorption of iodide, similar to several other monovalent ions, namely, sodium, potassium, and chloride. Very efficient absorption results in very low fecal iodide content. Iodide appears to dissolve freely into the blood and excessive iodide is primarily excreted by the kidneys.

Metabolism and Function of Iodide

An adult human contains roughly 15 to 20 mg of iodide. For the most part, iodide is concentrated in the thyroid gland as well as the salivary and gastric glands. The thyroid gland contains roughly 75 to 80% of body iodide. In thyroid gland parenchyma, the concentration of intracellular iodide may be 30-fold higher than the extracellular fluid. Thus, these cells must utilize aggressive active transport systems to acquire such a large concentration of iodide. The thyroid gland uses iodide to synthesize thyroid hormone. At least 60 μg of iodide must be taken up by the thyroid gland daily to produce adequate thyroid hormone. Salivary glands also utilize an active transport mechanism to accrue iodide.

The iodine in the thyroid gland is incorporated into a globulin protein, termed *"thyroglobin,"* which is the storage form of iodine. It can be removed from storage and react with the amino acid tyrosine. Iodination may occur on the 3, 5, 3′, and 5′ carbon positions of the six-member rings of the thyronine structure. When iodide is bound to all four positions, the compound is called *thyroxin* (T_4) (Figure 10.6). Iodination at the 3, 5, and 3′ ring positions results in a molecule called *triiodothyronine* (T_3). Collectively, T_3 and T_4 are referred to as "thyroid hormone," with T_4 predominating in the blood. Roughly 90% of the

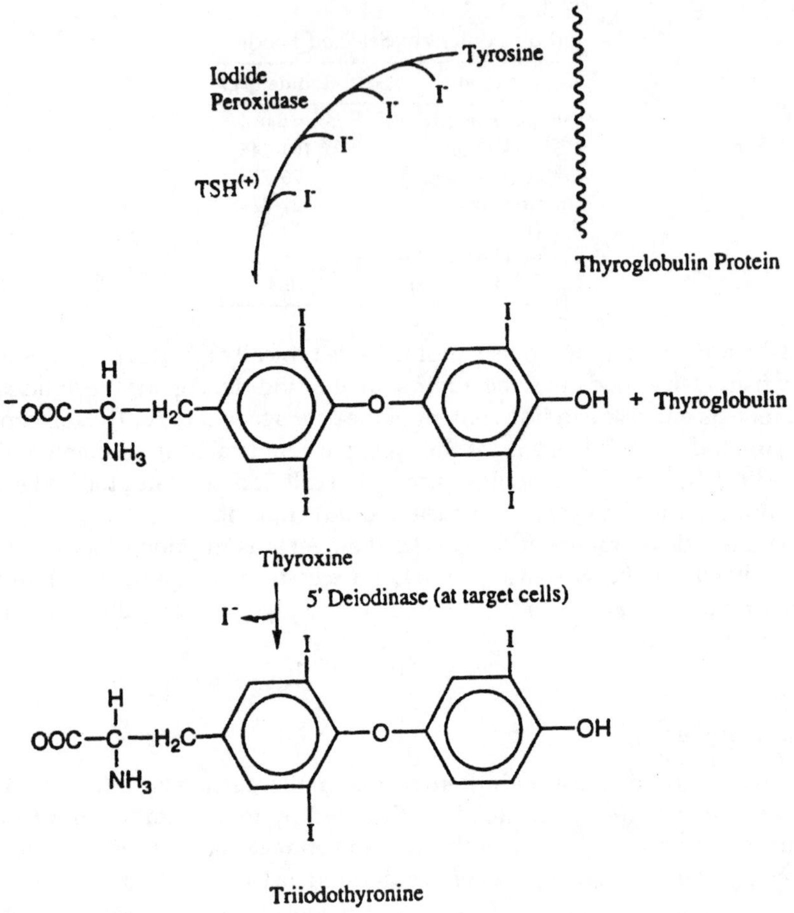

FIGURE 10.6
Thyroid hormone synthesis.

thyroid hormone released daily is T_4 and the remaining 10% is T_3. However, T_3 is about 5 to 10 times more potent than T_4. In the blood, about 80% of thyroid hormone binds to thyroxine-binding protein (TBP), about 10 to 15% binds to thyroxine-binding prealbumin, and the remainder to albumin.

There is a unique control mechanism regarding the production of these compounds. The hypothalmus releases a peptide known as *thyrotropin-releasing hormone (TRH)*, which in turn stimulates the pituitary to produce *thyroid-stimulating hormone (TSH)*, also called *thyrotropin*. TSH circulates to the thyroid gland and then initiates the production of thyroid hormone, which then enters the blood and circulates to peripheral tissue. Thyroid hormone output will increase and exert a negative feedback on the release of TRH. TSH may do the same, but to a lesser extent. Almost all of the thyroxine in the circulation may become converted (deiodinated) to the T_3 after entering peripheral tissue. Thyroid hormone has its receptors in the nucleus of the cells; thus its activity is largely attributed to influence on gene expression. Thyroid hormone also undergoes some low-affinity binding in the cytoplasm. However, the binding is not to the same protein receptor as is found in the nucleus.

Thyroid hormone affects virtually every cell in the human body, perhaps with the exception of the adult brain, testes, spleen, uterus, and the thyroid gland itself. Thyroid hormone promotes the activities associated with glucose breakdown and thereby increases metabolism and heat production. Thyroid hormone generally acts by inducing or suppressing the expression of certain genes. One outstanding function of thyroid hormone is the induction of expression of the gene for growth hormone. This explains why earlier studies demonstrated that animals deficient in thyroid hormone presented lower amounts of growth hormone in their pituitary gland. It also helps explain some of the general anabolic effects of thyroid hormone. More specific effects of thyroid hormone are listed in Table 10.6.

TABLE 10.6
Effects of Thyroid Hormone on Specific Human Mechanisms

Tissue/Mechanism	Effect of Thyroid Hormone
Carbohydrate metabolism	Stimulates glucose absorption as well as uptake by cells; enhances carbohydrate metabolism, especially glycolysis and gluconeogenesis; enhances insulin release
Fat metabolism	Enhances fat mobilization from adipocytes; increases FFA content of plasma and increases fatty acid oxidation in cells; decreases plasma cholesterol and triglycerides, probably by increasing bile cholesterol content and subsequent fecal loss
Protein synthesis	Increases general protein synthesis; however, excessive amounts result in protein catabolism
Basal metabolism	Increases general metabolism of most cells; lack of thyroid hormone results in a 50% reduction in basal metabolic rate
Cardiovascular system	Increase heart rate and stroke strength; increases blood volume slightly; blood pressure is generally unchanged while systolic pressure can be elevated and diastolic relatively decreased
Respiration	Increased respiration associated with increased cellular metabolism
Feeding/digestion	Increased appetite and food intake; increased rate of digestive juice secretion and motility of digestive tract; lack of thyroid hormone results in constipation
Skeletal muscle	Increases vigor of contraction
Central nervous system	Increases rapidity of elation; excessive amounts result in nervousness and anxiety
Endocrine glands	Increases rate of most endocrine secretions

Since a higher blood thyroid hormone concentration increases metabolic rate, synthetic thyroid hormone was once prescribed to treat morbidly obese people. However, the effects of thyroid hormone are not only limited to increasing cell metabolism and potentially deleterious side effects limited its use for this purpose. Therapeutic thyroid hormone therapy also affects blood pressure and heart activity, as well as producing nausea, sweating, diarrhea, anxiety, headaches, and insomnia. Today, thyroid hormone is prescribed mostly to treat hypothyroidism, a condition in which the thyroid gland fails to produce adequate thyroid hormone. During the growing years, thyroid hormone is very important because it promotes growth and maturation of the skeleton, CNS, and reproductive organs.

Recommended Levels for Iodide Intake

The RDA for adults is 150 μg/d. During pregnancy, the RDA is 175 μg/d, followed by an increase to 200 μg/d during lactation. Most individuals in developed countries receive at least the recommended amounts of iodide via iodized salt consumption. However, as mentioned above, iodide deficiency is still one of the most prevalent nutrition-based problems globally.

Iodide Deficiency

A deficiency of iodide limits the thyroid hormone synthesis in the thyroid gland. Thus, most of the signs and symptoms of iodide deficiency result from hypothyroidemia. An iodide deficiency in childhood can result in poor growth, poor maturing of organs and sexual maturity, along with mental deficits. A striking characteristic of iodide deficiency is an enlargement of the thyroid gland (Figure 10.7). Treatment of goiter usually begins with iodide-rich foods, including iodized salt, which will shrink the goiter with time but not necessarily correct any of the developmental problems (growth and mental aptitude) in children. Before the widespread use of iodized salt, various regions of the American midwest were referred to as the "goiter belt," due to a low soil iodide content and decreased availability of iodide-rich fish.

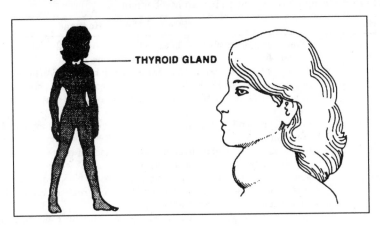

FIGURE 10.7
Goiter and the position of the thyroid gland

Infants born to mothers with low iodine in their diets, particularly in the third trimester of pregnancy, may suffer from a condition called *cretinism*, in which they often demonstrate stunted growth and present deficits in mental development. These individuals exhibit large heads relative to body size, are deaf, and have coarse features. This permanent condition is common in endemic goiter regions: Himilayas, central Africa, and central South America.

Certain foods contain substances called *goitrogens* that appear to block iodide entry into the thyroid gland. Foods containing goitrogens include broccoli, kale, cauliflower, rutabaga, turnips, brussels sprouts, and mustard greens. However, most individuals do not eat enough of these vegetables to pose a threat to normal iodide metabolism and thyroid gland activity. Routine blood tests include T_3 and T_4 concentrations, thus providing a screening tool for thyroid deficiency or other thyroid hormone-impacting diseases.

Copper

Copper in the human body shifts between two oxidation states, *cuprous* (Cu^{1+}) and *cupric* (Cu^{2+}) state. By and large, the cupric state predominates. Copper exerts much of its action by being a cofactor for several enzymes that are often referred to as cuproenzymes. Copper is fundamentally involved in iron metabolism. If a copper deficiency occurs, the signs and symptoms presented are similar to those of iron deficiency anemia. Copper is required for the proper synthesis of collagen and is needed to maintain the integrity of the connective tissue.

Dietary Sources

Dietary sources of copper are found in a wide variety of foods with very little in common (Table 10.7). Copper is found in foods such as nuts, shellfish, organ meats, dried fruits, seeds, and legumes. Grains and grain products, as well as chocolate, have appreciable levels of copper. While these food items are good-to-excellent sources of copper, the absolute amount of copper absorbed may be influenced by other dietary components. Furthermore, the origin of a food or the processing and handling of a food can greatly change the copper content. As with iodide and certain other minerals, the soil content in which plants were grown and feed content and water sources for livestock also will influence the copper content of the final food product. Surveys reveal that the copper consumption in the U.S. ranges between 0.7 to 7.5 mg daily.

TABLE 10.7
Copper Content of Selected Foods

Food	Copper (mg)
Liver, beef (3 oz)	3.8
Cashews, dry roasted (1 c)	3.0
Black-eyed peas (2 c)	0.9
Molasses, blackstrap (2 tbl)	0.8
Sunflower seeds (1 c)	2.5
V-8 juice (1 c)	0.5
Tofu, firm (2 c)	1.0
Beans, refried (2 c)	0.8
Cocoa powder (2 T)	0.4
Prunes, dried (10)	0.4
Salmon, baked (3 oz)	0.1
Pizza, cheese (1 slice)	0.1
Bread, whole wheat (1 slice)	0.1
Milk chocolate (1 oz)	0.1
Milk, 2% (1 c)	0.1

Absorption

Copper may be absorbed by both the stomach and small intestinal mucosa. However, most of the absorption is attributed to the latter. Both saturable active transport and passive uptake mechanisms are thought to be responsible for copper absorption. The percentage of copper absorption is decreased as the luminal content of copper increases. For instance, with intakes approximating 7.5 mg, about 10 to 20% of the copper is absorbed. Meanwhile, a much lower copper intake, approximating 1.0 mg, will result in as much as 50 to 75% absorption.

Several minerals will influence copper absorption. Excess dietary iron can decrease copper absorption, while contrarily, too much copper may cause an iron deficiency. Excessive zinc consumption will also decrease copper absorption. The mechanism by which dietary zinc inhibits the uptake of copper involves the intestinal protein thionein eluded to earlier.

As dietary zinc levels increase, thionein synthesis in mucosal enterocytes increases. This results in the binding and "trapping" of zinc within the mucosal cell via the formation of metallothionein. Metallothionein is not easily dissociated and, consequently, when enterocytes are sloughed off in the normal mucosal turnover, zinc is lost through the fecal compartment. However, thionein has a greater affinity for copper. Thus, when excess zinc is consumed, the increased thionein production will cause copper to be sequestered within enterocytes and eventually excreted in the feces. As little as 18.5 mg of zinc daily can decrease copper absorption while even higher intakes (25 mg) for several weeks can reduce the activity of key cuproenzymes such as *superoxide dismutase*.

The presence of certain amino acids, histidine in particular, can enhance copper absorption. In addition, binding ligands such as gluconate and citrate can assist in copper absorption as well. Also, the type of carbohydrate consumed may influence copper absorption efficiency, although more information is needed in this area. One interesting aspect of copper absorption is that it is not as strongly affected by the presence of phytate as are absorption of zinc and iron.

Metabolism and Function

Copper, once absorbed, is transported bound primarily to albumin and *transcuprin*. The half-life of the copper–albumin interaction is brief (10 min). Copper that is delivered to the liver may reenter circulation, however, this time in association with the α-macroglobulin *ceruloplasmin*. This compound will transport copper to other tissues and also assist with the transport of iron aboard transferrin as it functions as a *ferroxidase*. This activity converts iron to the appropriate oxidation state (ferric) for transport aboard transferrin.

Ceruloplasmin, which can carry up to six atoms of copper, has a molecular weight of approximately 160,000 and contains as much as 60 to 90% of the plasma copper. The remainder of copper in the systemic circulation is loosely bound to plasma albumin. A normal level of plasma copper is 0.9 µg/ml, and ceruloplasmin varies between 15 to 60 mg/100 ml.

An adult may contain 50 to 120 mg of copper with the most concentrated tissue being liver. The heart, brain, kidneys, and spleen are also concentrated with copper relative to other tissue. Interestingly, on a body weight basis, infants and younger children have a higher content than adults. For adults, bile represents the primary route of excretion. About 2 mg of copper is excreted via bile daily. Copper is also excreted from the human body in the urine (10 to 50 µg/d) and to a minor extent, through the loss of hair and skin.

Excess copper binds to liver thionein (metallothionein), thereby decreasing the potential for copper toxicity. It seems that copper, iron, and zinc are all involved in regulating the synthesis of metal-binding thionein proteins. Each of these minerals has specific metal-responsive elements that influence thionein expression. The metal-responsive element sensitive to copper is called CUPI.

Most of the functions of copper are mediated through its role as a component of key enzymes. Copper-containing *amine oxidases* are present in the plasma and catabolize some physiologically active amines such as tyramine, histidine, and polyamines (Figure 10.8). Monoamine oxidases break down catecholamines (norepinephrine, tyramine, dopamine, and serotonin). Diamine oxidase inactivates histamine, particularly in the small intestine where activity of the enzyme is high, as well as in the kidney. *Lysyl oxidase* is a cuproenzyme that catalyzes the posttranslational modification of lysine to hydroxylysine in collagen. This helps collagen proteins crosslink into larger fibers. The connective tissue strength is thus dependent on the activity of lysyl oxidase and therefore upon copper.

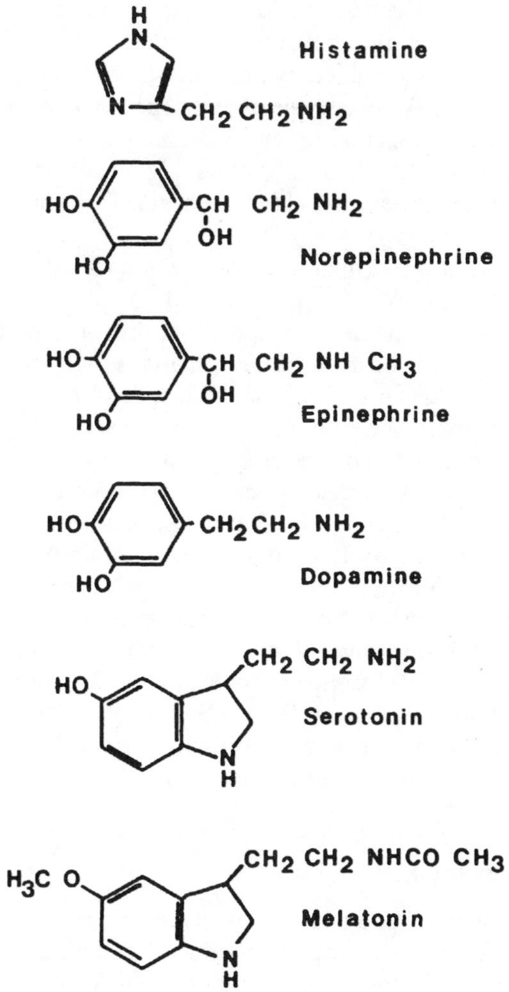

FIGURE 10.8
Biologically active amines.

Copper is utilized by most cells as a component of the enzyme *cytochrome c oxidase*, which is at the terminal end of the mitochondrial electron transport chain. This enzyme is involved with the reduction of oxygen to form water and is the rate-limiting enzyme in electron transport and its activity is dependent upon tissue copper content. The levels of cytochrome c oxidase are very high in tissue, such as the heart, where the oxidation of fatty acids and pyruvate are greater than in other tissue.

Dopamine hydroxylase is another significant enzyme in that it catalyzes the conversion of dopamine to norepinephrine. Cytosolic *superoxide dismutase* (SOD), which not only contains copper but zinc as well, is a powerful antioxidant that squelches superoxide radicals as depicted in the following reaction:

$$2\,O_2^- + 2\,H^+ \xrightarrow{\text{Cu/Zn–SOD}} H_2O_2 + O_2$$

Superoxide radicals can be destructive to cellular structures by causing peroxidative damage primarily to phospholipid components of membranes. The hydrogen peroxide formed by SOD can then be metabolized by peroxidases, such as glutathione peroxidase, a selenium-containing enzyme. Higher levels of cytosolic SOD are present in the brain, thyroid, liver, pituitary, erythrocytes, and kidneys. SOD has two atoms of copper per molecule. There is also an extracellular SOD which is found in higher concentrations in the lungs, thyroid, and uterus and in small amounts in blood plasma. This antioxidant does not contain copper.

Tyrosine metabolism involves copper at three reactions. First, the cuproenzyme *tyrosine hydroxylase* converts tyrosine to L-dopa (3,4-dihydroxyphenylalanine). L-Dopa can be metabolized further, serving as a substrate for dopamine or melanin synthetic processes. Dopamine can then be converted to norepinephrine which is catalyzed by dopamine hydroxylase, a cuproenzyme. Dopamine hydroxylase requires at least 8 atoms of copper and requires the redux potential of vitamin C.

Metabolism of L-dopa to melanin occurs in pigment cells called *melanocytes*. The color of skin, hair, and eyes is dependent upon the enzyme. In copper deficiency, tyrosinase activity is low and leads to decreased pigmentation. This is especially obvious in animals, as darker fur can begin to lighten or turn gray. Last, as a copper-containing hydroxylase, the enzyme is involved in tyrosine catabolism.

Copper is also a part of other proteins such as *transcuprin*, a plasma protein which may involve copper transport. Blood *clotting factor V*, while nonenzymatic, contains copper. Interestingly, however, copper deficiency is not known to impair blood clotting. Copper is also required for proper myelination of the CNS. Phospholipid synthesis depends upon cytochrome c oxidase, and this may be a reason why copper deficiency leads to decreased myelination, necrosis of nerve tissue, and neonatal ataxia in copper-deficient animals.

Recommended Levels of Intake

The results of nutrition surveys suggest that most Americans consume less than adequate amounts of copper. Some researchers speculate that over a lifetime a marginal diet copper may be a contributing factor in the development of heart disease. The estimated safe and adequate intake (ESADDI) for copper is 1.5 to 3.0 mg. Most survey studies show that Americans consume about 1.0 mg or less of copper per day.

Deficiency

Copper deficiency has been observed in premature infants and infants suffering from malnutrition. Overt symptoms in adults are rare but may occur in those who consume zinc supplements for a period of time. Animals that are fed diets deficient in copper often exhibit cardiac abnormalities such as blood vessel and heart rupture, abnormal EKG's, and have elevated serum cholesterol, triglycerides, and glucose.

Genetic Anomalies Influencing Copper Status

There are two well-known genetic diseases affecting copper metabolism. *Menkes' kinky-hair disease*, characterized and reported in the early 1960's, is an X-linked chromosomal disorder which manifests abnormalities in copper absorption. This results in a copper deficiency-like syndrome despite what may be adequate dietary copper consumption. Contrarily,

Wilson's disease, described in the early part of the 1900's is characterized by increased liver copper content, leading to severe hepatic damage, followed by increased brain copper levels and neurological aberrations. Thus, Wilson's disease results in a copper toxicity syndrome.

In Menke's syndrome, individuals experience depigmentation of the skin, kinky hair, central nervous system damage, and muscle and connective tissue abnormalities. Interestingly, anemia is not common, nor is neutropenia. The problem lies in the transport of copper from intestinal enterocytes. While parenteral copper administration is able to correct plasma levels, there remains a deficit in neurological tissue and infants with Menke's syndrome experience cerebral degeneration and generally do not survive beyond infancy.

Wilson's disease is an autosomal recessive disorder that is associated with excessive copper accumulation. Individuals presenting Wilson's disease typically experience premature death. Here the major flaw is a decreased ability to incorporate copper into ceruloplasmin as well as a decreased ability to excrete copper in the bile. This appears to be a manifestation of a defective gene for P-type ATPase cation transporters and results in excess accumulation in the liver and brain tissue. The defect occurs on chromosome 13 for humans. Preliminary signs of Wilson's disease include liver dysfunction, neurological disorders, and copper deposits in the cornea of the eye that result in a "halo" appearance around the pupil, which is referred to as the Kayser-Fleischer ring. Kidney stones and acidic urine can also occur. Wilson's disease is managed with copper chelators such as D-penicillamine as well as zinc supplements, which decrease copper absorption by promoting the synthesis of enterocyte thionein.

Selenium

Selenium achieved world attention as the nutritional deficiency responsible for Keshan disease. Lately, interest in selenium and disease prevention has included chemoprevention of cancers. Selenium primarily functions as part of the antioxidant complex *glutathione peroxidase*, although other functions are being revealed.

Dietary Selenium

Like other minor minerals, the amount of selenium in a food is highly dependent on the level found in the soil where crops are grown and animals grazed and drank. Therefore, the risk of deficiency as well as toxicity could be a concern if regional inhabitants subsisted upon crops and livestock from that area. However, in countries such as the U.S. the varying level of selenium in the soil is not that great a concern as in most regions inhabitants consume foods grown throughout the country as well as internationally. Better dietary sources of selenium include seafood, tuna, meat, and cereals, especially wheat-based cereals (Table 10.8). In areas where the soil is high in selenium, cow's milk may also be a more concentrated source.

Absorption

Selenium is efficiently absorbed in the gastrointestinal tract in several organic forms. However, the absorption of two distinct selenium forms (selenomethionine and selenite) has

TABLE 10.8
Selenium Content of Selected Foods

Food	Selenium (μg)
Snapper, baked (3 oz)	42
Halibut, baked (3 oz)	40
Salmon, baked (3 oz)	32
Scallops, steamed (3 oz)	69
Clams, steamed (20)	240
Oysters, raw (1 c)	257
Molasses, blackstrap (2 tbl)	8
Sunflower seeds (1 c)	87
Ground beef (3 oz)	12
Chicken, baked (3 oz)	23
Bread, whole wheat (1 slice)	10
Egg (1)	15
Milk, 2% (1 c)	5

been assessed the most in humans using stable isotopes. Selenomethionine is a selenium analog of a sulfur-containing amino acid. Selenium and sulfur are exchanged in methionine due to their chemical similarities. The major site of absorption is the duodenum, although some selenium is absorbed in the ileum and jejunum. Selenium absorption does not occur in the stomach. There is no known regulatory mechanism for selenium absorption. A range of 50 to 100% absorption of these two forms has been demonstrated.

Metabolism and Function

When selenium is absorbed as selenomethionine, it is incorporated into a plasma protein called *selenoprotein P*. This protein functions to transport and store selenium. As selenite, selenium becomes incorporated into the metalloenzyme glutathione peroxidase. About 50 to 60% of selenium excreted is through the urine, and 40 to 50% of excreted selenium is through the feces. Body stores of selenium greatly influence renal clearance of this mineral. Therefore, the kidneys appear to be the principal regulatory mechanism for selenium homeostasis. Endogenous selenium is also lost through the feces. This was demonstrated by showing that fecal selenium excretion remains the same regardless of dietary intake. At toxic intakes of dietary selenium, volatile selenium compounds such as dimethylselenide are exhaled and can escape through the skin.

Selenium exerts some of its physiological effects as a coenzyme for glutathione peroxidase, which is often abbreviate as GPX. Glutathione peroxidase functions to reduce organic and hydrogen peroxides (Figure 10.9). This is especially important for phagocytic cells such as leukocytes and macrophages. In these cells, peroxides are the by-products of the oxidative destruction of foreign matter; therefore, glutathione peroxidase protects these cells from being autodestructive.

Another site of glutathione peroxidase activity is platelets. Here, GPX acts in an antiaggregative capacity. This metalloenzyme reduces fatty acid peroxide formation and the ratio of prostacyclin (an antiaggregating factor) to thromboxane (a proaggregant) becomes increased. Through this mechanism, selenium is prophylactically linked to cardiovascular disease by decreasing platelet aggregation, which reduces the incidence of clots and atherosclerosis.

In general, glutathione peroxidase stablizes cell membranes since they are composed of unsaturated fatty acids that may be susceptible to oxidation. Free radical production has

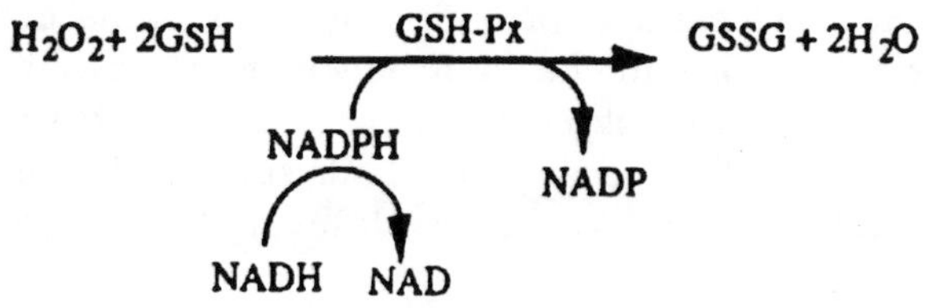

$$H_2O_2 + 2GSH \xrightarrow{\text{GSH-Px}} GSSG + 2H_2O$$

NADPH

NADP

NADH NAD

GSH-Px	glutathione peroxidase (Requires Se)
GSH	reduced glutathione
GSSG	oxidized glutathione
H_2O_2	hydrogen peroxide

FIGURE 10.9
The reduction of oxygen radicals in a red blood cell involving glutathione peroxidase.

been implicated in the aging process and as an initiating event in tumor development. Adequate levels of selenium assure that sufficient glutathione peroxidase will be available and protect against tumor development and the aging process. Glutathione peroxidase is important for the stability of red blood cells since oxygen is certainly abundant. The lack of mitochondria in RBCs further depletes these cells of antioxidants, making glutathione peroxidase much more important. There are also several isoforms of glutathione peroxidase that are indicated by numerals 1 through 4. The tissue distribution of these isoforms vary. For instance, while GPX1 and GPX4 are expressed in most tissue, RBCs contain more GPX1, liver more GPX2 and GPX3, kidneys more GPX1 and GPX3, and the testes more GPX4.

The enzyme *iodothyronine deiodinase* contains selenium. This enzyme converts thyroxine (T_4) to triodothyronine (T_3), a deiodination reaction. T_3 is an active thyroid hormone. There are other nonselenium-containing deiodinases, which may catalyze this reaction. Type 1 deiodinase is selenium-containing, and in selenium deficiency, the synthesis of this deiodinase is markedly diminished, resulting in the production of less T_3 and also causing an accumulation of T_4. The other deiodinases do not respond as an adaptation to selenium deficiency.

Relationships With Other Nutrients

Copper deficiency can possibly decrease glutathione peroxidase activity. While it is still unclear as to why this occurs, it is probable that the gene for glutathione peroxidase is not expressed to the same extent during copper deficiency.

Vitamin E has been shown in animals to spare selenium and reduce the amount necessary in the diet. Other factors with such a role have also been identified; these include: decreased food intake, high protein intake, high levels of vitamin A and vitamin C, and synthetic antioxidants. On the other hand, there are substances and situations which are known to antagonize dietary selenium, thereby increasing its need. These include heavy metals, sulfate, mercaptans, chlorinated hydrocarbons, and deficiencies of vitamin E, riboflavin, vitamin B_6, and methionine.

There are substances which are known to reduce the potential for selenium toxicity. These substances may act as methyl donors that will synthesize selenium metabolites that are simply excreted. The methyl donors include methionine, betaine, choline, creatinine, and amidinoglycine. Also, the heavy metals mercury, cadmium, lead, silver, and arsenic, along with the trace elements copper, zinc, and iron, substitute for selenium and reduce its toxic potential. Furthermore, antioxidants such as vitamin E, DPPD, and BHT help the antioxidant role of glutathione peroxidase and thereby reduce toxic effects of selenium.

Recommended Levels of Intake

The RDA for selenium varies by gender and age. In adult males, 70 µg of selenium is recommended, compared to 55 µg for females. Younger adolescent females have a higher RDA than their male counterparts, with 45 µg for ages 12 to 14. The RDA is 50 µg/d for both adolescent males and females from 15 to 18 years of age.

Deficiency

There are several signs of selenium deficiency in those cases documented in humans, mostly premature infants or patients receiving protracted total parenteral nutrition for extended periods of time. Cardiomyopathy, cataracts, increased RBC fragility, skeletal muscle degeneration, and impaired growth are some of the symptoms. Areas of poor soil selenium in China have a high incidence of Keshan disease that is essentially a cardiomyopathy. Keshan disease is characterized by marked cardiac hypertrophy and failure. Children are mostly affected by this condition.

Toxicity

There are three forms of selenium toxicity: acute selenosis, subacute selenosis, and chronic selenosis. Acute selenosis occurs when excess amounts of selenium are ingested over a short length of time. Symptoms of acute selenosis include an unsteady gait, cyanosis of the mucous membranes, and difficulty in breathing which can lead to death. Autopsy reports of acute selenosis describe liver congestion, endocarditis, myocarditis, and smooth muscle degeneration in the gastrointestinal tract, gallbladder, and bladder. Long bone erosion was also reported in these cases.

When large doses of selenium are ingested over a long time frame, subacute selenosis is observed. Symptoms of subacute selenosis include neurologic dysfunction such as vision impairment, ataxia, and disorientation; respiratory distress is often seen as well. Subacute selenosis is commonly seen in livestock which graze on selenium-accumulating plants. These seleniferous plants are concentrated in Western states such as Montana, Colorado, Wyoming, New Mexico, and Arizona.

Chronic selenosis occurs when moderate doses of selenium are ingested over a considerable length of time. This condition is characterized by skin lesions and dermatitis such as alopecia and hoof necrosis (in livestock), emaciation, chronic fatigue, anorexia, gastroenteritis, liver dysfunction, and spleen enlargement.

The most toxic forms of selenium are noted to be sodium selenite, sodium selenate, selenomethionine, and selenodiglutathione. However, there are wide variations in selenium toxicity with respect to the valence state of the molecule. Recently, a multitude of selenium compounds have been synthesized as chemopreventive/anticarcinogenic substances. These are being tested for their toxic effects.

There is an area of China which has unusually high concentrations of selenium in the soil. This becomes incorporated into the food supply, so the residents were evaluated for clinical and biochemical indications of selenium intoxication. The average daily selenium intake was estimated to be 1.4 mg for adult males and 1.2 mg for adult females. When comparing this group to those whose selenium intakes were 0.07 mg and 0.06 mg, respectively, for men and women, increased clotting time and reduced serum glutathione were observed. Clinical signs that were observed consisted of garlic odor in the breath and urine, brittle or lost nails, lowered hemoglobin levels, and nervous system problems such as peripheral anesthesia, acroparesthesia, and pain in the extremities.

In livestock, symptoms of selenium toxicity are seen in the nervous system, such as ataxia, tremors, hypersensitivity, and convulsions. In humans, nervousness, chills, numbness, impaired nerve conduction, and peripheral anesthesia occur. Mottled teeth have been seen in humans with selenium toxicity. The liver has been demonstrated in animals to have steatosis and necrosis when intoxicated with selenium. However, this has not been reported in humans.

Kidney problems such as congestion, necrotizing nephrosis, and calcinosis have only been reported in animals. The heart appears to be affected by selenium toxicity as myocarditis in rats, and bradycardia in humans. Only livestock have shown respiratory disturbances such as congestion, edema, respiratory distress, and hydrothorax. The skin is affected by selenium toxicity, and this is seen as thick, streaked, brittle nails; dry, brittle hair; hair loss; and red, swollen hands and feet. In animals, cracked hooves are noticed as well as dermatosis and alopecia. Anemia, increased prothrombin time, and decreased hemoglobin are hematological parameters seen in both humans and animals. Decreased immune function has been demonstrated in rats with selenium toxicity. In both animals and humans with selenium toxicity, loose stools, diarrhea, excessive salivation, and dyspepsia have been observed. Deformities of fetal chicks and ducks are seen in selenium toxicity.

Fluoride

In nature, the element fluorine exists primarily as a negatively charged ion. Thus, similar to iodide (iodine) and chloride (chlorine), fluorine is commonly referred to as *fluoride*. Fluoride was first recognized as a toxic element in animals in the 1920s when phosphate salts from rocks were used as a source of calcium and phosphorus for farm animals. Some of the rocks contained 1 to 2% fluoride. Animals had depressed growth and increased mortality from fluoride toxicity. On the contrary, in the late 1930s, it was observed that in areas where water supplies had higher levels of fluoride, there was a decreased incidence of dental caries. The link between fluoride and dentition soon followed.

Sources

Most foods are poor sources of fluoride and probably should not be used exclusively as such to meet human needs. However, the process of adding fluoride to drinking water (*fluoridation*) has greatly improved human fluoride consumption. Fluoridation, a practice which began in the 1940s in the U.S., typically utilizes sodium fluoride and sodium fluorosilicate at about 1 to 2 ppm. About 1 mg/d is consumed by Americans through fluoridated drinking water. Thus, fluoridated water and foods prepared with fluoridated water are among the best sources. Infant formulas and foods are made with fluoridated water, thereby improving an infant's intake. Also, fluoride-containing toothpastes, which typically use sodium fluoride, account for some fluoride ingestion.

Absorption

In general, fluoride is very well absorbed from most dietary sources. Soluble fluoride sources, such as the aqueous-dissolved sources in fluoridated water, are almost completely absorbed. Fluorides bound to proteins demonstrate moderate absorption. Unlike other minerals, fluoride is absorbed to a great extent in the stomach. Thus, ingested fluoride will be represented within the blood within minutes of consumption and achieve maximal levels within ½ hour or so. Fluoride is also absorbed along the length of the small intestine. Regardless of site of absorption, fluoride is probably absorbed by passive diffusion. Like sodium, potassium, and chloride, fluoride absorption does not appear to be hindered relative to physiological status, nor is it hindered competitively by its fellow halogen anion, chloride.

Metabolism and Function

Blood fluoride levels are rather low in the part per billion concentration range. As suggested above, fluoride is stored in calcified tissues (bones and teeth), where the levels are proportional to the intake through the diet. Excretion is primarily by way of the urine, with small levels appearing in the feces. Fluoride balance is usually positive in humans, with a slow increase with aging. However, fluoride is not efficiently transferred across the placenta. Therefore, a newborn infant will have relatively lower levels of fluoride. Fluoride accumulation occurs at the time teeth are being developed.

Fluoride is important for bone and dental health. Fluoride is incorporated into hydroxyapatite crystal at places that contain hydroxyl (OH^-) chemical groups. This can occur either at the point of initial crystalization or by displacement in mature hydroxyapatite crystals according to the following equation:

$$Ca_{10}(PO_4)_6(OH)_2 + xF^- \longrightarrow Ca_{10}(PO_4)_6(OH)_{2-x}F_x^-$$

Such a substitution will cause the crystal to become harder and more stable. Therefore, the general effect of fluoride will be a hardening of dental aspects such as enamel. This is the primary mechanism by which fluoride helps to prevent tooth decay.

Recommended Intake Levels and Toxicity Concerns

Currently, there is not an RDA for fluoride. The ESADDI for fluoride is 1.4 to 4.0 mg/d. Excess fluoride intake may occur, although its incidence is rather rare. If the level of fluoride in bones and teeth exceeds 3000 µg/g tissue, fluoride will begin to accumulate in the soft tissues. Such toxicities may lead to deformed bones and discolored to mottled teeth. This is called *fluorosis*. Fluoride may also inhibit fatty acid oxidation and the formation of acetyl CoA. Inhibition of glycogen breakdown has also been suggested. Signs of accelerated aging often appear, as well as loss of appetite, body weight loss, gastrointestinal enteritis, muscular weakness, convulsions, pulmonary congestion, and respiratory and cardiac failure.

Chromium

Chromium was first discovered to be essential in 1959 and can exist in several oxidation states ranging from −2 to +6, with the trivalent +3 being the most relevant to humans. The primary role of chromium is to serve as structural component of a complex compound called *glucose tolerance factor (GTF)*. This compound aides in the function of insulin and is thought to help in insulin binding to membranes. Deficiency may result in elevated blood glucose and cholesterol. The trivalent form of chromium is the most effective form. Chromium enhances protein synthesis, but this is probably the result of its synergetic influence upon insulin, where insulin increases the transport of amino acids across the cell membrane.

Dietary Chromium

It is only in more recent times that scientists have begun to investigate the chromium content of foods (Table 10.9). Egg yolks, whole grains, and meats, especially organ meats, are better sources. Cheeses, mushrooms, nuts, beer, and wine also make significant contributions. Dairy products are relatively poor chromium sources. Vegetation grown in chromium-rich soils may also make a significant contribution to the human diet. Many multivitamin–multimineral supplements include chromium. Most of the chromium in foods is as the trivalent form. Brewer's yeast is a good source of chromium because of its content of GTF.

Absorption

The absorption of chromium probably occurs via a carrier mediated system at lower intakes, which is complemented by passive diffusion at higher intakes. The jejunum is the

TABLE 10.9

Chromium Content of Selected Foods

Food	Chromium (μg)
Meat	
Turkey ham (3 oz)	10.4
Ham (3 oz)	3.6
Beef cubes (3 oz)	2.0
Turkey (3 oz)	1.7
Chicken (3 oz)	0.5
Grains	
Waffle (1)	6.7
English muffin (1)	3.6
Bagel, egg (1)	2.5
Rice, white (1 c)	1.2
Bread, whole wheat (1 slice)	1.0
Fruits and vegetables	
Broccoli (2 c)	11.0
Juice, grape (1 c)	7.5
Potatoes, mashed (1 c)	2.7
Juice, orange (1 c)	2.2
Lettuce, (1 c)	1.8
Apple, unpeeled (1)	1.4

primary site of absorption; however, it will occur along the length of the small intestine. If chromium is in an inorganic state, the absorption appears to be very low (<5%). However, chromium provided in the form of organic GTF demonstrates a much higher absorption (15 to 25%). Chromium associated with the molecule, picolinate, also demonstrates better absorption than inorganic chromium alone.

Metabolism and Function

Tissue levels of chromium are relatively high in infancy and decline with age. The adult body may contain 4 to 6 mg of chromium and more concentrated tissues include the kidneys, liver, spleen, pancreas, bone, and muscle, including cardiac muscle. The concentrations of chromium in the blood are not well regulated. It appears that the excretion of chromium in the urine provides the primary means of disposal. Inorganic chromium is transported in the blood primarily aboard transferrin as chromium competes with iron for binding sites. Also, chromium can be transported via albumin and plasma globulins and maybe lipoproteins.

Chromium as part of GTF appears to be absorbed intact and is available to cells as active GTF. Circulating inorganic chromium must first be complexed within GTF, which probably occurs in the liver. GTF then circulates to peripheral tissue. Glucose tolerance factor is formed via the coupling of chromium to nicotinic acid. It is believed that GTF establishes a disulfide interaction between insulin and insulin receptors on the plasma membrane of cells. Thus, the general physiological significance of chromium is to enhance the actions of insulin. Insulin enhances glycolysis, glycogen synthesis, fatty acid synthesis, and protein synthesis.

Chromium has had recent interest as a supplement with reports in animals and humans that increased lean body mass and reduced body fat result with chromium supplementation. Earlier investigation suggested that chromium supplementation increased lean body mass with a decrease in percent body fat in males and females undergoing resistance training. However, later human studies do not support a change in body composition. See Chapter 14 for a more detailed review of the efficacy of chromium supplementation.

Recommended Levels of Intake and Chromium Imbalance

No RDA has been established for chromium. The Estimated Safe and Adequate Intake for chromium is 50 to 200 µg/d. Chromium deficiency is not a readily recognizable nutritional disorder, although some scientist have suggested that mild chromium deficiency is a compounding factor in the development of several human diseases. The elderly may be especially susceptible to the development of chromium deficiency. Nutrition surveys have indicated that chromium levels decrease with age as well as that elderly populations in the U.S. are consuming less than the recommended levels of chromium.

Chromium deficiency can result in glucose intolerance, which is an inability to properly reduce blood glucose levels after a meal and throughout the day. One consequence in glucose intolerance is hyperinsulinemia. It has been suggested that mild chromium deficiency may be a risk factor for syndrome X, which places an individual at significantly higher risk of heart disease.

Little is known about the toxic effects of chromium in larger doses. Scientists have reported that supplementation as much as 800 µg daily is safe, while others question as to whether or not excessive chromium chronically consumed would deposit excessively in tissue such as bone, and have milder long-term effects.

Manganese

Manganese was first identified as an essential nutrient in the early 1930s. Despite its wide distribution in nature, manganese occurs in very low quantities in human tissue. However, its significance to human function can not be overlooked. It is both an activator and a constituent of several enzymes. In humans, manganese exists in either the +2 or +3 oxidation state.

Dietary Sources

Whole-grain cereals, fruits and vegetables, legumes, nuts, tea, and leafy vegetables are better food sources of manganese. Animal foods are generally poor contributors of manganese. Additional substances in plants, such as fiber, phytate, oxalate along with excessive calcium, phosphorus, and iron can decrease manganese absorption.

Absorption

Relatively little is known about the mechanisms of manganese absorption. It is likely that a saturable, active transport system is involved. It is clear, however, that manganese is absorbed along the entire length of the small intestine. About 2 to 15% of ingested manganese can be absorbed; however, the presence of dietary factors such as fibers, phytate, oxalates, calcium, and phosphorus can decrease the absorption percentage.

Metabolism and Function

The total amount of manganese in an adult is about 12 to 20 mg. It is widely and uniformly distributed in tissue. Within cells it is concentrated in the mitochondria, with relatively larger content in the nucleus as well. Bones, liver, kidney, pancreas, lactating mammary gland, and the pituitary gland contain higher than average levels, whereas the skeletal muscles are by comparison lower. In bone, manganese is found as part of hydroxyapatite. The level of manganese in bone and the liver are 3.5 and 2 mg/kg, respectively. Manganese is transported in the blood bound to transferrin or other proteins, notably α-2-macroglobin, at a level approximating 1 to 2 μg/100 ml of blood. Its primary route of excretion from the human body is via fecal elimination of unabsorbed manganese along with that incorporated into digestive secretions.

Manganese functions largely as either an activator of specific enzymes or it is a key component of metalloenzymes. Manganese is fundamentally important in cartilage tissue formation and remodeling, and in particular in chondroitin sulfate. UDP-Glucuronic acid and N-acetyl galactosamine are condensed in the presence of a polymerase enzyme, resulting in a polysaccharide chain and along with additional sulfate addition allows for the formation of chondroitin sulfate in cartilage. The polymerase is a manganese-dependent enzyme. Manganese is also involved with aspects of carbohydrate metabolism as it is a cofactor for pyruvate carboxylase as well as an activator for the gluconeogenic enzyme phosphenolpyruvate carboxylase (PEPCK). Manganese plays a role in the formation of prothrombin. Arginase, which is involved in urea synthesis, contains 4 atoms of manganese, while the dipeptidase, prolidase, is activated by manganese. Mitochondrial superoxide dismutase is a manganese-dependent enzyme (Mn-SOD). Last, manganese may function as a modulator of second messenger systems. For instance, manganese increases cAMP levels in stimulated cells as well as being an activator of guanylate cyclase.

Recommended Levels of Intake and Manganese Imbalance

There is no RDA for manganese, but an Estimated Safe and Adequate Intake of 2.0 to 5.0 mg/d has been established. In animals, manganese is important for both reproductive performance and for bone development. In chickens, for instance, slip tendon is a condition caused by manganese deficiency in which the ridges on the leg bones of chickens are diminished such that a tendon may slide over the ridge. Manganese deficiency in people is rare — however, nausea, vomiting, dermatitis, decreased growth of hair and nails, and changes in hair color can result. Manganese toxicity is also rare, although miners inhaling manganese-rich dust can experience Parkinson-like symptoms.

Cobalt

Cobalt occurs regularly in plant and animal tissues and is widely distributed. In humans cobalt is part of vitamin B_{12}. Therefore, cobalt's presence and function in tissue is really a reflection of vitamin B_{12}. Since humans are unable to synthesize vitamin B_{12}, cobalt itself is not viewed as an essential nutrient, but merely a component of an essential nutrient.

Cobalt is poorly absorbed as an inorganic element. If cobalt is injected, relatively small amounts are present in the urine. Small amounts are also found in the saliva. Traces may also be found in bile and pancreatic juices and some in the feces. A deficiency of cobalt can be experienced in ruminant animals. These animals need to ingest cobalt for the synthesis of vitamin B_{12} by their gut microflora. In such animals, emaciation, weakness, and anemia are common signs of cobalt deficiency.

Cobalt can be toxic in the range of 10 to 20 mg/kg body weight. Polycythemia, bone marrow hyperplasia, reticulocytosis, and increased blood volume are signs of toxicity. Excessive cobalt depresses oxidative phosphorylation and leads to tissue hypoxia, changes in the nervous system, thyroid hyperplasia, and myxedema. Congestive heart failure has been reported in humans.

Boron

There is a growing body of evidence to argue in favor of the essentiality of boron. Boron has been recognized as essential for plants since the 1920s. However, its essentiality for humans has not really been investigated until the 1980s. It appears at this time that boron does indeed influence the composition and mechanical properties of bone.

Dietary Sources and Absorption

Fruits, leafy vegetables, nuts, and legumes are rich sources of boron, while meats are among the poorer sources. Beer and wine also make a respectable contribution to human boron intake. Boron appears in foods primarily as sodium borate and boric acid, two forms that seem to be readily absorbed (>90%).

Metabolism and Function

While relatively little is known regarding boron transport in the blood, physiological levels appear to be regulated primarily by urinary excretion. Boron is found in many tissues; however, the bone contains the most. In plants, boron is an essential factor for cell maturation and differentiation. This role has not been determined in humans to date. Furthermore, flavonoid synthesis in plants is dependent upon boron, while flavonoid synthesis does not seem to occur in humans. Boron appears to either directly or indirectly affect the metabolism of calcium in bone and influences the composition and strength of bone. This is an area that has been receiving more and more attention as scientists try to address bone diseases. Interestingly, boron needs are increased during a vitamin D deficiency. Also, boron has been recognized to ameliorate many of the manifestations of magnesium deficiency in bone tissue.

Recommended Levels of Intake; and Boron Imbalance

Although not established to date, our requirement for boron is probably about 1 mg daily. Boron deficiency results in an increased urinary loss of calcium and magnesium, assumedly derived from storage primarily in bone. Conversely, taking large amounts of boron may induce nausea, vomiting, lethargy, and an increased loss of riboflavin.

Molybdenum

The essentiality of molydenum was first identified in 1958. However, much of the research has been difficult because it is an ultra-trace mineral. In human tissue, molybdenum is typically found in concentrations less than 1 ppm (<1 µg/g of wet tissue). Furthermore, researchers have had difficulty inducing molydenum deficiency in experimental animals because of its relatively small need compounded by the inability to purify experimental diets to reduce all traces of molybdenum.

Dietary Sources and Absorption

Most of the foods humans eat contain a respectable amount of molybdenum which ultimately reflects the soil content in which the plants were grown. Organ and other meats, legumes, cereals, and grains are among the better sources of molybdenum. Very little is known at this time regarding the absorptive processes for molybdenum. While the stomach does appear to be able to contribute to the absorption of molybdenum, most absorption probably occurs in the proximal small intestine. At lower intakes, molybdenum is probably absorbed by active carrier-mediated transport, which is complimented by passive diffusion at higher intake levels. Molydenum absorption has been estimated to range from 25 to 80%. Diets high in molybdenum decrease copper absorption and also increase copper loss in the urine.

Metabolism and Function

As mentioned above, the content of human tissue is typically less than 1 ppm. Tissues such as the liver, adrenal glands, kidneys, and bone are the most concentrated. Other tissues, such as muscle, lungs, brain, spleen, and small intestine also contain slightly higher concentrations as well.

Molydenum, as the constituent of molybdoenzymes, participates in certain oxidation–reduction reactions. Molybdenum is a component of a cofactor for the *molybdopterin* structure that is at the catalytic site of the enzymes (Figure 10.10). Xanthine oxidase and xanthine dehydrogenase are found in a variety of tissue and the dehydrogenase form can be converted into the oxidase form in tissue. These enzymes are fundamental in hydroxylating various purines and pyrimidines, pteridines, and other heterocyclic nitrogen-containing compounds. In this sense, molybdenum is necessary for the transformation of hypothanine to xanthine as well as xanthine to uric acid.

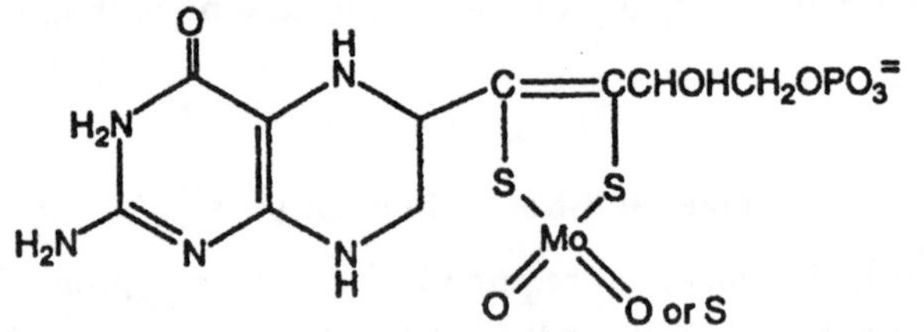

FIGURE 10.10
Pterin structure containing an atom of molybdenum

The molybdoenzyme sulfite oxidase catalyzes the conversion of sulfite to sulfate. This is a mitochondrial enzyme located in several tissues and is responsible for the terminal step in the metabolism of sulfur-containing amino acids (cysteine and methionine). Last, the molybdoenzyme aldehyde oxidase may be important in the metabolism of certain drugs.

Recommended Levels of Intake and Molybdenum Imbalances

The ESADDI for adults is 75 to 250 µg of molybdenum daily. Because of molybdenum's widespread availability in the diet, a deficiency is somewhat rare. However, people receiving intravenous (IV) feedings for several months are at risk. In contrast, molybdenum is fairly nontoxic. However, as molybdenum is involved in the breakdown of bases to the waste product uric acid, which is excreted via the urine, higher intakes of this mineral could place certain prone individuals at greater risk of kidney stones. Excessive uric acid production may also increase the risk of developing gout.

Vanadium

Vanadium exists in several oxidation states ranging from +2 to +5. In humans, as well as other organisms, vandium appears mostly in the pentavalent form vanadate (VO_3^- or $H_2VO_4^-$) or in the tetravalent state vanadyl (VO^{2+}). Recently, it has become a popular supplement for weight-training individuals who hope to increase their muscle mass.

Dietary Sources and Absorption

Although still only containing nanograms to micrograms of vanadium, breakfast cereals, canned fruit juices, fish sticks, shellfish, vegetables (especially mushrooms, parsley, and spinach), sweets, wine, and beer are better sources. While pertinent information is somewhat lacking, vanadium absorption appears to be relatively small (5 to 40%).

Metabolism and Function

Vanadium is present in trace concentrations in most organs and tissue throughout the human body and has long been questioned in regard to essentiality. It is important to realize that the presence of a substance does not necessarily indicate essentiality. Nevertheless, researchers have discerned that the absence of vanadium from animal diets reduces their growth rate, infancy survival, and hematocrit, despite the inability of researchers to identify specific functions for vanadium.

Vanadium administered in higher quantities exerts numerous effects upon human metabolism. However, these activities cannot be considered vanadium dependent since they are observed only when vanadium is administered in excessive amounts. In this manner vanadium acts as a pharmaceutical agent, not necessarily a nutrient. One such effect that is receiving a lot of research attention is vanadium's ability to mimic the activity of insulin. Thus, vanadium appears to be able to affect glucose metabolism in a manner similar to insulin. Promising research with diabetic animals has suggested that vanadium therapy may control high blood glucose levels (hyperglycemia).

Recommended Levels of Intake and Vanadium Imbalances

A dietary requirement for vanadium has yet to be established; however 10 to 25 µg of vanadium per day may be appropriate. As mentioned above, vanadium deficiency may result in reductions in growth rate, infancy survival, and hematocrit. Further, vanadium deficiency may alter the activity of the thyroid gland and its ability to properly utilize iodide. Contrarily, signs of vanadium toxicity such as a green tongue, diarrhea, abdominal cramping, and alterations in mental functions have been reported in individuals ingesting greater than 10 mg of vanadium daily over extended periods of time.

Nickel

In general, plants are more concentrated sources of nickel than are animal foods. Nuts are the most concentrated sources, while grains, cured meats, and vegetables offer respectable amounts. Fish, milk, and eggs are recognized as poorer nickel sources. The absorption of nickel from the gut is probably affected by varying the amounts of copper, iron, and zinc, and perhaps vice versa. Adult requirements for nickel are most likely about 35 µg daily.

The possible essentiality of nickel has not been seriously considered until the last 20 years or so. Furthermore, defining exact roles for nickel in humans remains somewhat elusive. However, nickel does seem to be involved in the breakdown of the amino acids leucine, valine, and isoleucine (branch-chain amino acids) and odd-chain-length fatty acids. Nickel research is relatively new, and more clear-cut roles for nickel will probably emerge within the next decade.

Arsenic

As a natural constituent of the earth's crust, arsenic can be found in most soils and is taken up by plants grown in them. However, the arsenic content of foods can also be affected by the arsenic content in pesticides and airborne pollutants. Among the most concentrated sources of arsenic are sea animals (fish, shellfish). Dietary requirements for arsenic have not been established, although 12 to 15 µg daily is probably sufficient.

Although arsenic has long been regarded as an undesirable substance, it may be an essential component of the human body after all. Although its involvement has not been clearly identified, arsenic is most likely important in the metabolism of two amino acids, methionine and arginine.

Arsenic deficiencies have resulted in a reduced growth rate in animals. Arsenic deficiency may also reduce conception rate and increase the likelihood of death in newborns. Perhaps no other constituent of the human body conjures up a stronger notion of toxicity than arsenic. It certainly is the only nutrient that can be fatal in milligram amounts. Arsenic, in the form of arsenic trioxide, can be fatal at doses greater than 0.76 to 1.95 mg.

Silicon

Not much is really known about the silicon content of various foods. Plants sources, including high-fiber cereal grains and root vegetables, seem to be better sources than animal sources. Silicon, in the form of quartz, is the most abundant mineral on the planet. However, silicon makes only a minuscule contribution to human body weight. Silicon seems to be involved in the health of connective tissue. In bone, silicon seems to improve the rate of both bone mineralization and growth. The manufacturing of collagen, a predominant protein found in connective tissue, relies upon an adequate supply of the nonessential amino acid proline and a slightly modified form of proline called hydroxyproline. Silicon is probably required for the optimal synthesis of both proline and hydroxyproline. Silicon is also important for the manufacturing of other proteins and substances vital to proper connective tissue. Silicon deficiency can result in poor growth and development of bone, including a decreased mineralization. Not much is known at this time regarding silicon toxicity.

11

Energy Metabolism

Every moment of every day the human body is engaged in a myriad of metabolic reactions in efforts to maintain homeostatic operations and other human functions and activities. The metabolic cost or energy expenditure is very large, easily 1500 to 3000 kcal or more in most adults. The total energy cost or total energy expenditure (TEE) is the sum total of all energy-releasing operations within the trillions of cells that comprise the human body. Adenosine triphosphate, along with other high-energy molecules, powers these operations. These molecules, principally ATP, are derived from the catabolism of energy substrate molecules such as carbohydrates, proteins (amino acids), fat, ethanol, and their metabolic intermediates such as pyruvate and lactate. These substrates are initially provided by the diet whereby they can either be used immediately or incorporated into storage forms such as glycogen, triglyceride, and even protein. All energy-requiring operations in human cells can fall into three broad groups: membrane transport, synthesis of molecules, and mechanical work.

Human cells are tireless in their efforts to maintain ATP levels to support homeostasis and other functions. Furthermore, most cells are generally indiscriminate in their selection of energy substrates for ATP production. Cells merely utilize energy substrates as dictated largely by their availability and hormonal and central influences upon metabolic pathways. Perhaps only erythrocytes (red blood cells; RBCs) are completely discriminate in their fuel substrate. Discussion in this chapter will provide an overview of total tissue, and cellular level energy metabolism

---

Total Energy Expenditure

The amount of energy released from the human body is directly or indirectly quantifiable. With the exception of small amounts of energy transferred to other entities during skeletal muscle operations, energy released from the human body is or will ultimately become heat energy. As body temperature is generally maintained within a narrow range, typically around 37°C (98.6°F), excessive heat must be dissipated. Measurement of that energy liberation within a given period of time, such as a minute, hour, or day, is called *metabolic rate*. Metabolic rate becomes a more accurate reflection of human energy metabolism as the time period is extended. This will take into account stretches during a 24-hour period when our metabolic rate is greater, such as in more active times of the day, or lower, as in less active times of the day or when sleeping.

Direct or Human Calorimetry

Metabolic rate can be measured directly using a *human calorimeter*. "Calorimeter" literally means the measurement of heat. This device is in essence an insulated chamber, and heat dissipated from a human is measured by the warming of a layer of water associated with the wall of the chamber. Heat lost from the body in the form of water vapor is also measured as it interacts with sulfuric acid. All environmental factors are controlled. Facilities of this nature are expensive to maintain and are only available at a handful of universities and research institutions.

Indirect Calorimetry

While human calorimetry directly measures heat production and is often referred to as *direct calorimetry*, there is an indirect method more commonly used to estimate human energy expenditure. This is called *indirect calorimetry*. Because ATP is generated from the combustion of energy molecules, and because combustion requires O_2 and produces CO_2, it is possible to estimate energy expenditure based upon the exchange of these gases with the environment. Representative chemical reactions for the combustion of carbohydrates, protein, and fat are shown below. Molecular oxygen (O_2) is used as a reactant for each reaction, while carbon dioxide (CO_2) is a product. Thus, utilizing mathematical equations generated from direct calorimetry, it is possible to estimate the amount of heat produced in a given period of time based upon the amount of O_2 inhaled or the amount of CO_2 expired. Indirect calorimetry is an accurate indicator of metabolism and can also be applied to estimate the energy of substances being utilized during the time of measurement.

$$\text{A Carbohydrate}$$
$$C_6H_{12}O_6 + 6O_2 \longrightarrow 6\,CO_2 + 6\,H_2O$$

$$\text{A Triglyceride (fat)}$$
$$2\,C_{57}H_{110}O_6 + 163\,O_2 \longrightarrow 114\,CO_2 + 110\,H_2O$$

$$\text{A Protein}$$
$$C_{72}H_{112}N_2O_{22}S + 77\,O_2 \longrightarrow 63\,CO_2 + 38\,H_2O + SO_3 + 9\,CO(NH_2)_2$$

Balanced chemical equations like those above can be used to calculate the *respiratory quotient (RQ)* for energy substrates. RQ is equal to the amount of CO_2 exhaled divided by the amount of O_2 inhaled. Gas exchange is measured with a spirometer.

$$RQ = CO_2/O_2$$

RQ of glucose	$6\,CO_2/6\,O_2 = 1.0$
RQ for the triglyceride	$114\,CO_2/163\,O_2 = 0.70$
RQ for the protein	$63\,CO_2/77\,O_2 = 0.82$

Once the gas exchange quantities and RQ are known for a given period of time then the energy expenditure can be calculated, using the thermal equivalent of the gas quantities (Table 11.1). For instance, if an individual consumed 15 l O_2 and expired 12 l of CO_2, in a 1-hour period of time, one could first calculate the RQ for that hour

$$RQ = 12/15 = 0.80$$

TABLE 11.1
Thermal Equivalents of O_2 and CO_2 for Nonprotein RQ

Nonprotein RQ	Caloric Value $1 l O_2$	Caloric Value $1 l CO_2$	Carbohydrate (%)	Fat (%)
0.707	4.686	6.629	0	100.0
0.71	4.69	6.606	1.1	98.9
0.72	4.702	6.531	4.76	95.2
0.73	4.714	6.458	8.40	91.6
0.74	4.727	6.388	12.0	88.0
0.75	4.739	6.319	15.6	84.4
0.76	4.751	6.253	19.2	80.8
0.77	4.64	6.187	22.8	77.2
0.78	4.776	6.123	26.3	73.7
0.79	4.788	6.062	29.9	70.1
0.80	4.801	6.001	33.4	66.6
0.81	4.813	5.942	36.9	63.1
0.82	4.825	5.884	40.3	59.7
0.83	4.838	5.829	43.8	56.2
0.84	4.85	5.774	47.2	52.8
0.85	4.862	5.721	50.7	49.3
0.86	4.875	5.669	54.1	45.9
0.87	4.887	5.617	57.5	42.5
0.88	4.899	5.568	60.8	39.2
0.89	4.911	5.519	64.2	35.8
0.90	4.924	5.471	67.5	32.5
0.91	4.936	5.424	70.8	29.2
0.92	4.948	5.378	74.1	25.9
0.93	4.961	5.333	77.4	22.6
0.94	4.983	5.29	80.7	19.3
0.95	4.985	5.247	84.0	16.0
0.96	4.998	5.205	87.2	12.8
0.97	5.010	5.165	90.4	9.58
0.98	5.022	5.124	93.6	6.37
0.99	5.035	5.085	96.8	3.18
100	5.047	5.047	100	0

At an RQ of 0.80, the individual would have need approximately 33% carbohydrates and 66% fat to fuel their metabolism. Under typical situations, the contribution of amino acids to energy production during rest is assumed to be minimum. Protein should be considered significant during extended fasting and/or prolonged exercise, or during and after a high protein meal. The metabolic rate is estimated by multiplying the amount of O_2 consumed (15 l) by the caloric value for $1 l O_2$ for an RQ = 0.80.

$$15 * 4.801 = 72 \text{ cal/h}$$

Components of Energy Metabolism

Total energy metabolism is a reflection of all cellular activities. However, human metabolism can fluctuate during a given period of measurement. A primary reason for the fluctuations are variations in human function and operations is based primarily upon activity, environmental conditions, and the digestion, absorption, and processing of ingested substances. Therefore *total energy expenditure* (TEE) can be subdivided into four principal components that are for the most part distinct. These are *basal metabolism* (BM), *thermal effect of activity* (TEA), the *thermal effect of food* (TEF), and *adaptive thermogenesis* (AT).

$$TEE = BM + TEA + TEF + AT$$

Basal Metabolism

Basal metabolism is the energy expended by internal processes during a period of complete rest (nonactive) in a climate-controlled environment (not unusually cold or warm) and at least 10 to 12 h after the consumption of the most recent meal. Basal metabolic rate (BMR) is simply basal metabolism within a specific time period such as a minute, hour, or day. The processes that take place during basal metabolism include those that fundamentally support life. They are those that support fundamental homeostasis, for example, the energy expended to support resting heart rate and respiration; the active processes of urine formation; cellular turnover; and the synthesis of proteins, nucleic acids, and other substances; and the tight regulation of ion concentrations across cellular membranes.

Basal metabolism is in essence identical to *resting energy expenditure* (REE). However, an individual does not have to be in a fasting state. The consumption of a meal within 2 to 4 h prior to measurement is typical of REE. Thus REE will be slightly greater than BM. Typically 50 to 75% and 65 to 75% of TEE is attributable to BMR and REE, respectively.

In light of the differing operations and masses of various tissues and organs in the human body, their contribution to basal metabolism will differ. For instance, the most metabolically active tissues are organs such as our heart, kidneys, lungs, brain, and the liver. Collectively these organs only contribute about 5% to adult body weight; however, the energy expended by these organs accounts for as much as 50 to 60% of BM. Skeletal muscle, which makes up about 36% and 45% of a woman's and man's body weight, respectively, is not as metabolically active as the organs just mentioned. However, skeletal muscle metabolism, which is largely remodeling operations, contributes about 25% to BM. Meanwhile, adipose tissue contributes relatively little unless its total mass is excessive.

As most other aspects of BM are generally static, increasing the skeletal muscle/fat ratio is perhaps the most significant, nonpharmacological way of greatly increasing BM. For example, it would be expected that a 90-kg (~200 lb) man with 12% body fat would have a higher BM than another man of the same weight yet with 25% body fat. On the basis of gender, men tend to have a greater skeletal muscle:adipose tissue ratio; thus the BM for men is on average greater than for women on a per weight basis. This concept is easily supported by the difference in O_2 consumption for women vs. men. On average, women tend to consume only about 80% of the O_2 (ml/min/kg) as men. Based on age, BM/kg body weight is highest during infancy and declines with age.

Without the assistance of a human calorimeter unit or a respirometer to measure gas exchange, there are several equations available to quickly estimate BMR for a day. A limitation of these calculations is that they tend to overestimate basal metabolism in heavier individuals with a higher percentage of body fat.

A. Rule of thumb

$$BMR = BW * 24 \text{ hours}$$

B. Body weight raised to the power of three fourths

$$BMR = 70 * BW^{.75}$$

C. Harris and Benedict equation

Men

$$BMR = 66 + (13.7 * BW) + (5 * Ht) - (6.8 * age)$$

Women

$$BMR = 655 + (9.6 * BW) + (1.7 * Ht) - (4.7 * age)$$

where: BMR (calories)
Wt (weight) = kilograms
Ht (height) = centimeters

Thermal Effect of Activity

The events of skeletal muscle activity are extremely costly from an ATP standpoint. Both the events of sarcomere contraction and relaxation require the hydrolysis of ATP. Myosin ATPase activity that powers the "power stroke" of sliding myofilaments and Ca^{2+} pumping across the sarcoplasmic reticulum and plasma membranes account for most of the energy expenditure. The TEA includes not only skeletal muscle activity during obvious movements such as walking, running, bicycling, climbing stairs, or vacuuming the floor, but also skeletal muscle activity associated with the maintenance of position and posture. While the contribution of the latter skeletal muscle effort may at first thought seem minor, sitting on a stool without back-support increases heat production by 3 to 5%. The increase in metabolism is even greater standing. To estimate TEA, an individual can maintain an activity log over a 24-h period and then apply energy equivalent coefficients, such as Table 11. 2 to the time involved in various activities. TEA can also be estimated for a given activity (Table 11.3). What is not always clear is the classification of recovery and adaptive mechanisms within skeletal muscle cells. For instance, resistance training can result in the expenditure of a several hundred calories during an intense training bout. However, energy expenditure by skeletal muscle is increased for 24 to 36 h after the intense bout as the tissue repairs and remodels. Is this TEA even though there is no activity, or is it considered BM?

TABLE 11.2
Energy Expended (Cal/kg body weight per min)

Type of Activity	Female	Male
Sleep or lying still	0.00	0.00
Sitting or standing still (i.e., sewing, writing, eating)	0.001–0.007	0.003–0.012
Very light activity (i.e., driving, walking slowly)	0.009–0.016	0.014–0.022
Light activity (i.e., sweeping, walking moderately, carrying objects)	0.018–0.035	0.023–0.040
Moderate activity (i.e., fast walking, dancing, biking, cleaning vigorously)	0.036–0.053	0.042–0.060
Heavy activity (i.e., fast dancing, swimming, tennis)	0.055	0.062

Note: Calculated activity associated quantities are in addition to basal metabolism during that time period. Modified from E. Whitney and C. Cataldo, *Understanding Normal and Clinical Nutrition*, West Publishing, St. Paul, MN, 1983.

TABLE 11.3
Calories per Minute Expended During Various Activities

Activity	Weight in pounds					
	100	120	140	160	180	200
Bicycling						
5 mph	1.9	2.3	2.7	3.1	3.5	3.9
10 mph	4.2	5.1	5.9	6.8	7.6	8.5
15 mph	7.3	8.7	10.0	11.6	13.1	14.5
20 mph	10.7	12.8	14.9	17.1	19.2	21.3
Running						
6 mph	7.2	8.7	10.2	11.7	13.1	14.6
7 mph	8.5	10.2	11.9	13.6	15.4	17.1
8 mph	9.7	11.6	13.6	15.6	17.6	19.5
9 mph	10.8	12.9	15.1	17.3	19.5	21.7
Skiing (X-country)						
2.5 mph	5.0	6.0	7.0	8.0	9.0	10.0
4.0 mph	6.5	7.8	9.2	10.5	11.9	13.2
5.0 mph	7.7	9.2	10.8	12.3	13.9	15.4
Skiing (downhill)						
	6.5	7.8	9.2	10.5	11.9	13.2
Soccer						
	5.9	7.2	8.4	9.6	10.8	12.0
Tennis						
	5.0	6.0	7.0	8.0	9.0	10.0
Walking						
3 mph	2.7	3.3	3.8	4.4	4.9	5.4
4 mph	4.2	5.1	5.9	6.8	7.6	8.5
5 mph	5.4	6.5	7.7	8.7	9.8	10.9
Weight training						
	5.2	6.0	7.3	8.3	9.4	10.5

Thermal Effect of Food

TEF is an increase in energy expenditure associated with food and has been called several names, including the specific dynamic action (SDA) of food and diet-induced thermogenesis (DIT). It represents an augmentation in metabolism attributable to the digestion, absorption, processing, and storage of food and its components. TEF increases metabolism above BM by 5 to 15%, depending upon the size and composition of a meal. Generally TEF is estimated as 10% of total energy intake during that same period. For instance, TEF can be estimated at 250 kcal for an individual who ingests a mixed diet containing 2500 kcal over a 24-h period. A high carbohydrate and/or protein:fat ratio provides a greater TEF.

TEF can begin even prior to the digestion and absorption of food. As mentioned previously, the mere thought, sight, smell, and taste of food results in a cephalic phase of digestion. This cephalic phase, mediated autonomically, can result in several secretory and motile operations. TEF appears to peak approximately 1 h after ingestion of the meal and wanes after 3 to 5 h. The events include smooth muscle operations, active transport release of various digestive and endocrine secretions, active transport at the apical and basilateral membranes of enterocytes, and processing and storage of absorbed substances.

Adaptive Thermogenesis

Changes in environmental temperature and radiant energy (i.e., solar radiation) can influence metabolic rate. It is a homeostatic objective of man to maintain constant or near constant core body temperature. This is because several aspects of human physiology are temperature based, such as the activity of enzymes. Thermal sensors are located at the skin level as well as deeper towards the body *core*, mainly in the spinal cord, the abdominal viscera, and in and around the great veins. Both skin and deep receptors are more sensitive to cold vs. warmth. Most effects to regulate body core temperature are initiated in the posterior hypothalamus.

As environmental temperature increases, heat production decreases until a "lower critical" temperature is reached. As environmental temperature continues to rise, metabolic heat production demonstrates a plateau until an "upper critical" environmental temperature is reached. Despite a reduction in the energy gradient for convection and radiation losses in a hotter environment, the body is still able to maintain core temperature by increasing evaporative loss. Under more comfortable temperatures, radiation and convection can account for as much as 60% and 15% of heat loss. Evaporation accounts for the majority of the remaining heat loss and conduction accounts for only about 2 to 3%. The upper critical temperature is a point at which core body temperature begins to rise and the well-being of the body is thus placed in jeopardy. Metabolic heat production increases at this point in an all-out survival effort to increase cardiac output and circulation to the periphery for heat removal.

As environmental temperature decreases, heat-conserving and heat-producing operations are increased. Less blood is circulated to the periphery, thereby reducing heat loss as well as causing a decrease in the production of sweat for evaporation. This is regulated by the hypothalamus. In addition, piloerection occurs. Piloerection is the standing on end of body hair. This has very little impact in humans, but in other animals it allows for the creation of a layer of insulator air close to their skin. As environmental temperature continues to fall, man can maintain body temperature to a point. This point, called "summit metabolism," is defined as the maximal rate of metabolism which occurs in response to cold without a decline in body temperature. Increases in metabolism are accounted for by either *shivering* or *nonshivering thermogenesis*. Shivering is the visible contraction and generated tension of subcutaneous skeletal muscle. ATP is hydrolyzed and heat liberated.

Nonshivering thermogenesis may result from epinephrine- or norepinephrine-promoted uncoupling of oxidative phosphorylation in certain cells such as brown adipose tissue. The mitochondria in these cells are engineered to perform this operation. This is perhaps more significant in infants. By adulthood, only negligible amounts of brown adipose tissue remain and nonshivering thermogenesis by this means is minimalized. Increased thyroid hormone secretion is stimulated by a cooling of the body. The hypothalamus releases thyrotropin-releasing hormone, which stimulates the anterior pituitary gland to release thyroid-stimulating hormone, which itself stimulates the release of thyroid hormone from the thyroid gland. Thyroid hormone increases the general metabolic rate of many cells. However, this response may be due to chronic exposure to cold, not necessarily an acute response to cold.

Integrated Energy Metabolism

In order for ATP to be available, cells must have a constant supply of energy substrates. Carbohydrates, proteins (amino acids), fat, ethanol, as well as intermediate molecules of their metabolism (i.e., pyruvate, lactate), are catabolized in energy metabolic pathways and their inherent energy transferred to the high-energy bonds of ATP and to a lesser degree

GTP. These energy substrates can be derived directly from the diet during a fed period (external eating) or they can be derived from endogenous stores of carbohydrate, protein, and fat (internal eating). Several factors, such as hormonal and neurological aspects, as well as availability of these substrates, are involved in the utilization of the different sources and will be briefly reviewed.

Insulin

In the mid 19th century, a German medical student named Paul Langerhans identified the "islet" structure of pancreatic tissue. Almost 3 decades later, von Mering and Minkowski demonstrated that pancreatectomy induced diabetes. However, it wasn't until the early 20th century with the work of de Mayer (1909), Sharpey-Schaffer (1917), and Banting and Best (1921) that the link between diabetes and the pancreatic islets became more clear. Using an acid–ethanol extraction procedure, a factor named "insulin," was derived from human islet cells and proved to have a hypoglycemic influence. Insulin was also found in bovine (cow) and porcine (pig) islet tissue as well. Shortly thereafter, the treatment of diabetes took a positive and life-saving turn. Interestingly, insulin was the first protein that proved to have hormonal activity.

Insulin is a polypeptide synthesized in β cells of pancreatic islets and consists of two chains (A and B) linked by disulfide bonds (Figure 11.1). The A-chain consists of 21 amino acids, while the B-chain consists of 30 amino acids. The disulfide bonds arising from cysteine residues are located at A7-B7 and at A20-B19. A disulfide bond also exists between cysteine residues between A6-A11. While there is some variation in the insulin amino acid sequence between mammalian species, the positioning of the three disulfide bonds seems invariant. For instance, the threonine residue at position 30 on the B-chain is alanine for pigs, dogs, and the horse, and serine for the rabbit. All amino acids of the A-chain are the same. Conversely, differences are found at the 8 to 10 position on the A-chain in cattle, goats, sheep, and horses, while alanine occupies position 30 on the B-chain. Despite variation in the amino acid sequencing of insulin between species, the general activity for all insulins is about 25 to 30 IU/mg dry weight.

Insulin is synthesized (translation) in a form referred to as *preproinsulin*, which has a molecular weight of 11,500. Posttranslational modification begins with the cleavage of the 23-amino acid *pre-* or *leader* sequence, resulting in a proinsulin molecule of approximately 9000 mol wt. The cleaved leader sequence is necessary for guiding preproinsulin into the endoplasmic reticulum during synthesis. Cleavage of the leader group also allows for the appropriate conformation for the formation of disulfide linkages.

Proinsulin is then translocated to the Golgi apparatus. In the Golgi apparatus, proinsulin begins conversion to mature insulin. The removal of a stretch of amino acids in the central portion of the proinsulin polypeptide creates mature insulin or just insulin. The removed amino acid sequence is called *C-peptide* and the remaining, once flanking, amino acid sequences are the A-chain and B-chain. Disulfide bonds now secure these two chains. This process continues after vesicles bud from the Golgi apparatus and traverse the cytoplasm towards the plasma membrane. Conversion of proinsulin to insulin is typically about 95% complete. Insulin and proinsulin combine with zinc within secretory granules and form hexamer structures. The secretory vesicles then fuse with the plasma membranes of β cells, releasing insulin, proinsulin, and C-peptide into the extracellular space. These structures are then free to diffuse into the blood. Proinsulin has less than 5% of the bioactivity of insulin while C-peptide has none. The half-life of insulin is 3 to 5 min while the half-life of proinsulin is much longer. Insulin is metabolized primarily in the liver, kidneys, and placenta. About 50% of circulating insulin is removed in a single pass through the liver.

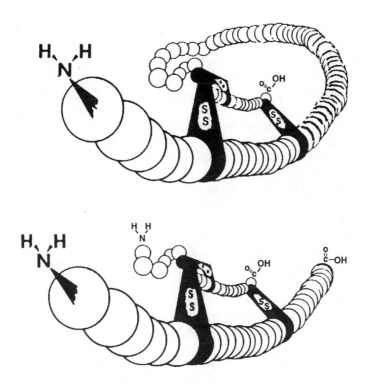

FIGURE 11.1
Disulfide bonding between the A- and B-chains of insulin. Mature insulin (bottom) has the C-peptide removed.

On a daily basis, the adult pancreas secretes about 40 to 50 units of insulin, which represents about 15 to 20% of that which is available in secretory vesicles. The release of insulin is an energy-dependent process and the strongest stimulus is an elevation in plasma glucose concentration. The threshold concentration for secretion is about 80 to 100 mg/100 ml, and a maximal response occurs when blood glucose is approximately 300 to 500 mg/100 ml of blood. While the exact mechanism(s) of glucose-stimulated insulin release are not clear, possible explanations include (1) an increased interaction of glucose with β cell plasma membrane glucose receptors; and (2) an increase in glucose metabolites in β cells or the rate of flux through metabolic pathways, such as the pentose phosphate pathway, Krebs cycle or glycolysis.

Secretion of insulin is influenced by several factors. For instance, α-adrenergic agonists such as epinephrine inhibit glucose stimulation of insulin release. β-Adrenergic agonists stimulate insulin release, most likely by increasing the intracellular concentration of cAMP. In addition, insulin secretion is increased by chronic exposure to growth hormone, estrogens, and progestins. Thus, it is not surprising to find insulin secretion elevated during the last trimester of pregnancy.

Insulin promotes the lowering of blood glucose concentration by several means. In adipose tissue and skeletal muscle, which collectively approximate 50 to 60% of the tissue in the adult body, it increases the number of glucose transporters at the plasma membrane face. Assumably, these transporters, particularly GLUT4, are translocated from an inactive intracellular pool. Increased glucose entry into hepatocytes appears to occur for a different reason. Insulin increases the activity of glucokinase primarily by induction. Glucokinase phosphorylates glucose diffusing into hepatocytes, thus maintaining a concentration gradient that favors further influx of free glucose. Similarly, the activity of skeletal muscle hexokinase II, which also causes the phosphorylation of glucose, is increased due to insulin.

The effect of insulin upon increased glucose entry is somewhat unique to certain cell types, such as adipocytes, skeletal and cardiac myocytes, and hepatocytes. Most other cells in the body will demonstrate a more consistent uptake of glucose from circulation, based upon their metabolic needs. This is explained by the variety of glucose transporter proteins describe below. Insulin also promotes the uptake of amino acids into cells, especially muscle cells.

Insulin will not only increase the uptake of glucose and amino acids into certain types of cells, but also strongly influences energy nutrient metabolic pathways within cells as well. As will be addressed in detail later, insulin promotes increased activities of glycolysis, the *pentose phosphate pathway,* glycogen formation (*glycogenesis*), and fatty acid synthesis (*lipogenesis*). Insulin also promotes the inhibition of glucose formation via the breakdown of glycogen (glycogenolysis) and conversion from noncarbohydrate molecules (gluconeogenesis). Furthermore, insulin will promote the inhibition of fat breakdown (lipolysis) and fatty acid oxidation, especially in adipocytes and hepatocytes, while at the same time promoting general protein synthesis, especially in muscle cells. Insulin will influence these pathways by either activating or deactivating key enzymes or influencing events of transcription and/or translation. In these ways, insulin is believed to influence either the quantity or activity of at least 50 different enzymes. The net effect of insulin is to decrease the circulatory concentration of glucose. In this sense, insulin stands alone and its general actions are opposed by several hormones such as glucagon, epinephrine, and cortisol. Also the net effect of insulin is to promote storage of exogenous energy. Because the liver receives portal blood that has drained from the pancreas, it is exposed to insulin concentrations that can be 3 to 10× greater than in the peripheral circulation. The liver binds and removes a substantial portion of insulin on this pass. The liver is also more sensitive to insulin, assumably via greater receptor concentrations than peripheral tissue as well.

Insulin acts by first binding with an insulin receptor on the plasma membrane, and its indirect actions can arise within seconds to minutes (nutrient transport, activation/inhibition of enzymes, RNA transcription) or hours (protein and DNA synthesis and cell growth). The insulin receptor is a heterodimer transmembrane glycoprotein. Its cytoplasmic region has tyrosine kinase activity and an autophosphorylation site. Insulin receptors undergo constant turnover as the half-life is only 7 to 12 h. The insulin receptor gene is located on chromosome 19. Most human cells will synthesize insulin receptors, with the average concentration being about 20,000 per cell. This is because insulin not only governs metabolic activity, but is also involved in cell growth and reproduction. Once insulin binds to a receptor, there is a conformational change and the receptor is internalized and one or more signals are produced. The internalization of cells may be important in cell turnover and in regulating receptor concentration. Furthermore, in hyperinsulinemic situations, such as in obesity, there is a down-regulation of insulin receptors. Fewer receptors are produced and those cells become less sensitive to insulin. This is sometimes the case in obesity-related type II diabetes mellitus.

Insulin elicits a second messenger action that culminates in a variety of intracellular events. These events begin with the activity of tyrosine kinase, which results in an increase of tyrosine phosphorylation in both the receptor itself as well as key intracellular proteins. This generally activates key enzymes such as GTPases, lipid kinases, and protein kinases, which mediate much of insulin's metabolic impact.

Glucagon

Glucagon is produced by α cells of pancreatic islets. It is a single-chain polypeptide consisting of 29 amino acids. Like insulin, glucagon is also synthesized in a larger prohormone form. Glucagon circulates in the plasma unbound and has a half-life of about 5 min. The liver is the primary site of glucagon inactivation. Since pancreatic endocrine secretions drain into the hepatic portal vein, much of the secreted glucagon is actually metabolized without ever reaching the peripheral circulation. Glucagon secretion is associated with hypoglycemia and inhibition of secretion is associated with hyperglycemia. The exact inhibitory mechanisms are unclear. It could be a more direct inhibition, via increased glucose reception, or more indirect via insulin or insulin-related events, or a combination of these or related events. Other stimulators may include some amino acids, particularly glucogenic amino acids such as alanine, serine, glycine, cysteine, and threonine. These amino acids will be important sources of glucose via gluconeogenesis. This also means that a protein-containing meal can in theory stimulate glucagon release, concomitant to stimulating insulin release.

While the influence of insulin is diverse, glucagon focuses its actions mainly upon the liver and adipose tissue. The binding of glucagon to glucagon-receptors on the plasma membrane of hepatocytes results in an increase in intracellular cAMP. The activation of phosphorylase by cAMP promotes glycogen degradation while also inhibiting glycogen synthesis. Furthermore, glucagon promotes the conversion of noncarbohydrate molecules to glucose in hepatocytes as well. In adipose tissue, glucagon promotes lypolysis principally by activating the enzyme hormone-sensitive lipase. As with hepatocytes, the binding of glucagon to receptors on the plasma membrane of adipocytes initiates a 2nd messenger cascade that begins with the activation of adenylyl cyclase through a G-protein-linked mechanism and produces increased cAMP levels.

Skeletal muscle cells do not express glucagon receptors. Thus, glycogenolysis in skeletal muscle is not influenced by glucagon but primarily by epinephrine and to a lesser degree norepinephrine. In general, glucagon is gluconeogenic, glycogenolytic, and ketogenic in hepatocytes, while it is lipolytic in adipocytes.

Insulin:Glucagon Molar Ratios

As many aspects of energy nutrient metabolism promoted by either insulin and glucagon are antagonistic in nature, the molar ratio of these two hormones becomes the predominating factor in determining net metabolic activity. For instance, the synthesis of glycogen can and will occur concomitantly to the breakdown of glycogen in hepatocytes and skeletal muscle. However, the algebraic net effect is dictated largely by the relative influences of insulin and glucagon and to a lesser degree by other hormones such as epinephrine and cortisol. An insulin to glucagon ratio of 2.3:1 may be expected from the consumption of a balanced diet. Meanwhile, the infusion of arginine also increases the secretion of both hormones, but more so for insulin, resulting in a ratio approximating 3:1. Conversely, if a glucose solution is infused in circulation, a ratio of 25:1 can be expected.

Epinephrine

Epinephrine (adrenalin) is synthesized in the adrenal medulla from the amino acid tyrosine, which itself can be synthesized from the essential amino acid phenylalanine. Intermediates of the synthesis of epinephrine include dopa, dopamine, and norepinephrine (noradrenaline). Epinephrine, norepinephrine, and dopamine are important molecules in the response to stress. They are synthesized in chromaffin cells and stored in secretory granules. Epinephrine is the principal catecholamine synthesized in chromaffin cells of the adrenal medulla, constituting 80% of the total catecholamine production.

However, epinephrine is not produced in extramedullary tissue. The conversion of dopamine to norepinephrine is catalyzed by the enzyme *dopamine β-hydroxylase (DBH)*. DBH requires ascorbate, an electron donor, and copper at the active site. Meanwhile, *phenylethanolamine-N-methyltransferase (PNMT)* catalyzes the production of epinephrine from norepinephrine (Figure 11.2). Synthesis of PNMT is induced by glucocorticoid hormones that reach the medulla via a portal vein from the adrenal cortex. As preganglionic nerve fibers from the splanchnic nerve synapse in the adrenal medulla, this region can be viewed as a ganglion without axonal extrusions.

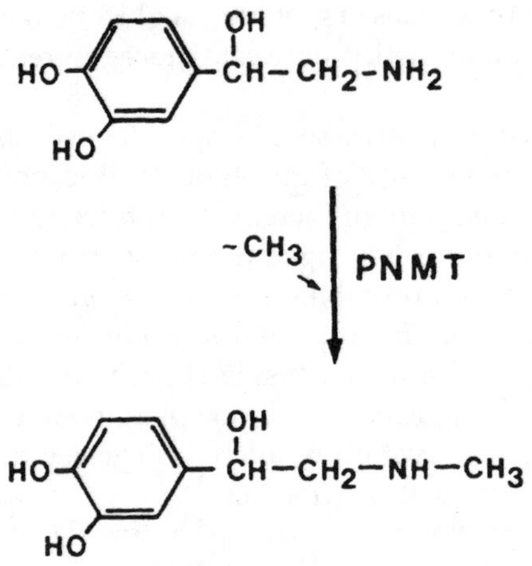

FIGURE 11.2
Production of epinephrine via the methylation of the primary amine group of norepinephrine.

The incorporation of catecholamines into secretory granules is an ATP-dependent transport mechanism. The granules also contain ATP-Mg^{2+}, Ca^{2+}, and DBH. Once inside the granule, epinephrine complexes with ATP in a 4:1 ratio. Secretory granules will fuse with the plasma membrane upon appropriate neural stimulation. β-Adrenergic and cholinergic agents stimulate fusion, while α-adrenergic agents inhibit it. Catecholamines circulate loosely bound to albumin. They have a half-life of about 10 to 30 sec. Catecholamines are metabolized by *catechol-O-methyl tranferase (COMT)* and *monoamine oxidase (MAO)*, which are found in many tissues.

The effects of epinephrine is mediated via its reception to two classes of receptors: α- and β-receptors are subdivided into α_1 and α_2 and β_1 and β_2. This classification system is based upon binding affinity of the different receptors for catecholamines. When epinephrine binds to β_1 on cardiac tissue, the force and rate of contraction are increased. Furthermore, the binding of epinephrine to β_2 receptors elicits smooth muscle relaxation and thus vasodilation in skeletal muscle and the liver.

Cortisol

Synthesized in the adrenal cortex, cortisol is the principal glucocorticoid in humans. It is derived from cholesterol and circulates in the blood bound predominately to corticosteroid-binding globulin (CBG), which is produced in the liver. Cortisol is also transported in the blood to a minor degree loosely associated with albumin. The binding of cortisol to a plasma protein allows for a longer half-life (60 to 90 min) than the polypeptide hormones discussed above. Cortisol is principally metabolized in the liver.

Cortisol has widespread effects in the human body and greater secretion is associated with stress and fasting where it mediates adaptive processes. Cortisol then plays a significant role in carbohydrate, protein, fat, and nucleic acid metabolism. Cortisol or structural analogs (hydrocortisone) is also applied clinically as an antiinflammatory agent as it will inhibit the migration of polymorphonuclear leukocytes, monocytes, and lymphocytes at the site of inflammation.

In the liver, the effects of cortisol are anabolic. Cortisol promotes gluconeogenesis in hepatocytes by binding to intracellular receptors and inducing the expressing of a number of enzymes involved in gluconeogenesis as well as amino acid transamination. Cortisol also promotes glycogen synthesis in the liver. This effect most likely occurs to maintain at least basal levels of glycogen stores during times when it could easily become exhausted (i.e., fasting, stress). Also, glucose 6-phosphatase activity is increased, allowing for more glucose to leave the liver.

In peripheral tissue, cortisol-induced activity appears to antagonize insulin activity. Protein and nucleic acid synthesis are inhibited, while protein breakdown is promoted by cortisol. Free amino acids in skeletal muscle, especially alanine, become resources for gluconeogenesis in the liver. Cortisol also inhibits the uptake of glucose and amino acids in skeletal muscle and promotes lipolysis in adipose tissue. Cortisol promotes a net protein catabolism in connective tissue and skin. The total white blood cell count of the blood is increased when cortisol levels are elevated. However, this is a net effect, as eosinophils, basophils, and lymphocytes are decreased while monocytes and polymorphonuclear leukocytes are increased.

Major Metabolic Pathways

Flux of metabolic pathways is regulated in several ways. First, hormonal influences such as insulin and glucagon can alter the activity of key enzymes by phosphorylation/ dephosphorylation. Second, hormonal influences can either induce or repress transcription and/or translation of key enzymes. Third, intermediates and products of the metabolic reactions as well as other substances can elicit allosteric influences upon the flux of metabolic pathways.

Most cells will use a variety of fuel sources (Table 11.4) — again, red blood cells are the only true obligate glucose users. The brain also is limited in its energy substrate. Under normal metabolic conditions the brain will derive nearly all of its energy from glucose. However, as discussed later, the brain can adapt to utilize more ketone bodies during starvation to spare blood glucose. Conversely, tissues such as muscle, liver, and kidney are omnivorous in their energy substrates. Here, substrate availability and hormonal influences are the greatest consideration.

Glucose Transport into Cells

Glucose metabolism for energy occurs in every cell in the human body and begins with glycolysis. As the intracellular concentration of free glucose is very low in most cells, glycolysis can not become physiologically significant until glucose either enters cells or becomes available from glycogen stores in some cell types. The facilitative diffusion of glucose across human cell plasma membranes occurs via *glucose transport proteins (GLUT)*. About

TABLE 11.4
Fuel Sources for Selected Organs and Tissue

Tissue or Cell Type	Energy Substrate	Metabolic or Cellular Considerations
Erythrocyte (RBC)	Glucose	Lacks mitochondria Obligatory lactate production
Hepatocytes	Glucose, fatty acids, amino acids, lactate, fructose, galactose ethanol	Primary site of ketone body synthesis Primary site of fatty acid synthesis Primary site of gluconeogenesis
Skeletal muscle	Glucose, fatty acids, certain amino acids, ketone bodies, some fructose	Availability of substrates Metabolic state
Cardiac muscle	Glucose, fatty acids, certain amino acids, ketone bodies, lactate	Availability of substrates Metabolic state
Smooth muscle	Primarily glucose	Produces some lactate
GI tract	Primarily glucose, certain amino acids especially glutamine	Produces some lactate
Retina	Primarily glucose	Produces some lactate
Kidneys	Primarily glucose, some lactate, glycerol and ketone bodies	Produces some glucose
CNS	Glucose, will adapt to use ketone bodies	
Adipose tissue	Glucose, fatty acids, some fructose	

six GLUT proteins have been described at its time, each varying in their operational properties as well as the types of cells in which it is expressed. GLUT1 is the most widely expressed isoform and provides most cells with their basal glucose requirements. GLUT1 is expressed at higher amounts in epithelial cells and the endothelium of barrier tissue such as the blood–brain barrier. GLUT2 is a high K_m isoform expressed in higher amounts in hepatocytes, pancreatic β cells, and basolateral membranes of intestinal and renal epithelial cells. GLUT3 has a relatively low K_m and is responsible for glucose transport in neurons. GLUT4 is expressed in insulin-sensitive cells such as adipocytes and cardiac and skeletal myocytes, and is primarily responsible for reducing elevated blood glucose levels (Figure 11.3). GLUT5 is a fructose transporter expressed in greater amounts in spermatazoa and the apical membrane of intestinal enterocytes. GLUT7 is a glucose transporter found on the endoplasmic reticulum membrane and transports free glucose out of the organelle after the action of glucose 6-phosphatase upon glucose 6-phosphate. This is of particular importance to hepatocytes during glycogen breakdown as it allows for glucose liberation for subsequent release into circulation.

Glucose is the principal energy source of the brain, and delivery of glucose to brain tissue requires transport across the endothelial cells of the blood–brain barrier and then into neurons and glia cells. GLUT1 has been determined to be in higher concentration in the brain with a less glycosylated form (45 kDa) of the glycoprotein found in the parenchyma,

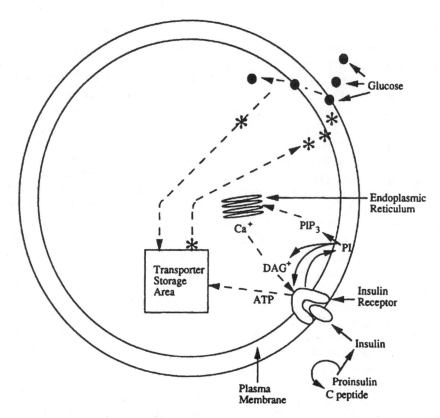

FIGURE 11.3
GLUT4 translocation via the binding of insulin to plasma membrane receptors.

predominantly glia and a highly glycosylated form (55 kDa) present in the blood–brain barrier. GLUT3 is also concentrated in neurons and GLUT5 in microglia. GLUT2, GLUT4, and GLUT7 have also been detected in the brain, but at lower concentrations.

Glucose transport across the plasma membrane (sarcolemma) of muscle has additional considerations beyond the presence of insulin and the mobilization of GLUT4 transporters. Glucose transport is increased by alterations in the metabolic condition of muscle cells. In the heart, increased inotropic activity, increased levels of epinephrine and growth hormone, and increased intracellular AMP and ADP can also increase glucose transport. It has been suggested that contraction of skeletal muscle elicits an increase in glucose transport that is independent, yet overlapping with the insulin effect. Contraction of skeletal muscle results in an increased blood flow to working muscle tissue. This supplies more glucose and insulin to that tissue. Also, insulin receptors may be more sensitive or have a greater binding affinity to insulin. Furthermore, muscle cell contractile activities result in an increase in intracellular Ca^{2+} content, which has been suggested to be associated with the translocation of GLUT4 from the intracellular pool to the sarcolemma.

Increased fatty acid oxidation can inhibit glucose transport. This occurs primarily by the inhibition of PFK1 by increased cytosolic citrate and ATP derived from fatty acid oxidation. This keeps glucose 6-phosphate from being utilized, and glucose 6-phosphate elicits a feedback inhibition on hexokinase.

Glycolysis

Glycolysis is a series of ten enzyme-catalyzed reactions that converts one 6-carbon glucose molecule to two 3-carbon pyruvate molecules (Figure 11.4). The net ATP yield of glycolysis is 2 ATP with the potential for 2 more ATP via the glycerol phosphate shuttle which allows for the reducing equivalents in the created cytosolic NADH to be transferred to mitochondrial $FADH_2$. Glycolysis also allows entry for the catabolism of other monosaccharides such as fructose (Figure 11.5) and galactose (Figure 11.6).

Glucose flux through glycolysis is governed by several key enzymes. The first influential enzymes are hexokinase in all tissue and glucokinase in hepatocytes (Table 11.5). Both enzymes phosphorylate glucose, forming glucose 6-phosphate. Hexokinase has a relatively low K_m and is inhibited by its product glucose 6-phosphate. This assures all cells glucose initiation through glycolysis, even when blood glucose concentrations are low, such as during fasting. However, the feedback inhibition helps regulate glucose flux relative to the ability of a cell to further metabolize glucose. Glucokinase, produced in hepatocytes, has a relatively high K_m and is not inhibited by its product. Glucokinase synthesis is induced by insulin. Glucokinase allows for large quantities of glucose to enter hepatocytes during hyperglycemic states, such as a fed state. This makes sense as the liver is a major metabolizing site for glucose during a fed state. About 50% of glucose will be converted to energy in the liver, while the remaining carbohydrate will be converted to glycogen and fatty acids. Because both secreted insulin and absorbed glucose perfuse the liver before entering the general circulation, a large proportion of glucose is transported into hepatocytes and never reaches the general circulation.

The activity of phosphofructokinase 1 (PFK1), which catalyzes the conversion of fructose 6-phosphate to fructose 1,6-bisphosphate, is regulated by several factors. In the liver one of the predominant factors is the activity of phosphofructokinase 2 (PFK2), an enzyme that catalyzes two opposite reactions, depending upon whether it is phosphorylated or not phosphorylated. PFK2 is phosphorylated when glucagon levels are elevated. Increased intracellular cAMP activates protein kinase A which phosphorylates PFK2. Conversely, the phosphate group is removed, via intracellular phosphatases, when insulin levels are elevated. The non-phosphorylated form of PFK2 catalyzes the conversion of fructose 6-phosphate to fructose 2,6-bisphosphate, which has an activating effect upon PFK1. This makes sense as elevations of both circulating insulin and hepatocyte intracellular fructose 6-phosphate would be observed in a fed state. The phosphorylated form of PFK2 catalyzes the conversion of fructose 2,6-bisphosphate back to fructose 6-phosphate, thus removing the activating influence of fructose 2,6-bisphosphate upon PFK1.

As glycolysis continues, the 6-carbon fructose 1,6-bis-phosphate molecule is split into two 3-carbon molecules, dihydroxyacetone phosphate and glyceraldehyde 3-phosphate. Dihydroxyacetone can then be converted to glyceraldehyde 3-phosphate. Therefore, 2 glyceraldehyde 3-phosphate molecules can result from 1 molecule of fructose 1,6-bisphosphate. The conversion of glyceraldehydate 3-phosphate to 1,3-bisphosphoglycerate reduces NAD^+ to NADH. Therefore, 2 NADH can be created in glycolysis from a single glucose molecule. In the next reaction, the phosphate at the number 1 position of 1,3-bisphosphoglycerate is transferred to ADP to form ATP. This reaction can potentially happen twice for every glucose molecule that enters glycolysis. This reaction is catalyzed by phosphoglycerate kinase and it produces 2-phosphoglycerate, which is subsequently converted to phosphoenolpyruvate (PEP) by enolase.

In the last reaction of glycolysis, PEP is converted to pyruvate by pyruvate kinase. Pyruvate kinase is activated by insulin. The binding of insulin to insulin receptors increases

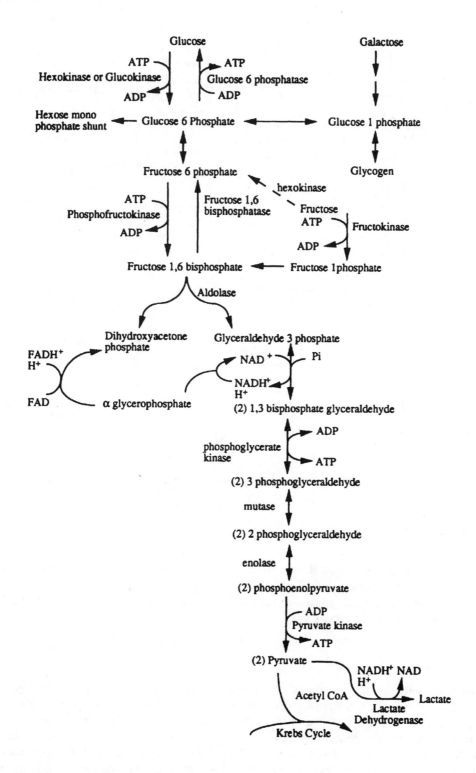

FIGURE 11.4
Glycolysis with entry of fructose and galactose.

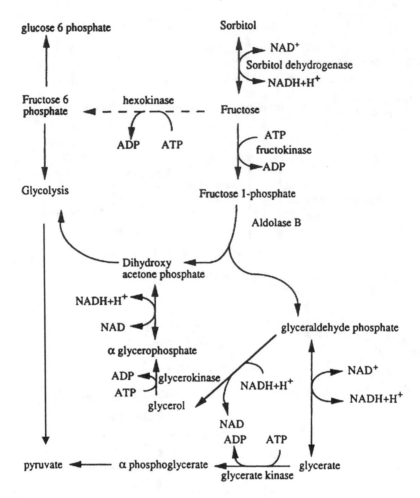

FIGURE 11.5
Metabolism of fructose.

phosphatase activity which dephosphorylates and thus activates pyruvate kinase. Conversely, the increased intracellular cAMP levels activate protein kinase A, which phosphorylates and deactivates pyruvate kinase. Increased cAMP can result from the binding of glucagon to glucagon receptors.

Fate of Pyruvate

Pyruvate is situated at a metabolic crossroads. Depending upon the type of cell and hormonal and metabolic influences, pyruvate can either be converted to the amino acid alanine or lactate in the cytosol or enter mitochondria and be converted to acetyl CoA or oxaloacetate. The conversion of pyruvate to lactate is a reduction reaction, and in the process NADH is oxidized to NAD^+ (Figure 11.4). This would negate the NADH created in glycolysis. This reaction is catalyzed in both directions by lactate dehydrogenase (LDH) which itself has five isoforms. LDH is composed of four subunits of either the heart (H) or muscle (M) type (i.e., MMMM, MMMH, MMHH, MHHH, HHHH), and different tissue will

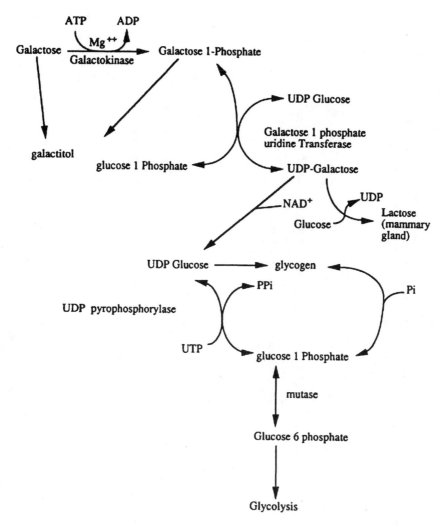

FIGURE 11.6
Metabolism of galactose.

express different forms. Lactate is produced in larger amounts in muscle and erythrocytes and can diffuse into the blood and serve as a gluconeogenic precursor in the liver or as an energy source for other cells.

Pyruvate in the mitochondria can be converted to acetyl CoA. Pyruvate dehydrogenase catalyzes this reaction and NAD^+ is reduced to NADH in the process. NADH can then transfer electron to the electron transport chain, enters the mitochondria and is converted to acetyl CoA; then NAD^+ is reduced. Pyruvate dehydrogenase exists in either a phosphorylated (inactive) or dephosphorylated (active) form. The products of pyruvate dehydrogenase, acetyl CoA and NADH, activate the kinase that phosphylates and inactivates pyruvate dehydrogenase. Conversely, CoASH (coenzyme A), NAD^+, and ADP inactivate the kinase, which keeps pyruvate dehydrogenase in an active state. Therefore, pyruvate dehydrogenase activity is controlled more by the metabolic state within the cell than directly by hormones.

TABLE 11.5
Reactions of Glycolysis

Reaction	Enzyme	Hormonal or Metabolic Influences	ATP or NADH
Glucose → glucose 6-phosphate	Glucokinase (liver)	Low K_m for glucose (~0.1 mM), induced by insulin	−1 ATP/glucose
	Hexokinase (all tissue)	High K_m for glucose (~10 mM), inhibited by glucose-6-phosphate	
Glucose 6-phosphate → fructose 6-phosphate	Phosphoglucose isomerase		
Fructose 6-phosphate → fructose 1,6-bisphosphate	Phosphofructokinase 1 (PFK1)	Activated by phosphofructokinase 2 (PFK2) in hepatocytes; PFK2 is activated by insulin and deactivated by glucagon; AMP activates PFK1 while citrate and ATP inhibit PFK1	−1 ATP/glucose
Fructose 1,6-bisphosphate → glyceraldehyde 3-phosphate + dihydroxyacetone phosphate	Aldolase		
Dihydroxyacetone phosphate → glyceraldehyde 3-phosphate	Triose phosphate isomerase		
Glyceraldehyde 3-phosphate → 1,3-bisphosphoglycerate	Glyceraldehyde 3-phosphate dehydrogenase		2 NADH/glucose
1,3-Bisphosphoglycerate → 3-phosphoglycerate	Phosphoglycerate kinase		2 ATP/glucose
3-Phosphoglycerate → 2-phosphoglycerate	Phosphoglyceromutase		
2-Phosphoglycerate → phosphoenolpyruvate	Enolase		
Phosphoenolpyruvate → pyruvate	Pyruvate kinase	Inhibited when glucagon is elevated, activated by insulin	2 ATP/glucose

Glycogen Synthesis

Like other bidirectional metabolic events, glycogen metabolism can be viewed as the alegebraic net product of the opposing operations: glycogen synthesis and glycogenolysis. It is possible, and often reality, for these two mechanisms to operate at the same time. Thus, the governing factor becomes the relative influences of all of the factors related to these operations. Some of the influences, such as metabolic products and intracellular factors (i.e., AMP, CA^{2+}) may primarily exert their influence only on one of the two pathways, while others, such as hormones, can exert their influence on both pathways. For example, AMP increases glycogen degradative operations only, while epinephrine and glucagon both activate glycogen-degradative mechanisms as well as inactivate glycogen-synthetic mechanisms.

Glycogen is a large branched polymer consisting of D-glucose, linked by α1-4 bonds in straight portions and α1-6 linkages at branch points (Figure 4.8). Glycogen contains more branching than plant starch, with points of branching occurring every 8 to 10 residues. One glucose unit with an exposed anomeric carbon is located at the "reducing end" of each glycogen molecule, and this monomer is attached to the protein *glycogenin*. This glucose unit functions as perhaps the anchoring and initiating point for the glycogen molecule, and it is believed that this glucose molecule is not readily available. The straight-chain oligosaccharide that extends from the reducing glucose monomer is the glycogen "primer." The glucose monomers at the ends of the initial straight chain as well as branch-chains are called "nonreducing" units which serve as either points of attachment for new monomers during synthesis or removal during glycogen breakdown.

The building block for glycogen is uridine diphosphate glucose (UDP-glucose), which is formed from glucose 1-phosphate, which itself is synthesized from glucose 6-phosphate (Figure 11.7). Insulin activates *glycogen synthetase*, the key regulatory enzyme in this process. When a growing straight chain contains 11 or more glucose monomers, another enzyme called branching enzyme or glucosyl 4,6-transferase relocates an oligomer of about 6 to 8 monomers and reattaches them at what becomes a branch point, via an α1-6 linkage.

Glycogen Degradation

Glycogen degradation or glycogenolysis is catalyzed by the active *phosphorylase* (phosphorylase a) enzyme. This enzyme is activated by epinephrine and increased intracellular AMP levels in muscle cells. The increased presence of AMP is mostly associated with muscle cell contraction and the hydrolysis of ATP to ADP. As a means of regenerating ATP, a phosphate from one ADP can be transferred to another ADP via adenylate kinase, producing ATP and AMP. Glucagon and epinephrine both participate in the activation of phosphorylase in hepatocytes. As mentioned above, both epinephrine and glucagon elicit a second messenger cascade, which culminates in an increased intracellular concentration of cAMP. In a chain of events, cAMP allows for the activation of cAMP-dependent protein kinase, which activates phosphorylase kinase a, which then converts glycogen synthase a (active form) to glycogen synthase b (inactive form). The events involved in glycogenolysis are presented in Figure 11.8.

Phosphorylase a, with the assistance of vitamin B_6, detaches glucose monomers from glycogen, forming glucose 1-phosphate, which is subsequently converted to glucose 6-phosphate by phosphoglucomutase. Phosphorylase a can liberate about 90% of glucose residues from glycogen as it splits the α1-4 links (straight chain). Glucose 6-phosphate in hepatocytes can be dephosphorylated by glucose 6-phosphatase in the endoplasmic reticulum. Glucose is transported out of the endoplasmic reticulum by GLUT7 and can diffuse from

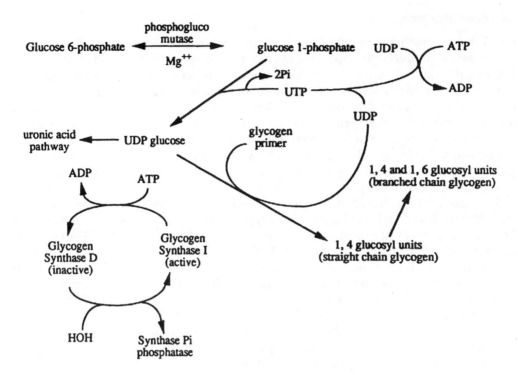

FIGURE 11.7
Glycogen synthesis.

the hepatocyte via GLUT2. A debranching enzyme is responsible for catalyzing the liberation of glucose units at branch points (~10% of total glucose). The product of this activity is free glucose, which can be transported out of the cell in the liver, again by GLUT2.

Pentose Phosphate Pathway

The primary importance of the pentose phosphate pathway (Figure 11.9) is the reduction of NADP+ to NADPH, which can be used for reducing equivalents for the synthesis of certain molecules (i.e., fatty acids), glutathione reduction, or other reactions. Also, this reaction pathway allows for the creation of ribulose 5-phosphate, which may be isomerized to ribose 5-phosphate and used in nucleotide biosynthesis. The reactions of the pentose phosphate pathway can be described as either oxidative or nonoxidative in nature. The oxidative enzymes include the conversion of glucose 6-phosphate to glucophoglucono-lactonolactone via glucose 6-dehydrogenase and conversion of 6-phosphogluconate to ribulose 5-phosphate. Both reactions reduce NADP+ to NADPH, while the latter reaction also produces CO_2. The nonoxidative reactions allow for the regeneration of glycolytic intermediates glyceraldehyde 3-phosphate and fructose 6-phosphate.

Krebs Cycle

The Krebs cycle (Figure 11.10), which occurs in the mitochondrial matrix, consists of eight sequential reactions whereby the final reaction produces a potential reactant for the first reaction. Therefore, this pathway is considered cyclic. In the reaction, acetyl CoA, which

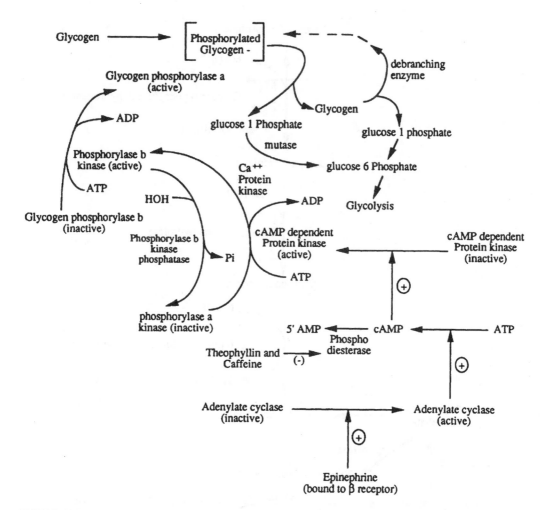

FIGURE 11.8
Glycogenolysis.

can be derived from a variety of sources, condenses with oxaloacetate forming citrate. Citrate synthase is the catalyzing enzyme and its activity is inhibited by its product. Aconitase catalyzes the conversion of citrate to isocitrate. Aconitase is bidirectional in activity, but favors citrate formation. Isocitrate dehydrogenase then converts isocitrate to α-ketoglutarate in the first oxidative reaction of the Krebs cycle. NAD^+ is reduced to NADH, and CO_2 is produced. The next reaction is also oxidative, as α-ketoglutarate is converted to succinyl CoA by α-ketoglutarate dehydrogenase. Here again, NAD^+ is reduced to NADH and CO_2 is produced. In the next reaction, the energy liberated by the cleavage of the high-energy thioester bond of succinyl CoA to form succinate and coenzyme A is sufficient to phosphorylate GDP, forming GTP. Next, succinate is converted to fumarate by succinate dehydrogenase in the third oxidizing reaction of the Krebs cycle. However, here FAD is reduced to $FADH_2$. Then fumarase catalyzes the conversion of fumarate to malate. Malate is subsequently converted to oxaloacetate in the fourth oxidizing reaction, one that reduces NAD^+ to NADH. This is an eqilibrium reaction that favors malate. The products of the Krebs cycle are 3 NADH, 1 $FADH_2$, and 3 CO_2. Thus, 12 ATP can be generated from each citrate formed in the initial reaction.

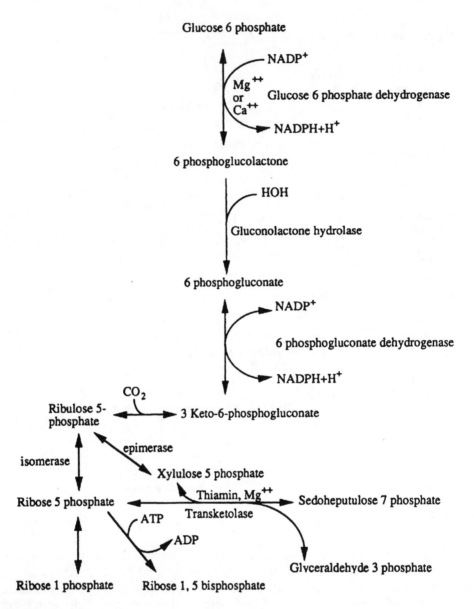

FIGURE 11.9
The pentose phosphate pathway.

The events of the Krebs cycle are influenced primarily by the redox state of $NAD^+/NADH$, the cellular level of intermediates, and the energy level (ADP/ATP) of a cell. For instance, if the ratio of NADH to NAD^+ is high, then the activities of isocitrate dehydrogenase, α-ketoglutarate dehydrogenase, and malate dehydrogenase slow due to relative lack of a reactant. High NADH to NAD^+ dictates that the reversible malate dehydrogenase catalyzes in the direction of malate, thus reducing the concentration of oxaloacetate, a reactant in the first reaction. Also, inhibition of isocitrate dehydrogenase by increased NADH to NAD^+ results in the accumulation of isocitrate, which is converted back to citrate by aconitase. Citrate inhibits citrate synthase, and thus citrate accumulates in the mitochondria. This will be important later when fatty acid synthesis is discussed.

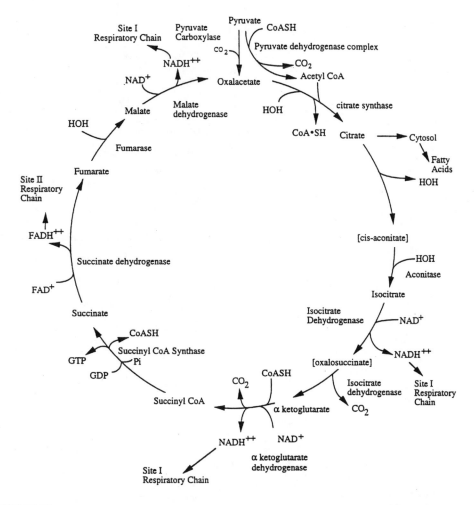

FIGURE 11.10
The Krebs cycle.

Increased ADP to ATP will speed up the Krebs cycle in general in two ways. Increased ADP indicates a need for cellular energy, and thus the electron transport chain will operate at a greater rate, thereby creating a higher NAD^+ to NADH ratio. Second, ADP allosterically increases isocitrate dehydrogenase activity.

Gluconeogenesis

Gluconeogenesis (Figure 11.11), the production of glucose from noncarbohydrate substrates, occurs mainly in the liver. The major precursors are lactate, glycerol, and certain amino acids. Gluconeogenesis utilizes several reversible reactions of glycolysis but must create chemical reaction bipasses around several unidirectional reactions, whereby the enzyme only catalyzes the reaction in the direction of glycolysis. Thus, gluconeogenesis can not be viewed simply as the reversal of glycolysis. The amino acid alanine and lactate are major gluconeogenic precursors and both are converted to pyruvate in the liver. In order for pyruvate to be converted to phosphoenolpyruvate it must first diffuse into the

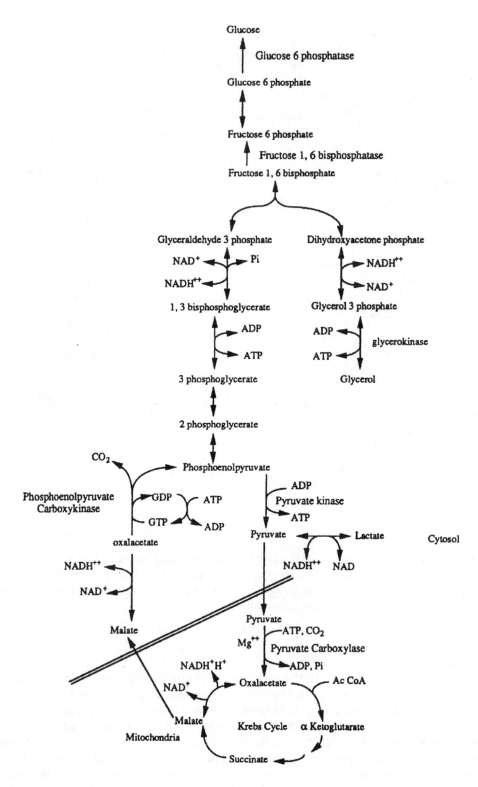

FIGURE 11.11
Gluconeogenesis.

mitochondria and undergo conversion to OAA and then malate. Pyruvate carboxylate catalyzes the conversion to OAA and then malate dehydrogenase converts OAA to malate.

Fatty Acid Oxidation

Fatty acids are a major source of energy for humans. Most cells, with the most notable exceptions being erythrocytes and cells of the brain, will utilize fatty acids. Fatty acids primarily undergo oxidation in the mitochondria and to a lesser degree in peroxisomes. β-Oxidation reduces even-chain-length fatty acids to acetyl CoA and odd-chain-length fatty acids to propionyl CoA. β-Oxidation involves four sequential steps and the products are $FADH_2$ and NADH and acetyl CoA. The latter product is available to either condense with oxaloacetate to form citrate and engage in the Krebs cycle or to form ketone bodies in the liver. Unsaturated fatty acids, which may account for as much as half the fatty acids humans oxidize, require additional enzymes.

Before a fatty acid can be oxidized, it must first be available in the cytosol. Fatty acids can either be liberated from intracellular pools, such as triglycerides in lipid droplets, or they can diffuse across the plasma membrane from the extracellular fluid (i.e., circulation). Circulatory fatty acids are primarily derived from triglycerides hydrolyzed in lipoproteins, such as VLDL and chylomicrons, by *lipoprotein lipase* or they are loosely bound to albumin. Once in the cytosol, fatty acids are found associated with a *fatty acid binding protein* (FABP) or Z-protein, which may help guide the fatty acid towards mitochondria.

Cytosolic long-chain fatty acids are activated in the cytosol by the attachment of coenzyme A via long-chain acyl CoA synthetase. This enzyme is associated with the outer mitochondrial membrane. The fatty acid–coenyme A complex is called *acyl-CoA*. This reaction requires energy which is provided as ATP is split to AMP and pyrophosphate (PP_i). The latter complex is cleaved into 2 phosphate molecules (2 P_i) by pyrophosphatase, thus regenerating the intracellular phosphate pool. Since AMP and 2 P_i are produced in the production of acyl-CoA, the equivalent of 2 ATP are required before fatty acid oxidation can begin. Shorter-chain-length fatty acids also undergo activation, but not until they are inside mitochondria.

While shorter-chain fatty acids can diffuse across the inner membrane of the mitochondria, longer-chain fatty acids, in the form of acyl-CoA, must be transported across the inner membrane. This requires the assistance of carnitine transport systems. Acyl CoA diffuses through the porous outer mitochondria membrane and carnitine is attached to acyl CoA in the intermembrane space by the actions of *carnitine-palmitoyl tranferase I*. CPTI is an integral protein associated with the outer mitochondrial membrane whose catalytic site is exposed on the intermembrane side of this membrane (Figure 11.12). This enzyme is inhibited by malonyl CoA, an intermediate of fatty acid synthesis.

Acyl carnitine is then transported across the inner membrane by carnitine acylcarnitine translocase, a symport protein that transports one carnitine molecule out of the mitochondrial matrix for every carnitine acylcarnitine it transfers into the matrix. Once inside the inner membrane, carnitine is split from the transferred fatty acid which is reactivated with coenzyme A. This reaction is catalyzed by *carnitine-palmitoyl transferase II*.

Mitochondria contain three somewhat identical FAD-dependent acyl CoA dehydrogenases, enzymes that act upon short-chain, medium-chain, and long-chain fatty acids. FAD is reduced to $FADH_2$ in a reaction that produces trans-Δ^2-enoyl CoA, which is hydrated to form L-3-hydroxyacyl CoA. L-3-hydroxyacyl CoA is then oxidized by NAD^+, forming NADH, and the product 3-ketoacyl CoA. Thiolase then splits 3-ketoacyl CoA to acetyl CoA and a fatty acyl CoA. The fatty acyl CoA is 2 carbons shorter than the fatty acyl CoA that began β-oxidation. Thus, if the original fatty acyl CoA was palmitoyl CoA, then the result

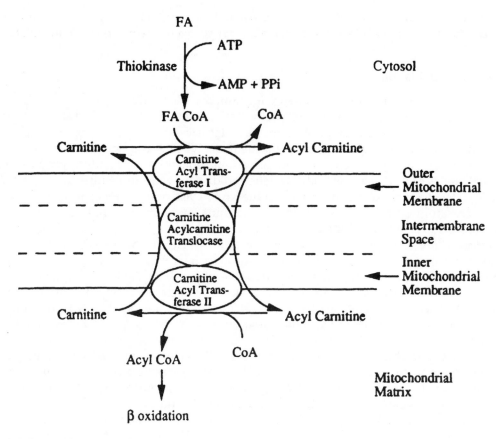

FIGURE 11.12
Carnitine acyl transferase system associated with the mitochondrial inner membrane.

is myristoyl CoA. For each "turn" of β-oxidation, or liberation of acetyl CoA, 1 $FADH_2$ and 1 NADH are generated. They are the equivalent of 5 ATP (Figure 11.13).

Ketone Body Production

Ketone bodies (acetoacetate, D-3-hydroxybutyrate, and acetone) are generally misunderstood and considered detrimental to human health. While they can present a health concern, it should be understood that it may only occur in atypical metabolic scenarios such as uncontrolled diabetes. There are two primary sources for ketone body production: fatty acid oxidation and amino acids (leucine, isoleucine, lysine, phenylalanine, tyrosine, and tryptophan). Alcohol oxidation can also result in ketone body formation. The formation of ketone bodies is presented in Figure 11.14.

Ketone bodies are formed in the liver to a limited degree daily. The most significant precursors for ketogenesis are fatty acids. During uncontrolled diabetes and starvation, the rate of ketone body production can increase significantly to reach levels that may have health consequences. While produced in the liver, hepatocytes will not utilize ketone bodies as an energy source. They will diffuse out of the liver and circulate to other tissue such as the heart, skeletal muscle, and the kidneys, and be combusted as fuel. During starvation the brain can adapt to utilize more and more ketone bodies as an energy source. As much as 50% of the brain's energy demands may be met by ketone bodies after several weeks of

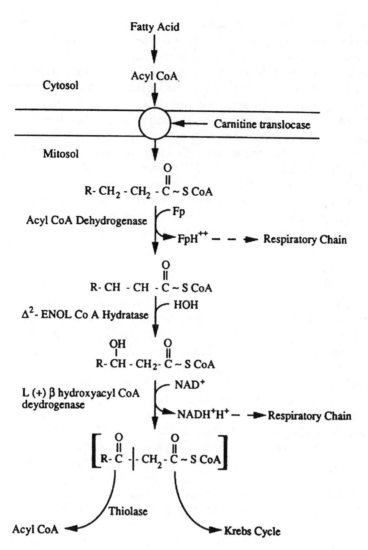

FIGURE 11.13
Fatty acid oxidation.

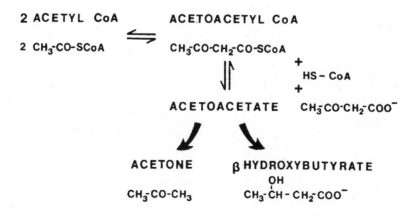

FIGURE 11.14
The formation of ketone bodies.

starvation. As an adult brain may utilize 140 to 150 g of glucose daily, reducing its glucose demands will slow the rate of body protein catabolism to serve gluconeogenesis.

Fatty acids, made available by hormone-sensitive lipase catabolism of adipocyte triglycerides, are oxidized in liver mitochondria to acetyl CoA. During periods of gluconeogenic operations, such as starvation, oxaloacetate is utilized as a glucose precursor, thereby decreasing its availability to condense with acetyl CoA to form citrate. This increases the flux of acetyl CoA through acetoacetyl CoA thiokinase in the direction of ketogenesis. Acetoacetyl CoA thiokinase condenses 2 molecules of acetyl CoA to form acetoacetyl CoA. This product molecule can then be condensed with a third acetyl CoA, via HMG CoA synthase, to form hydroxy-3-methylglutaryl CoA (HMG CoA), which is then cleaved by lyase to form *acetoacetate* and acetyl CoA. Acetoacetate can undergo reduction by NADH to form β-*hydroxybutyrate*. *Acetone* can be formed by a nonenzymatic decarboxylation of acetoacetate. Acetone production is relatively small and much of what is created is volatilized in the lungs and expired. The creation of ketone bodies from amino acids is discussed in Chapter 6.

Fatty Acid Synthesis

Fatty acid synthesis or *de novo lipogenesis* is depicted in Figure 11.15. It is a series of cytosolic reactions beginning with the 2-carbon acetyl CoA. In the preliminary reaction, bicarbonate (a source of CO_2) provides a carbon to acetyl CoA, resulting in malonyl CoA. Acetyl CoA carboxylase is a multienzyme complex that catalyzes the reaction and it is the first committed step. ATP and biotin are necessary for the reaction to occur. The ensuing reactions propagating fatty acid synthesis are complexed together and are referred to collectively as *fatty acid synthase (FAS)*. The first FAS reaction is catalyzed by malonyl transacylase (malonyl transferase) whereby a second acetyl group, associated with a carrier protein and phosphopantethine, is utilized and attached to malonyl CoA. CO_2 is removed in a subsequent reaction and the remaining 4-carbon molecule engages with further enzymes that comprise FAS. In addition to malonyl transacylase, FAS also includes ketoacyl synthase, acetyl transferase, hydratase, enoyl reductase, ketoacyl reductase, and thioesterase enzymes as well as acyl carrier protein (ACP) which contains pantothenic acid in the form of 4′-phosphopantetheine. ACP takes over the role of CoA. While these proteins are complexed together in humans, as well as other mammals, birds, and yeast, they are independent proteins in bacteria and plants. Fatty acids under construction derive their carbons from malonyl CoA, via acetyl CoA. The end product is the 16-carbon saturated fatty acid palmitate with the original "primer" acetyl CoA representing carbons 15 and 16. If the 3-carbon fatty acid propionate is available, it, too, can be used as the primer in fatty acid synthetase. This results in longer fatty acid chains of uneven numbers. This is more common in ruminants as propionate is formed to by microbes inhabiting their rumen.

Fatty acid synthesis is regulated at several levels. For instance, the expression of acetyl CoA carboxylase may be induced by insulin, while elevated levels of insulin and cytosolic citrate increase its activity. Long-chain acyl CoA, cAMP, and glucagon all decrease its activity. Citrate probably acts as an activator by forming an aggregate with an inactive acetyl CoA protein, thereby activating it. Many of the same influences upon acetyl CoA carboxylase also exist for FAS. Also, it has recently become clear that PUFAs can actually decrease the expression of FAS complex enzymes. It appears that there may be a nuclear binding protein that selectively binds ω-3 and ω-6 PUFA. ω-3 PUFA are believed to be more potent at this task. The proteins complexed within FAS appear to be coded by a single gene; thus transcription results in the formation of all components. Increasing levels of plasma FFA are associated with decreased lipogenesis, while high-carbohydrate diets, especially sucrose, are associated with increased lipogenesis.

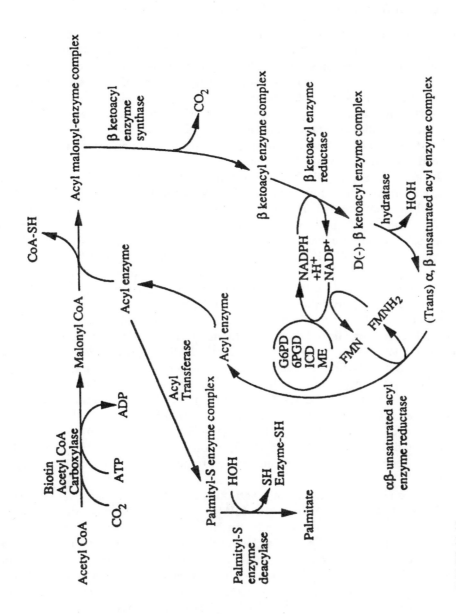

FIGURE 11.15
Fatty acid synthesis.

NADPH provides the reducing hydrogens for fatty acid synthesis. Most of the NADPH is derived from the pentose phosphate pathway or hexose monophosphate shunt. Cytosolic malic enzyme and isocitrate dehydrogenase are also sources of NADPH; however, the significance of the latter enzyme is believed to be minor.

Molecular Control Mechanisms of Fat Metabolism

Lipid metabolism is under control of a superfamily of nuclear hormone receptors. These receptors are transcription factors that mediate nuclear-acting hormones such as glucocorticoids, mineralcorticoids, estrogens, progestins, androgens, thyroid hormones, vitamin D, and retinoic acid. One type of nuclear receptor that has profound effects upon lipid metabolism is the *peroxisome proliferator-activated receptors (PPARs)* that belong to the steroid/thyroid/retionid receptor superfamily. PPARs were first shown to be activated by substances that induce peroxisomal proliferation. These are termed *orphan receptors,* since no known hormone specifically binds to these receptors. However, such orphan receptors, such as the PPARs, are activated by a number of compounds.

The PPARs are important in the control of fatty acid oxidation and synthesis. Three subtypes have been identified thus far: PPARα, PPARδ, and PPARλ. PPARα was the first discovered and the most studied. These receptors bind to promoter regions of genes that play a critical role in fat metabolism. Induction of this receptor results in the proliferation of peroxisomes, which are involved in the metabolism of longer-chain fatty acids. Subsequently, it was discovered that PPARα could induce enzymes associated with fatty acid catabolism, such as medium-chain acyl dehydrogenase and carnitine-palmitoyl transferase I. Furthermore, it was discovered that for these receptors to function, they had to be activated by the binding of particular compounds (however, not hormones). Many such agents, termed ligands, have been identified. In the case of PPARα, it was discovered that several naturally occurring fatty acids could activate this receptor. A large number of unrelated compounds have been discovered that activate PPARα, including various fatty acids such as oleate, eicosanoids, fibrates, peroxisome proliferators, and inhibitors of mitochondrial β-oxidation. At the promoter level, however, it was determined that the PPAR/ligand complexes could not act by themselves. They need to interact with a retinoic acid receptor (RXR), which itself is first activated by a retinoic acid derivative, such as 9-*cis* retinoic acid. Together the entire complex must bind to the promoter 5′ at specific recognition or response elements (nucleotide base pairs). Thus, PPARs function as heterodimers with RXRs and are separated from each other by one base pair on the promoter regions of candidate enzyme genes.

PPARα have been identified in a variety of tissues including liver, heart, and kidney. It was later discovered that other isoforms of PPARs existed. PPARγ has received a lot of interest and is found in appreciable amounts in fat cells. It is thought to be activated by such compounds as prostaglandins and a class of diabetic drugs termed "thiazolidinediones." In the case of PPARγ, this receptor, again with its heterodimeric partner RXR, stimulates fat synthesis. PPARγ appears to increase insulin sensitivity in adipose and skeletal muscle when a thiazolidinedione is administered; however, the exact mechanism in unknown. PPARγ can increase the expression of phosphoenolpyruvate carboxykinase (PEPCK), which catalyzes the conversion of oxaloacetate to phosphoenolpyruvate, which is the rate-limiting enzyme in gluconeogensis. It can also stimulate the peroxisomal acyl CoA oxidase gene. Fibroblasts that overexpressed PPARγ using transfection techniques developed adipocyte-like characteristics once an appropriate ligand was added.

PPARδ does not have a known function at the moment. Nonetheless, the PPARs present a newer piece to the puzzle in understanding how lipid metabolism is controlled at the molecular level. In some fashion, fatty acids, acting as ligands to these receptors, are acting as hormones and allow an entire new area of research to pursue metabolic control mechanisms related to fat metabolism and adoposity. It would appear that PPARα favors fat catabolism and PPARγ fat synthesis.

Alcohol Oxidation

The oxidation of alcohol (ethanol) primarily takes place in the liver by three enzyme systems (Figure 11.16). All three systems produce *acetaldehyde*, which can be further metabolized to acetate. The accumulation of acetaldehyde, as in chronic abusive alcohol consumption, is believed to be toxic to hepatocytes.

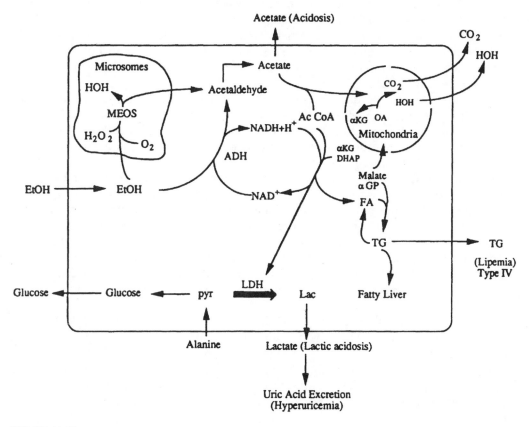

FIGURE 11.16
Ethanol metabolism in liver cells.

The major alcohol-metabolizing enzyme is *alcohol dehydrogenase*, which may have as many as 20 different isoenzyme forms. One of the biggest determinants for the rate of this reaction is the availability of NAD^+. Alcohol dehydrogenase is cytosolic and generates acetaldehyde, which must then enter mitochondria for further oxidation by aldehyde dehydrogenase to acetate. *The microsomal ethanol-oxidizing system (MEOS)* is located in the smooth endoplasmic reticulum and involves the cytochrome P_{450} enzyme system. This monooxygenase enzyme complex is also involved in the detoxification of drugs and xenobiotics. Last, peroxisomal oxidation of ethanol occurs as catalase uses hydrogen peroxide to convert ethanol to acetaldehyde. As with the acetaldehyde created in the cytosol by alcohol dehydrogenase, the acetaldehyde produced within the smooth endoplasmic reticulum and peroxisomes must enter mitochondria for further oxidation to acetate. Most of the acetate will diffuse from the liver and be metabolized by extrahepatic cells.

Energy Substrate Utilization

On a daily basis, the utilization of energy substrates fluctuates in various cell types, based upon availability, presence of hormones, and physiological state. While the consumption of substrates in some tissue can go unchanged throughout the day or for longer periods, some cell types can adapt to utilize alternative substrates. As discussed previously, cellular substrate metabolism is influenced by the presence and quantity of mitochondria, the rate of expression of enzymes and transporters, the presence of allosteric influences, and the energy and redox state of the cell.

As nutritional state is perhaps the single most influential factor in energy nutrient utilization, it seems that the most logical way to investigate energy metabolism is by way of fluctuating or adaptive nutritional state. The major organs involved in the metabolism of energy molecules in the human body are the liver, adipose tissue, and skeletal muscle. The heart should also be recognized as well. These organs will accommodate greater energy influx during periods of nutrient absorption from the digestive tract than can immediately be utilized as fuel or be used in the development of energy stores. Other tissue can also do this, but not to the extent shown by these organs. Other organs and tissues, such as the CNS, RBCs, and renal parenchyma will also be pivotal in considering integrated energy utilization. The primary metabolic objective during fluctuating daily nutritional states is the maintenance of blood glucose. Even during fasting periods lasting several days, this is still the primary objective. However, as starvation becomes more protracted, the preservation of body protein stores becomes a strong consideration as well.

One last consideration must be made with regard to metabolic states. While it is often easier to discuss metabolic states as definitive situations such as a fed state or a fasting state, there are transitional periods where opposing influences overlap. This is largely due to the molar concentration of insulin:glucagon and the residual effects of hormones. For example, during the first hour or so after eating a meal, some of the residual effects of fasting still linger and, conversely, the transition from a fed to fasting state is not easily defined either.

The fact that several intermediates of energy pathways sit at metabolic crossroads provides coordination of energy pathways. Therefore, while the energy pathways are often taught as if they were separate entities, they do indeed feed in and out from each other. For instance, acetyl CoA, which can be formed by beta oxidation or from pyruvate, can be used to make ketone bodies or in the production of citrate which can continue through the Krebs cycle for immediate energy or become involved in fatty acid synthesis. Pyruvate is another crossroad intermediate. It can be produced via glycolysis or from lactate and catabolism of certain amino acids. Pyruvate can be used to produce acetyl CoA or oxaloacetate in mitochondria or used to synthesize alanine or lactate in the cytosol.

Early Refeeding and a Fed State

While size of a meal and its composition can be influential, the following discussion will assume a typical mixed diet. Ingestion of food leads to the absorption of energy molecules into both the lymphatic circulation (i.e., chylomicrons) and the hepatic portal vein (i.e., amino acids, monoglycerides, glycerol, shorter-chain-length fatty acids, and medium-chain triglycerides). Both of these circulations will flow into the systemic circulation after passing through the thoracic duct and perfusing the liver, respectively. The liver will remove more than half of the absorbed amino acids and glucose and nearly all of the galactose and fructose during the primary perfusion. The remaining amino acids and glucose, along with select amino acids (mostly BCAA) released by the liver, serve to increase the levels of these energy sources in the blood. The augmented levels of glucose and amino acids become the primary stimuli for insulin release and the resulting increase in the insulin:glucagon ratio that will dictate the majority of the ensuing metabolic events. The release of insulin, as strongly stimulated by glucose and less strongly by amino acids, is actually "primed" or amplified by circulating digestion-related hormones such as gastrin, CCK, secretin, and gastrin inhibitory polypeptide.

Insulin promotes the translocation of GLUT4 receptors to the plasma membrane of muscle and adipose tissue. Insulin also promotes the increased uptake of glucose in the liver. All three tissue types will play primary roles in storing excess energy. During the period of early refeeding, the liver is still engaged in gluconeogenic operations, which will linger for some time. Thus, some of the glycogen synthesized early in refeeding is actually derived from gluconeogenic precursors. Dietary glucose is phosphorylated to glucose 6-phosphate and, along with glucose 6-phosphate derived from gluconeogenesis, is used to synthesize glycogen. Some glucose 6-phosphate will also continue through glycolysis as glycolytic enzymes become activated by the increasing insulin:glucagon ratio. However, glucose flux through glycolysis in early refeeding is not as great as perhaps expected. The primary reason is because the gluconeogenic and lypolytic effects of fasting are still lingering and hepatocytes are still oxidizing fatty acids. As a result, increased quantities of acetyl CoA are available in the cell and inhibit pyruvate dehydrogenase, thereby favoring gluconeogenesis and slowing glycolysis upstream. Also, some diet-derived amino acids as well as amino acids delivered to hepatocytes during fasting can be used to produce glucose 6-phosphate and subsequently glycogen. This notion is easily supported by experimental findings that a lot of liver glycogen monomers are derived from the carbon skeletons of amino acids. Thus, in the liver, gluconeogenic and glycolytic operations coexist for an hour or two as the former wanes and the latter increases. The slowing of glycolysis in early refeeding also allows for more glucose 6-phosphate to be used as a reactant for the pentose phosphate pathway. The primary significance to energy metabolism is that the oxidative reactions of the pentose phosphate pathway produce NADPH that is necessary for subsequent fatty acid synthesis.

In the early refeeding state, fatty acid oxidation also continues in skeletal muscle and wanes slowly with time. Again, pyruvate dehydrogenase is inactivated by increased levels of mitochondrial acetyl CoA and ATP, as well as relatively higher amounts of NADH/NAD$^+$. Therefore, pyruvate generated from glycolysis will be converted to lactate. This lactate can diffuse from the cell, circulate to the liver, and be used in gluconeogenesis or other operations. Muscle cell glucose 6-phosphate is also used to resynthesize glycogen within muscle cells. The pentose phosphate pathway is not a consideration in muscle, primarily due to its lack of fatty acid and steroid synthesis.

While small amounts of glycogen exist in adipose cells, most of the glucose entering these cells will be oxidized for energy and to generate glycerol 3-phosphate which is necessary in the synthesis of triglyceride, along with fatty acids which are derived from the blood. Therefore, these cells use the increased intracellular pool of glucose 6-phosphate to synthesize fatty acids and a little glycogen as well as an immediate source of energy to drive the synthetic and homeostatic operations.

As the fed state continues, the anabolic effects of the elevated insulin:glucagon ratio dominate. Gluconeogenesis becomes inhibited in the liver and fatty acid oxidation trickles to a stop. At this time, glucose becomes the primary source of fuel in skeletal muscle cells, which are also fully engaged in glycogen synthesis operations. The extent to which muscle cells will take up glucose from the blood is strongly influenced by its ability to store glucose as glycogen as well as its ability to metabolize glucose as an energy source. Skeletal muscle will not be a site of lipogenesis. The skeletal muscle triglyceride pool is derived from lipoproteins, via lipoprotein lipase, and circulating fatty acids loosely bound to albumin.

Most other cell types will be oxidizing glucose in the fed state. The glucose will be a mixture of premeal circulating glucose and absorbed glucose. The net effect will be a reduction in circulatory glucose as promoted by a relatively high molar ratio insulin to glucagon.

Fasting

After several hours, depending upon the size and composition of the meal, the metabolic picture of the human body slowly slips into early fasting. Here the anabolic effects of insulin will linger as the catabolic effects of glucagon begin to become more prominent. As less and less absorbed glucose enters the circulation and the concentration of glucose normalizes and even begins to move in the direction of hypoglycemia, more glucagon will be secreted. Homeostatic efforts swing in favor of providing glucose to the blood from energy stores, while at the same time making other energy substrates available to reduce glucose utilization in tissue throughout the body. The needs of the CNS and RBCs alone account for about 100 to 125 g and 45 to 50 g of glucose daily in an adult. These high requirements continue in early fasting but will decrease as the fasting continues.

Glucagon promotes the activation of phosphorylase in liver cells, while concurrently the inactivating influence of insulin upon this enzyme decreases. At the same time that glucagon would act as a repressor of glucokinase in the liver, the inducing influence of insulin upon the synthesis of this enzyme diminishes. In addition, insulin's positive influence on the glycogen synthase system enzymes decreases. Thus, the net effect of these activities is that glucose entry into hepatocytes becomes minimized and glycogen metabolism strongly favors breakdown. Also, at the same time glucose 6-phosphatase is induced by glucagon, which will liberate glucose from glucose 6-phosphate derived from glycogen and gluconeogenesis. The substrates for gluconeogenesis include glycerol from fat-mobilizing processes and circulating blood lactate.

Perhaps the most significant of substrate for gluconeogenesis is amino acids, primarily alanine from skeletal muscle. Cortisol is the principal stimulus for the catabolism of muscle protein and pyruvate serves as the recipient for transaminated nitrogen forming alanine. Interestingly, increased circulating alanine levels serve as a stimulus of glucagon release. This makes sense, as glucagon promotes liver gluconeogenesis. Pyruvate is reformed in hepatocytes and enters mitochondria. Pyruvate carboxylase converts much of the pyruvate to oxaloacetate some of which can condense with beta oxidation-derived acetyl CoA to satisfy hepatocyte energy demands. The remaining pyruvate is available for gluconeogenesis. Figure 11.17 provides an overview of energy flux after 24 h of fasting.

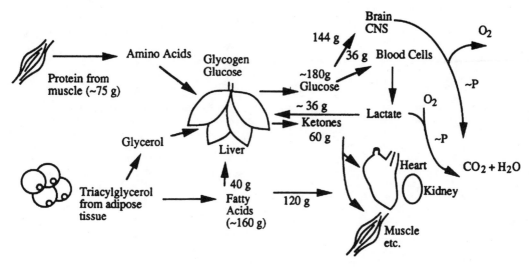

FIGURE 11.17
Energy metabolism during early adaptive starvation.

Prolonged Fasting (Starvation)

As starvation continues beyond 1 day, several events take place. First, hepatic glycogen stores become exhausted within the first 24 to 36 h. Thus, the reliance upon skeletal muscle amino acids and other gluconeogenic precursors increases. Second, the production of ketone bodies increases as more and more fatty acids are mobilized and oxidized in the liver. And third, as fasting continues for many days to weeks, tissues in the body adapt to utilize more ketone bodies in efforts to spare body protein.

12

Body Composition and Obesity

The composition of the human body can be assessed at several levels. As briefly discussed in Chapter 1, body composition can be assessed at the elemental level. Here oxygen, hydrogen, carbon, and nitrogen are recognized as the greatest contributors to human mass. This is easily understandable, because these four elements are the primary atomic building blocks for key organic molecules and water (Table 12.1). Next, human body composition can be assessed at the molecular level, with minerals grouped together to represent that which is not molecular. For instance, in a lean adult male, water provides about 60% (56 to 64%) of his mass, and both protein and fat will each account for roughly 15 to 16% of his total mass (Table 1.2). About 4 to 6% of human mass can be attributed to minerals while the remaining 1% or so is attributable to substances like carbohydrates and nucleic acids.

TABLE 12.1
Theoretical Contributors to Body
Weight for a Lean Man and Woman

Component	Man	Woman
Water	62%	59%
Fat	16%	22%
Protein	16%	14%
Minerals	6%	5%
Carbohydrate	<1%	<1%
	100%	100%

At the molecular level, the substance which can provide the greatest degree of fluctuation is body fat. Body fat can account for as little as 5% of mass in excessively lean adults or as much as 65 to 70% of the total mass in excessively (morbidly) obese individuals. Adipose tissue is approximately 86% triglyceride. The remaining 14% of adipose tissue mass is largely water, protein, carbohydrate, and minerals. These substances are associated with the intracellular and extracellular fluids, connective tissue, and enzymes as well as structural cell aspects such as membranes. Because of the disproportion of major substances found in adipose tissue, as an individual accumulates larger fat stores, the body fat percentage increases while the percentage of the other substances decreases. Figure 12.1 presents the percentage contributions of fat, muscle, bone, and organs to total body mass for a reference man and woman.

Typically, body composition is assessed to determine percentage of body fat and lean body mass (LBM) or fat-free mass (FFM). While FFM and LBM are often used interchangeably, LBM includes not only all nonfat portions of the human body but also *essential fat deposits* as well. Essential fat is found associated with the bone marrow, the CNS, and internal organs. Women also have essential body fat associated with mammary glands and the pelvic region. Essential body fat for a normal adult male and female may be 3% and 12% of their body weight, respectively.

TABLE 12.2

Select Techniques for Body Composition Assessment

Technique	Advantages of Application	Disadvantages of Application
Anthropometry (skinfold thickness, circumferences)	Inexpensive; estimation of total body fat and regional muscle	Inaccuracy increases with obesity and individuals with firm subcutaneous tissue
CAT scan	Assesses organ size and fat distribution and bone size	Expensive equipment; limited availability; small radiation exposure
Bioelectrical impedance analysis (BIA)	Estimates LBM via total body water; inexpensive equipment, nonhazardous	Several prediction formulas; fluid and electrolyte inconsistancies can produce error
Creatinine excretion	Estimation of muscle mass; nonhazardous	Influenced by diet; several factors can decrease accuracy; participant cooperation is vital
Densitometry	Provides estimation of LBM and body simultaneously; generally nonhazardous	Participant cooperation is vital; unsuitable for children and elderly individuals; intestinal gas may induce element of error
DEXA	Estimates total body fat-free soft tissue and body fat; can provide bone mineral estimation if desired	Expensive equipment; limited availability; radiation (X-ray) exposure
Infared interactance	Safe, noninvasive, rapid	May overestimate body fat in very lean individuals; may underestimate body fat in very obese
MRI	Provides estimation of organ sizes, muscle, fat, fat distribution, total body water	Expensive equipment; limited availability
Total body potassium (TBK)	Nonhazardous; minimal participant cooperation necessary	Expensive equipment with limited availability; potassium imbalance affects accuracy

Modern techniques for the assessment of body composition range from simple use of calipers to measure skinfold (fatfold) thickness to the utilization of complex instrumentation such as computerized axial tomography (CAT), dual-energy X-ray absorptiometry (DEXA), and magnetic resonance imaging (MRI). Discussion below focuses upon three of the more common methods, while Table 12.2 describes several of the techniques advantages, and shortcomings.

Methods for Assessing Body Composition

Densitometry

The Greek mathematician Archimedes is often credited with the original concept of densitometry, which is the basis for hydrostatic or underwater weighing. He concluded that the volume of an object submerged underwater was equal to the volume of water displaced by an object. He hypothesized further that an object's density can be calculated simply by dividing the object's weight on land by its loss of weight submerged in pure water. This concept can be applied to humans; however one must account for residual lung air and

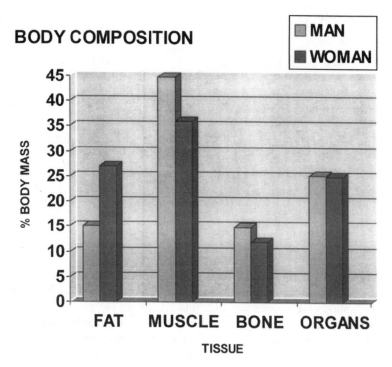

FIGURE 12.1
Percentage contribution of fat, muscle, bone, and organs to total body mass.

gases in the lumen of the gut. For instance, for a man weighing 80 kg on land and 3.5 kg underwater, 76.5 kg represents the loss of body weight and the weight of water displaced. Again, the buoyancy influence of the residual lung gas must be mathematically accounted for as well as the gas in the gastrointestinal tract. Body density can then be estimated using the following calculation:

$$\frac{\text{weight of body on land}}{\dfrac{(\text{weight of body on land} - \text{weight underwater})}{\text{density of water}} - \text{residual lung gas} - \text{gastrointestinal gas}}$$

Residual lung gas is estimated to be approximately 24% of vital lung capacity, while the residual gas in the gastrointestinal tract is typically 50 to 300 ml. Many researchers choose to either ignore residual gastrointestinal gas or simply use 100 ml. In addition, the density of water with relation to temperature needs to be known and taken into account.

Once body density is known, then the percentage of body fat and total fat and lean body mass can be estimated using equation A (below). Estimations of body density are based upon assumptions that the density of body fat is 0.9 g/cm³ and that of fat-free mass is 1.1 g/cm³. Also, it is assumed that fat-free mass is composed of 20.5% protein, 72.4% water, and 7.1% bone mineral. Underwater weighing is considered a noninvasive tool for assessing body fat, and the error of estimation of body fat by this means is about 2.7% for adults and 4.5% for children and adolescents. Once the percentage body fat is estimated, then the weight attributable to body fat and lean body weight can be estimated using calculations B and C (below).

A. Percentage body fat

$$\% \text{ body fat } = \frac{495}{\text{body density}} - 450$$

B. Weight of body fat

body weight × % body fat = weight of body fat

C. Weight of lean body weight

body weight – weight of body fat = weight of lean body weight

Anthropometry

Anthropometry literally means "the measurement of man." Body composition is estimated by measuring various limb circumferences and obtaining skinfold thickness measurements to assess subcutaneous fat deposition. Skinfold thickness estimation of body fat requires that several assumptions are made, including that: (1) a direct relationship exists between the quantity of fat deposited just below the skin and total body fat and does not vary within and between individuals; (2) the thickness of the skin and subcutaneous adipose tissue has a constant compressibility throughout; and (3) the thickness of skin is negligible and a constant fraction of skinfold measurements. Skin thickness tends to vary between 0.5 to 2.0 mm.

Skinfold thickness measurements are obtained with calipers at several anatomical locations. Primary sites of measurement are the triceps, abdomen, subscapular, thigh, and suprailiac (Figure 12.2 and Table 12.3). Secondary sites include the chest, midaxillary, and the medial calf. The use of skinfold calipers requires training and precision in measurement technique. Several factors much be taken into consideration. First, when a caliper is initially applied to a skinfold, a brief period of time is necessary prior to the reading of the thickness. About 4 sec will allow the tips of the caliper to appropriately compress the skinfold. The reading will become smaller with time as the calipers compress the skinfold and fluids are forced out of the area. This increases error to the measurement. Therefore, if an accurate measurement is not obtained after 4 to 5 sec, the skinfold should be released and measurement can be attempted again momentarily. Also, error is typically introduced when different individuals perform the skinfold measurements.

It should not matter from which side of the body skinfold measurements are obtained. It seems that many North American investigators prefer the right side, while many European investigators prefer the left. It is recommended that inexperienced skinfold technicians should mark the subjects body at points of measurement, especially if tape measures are used to locate midpoints. The caliper is most easily used by holding it in the right hand so that the dial is exposed for reading during measurement. The caliper tips should be placed 1 cm (~½ inch) distal to the fingers holding the skin (Figure 12.2).

Bioelectrical Impedance

Bioelectrical impedance (BEI) or total body electrical conductivity (TOBEC) assessment is based upon the conductivity properties of electrolyte-based medium. An individual rests

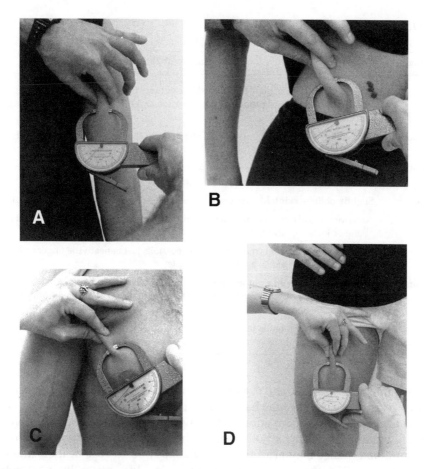

FIGURE 12.2
Common sites of skinfold measurements. Tricep (a), suprailiac (b), pectoral (c), thigh (d).

in a supine position, and BEI is measured by passing a weak electric current through the body from one electrode to another placed on peripheral extremities (hands and feet). The current is painless and the rate of conductivity represents proportions of LBM and fat mass. LBM will have more water and associated electrolytes and therefore will demonstrate greater electrical conductivity. Some bathroom scales today have built in BEI system.

Variations in Body Composition

Lean Body Mass and Fat

Several factors such as age, gender, stature, heredity, and pregnancy will influence body composition. At birth and during infancy and early childhood, minimal but evident differences exist between males and females with regard to body composition. Males tend to have a little more total body mass and a slightly higher percentage of LBM. However, at the onset of puberty males experience a burst in the development of LBM. Meanwhile, at

TABLE 12.3
Sites of Skinfold Measurements

Location	Measurement Technique
Tricep	Vertical skinfold measurement on the back of the arm at the midpoint between the tip of the shoulder or lateral process of the acromion and the tip of the elbow or the olecranon process of the ulna
Subscapular	Oblique skinfold measurement made just beneath the tip of the scapula or inferior angle of the scapula bone
Abdominal	Vertical skinfold measurement made approximately 3 cm to the right and 1 cm below the midpoint of the umbilicus or "belly button"
Suprailiac	Slightly oblique skinfold measurement just above the iliac crest at the midaxillary line
Thigh	Anterior vertical fold measured at the midpoint between the superior border of the patella bone or knee cap and the inguinal crease
Pectoral (chest)	Skinfold measurement is made as high as possible, just beneath the fingers, along the line from the anterior axillary fold to the nipple
Medial calf	Subject is sitting with right leg flexed approximately 90° at the knee. Vertical skinfold measurement is made at the medial region of maximum calf circumference.
Midaxillary	Skinfold measurement is made at the right midaxillary line at the level of the superior aspect of the xyphoid process

roughly the same time, females tend to experience a similar burst in body fat accumulation. At about 10 years of age, a male may have a body fat percentage of 13% vs. 19% in a female of the same age. Then, throughout adolescence and into early adulthood the percentage of body fat will typically increase for both genders, however, disproportionately for females. In early adulthood, males may attribute approximately 15 to 16% of their mass to fat in comparison to 22 to 24% for females. Also, females tend to achieve the maximal LBM by age 18, while males tend to continue to demonstrate increases in LBM into their early 20s.

Body Water and Minerals

The water content of the human body is never higher than at birth — about 70% of a term newborn infant's weight may be water. Even higher body water percentages, as much as 83%, are possible in premature infants. During the first year of life, an infant's body water content will decrease slightly as more body fat is accumulated. However, during the next 5 to 6 years, a child's body water percentage will increase slightly only to then demonstrate a minor decline during the ensuing 2 to 3 years. By about the age of 10, a child's body water content is still roughly 62 to 65%. Furthermore, at this point males generally possess a slightly higher percentage of body water than females. By adulthood, body water content is generally 56 to 64%. As the water content of the extracellular fluid is by and large controlled hormonally, the greatest influence upon tissue water content remains the ratio of skeletal muscle to adipose tissue.

While body water content, as a percentage of total mass, seems to decrease from birth to adulthood, the opposite appears to be true for mineral content or ash percentage. A typical term newborn may only be about 3.2% mineral, while an adult may be roughly 4 to 6% minerals, by mass. While many general statements can be made regarding body composition, gender, and aging, it is very likely that heredity plays a role as well. For example,

African-Americans tend to have more LBM than European-Americans. African-Americans also have more dense bones, allowing for a greater total body calcium content.

Adipocytes

Adipocytes, classically viewed as simple and inert containers of stored energy, are now beginning to be recognized as more complex tissue, having both endocrine function and involvement in the regulation of energy homeostasis and body composition. As adipose tissue is the most manipulative human tissue from an energy perspective, it only makes sense that this tissue might function as a gauge for energy storage, as well as possess the ability to respond to varying levels of storage. For some individuals, body fat can represent as little as 4 to 5% of body mass, while in morbidly obese individuals it can account for as much as 65 to 70% of human mass. While not all body fat is found within adipocytes, the majority of it is, and thus increases in human body fat occur by expansion of adipose tissue mass. Therefore, the function of adipose tissue, either as a whole or regionally, may be adaptive to varying degrees of adiposity.

The notion that adipocytes play a role in human energy homeostasis via secretion of endocrine factors probably dates back to the 1950s. During that time, it was proposed that adipocytes possess the capability of registering excessive energy stores and respond by secreting an endocrine factor, called *adipostat*, which would limit food intake. However, interest waned in the years that followed and was not reawakened for several decades. In the 1980s, a serine protease called *adipsin* was reported to be secreted by cultured adipocytes. Because subsequent investigations revealed that adipsin secretion was markedly reduced in various obese rodent models, scientists speculated that this chemical may be the underlying factor involved in human obesity. However, it was soon determined that adipsin is not reduced in obese humans and thus could not be the causative factor. As researchers continued to investigate the endocrine properties of adipocytes it became known that this tissue could secrete a variety of interesting factors, including angiotensinogen and tumor necrosis factor α (TNFα). TNFα is a cytokine expressed in cell types such as macrophages. Subsequent investigations indeed determined that TNFα is overexpressed in obese animals and humans. Furthermore, there is also some evidence to suggest that another secreted substance, *leptin*, may also be involved in the development of obesity-linked insulin resistance.

Hypertrophy and Hyperplasia

Adipose tissue can expand by both *hypertrophy* and *hyperplasia*, although, more than likely, once a adipocyte has matured it has minimal capacity for cell division. This means that the majority of adipose tissue expansion, resulting from excessive energy intake, occurs by hypertrophy of mature, terminally differentiated adipocytes. However, the presence of new adipocytes has been observed as adiposity increases. Therefore, the potential for hyperplasia must reside in precursor forms of adipocytes.

Within adipose tissue there appears to be pockets of fibroblast-like adipocyte precursor or *stem cells* which can reproduce and differentiate into adipocytes. More than likely, growth factors regulate the process of adipocyte development from the early commitment of stem cells to the terminal stages of differentiation. Of the different growth factors investigated, perhaps the ones receiving the most attention at present are the *bone morpho-genetic proteins* (BMPs). While present in many tissues, as well as having a variety of functions, BMPs were named so as they induced endochondral bone formation when implanted subcutaneously in rats.

While the genetic factors involved in committing the stem cells to the adipocyte lineage are still elusive, some potential clues have been discovered. For instance, a lipid-activated transcription factor, called *PPARγ2*, may be involved. The expression of this factor may be unique to adipocytes. Furthermore, another factor called *preadipocyte factor-1* (Pref-1) may also be involved in adipocyte stem cell commitment. Pref-1 is a transmembrane protein that contains several epidermal growth factor-like repeats. Pref-1 is only expressed in proliferating preadipocytes. Insulin-like growth factors (IGFs) have also been shown to be involved in the regulation of proliferation and differentiation of adipocyte stem cells. For instance, at least in chicks, both IGF-I and IGF-II stimulate stem cell proliferation. IGFs may be autocrine, paracrine, or endocrine. IGF-I is expressed in chick adipocyte precursor cells as well as certain mammals. Furthermore, the involvement of IGFs is probably regulated via the expression of IGF-binding proteins. To make the events of adipocyte stem cell proliferation and differentiation even more complicated, several other factors appear to be involved, including a number of fibroblast growth factors (FGFs) and their receptors, transforming growth factors α and β (TGF-α and TGF-β), and epidermal growth factor (EGF). More likely than not, these various growth factors work synergistically in the complicated process of adipogenesis.

Obesity

Obesity is a worldwide epidemic. European nations (e.g., Finland, Greece, the Netherlands, and Spain), Pacific and Indian Ocean island populations, Canada, and the U.S. have witnessed an increase in the prevalence of obesity over the past decades. The National Center for Health Statistics in the U.S. estimates the prevalence of obesity to be 35% for Americans. A 1995 commentary in the medical-based journal *Lancet* indicated that if weight gain continues at the current rate, by the year 2230, 100% of adults in the U.S. will be defined as overweight. However improbable this may be, it is indeed an intriguing extrapolation of a current trend.

A number of ideas have been proposed to explain this increased weight gain. Researchers continue to debate the role of dietary fat in the development and maintenance of obesity. A body of current literature suggests that under isoenergetic conditions the proportion of calories from fat neither influences the development of obesity nor is it the solution to the problem. However, health professionals are generally in agreement that it is excess energy intake relative to energy expenditure that promotes weight gain and increasing adiposity.

An increased occurrence of disease accompanies the rising obesity rate. Research supporting a positive correlation between obesity and mortality has been well established during the past decade by large American cohort studies such as the Framingham Heart Study, National Health and Nutrition Examination Survey (NHANES) I Epidemiologic Follow-up Study, and the Nurses Health Study. Many ailments, such as hypertension, dyslipidemia, diabetes mellitus, osteoarthritis, gastrointestinal disorders, and respiratory anomalies seem to occur secondary to obesity and will be discussed below.

The many social and psychological aspects of appetite also seem to influence weight gain or the efficacy of weight loss efforts. In modern times, the general availability of food in developed countries allows for the consumption of food for reasons other than the relief of hunger. For many individuals, food enhances celebration or entertainment, suppresses stress/anxiety, and alleviates boredom. Further, convenient and efficient meals are extremely popular in today's Western society.

Financial Implications of Obesity

Obesity financially impacts society. Reports have indicated that the various treatments of obesity utilize an estimated 5 to 7% of annual health care costs. Pharmacological companies annually invest millions of research dollars into developing drugs (primarily appetite regulation) that will combat obesity. From a consumer perspective, the American population spends several million dollars yearly on exercise equipment and nutrition supplements that claim to prevent obesity or promote weight loss.

History of Obesity

Evidence of obesity exists as far back as 25,000 years ago. Drawings and artifacts from the Paleolithic period (early Stone Age) depict stout women with large pendulous breasts and primarily female-pattern (gynoid) obesity. Treatment for obesity can be traced back as early as 5th century BC. Hippocrates prescribed the following therapy for the obese individuals in his day:

> Obese people and those desiring to lose weight should perform hard work before food. Meals should be taken after exertion and while still panting from fatigue and with no other refreshments before meals except only wine, diluted and slightly cold. Their meals should be prepared with a sesame or seasoning and other similar substances and be of a fatty nature as people get thus, satiated with food. They should, moreover, eat only once a day and take no baths and sleep on a hard bed and walk naked as long as possible.

The American-based NHANES data has documented this century's obesity explosion, at least in the U.S. Indication that obesity has been on the rise since the 18th century exists in a monograph written by Thomas Short, "I believe no age did ever afford more instances of corpulence than our own." Various diets had also been published throughout history, with "fad diets" and diet books in general publication since the 1850s. In modern times, numerous books on dieting are available to the population at large and at least one book of this nature can be found on the *New York Times* Best-Seller List for at least 2 decades now.

Although some early scientists expressed medical concern, the society at large viewed obesity as a sign of wealth and prosperity. Even current perception of ideal body weight varies by culture. As the study of obesity, adipose tissue, and metabolism increased with the advent of modern medicine, it was in the 20th century that concern arose in regards to obesity and disease risk. Availability of research funding for obesity has increased in the past 50 years, with a greater allowance invested in the genetic influence of its onset and appetite regulation.

Definitions and Prevalence

Obesity has been defined in several manners. The truest definition is also perhaps the most simple. Obesity is a physical state of excessive body fat or over-fatness. Here, body fat mass is best estimated by underwater weighing or one of the other techniques mentioned above. The term *overweight* specifies excess mass of all body tissue: fat mass and fat-free mass (i.e., muscle tissue, bone, and water). Therefore an individual is overweight but not obese if, for example, excess muscle mass is present. This is often the situation for body builders and muscular, yet lean athletes. However, numerical classifications, such as body mass index (BMI) and ideal weight ranges, of obesity often define overweight as a condition preceding obesity, or the terms are often used interchangeably.

Throughout history, various standards have determined the ideal weight of an individual. Perhaps the most widely published are the Metropolitan Life Weight for Height Tables. First published in 1942 for women and 1943 for men, these tables documented the first guidelines for a "desirable weight" based on the lowest mortality rate for each height category. In 1959 the Metropolitan tables were adjusted to account for frame size. Ideal weight ranges were now available for men and women based on small-frame, medium-frame, or large-frame. Table 12.4 presents a more modern revision which came in 1983 as a result of data from the 1971 to 1974 National Health and Nutrition Examination Survey (NHANES I). According to these tables, obesity is defined as greater than 124% of ideal body weight for men and 120% of ideal body weight for women. In a 1995 publication, the U.S. Department of Agriculture (UDSA) and Department of Health and Human Services (DHHS) graphically established ideal weight ranges in the *Dietary Guidelines for Americans*, 4th edition.

TABLE 12.4
Metropolitan Life Insurance Company Height and Weight Tables

MEN					WOMEN				
		Weight[a]					Weight[a]		
Height		Frame Size			Height		Frame Size		
Feet	Inches	Small	Medium	Large	Feet	Inches	Small	Medium	Large
5	2	128–134	131–141	138–150	4	10	102–111	109–121	118–131
5	3	130–136	133–143	140–153	4	11	103–113	111–123	120–134
5	4	132–138	135–145	142–156	5	0	104–115	113–126	122–137
5	5	134–140	137–148	144–160	5	1	106–118	115–129	125–140
5	6	136–142	139–151	146–164	5	2	108–121	118–132	128–143
5	7	138–145	142–154	149–168	5	3	111–124	121–135	131–147
5	8	140–148	145–157	152–172	5	4	114–127	124–138	134–151
5	9	142–151	148–160	155–176	5	5	117–130	127–141	137–155
5	10	144–154	151–163	158–180	5	6	120–133	130–144	140–159
5	11	146–157	154–166	161–184	5	7	123–136	133–147	143–163
6	0	149–160	157–170	164–188	5	8	126–139	136–150	146–167
6	1	152–164	160–174	168–192	5	9	129–142	139–153	149–170
6	2	155–168	164–178	172–197	5	10	132–145	142–156	152–173
6	3	158–172	167–182	176–202	5	11	135–148	145–159	155–176
6	4	162–176	171–187	181–207	6	0	138–151	148–162	158–179

Note: Weights at ages 25 to 29 based on lowest mortality. Weight in pounds according to frame, in clothing weighing 5 pounds for men and 3 pounds for women with 1 inch heels.

[a] Measured in pounds.

Source of basic data: *1979 Build Study,* Society of Actuaries and Association of Life Insurance Medical Directors of America, 1980. Reproduced with permission from Metropolitan Life Insurance Company.

TABLE 12.5
The Life Insurance Study Weight Classification and
Associated Mortality Risk

Weight Classification	BMI Range	Mortality Risk
Underweight	19.9 or less	Increased risk
Normal weight range	20.0–24.9	Very low risk
Pre–obesity or overweight	25.0–29.9	Slight risk
Class I obesity	30.0–34.9	Moderate risk
Class II obesity	35.0–39.9	High risk
Class III obesity	40.0 and greater	Very high risk

TABLE 12.6
World Health Organization Weight Classifications

Weight Classification	BMI Range
Underweight	18.49 or less
Normal range	18.5–24.99
Grade I obesity	25.0–29.99
Grade II obesity	30.0–39.99
Grade III obesity	40.0 and greater

The more common and accurate determinant of obesity based upon body weight is the body mass index (BMI) (kilograms body weight/meters of height^2). Classification of obesity by this method varies, depending on the referenced standards and definitions. The National Center for Health Statistics, the World Health Organization, and NHANES all use different cut-off points to derive the percentage of obese Americans. Although a universal cut-off point does not exist, a BMI ≥ 30.0 is a common indicator for obesity and a BMI of 25.0 to 29.9 defines overweight. The World Health Organization (WHO) defines obesity at a BMI of ≥ 25.0, arguably to be consistent with the scientific definition and avoid an "overweight category." Thus, by this definition of obesity, the WHO reports the prevalence of obesity to be 58.7% in America. According to NHANES III results, 59.4% of men have a BMI ≥ 25.0 as do 50.7% of women in America, an estimated total of 97.1 million Americans. However, data from NHANES III determined the prevalence of obesity in America, using a BMI of ≥ 27.8 for men and ≥ 27.3 for women. Thus, according to NHANES III calculations, only 33.4% of Americans are obese.

Obesity may also be classified according to degree of severity. Tables 12.5 and 12.6 illustrate the correlation between obesity classification and the risk of mortality associated with each. One of the primary inconsistencies, especially in North America, is the discrepancy between organizations and the BMI cut-off points published to define obesity. For example, the International Obesity Task Force uses identical BMI ranges for pre-obesity, class I, class II and class III obesity as presented on Table 12.5. However, what they classify as pre-obesity or overweight (BMI of 25.0 to 29.99) is considered grade I obesity by WHO (Table 12.6). WHO eliminates the pre-obesity/overweight class with their guidelines. NHANES III guidelines are more generous than the WHO and, as previously stated, define obesity at BMI of 27.8 for men and 27.3 for women.

Distribution of Adipose Tissue

Two patterns of obesity exist: *android* obesity and *gynoid* obesity. Android obesity is more associated with males, and excess fat stores accumulate in the torso area. This type of obesity is a public health concern because of its association with disease states such as hypertension, insulin resistance, breast cancer, stroke, diabetes, and cardiovascular disease. Gynoid obesity is more associated with females, and excess fat stores accumulate in the periphery, specifically hips and thighs. Peripheral fat stores seem to release free fatty acids more readily than do truncal fat stores. Throughout history, women have relied upon the accessibility of these fat stores during pregnancy and lactation.

The location of adipose tissue relative to other body tissue is also a health risk concern. Fat tissue located just beneath the skin tissue is defined as subcutaneous fat. Adipose tissue within muscle and associated with organ tissue is defined as visceral fat. To some extent, fat is located in both areas; however, visceral fat obesity, which is highly correlated with android obesity, is of a greater health concern. Because of its association with impaired glucose metabolism, dyslipidemia, and hypertension, increased accumulation of visceral fat is considered a risk factor for heart disease.

Distribution of adipose tissue can be assessed by calculating the waist-to-hip ratio. Waist-to-hip ratio represents the differentiation between the circumference of the waist at its narrowest point and circumference of the hips at their widest point, including the buttocks. Abdominal obesity and increased risk of heart disease are indicated by a larger ratio. Table 12.7 depicts the rating scale for health risks associated with waist-to-hip ratio measurements.

TABLE 12.7
Waist-to- Hip Ratio Ratings for
Increased Health Risk

Risk	Men	Women
Highest	>0.95	>0.85
Moderate	0.90–0.95	0.80–0.85
Lowest	<0.90	<0.80

The American Paradox

One might infer that the 8% increase in the prevalence of obesity during the last decade indicates that Americans are consuming more calories and that a greater proportion of these calories is derived from fat. However, according to a recent review of data from the NHANES studies and food consumption surveys, this may not the case. The most rapid rise in obesity occurred during a period in which caloric intake and fat intake were reported to have decreased. The only consistent factor during the past 20 years was the sedentary lifestyle led by nearly 60% of the population. It is estimated that only one-fifth of Americans consistently participate in regular exercise. These factors have suggested that increasing energy expenditure through regular exercise may be the most influential aspect in preventing and correcting obesity.

Genetic influences

Information gathered by studying twins, adoptees, and families suggest that genetics may account for as much as 80% of the variance in BMI. Furthermore, heredity may possibly account for as much as 40% of obesity-related factors such as inactivity, regional adipose tissue deposition (i.e., above the waist vs. below the waist), resting metabolic rate, rate of lipolysis, alterations in energy metabolism in response to overeating, food preferences, LPL activity, maximal insulin-stimulated lipogenesis, and various aspects of eating behavior.

Without doubt, the human genome favors the development of fat storage as a survival mechanism in comparison to energy expenditure. The accumulation of moderate energy stores allowed for extended periods of fasting between energy intake. However, the influence of modern environmental factors, such as the high availability of food and energy-dense foods in developed countries in combination with a reduction in activity, has lead to a maladaption of human genetic intentions. With the exception of single-gene disorders that directly result in obesity, such as Prader-Willi, Bardet Biedl, and Cohen syndromes, obesity is more likely the result of subtle alterations in the interactions of genetic and environmental factors, these alterations, of course, favoring the accumulation of energy stores.

With the recent advances in human gene cloning, researchers have examined the genetic influences of the body's regulatory mechanisms for storing fat. Mutations in the *ob* (obese) gene influence the degree of obesity through abnormal regulation of energy balance. In 1995, the expression of the *ob* gene in human adipose tissue was first demonstrated. Since 1950, five mutations have been discovered that may interfere with body regulation of energy and fat stores. Over the years, researchers theorized that energy balance in mammals is controlled in one of three different ways, all feedback loops. The *lipostasis* theory suggested that a product of fat metabolism circulates in the blood and signals the hypothalamus to regulate the amount of triglyceride stored in adipose tissue. The *glucostasis* theory suggested that plasma glucose is the substrate that signals the regulation mechanism of the hypothalamus. The final theory suggested that body temperature (dietary induced thermogenesis) is a signal to the hypothalamus to control energy intake. However, all of the postulated theories do not demonstrate regulation of food intake *in vivo*. The circulating factor now thought to primarily regulate the feedback mechanism to the hypothalamus is a product of the *ob* gene itself — *leptin*. In fact, various hormonal factors influenced by gene expression regulate appetite feedback controls, as will be described.

Regulation of Energy Intake, Storage, and Expenditure

With the exception of a limited amount of energy stored as glycogen, it has become very clear that fat is the means by which excessive energy is stored in the human body. Also, in accordance with the first law of thermodynamics which, when applied to humans, states that the amount of energy stored is equal to the amount in excess of that utilized for metabolic operations. Although subtle homeostatic mechanisms attempt to keep minimal imbalances close to zero, even a small imbalance over a protracted period of time can result in significant gains in body weight. For instance, a healthy, nonobese adult may ingest as much as 900,000 kcal during a year and not experience a change in body weight. However, in theory if energy intake exceeds expenditure by as little as 2% daily, this can result in an accumulation of approximately 2.3 kg (5 lb) of fat over a year's time. There are at least two assumptions being made here. First, it is assumed that 0.45 kg (1 lb) of fat uniformly contains 3500 kcal, and second, that an increase in energy storage results in only an expansion of adipocytes. With respect to the latter assumption, it is clear that not all of mass accumulated during an increase in body weight is actually triglyceride. Adipocyte hypertrophy, and perhaps hyperplasia, have to allow for an expansion of the plasma membrane and nonfat cellular components as well. Furthermore, increases in bone density, muscle, and associated connective tissue are enhanced to physically support a greater mass against the force of gravity. Thus, the average 9.1 kilogram of body weight increase experienced by Americans between the ages of 25 and 55 would only represent an average daily imbalance of 0.3% of kilocalories, and once nonfat gains are taken into consideration, the imbalance would become smaller still.

Contrary to scientific and medical hope, the physiology associated with feeding is complex and involves numerous factors. The hypothalamus, and more specifically local hypothalamic regions, is responsible for the eating and body weight regulation. These regions include the paraventricular nucleus (PVN) in the dorsomedial region, the arcuate (ARC), suprachiasmatic (SCN) and ventromedial nuclei (VMN), and medial eminence (ME) in the basomedial region, and the medial preoptic area (MPO) just anterior to the PVN. These regions form the primary components of a system that integrates information regarding body composition and energy intake and expenditure. Information via vagal and catecholaminergic impulses and hormonal factors such as CCK, leptin, glucocorticoids, and insulin are all received by the hypothalamus. The hypothalamus can then release peptide factors and initiate efferent signals that affect food intake and deposition. In addition, autonomic impulses influence energy expenditure and insulin release. Lesions within the ventromedial hypothalamus are known to result in hyperinsulinemia, hyperphagia, and hypometabolism.

Futile Cycle Systems

At least in animals, such as the rat, there are present metabolic futile cycling systems that regulate energy expenditure to allow for weight maintenance despite fluctuations in energy intake. Brown adipose tissue (BAT) is a specialized form of adipose tissue that is highly vascularized. This provides its darker color. It is innervated by the sympathetic nervous system. BAT is present in other animals and in human neonates. When stimulated, BAT becomes involved in thermogenesis via an uncoupling of the oxidative and phosphorylative activities of the electron transport chain. The mitochondrial protein involved is called *thermogenin*, or uncoupling protein, which allows electrons to move down their concentration gradient across the inner mitochondrial membrane without coupling the liberated energy with ATP generation. The net result is an increased flux of energy nutrients through oxidative pathways without the associated generation of ATP. Thus, there is a continuation of an ADP to ATP ratio that favors further oxidation and a continued generation of heat. Typically, the content of BAT in humans decreases with age and the significance of this futile cycle in adults is negligible. Therefore, BAT differences between obese and lean individuals are not necessarily a factor.

Another futile cycle-inducing factor is *uncoupling protein 2*, which has been identified in mice and up-regulated when they are fed diets rich in fat. Unlike the similar protein in BAT, this protein is believed to uncouple substrate oxidation from the generation of ATP in white adipose tissue and skeletal muscle. However, whether or not this gene is expressed in humans remains the topic of investigation.

Chemical Mediators of Energy Homeostasis

Insulin

Barring anomaly, the level of circulating insulin appears to be proportionate to volume of adipose tissue. In addition to the effect of insulin upon energy substrate metabolism, it also influences appetite and food intake. Insulin is able to cross the blood–brain barrier by way of a saturable transport system and may reduce feeding by inhibiting the expression of neuropeptide Y (NPY), enhancing the effects of cholecystokinin (CCK), and inhibiting neuronal norepinephrine reuptake. Thus, teleologically, the correlation between adiposity and plasma insulin levels may be an adaptive mechanism to support decreased caloric consumption. Interestingly, the influence of insulin upon NPY expression is not seen in the genetically obese Zucker (*fa/fa*) rats. Because the *fa* gene codes for the leptin receptor, it is likely that some of the effects of insulin upon reducing appetite are leptin mediated.

Cholecystokinin

Cholecystokinin, as discussed in Chapter 3, is secreted by mucosal cells of the proximal small intestine in response to the presence of food components. Postprandial circulating CCK levels are related to satiety and feeding in humans. There appear to be two types of CCK receptors (A and B) and both may be involved in regulating food intake. CCK-A receptors are present within the gastrointestinal system, while CCK-B receptors are present in the brain. By way of interaction with CCK-A receptors in the pylorus, CCK promotes contraction of the pyloric sphincter, which increases gastric distention. This initiates vagal afferents from the stomach that terminate in the nucleus of the solitary tract within the brain stem. Impulses are then transmitted to the parabrachial nucleus, which are then connected to the ventromedial hypothalamus, resulting in decreased food intake. This mechanism is diminished by vagotomy.

While CCK-B receptors are found in the brain, CCK circulating in the systemic circulation does not cross the blood–brain barrier. Therefore, it has been suggested that since the brain can also produce some CCK, afferent neural signals may result in the release of CCK in the cerebral spinal fluid which binds with CCK-B receptors and decreases feeding.

Neuro-Endocrine Influences

Leptin and Leptin Receptor-Related Obesity

In 1995, leptin, a protein chain of 167 amino acids, was discovered as a product of the obese (*ob*) gene. Its receptor was cloned shortly thereafter. The name "leptin" is derived from the Greek word "leptos" meaning thin. In obese hyperphagic homozygote *ob/ob* mice, two prominant mutations have been identified that either lead to a lack of mRNA expression or production of an ineffective product. Leptin has been shown to reduce food intake and increase energy expenditure in both obese and lean animals. In humans, adipose cells also synthesize and secrete this protein relative to the amount of body fat stores. Leptin receptors have been found in various body tissues, for example: the kidneys, liver, heart, skeletal muscle, hypothalamus, pancreas, and anterior pituitary. Leptin receptors found in the arcuate nucleus of the hypothalamus have led researchers to hypothesize that leptin may somehow regulate satiety. Leptin appears to also decrease NPY synthesis and release from that same region. In addition, leptin has been shown to increase corticotropin-releasing factor (CRF) expression and release from the hypothalamus.

It is possible that serum leptin levels are elevated in some obese subjects, due to the receptor's resistance to leptin's action. This is supported by another model of genetic obesity in mice. The so-called obese diabetic mouse has a mutation in the diabetes (*db*) gene. It is typical for these mice to have a ten-fold greater level of leptin in comparison to lean control mice. Further, as it has not been determined that there is an anomaly in the *ob* gene in these animals, a defect in the receptor is suspect at present. Some human cross-sectional studies have revealed that obese individuals may also have elevated levels of leptin. However, recent efforts have not determined a defect in the hypothalamic leptin receptor in these individuals. It is speculated that there may be leptin resistance, while the mechanism has not been resolved.

The presence of receptors in the pancreas has also led researchers to hypothesize that serum leptin may somehow regulate insulin metabolism; whether this is indeed the case is also unresolved. *In vitro* investigative efforts have demonstrated that leptin did not alter the uptake of glucose in the absence of insulin nor was the glucose sensitivity to insulin influenced by leptin. Other studies appear to strongly correlate a counterregulatory effect of leptin with insulin resistance.

Leptin may also play a role in energy substrate metabolism as there may very well be an inverse correlation between leptin and energy intake, fat intake, resting energy expenditure, carbohydrate oxidation, and respiratory quotient (RQ). Therefore, those resistant to leptin may encounter two metabolic obstacles: (1) the link between the CNS and appetite regulation is disturbed and (2) resting energy expenditure is decreased, facilitating weight gain. Also, there is evidence to suggest that leptin levels decrease in response to weight loss and remain decreased as long as the weight loss is maintained. Furthermore, increased levels of leptin have been found in normal weight and obese women when compared to their male counterparts, as well as female-patterned obesity (or peripheral fat stores). This is an expected finding, because females have a greater percentage of body fat mass.

Neuropeptide Y

Neuropeptide Y (NPY) is a peptide synthesized and secreted by the neurons of the arcuate nucleus of the hypothalamus, partially regulated by leptin. Increased activity of these neurons has been demonstrated in animal studies during periods of energy deficit, and therefore obesity may develop in response to abnormal increased production. NPY appears to stimulates food intake, especially carbohydrate sources. The paraventricular nucleus appears to be particularly sensitive to NPY. Interestingly, NPY is also synthesized and released by adrenal gland and sympathetic nerves into circulation, but, it does not cross the blood–brain barrier.

Feeding is stimulated when NPY is injected directly into the medial hypothalamus of satiated animals. Furthermore, there is a preference for carbohydrates. NPY seems to increase RQ while simultaneously being associated with a reduction in energy expenditure. It is believed that the NPY-induced increased utilization of carbohydrate allows for the production of more acetyl CoA for lipogenesis. NPY also seems to support fat storage in white adipose tissue, while decreasing BAT activity. Interestingly, NPY may have a stimulatory effect on the secretion of insulin, vasopressin, and leutinizing hormone.

Galanin

Galanin is another peptide factor whose concentration and receptor concentration are found in greater amounts in the hypothalamus. Galanin increases feeding and also increases the preference for carbohydrate and fat. While galanin does not appear to effect RQ it is associated with a reduction in energy expenditure since it inhibits sympathetic nervous system activity.

Two subclasses of receptors have been identified in rats, but only one in humans. Unlike leptin and NPY, plasma galanin concentrations and activity do not appear to be regulated by weight. It also has an inhibitory effect on insulin secretion, and synthesis of galanin is inhibited in response to increased serum insulin.

Obesity: Gender and Age

Gender

Obesity impacts women to a greater extent than men, apparently even during the Paleolithic period as discovered artifacts and sketches depicted only women as obese. Since the beginning of time, women have relied on fat stores more than men have for reproduction. In women, essential body fat may account for 12% of total body weight vs. 3% for men. Also, on average, storage fat accounts for a much greater percentage of total body weight for women versus men.

According to American-based NHANES III data (1988 to 1994), 24.9% of women are defined as obese (BMI ≥ 30) compared to 19.9% of men. This figure has increased slightly more than 8 percentage points (from 16.5%) since NHANES II data (1982 to 1984). Women exceeding ideal weight ranges (BMI ≥ 25) constitute 50.7% of American females. All age groups of women, as well as Americans as a whole, have demonstrated a rise in the prevalence of obesity. However, the age group 50 to 59 years old expresses the highest percentage of obesity as well as the greatest increase in the occurrence of obesity between NHANES II and NHANES III data.

For more than two thirds of American women, the struggle with weight gain begins in adulthood. Weight gain commonly occurs at the end of puberty or following menopause. Pregnancy may lead to obesity, as researchers have demonstrated that excessive weight gain is often maintained postpartum. Menopause is also a significant contributor to weight gain as fat mass increases due to estrogen losses. Decreased fat metabolism and increased sedentary lifestyle may explain the high rates of obesity in the 50- to 59-year-old cohort. Prevalence of obesity may decrease beyond these years, due to losses of lean body mass.

Obesity in Children

As much as 30% of obese adults were overweight as children. According to NHANES III data, 10.9% of American children and adolescents exceed optimal BMI levels with the current cut-off point at the 95th percentile. At the 85th percentile, 22% of American children are considered to be overweight. Children and adolescents are commonly measured using weight-for-height tables; however BMI is a more consistent and accurate predictor of adiposity. Recently, it has been suggested that the Ponderal index (PI) (weight/height^3) may be a better indicator of childhood obesity, and an easier method of establishing guidelines, since it is less affected by age and race.

As children reach puberty, the percentage of adipose tissue changes, but oppositely for males vs. females. As mentioned above, while the fat percentage decreases in males, female bodies begin to deposit fat in preparation for reproduction and lactation. Although a natural growth pattern for young girls, the increased fat deposition contradicts the "American ideal" and enhances preoccupation with body image. It has been estimated that as many as one third of American females ages 14 to 16 years attempted "extreme" diet method (i.e., use of laxatives, fasting, diuretics), and more than 75% have a desire to lose weight.

Although eager to lose weight, decreased physical activity is evident among today's youth. A recent study examining the activity levels of third and fourth graders found that most reported their leisure time focused around sedentary activities. Boys reported that playing video games (33%) was their primary leisure time activity, and girls reported doing homework (39%). In effort to increase physical activity among children, the Center for Disease Control in the U.S. has championed a set of guidelines for schools and community programs to encourage physical activity among children and an appreciation for it so that it becomes integrated into their lifestyle. This effort was extended as a means to prevent childhood and, in the long term, adulthood obesity.

Obesity and Related Diseases

Dyslipidemia

It is clear that excessive accumulation of body fat, especially deposited within the abdominal region, has an adverse effect upon blood lipids. The dyslipidemia associated with obesity is characterized by elevated fasting plasma triglycerides, decreased HDL-cholesterol, and moderate elevations in total cholesterol and LDL-cholesterol. It appears that fat deposition in the abdominal region presents more atherogenic lipid profiles than does excessive fat accumulation in the gluteofemoral region. Lifestyle modifications such as exercise and hypocaloric diet therapy are effective strategies not only for promoting weight loss and decreases in body fat percentage, but also provide favorable changes in plasma lipid profiles. Numerous research efforts have indicated that lower-fat diets are effective in reducing serum concentrations of total cholesterol and LDL-cholesterol, irrespective of calorie level. However, reductions in total cholesterol and LDL-cholesterol are typically accompanied by reductions in HDL-cholesterol as well. Therefore, exercise is an important component of a weight loss program to improve HDL-cholesterol levels.

Hypertension

As many as 50 million adult Americans present hypertension. Obesity is perhaps the most important controllable risk factor in the development and maintenance of hypertension. Obesity is correlated to not only with the risk of new onset hypertension but the severity of existing hypertension as well. The development of obesity-related hypertension is often coupled with the development of other heart disease risk factors such as dyslipidemia. Weight loss results in rapid reductions in blood pressure that are maintained with a stabilized lower body weight. More than 80% of obese adolescents have an elevated blood pressure and most have at least one cardiovascular disease risk factor. Much of the problem is related to the high-fat, high-saturated fat and cholesterol diet and reduced physical activity common to obese adolescents in comparison to nonobese adolescents.

The mechanisms involved in causing obesity-related hypertension are multifactorial. Potential factors involved in the pathogenesis of obesity-related hypertension can be separated into volume-related factors, neurohumoral factors, and others. Volume-related factors can include increased sodium sensitivity, increased renal sodium reabsorption, and increased plasma volume; meanwhile neurohumoral factors may include insulin resistance syndrome, increased aldosterone levels, increased renin levels, increased norepinephrine levels, and increased sympathetic activity. Outside of these two categories, obesity-related hypertension may result from left ventricular hypertrophy (independent of blood pressure) and sleep apnea.

Diabetes Mellitus

More than 16 million individuals in the U.S. alone have been diagnosed as afflicted with diabetes mellitus. Of these individuals, about 90% have type 2 diabetes mellitus, and of these individuals, as much as 80 to 90% are overweight or obese. The risk factor for the development of type 2 diabetes mellitus is relative to the severity and duration of the obesity and further amplified by the centralized deposition, especial visceral, of adiposity. Thus, managing obesity is a first-line therapy for diabetes mellitus. It is well established that even modest reductions in weight loss can reduce hyperglycemia in type 2 diabetes mellitus.

There are several physiological mechanisms involved in the improved glycemic control that results from weight loss. Perhaps one of the most clear effects is a reduction in hepatic glucose production. Hepatic glucose production is associated with the level of hyperglycemia in type 2 diabetes mellitus, and in fact, hepatic glucose production is one of the most significant supportive factors in hyperglycemia. Perhaps as significant as the reduction of hepatic glucose production is the return of insulin sensitivity in skeletal muscle and adipose tissue. Again, the severity of insulin resistance is directly related to the severity of the obesity, and, furthermore, there is evidence that a centralized visceral obesity is a correlate of insulin resistance in type 2 diabetes mellitus. This effect of reduced body weight and fat is paramount, because insulin resistance is at the hub of interrelated cardiovascular risk factors such as dyslipidemia, hypertension, and impaired fibrinolysis.

One of the cellular mechanisms involved in the improvement in insulin resistance induced by weight loss is improved tyrosine kinase activity of the transmembrane insulin receptor. Researchers have shown that tyrosine kinase activity in insulin-resistant type 2 diabetes mellitus is only half of that obese nondiabetic individuals, and that following significant weight loss of 13 kg, tyrosine kinase activity returned to normal. Interestingly, those individuals were still overweight and were still diagnosed with diabetes mellitus; however, insulin sensitivity had increased fourfold.

Diet Therapy

Very Low Calorie Diets

The very low calorie diet (VLCD) is a controversial treatment, but under supervision by a team of health care professionals it is accepted as a means to promote weight loss in the obese patient. VLCDs promote significant weight loss (maybe 1/3 to 1/2 lb/d) in the short term, but their long-term efficacy remains inconsistent. The American Dietetic Association (ADA) recommends that these diets only be implemented into an individual's weight loss strategy under certain conditions:

- The individual should exceed at least 30% of the ideal body weight or possess a minimum body mass index of 32.
- The individual should not suffer from the following contraindicated medical conditions: pregnancy or lactation, active cancer, hepatic disease, renal failure, active cardiac dysfunction, or severe psychological disturbances.
- Behavior modification training should be a component to the therapy, training the individual to commit to establishing new eating and life-style behaviors that will assist the maintenance of weight loss.
- The individual should be committed to taking the time to complete both the treatment and the maintenance components of a program.

Since caloric intake is kept to a minimum, typically 400 to 600 cal/d, the ADA also recommends carefully monitored vitamin and mineral supplementation to ensure adequate nutrient consumption. To prevent excess loss of lean body mass, protein intake should account for 0.8 to 1.0 g/kg body weight per day or a minimum of 70 g daily. Certain diet therapies provide greater amounts of protein, such as 1.2 to 1.5 g of protein per kilogram body weight per day, or up to 100 g/d. These diets are referred to as *protein-sparing modified fasts (PSMF)*. Carbohydrate intake on the VLCD can range from 50 to 70 g daily. Carbohydrate consumption on the PSMF is lower because of the excess protein, but enough to minimize ketosis at 45 to 50 g daily. If exercise is incorporated into the weight loss plan, the carbohydrate allotment may increase. Essential fatty acids are usually provided in the amount of 10 grams daily.

Macronutrient Distribution

The efficacy of reducing dietary fat to rectify obesity remains controversial. However, current recommendations from professional health organizations continue to advise that fat calories should be monitored to prevent and treat obesity. Since obesity is a result of excess energy intake relative to energy expenditure, dietary fat may be a contributor as an energy-dense macronutrient. Although epidemiological studies cannot determine a positive correlation between dietary fat and obesity under isoenergetic conditions, clinical studies continue to investigate this hypothesis due to inaccuracies in participants' recollections of food consumption and energy expenditure. Epidemiological studies have demonstrated a positive correlation between increased dietary fat and increased prevalence of obesity. Concern regarding compliance has arisen in this crusade to lower the dietary fat content. Researchers continue to conclude that satiety is not sacrificed if fat consumption is lowered. Carbohydrates contribute significantly to satiety and have been demonstrated to maintain weight loss.

Pharmacological Treatment of Obesity

The U.S. Food and Drug Administration (FDA) states that individuals with a BMI ≥ 30 or those with a BMI of 27 or greater with a co-morbid factor such as hypertension or type 2 diabetes mellitus are candidates for drug therapy. Drug therapy alone has not been found to be very successful. Furthermore the National Task Force on the Prevention and Treatment of Obesity has stated that:

Pharmacotherapy for obesity, when combined with appropriate behavioral approaches to change diet and physical activity, helps some obese patients lose weight and maintain weight loss for at least 1 year. There is little justification for the short-term use of anorexiant medications, but few studies have evaluated their safety and efficacy for more than 1 year. Until more data is available, pharmacotherapy cannot be recommended for routine use in obese individuals, although it may be helpful in carefully selected patients.

One of the more prevalent types of agents used for weight loss are amphetamine-like substances such as *phenteramine* (Fastin, Apipex-P). These substances prolong the activity of the catecholamines epinephrine and norepinephrine in the brain. This leads to appetite suppression. Moderate effectiveness is experienced with these agents; however, it is generally advised not to continue use beyond 12 weeks.

Sibutramine (Meridia) inhibits the reuptake of both norepinephrine and serotonin in neurons from synaptic gaps, thereby prolonging and increasing their activity. As a result appetite is reduced. The results of animal studies have been encouraging in that food intake was reduced and thermogenesis was increased. Human trials have demonstrated that as much as two thirds of patients treated with 15 mg daily experienced a reduction of at least 5% of their body weight, with as many as 39% losing greater than 10% of the body mass. As with most medications, side effects are commonly experienced. Dry mouth, constipation, increased blood pressure, tachycardia, and insomnia are among the side effects reported. There appears to be minimal risk of cardiopulmonary anomalies such as valvular aberrations or primary pulmonary hypertension (PPH).

The weight loss experienced with sibutramine typically results in favorable changes in a patient's lipid profile similar to that observed in weight loss without pharmacological assistance, so the improved lipid profile, decreased triglycerides, total cholesterol and LDL-cholesterol, and increased HDL-cholesterol are related more to the weight loss itself rather than the drug.

Orlistat (Xenical) is a gastrointestinal lipase inhibitor. Its actions are localized to the gut and it does not impact the CNS and decrease appetite. Orlistat, at a dose of 120 mg 3 times daily, can inhibit the absorption of as much as 30% of ingested fat. Clinical trials have demonstrated that more than half of patients receiving Orlistat lost more than 5% of their total body weight after 1 year, and 25% of the patients lost as much as 10% of their body weight. In conjunction with the weight loss, patients receiving Orlistat also demonstrated reductions in blood pressure and desirable changes in their lipid profiles. Interestingly, while the reduction in blood pressure experienced by those receiving Orlistat was dependent upon weight loss, the favorable changes in lipid profiles were independent of weight loss. While some gastrointestinal distress may be experienced with the use of Orlistat, there are not cardiovascular or CNS side effects.

Pharmaceuticals such as *fenfluramine* (Pondimin) and dexfenfluramine (Redux), which increase serotonin release in the brain were extremely popular in the early 1990s, especially in America. The combination of fenfluramine and phentermine was commonly called "fen-phen." However, the Food and Drug Administration (FDA) pulled these drugs from the market in 1996 after enough evidence was mounted demonstrating that their use was associated with PPH. Subsequently, the popularity of so-called "herbal fen-phen," a combination of ephedrine (ma huang) and St. John's Wort, was popularized. Ma huang utilization should include caution, as over 800 reports of illness and 38 deaths were reported in the U.S. alone. The pharmacological properties of ma huang's ephedrine alkaloids are undetermined at this time. Meanwhile, the FDA has recommended that daily doses not exceed 24 mg and the length of utilization not exceed 7 days.

Surgical Treatment

Gastroplasty, or stomach stapling, is at this time the most common surgical procedure for the treatment of severe obesity. Typically, gastroplasty is reserved for individuals who are at least 100% above ideal weight (BMI ≥ 45). Rows of stainless steel staples applied across the top of the gastric chamber reduce the size of stomach. Only a small opening, approximating 1 cm, is provided as an outlet to the distal stomach. The new stomach may have only a volume of 20 to 40 ml, and minimal amounts of foods resulting in gastric distention will produce satiety.

Liposuction

Liposuction involves the suctioning of adipose tissue through a tube inserted through a 1- to 2-cm incision. Successful recovery of skin turgor is more evident in younger individuals and those individuals with smaller amounts of fat removed. This procedure is not necessarily considered a weight reduction technique, but cosmetic surgery. Typically only about 2.5 kg or less of fat is removed during a single procedure.

Suggested Readings

Rosenbaum, M., Liebel, R.L., and Hirsch, J., Obesity, *N. Eng. J. Med.*, 337(6), 396, 1997.

Hirschberg, A.L., Hormonal regulation of appetite and food intake, *Ann. Med.*, 30, 7, 1998.

Leibowitz, S.F., Brain peptides and obesity: pharmacologic treatment, *Obes. Res.*, 3(4), 573S, 1995.

Flier, J.S., The adipocyte storage depot or node on the energy information superhighway?, *Cell*, 80, 15, 1995.

13

Nutrition and Activity

Exercise and exercise training demand the involvement of several organ systems, not only to support bouts of acute activity but also to adapt in response to training, thus providing an improvement of performance. The skeletal-muscular system, under the command of the motor cortex of the brain, provides the locomotion of the human body. The coordinated and concerted contraction of skeletal muscle cells pulls upon bones to provide movement. Contraction of skeletal muscle cells is powered by ATP which itself is generated from a mixture of carbohydrate, fat, and amino acids, which themselves can be derived from several endogenous storage facilities as well as from exogenous resources. The cardiovascular system provides transportation of hormones, nutrients, and oxygen to support an exercise bout, while also providing an avenue for waste removal from muscle (i.e., heat and CO_2). Hormones, such as epinephrine, glucagon, cortisol, and thyroid hormone and growth hormone, create a metabolic scenario supportive of activity and in conjunction with whole-body homeostasis. The exocrine activity of sweating allows for excessive heat removal and the renal system helps regulate fluid and electrolyte balance as well as blood pressure.

The increase in total energy expenditure (TEE) during and after exercise is mostly attributable to an increased metabolism within working muscles themselves. For example, stimulated quadriceps femoris muscle working at maximal exertion may increase its metabolism 300-fold. Furthermore, depending upon the intensity and duration of an exercise, along with the mass of skeletal muscle involved, TEE may be augmented by several hundred kilocalories to power postexercise recovery and adaptation mechanisms. While most of the increased energy expended during exercise is attributed to exercising muscle, metabolism within various supporting organs (i.e., heart, lungs) must also increase to support exercise as well.

Muscle and Fiber Types

The body contains over 215 pairs of skeletal muscle which approximates 40% of human mass. These muscle vary in their size, origin, and insertion. All skeletal muscle is comprised of numerous skeletal muscle cells (*myocytes* or *muscle fibers*), which range between 10 to 80 μm in diameter and generally extend the length of the muscle. Almost all muscle fibers are innervated by only one nerve fiber or motor neuron. The motor neuron terminates at the neuromuscular endplate or junction, typically located in the central region of the muscle fiber. Conversely, a single motor neuron can innervate several muscle fibers. A motor neuron plus all of the muscle fibers it innervates is called a *motor unit*. It is the nature of movement that generally defines the number of muscle fibers innervated by a single motor neuron. For example, motor units of extraocular muscle controlling the "fine movement" of the eyes have a fairly low 1:15 (motor neuron to muscle fiber) innervation ratio.

Oppositely, motor units associated with the gastrocnemius and tibialis anterior muscles of the legs, controlling "gross movement," have an innervation ratio as high as 1:2000.

Acetylcholine (Figure 13.1) is the neurotransmitter released by motor neurons into the synaptic gap at neuromuscular junctions, as depicted in Figure 1.21. Acetylcholine then elicits the "firing" of an action potential that radiates uniformly outward along the *sarcolemma* (plasma membrane) of the muscle fiber. Acetylcholine initiates the action potential by evoking the opening of acetylcholine-gated protein channels. The opening of specific channels allows sodium to traverse the sarcolemma from the extracellular fluid and depolarize the membrane to threshold.

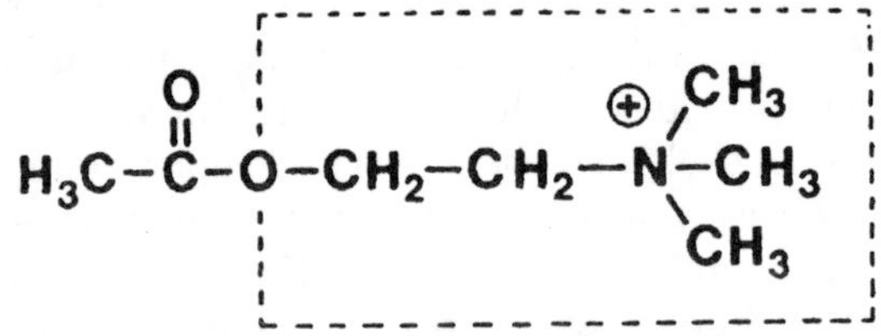

$$H_3C-\overset{\overset{\displaystyle O}{\|}}{C}-O-CH_2-CH_2-\overset{\oplus}{N}\overset{\displaystyle CH_3}{\underset{\displaystyle CH_3}{|}}-CH_3$$

FIGURE 13.1
Acetylcholine is the neurotransmitter at neuromuscular junctions. An ester bond connects acetic acid and choline (box).

Muscle fibers contain several unique features that are supportive of muscle contraction. First, muscle fibers are "excitable," as mentioned above. Quite simply, they can respond to a specific stimulus by initiating an action potential and then propagating the action potential along the sarcolemma. This sets in motion the activities that ultimately will allow for muscle fiber contraction as discussed below. Second, from a structural perspective, skeletal muscle fibers contain contractile fibrils, a relatively rich compartment of mitochondria, a specialized endoplasmic reticulum called the *sarcoplasmic reticulum*, a T-tubule system that invaginates the sarcolemma, and augmented glycogen and triglyceride stores. They also contain creatine phosphate, which helps maintain optimal levels of ATP in early activity (Figure 13.2).

Excited (stimulated) muscle cells are flooded with calcium primarily from the sarcoplasmic reticulum and to a lesser degree from the interstial space. Calcium evokes muscle fiber contraction by allowing sarcomeres to contract. Sarcomeres are the smallest contractile unit of muscle fibers and each one is a organization of overlapping thick (myosin) and thin (actin) filament (see Figures 1.22, 1.23, and 1.24). Sarcomeres are arranged in series (side by side), making up myofibrils. Actin filaments are attached at both ends of the sarcomeres and extend toward the center. Myosin is positioned between actin fibers in parallel. In a nonstimulated (resting or relaxed) state, binding sites for myosin upon actin fibrils are obscured by a long filamentous protein called tropomyosin. Also associated with actin and tropomyosin is a complex of proteins called troponins (C, T, I). When a muscle fiber is stimulated and the intracellular calcium concentration increases, calcium binds with the troponin complex and this interaction moves tropomyosin away from myosin binding sites on actin fibers (see Figure 1.25). Once myosin binds to actin, it pulls actin towards the center of the sarcomere, contributing to the shortening of the myofibril, which contributes to the shortening of the myofiber as a whole.

Human muscle fibers can be separated into two primary classes there are differentiated by their rate of tension development. Type I fibers take approximately 110 msec to

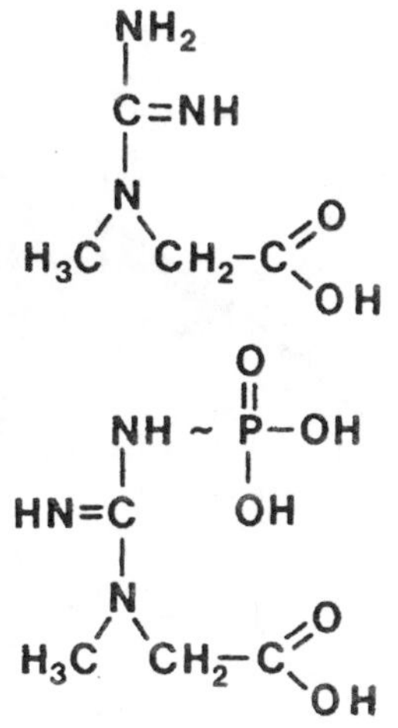

FIGURE 13.2
Creatine (top) and creatine phosphate (bottom).

generate peak tension, while type II fibers can generate peak tension in about 50 msec. With respect to this relative difference, type II fibers are also referred to as *fast-twitch* (FT) fibers and type I fibers are called *slow-twitch* (ST). The difference in the rate of tension development is largely attributed to the expression of different myosin ATPase isozymes. FT fibers produce the more rapid form of myosin ATPase in comparison to the ST fibers. Thus FT fibers can split ATP more rapidly and generate tension at a faster rate. There is only one recognized type of ST fiber, while there are three types of FT fibers (FT_a, FT_b, FT_c). On the average, most muscles contain about 50% ST fibers, 25% FT_a, 22 to 25% FT_b, and 1 to 3% FT_c. Furthermore, motor units will contain similar muscle fiber types. For example, if a certain motor unit innervates 100 muscle fibers then all 100 of the fibers will be of the same type.

When a muscle is stimulated, the percentage of contained muscle fibers actually contracting largely depends upon the force necessary to perform a specific movement. The motor cortex will call upon or *recruit* more and more motor units to contract a muscle, depending upon the perceived necessary force. It appears that there is a fixed order of recruitment of motor neurons and that the order may be associated with the size of motor neurons. For example, assuming a muscle contains 200 motor units, these units may be designated 1 through 200. Motor unit 1 would always be recruited first and 200 recruited last. Since ST twitch fibers tend to be innervated by smaller motor neurons, they will predominate those motor units recruited first (Figure 13.3). Thus for muscular movements requiring lesser amounts of force, slow twitch muscle fibers provide most of the contraction.

Beyond rate of tension development, FT and ST fibers can also be distinguished by other intracellular features, as well as some extracellular features. The ST fibers have a relatively higher blood flow capacity, greater capillary density, and a relatively greater mitochondrial and myoglobin content. The ST muscle fibers produce most of their ATP via the oxidation of energy substrates such as fatty acids and glycolysis-derived pyruvate. As long as blood flow is sufficient, ST fibers are generally resistant to fatigue. Contrarily, FT fibers are much more glycolytic and prone to early fatigue. While still inferior to ST muscle fibers in their oxidative capabilities, FT_a fibers will have more mitochondria, myoglobin, and associated capillarization than the other FT fibers.

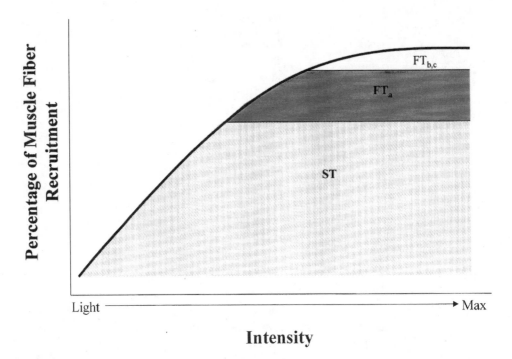

FIGURE 13.3
Recruitment of muscle fiber type based upon intensity.

Muscle Adaptations to Strength Training

Cellular hypertrophy, not hyperplasia, appears to be the primary cause of muscle enlargement produced by strength training. The increase in skeletal muscle mass developed during strength training is attributed to either comparable increases in cross-sectional area of both ST and FT muscle fibers or a disproportionate increase by FT fibers in relation to ST fibers. The hypertrophy is primarily the result of an augmentation of the number of myofibrils as the mitochondrial protein content tends to decrease. Thus, there is the suggestion that the endurance capacity of strength-trained muscle fibers decreases. However, strength-trained hypertrophied muscle appears to readily adapt to endurance cross-training and therefore compromised endurance performance can be avoided.

Muscle fiber hypertrophy is associated with gains in strength. However, increments in strength gain exceed what can be accounted for by increased muscle fiber area. For instance, strength training may result in a gain in force generation by 30 to 40% above what can be accounted for by muscle hypertrophy. In addition, the hypertrophic process associated with strength training may be complimented by a shift in myosin isoforms from the fast towards the slower isoform. Thus, training results in adaptive gene expression processes.

Muscle Adaptations to Endurance Exercise

The primary adaptations resulting from endurance training are metabolic and cardiovascular. Endurance training increases the ability of muscle cells to oxidize fatty acids and conserve carbohydrates. Mitochondrial protein, as well as oxidative activity of muscle homogenates, increases two-fold after endurance training, representing the potential for greater oxidative capacity. Furthermore, adaptation in the storage, transport, mobilization, and endogenous production of energy molecules occurs as a result of endurance training.

Endurance training elicits changes in muscle vasculature content as well as circulatory dynamics. The vascular density may increase 5 to 10% (capillary to muscle fiber) after endurance training. The augmentation in capillary density increases the opportunity for nutrient and gas exchange between blood and muscle fibers. At submaximal levels of exercise, blood flow to muscle may remain unchanged compared with flow prior to training. However, at higher intensities, active muscle blood flow is greater than at pretraining levels. Furthermore, endurance training results in a precise redistribution of blood flow within active muscle. The more oxidative portions of active muscle receive an increased portion of blood flow in comparison to more glycolytic regions. This occurs both in anticipation to and during an exercise bout.

The ability of muscle cells to adapt to endurance training by augmentation of the mitochondrial compartment is observed in both ST and FT fibers. Muscle mitochondrial content may reach a plateau or steady-state level after 4 to 5 weeks of training. In order for a muscle fiber to adapt, it must be recruited. Since ST fibers demonstrate an earlier recruitment, they will adapt at lower-intensity training levels, while both ST and FT fibers will adapt at higher intensities. Furthermore, training duration and the relationship between training intensity and duration influence adaptations in muscle fiber mitochondrial content. For instance, the greatest increase in mitochondrial content is observed at higher intensities, such as training bouts of 15 min at 100% VO_2max performed regularly for several weeks. Training at a level approximating 85% VO_2max for 30 min will result in similar mitochondrial increases as training at a level approximating 70% VO_2max for 90 min. At lower intensities, such as 50% VO_2max for 90 min, mitochondrial content increases linearly and plateaus at a level less than training at 70% VO_2max for the same length of time. Last, training at a level of about 40% VO_2max results in only minimal adaptation of mitochondrial content. Figures 13.4a and 13.4b present the effect of training on muscle fiber mitochondial content. However, it should be realized that many of the performance benefits associated with longer duration training sessions at lower intensity occur due to adaptations taking place outside muscle tissue, such as increased cardiovascular function, increased substrate availability, and other factors.

Oppositely, detraining or non-use of muscle reduces the level of trained muscle fiber mitochondria. In muscle fibers that have been trained to reach a steady state of mitochondrial content, it takes about 1 week to reduce the training gain by 50%. Furthermore, retraining of that muscle will allow a reestablishment of the steady-state mitochondrial content; however, the time involved will be longer than the detraining interval.

Hormonal Adaptation to Acute and Chronic Exercise

In a healthy human, exercise is the most powerful physiological perturbation. The endocrine system must adapt to not only the support the increased metabolic demands of exercising muscle but it must also maintain euglycemia and other aspects of homeostasis. The endocrine factors that are modified during a single bout of exercise, as well as those that potentially adapt as an effect of training, include catecholamines, insulin, glucagon, adrenocorticotropic hormone (ACTH), cortisol, growth hormone (GH), and endorphins.

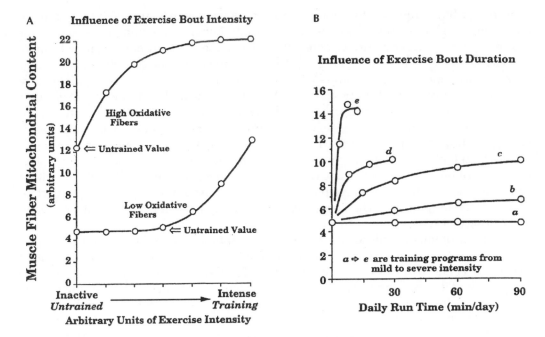

FIGURE 13.4
A. Effect of training and de-training upon muscle mitochondrial content. B. Influence of exercise intensity and duration upon muscle mitochondrial content.

These humoral factors greatly dictate energy nutrient metabolism during activity as well as during recovery and adaptation.

The circulatory concentration of epinephrine and norepinephrine increases during exercise proportiate to intensity and duration. However, catecholamine release from the adrenal glands during a bout of exercise can be dampened by elevated blood glucose levels. This is especially true for norepinephrine. For example, a fasting individual who has not consumed a carbohydrate-containing preevent meal will experience a greater catecholamine increase than an individual who consumed a carbohydrate-containing preevent meal or supplement. The presence of elevated concentrations of epinephrine will stimulate glycogen breakdown in hepatocytes and skeletal muscle cells as well as triglyceride breakdown in adipocytes and muscle fibers. Epinephrine appears to be a much more potent stimulator of muscle glycogenolysis and probably muscle fiber lypolysis than norepinephrine. Both epinephrine and norepinephrine are potent stimulators of lypolysis in adipocytes.

Circulating insulin levels decrease during exercise of higher intensities (>50% of VO_2max). This is largely attributed to α-adrenergic inhibition of pancreatic secretion of insulin. Glucagon secretion, on the other hand, does not seem to be influenced strongly by adrenergic activity. This makes circulatory glucose concentration the primary regulator of glucagon secretion during exercise. Circulatory levels of growth hormone and cortisol also increase during exercise, and levels are associated with intensity of exercise. While the exact mechanisms regulating the secretion of these hormones during exercise are unclear, it appears likely that there is central command.

Resting insulin levels appear to decrease as a result of endurance training. Whether or not endurance training alters resting levels of other hormones such as ACTH and cortisol has not been firmly established. While some researchers have found that training decreases resting levels of these hormones, others have reported that there is not a change.

While it is rather unclear as to whether endurance training reduces sympathetic activity at rest, it does seem that endurance training does not alter resting plasma epinephrine. However, there have been cross-sectional reports that resting plasma epinephrine levels of individuals engaged in endurance training for several years are higher than in untrained individuals. Conversely, even though catecholamine levels are increased during exercise relative to intensity levels, they appear to be reduced at a given work load as the result of endurance training. This effect begins after just a few days and may be complete after just a few weeks. It is likely that as muscle adapts, an individual's exercise intensity is actually decreased to achieve the same work load. However, there is evidence to suggest that with years of training the reduction in circulating catecholamine response at a given workload actually becomes similar to, or even greater than, untrained levels after years of hard endurance training. Other hormones such as ACTH, glucagon, and growth hormone have also been reported to decrease at a given work load after periods of training.

One possible explanation for the early hormonal adaptation to endurance training may be that as intramuscular glycogen and triglyceride stores increase and trained fibers become more oxidative, there is a decreased need for circulatory glucose by working muscle. Exercise training also appears to enhance insulin sensitivity. Thus, despite a reduction in the insulin response to a glucose load, glucose tolerance may be improved with training probably due to a significant increase in GLUT4.

Carbohydrate Metabolism and Exercise

Fuel sources for working muscle are derived from tissue-stores and circulating carbohydrate, fat, and amino acids. Furthermore, ingestion of energy nutrients such as glucose, glucose polymers, fructose, fat, and certain amino acids can indeed become an important source of fuel to support an exercise bout as well as preparation for and recovery from the bout. After accounting for water, the major mass of the human body can be viewed as an energy reserve, much of which is available to support physical activity. This notion is based upon the relatively higher contribution of adipose tissue triglyceride and skeletal muscle-based protein to human mass.

Carbohydrate stores are largely found in hepatocytes and muscle fibers. Typically hepatocytes attribute about 6 to 8% of the their mass and muscles about 1 to 2% of their mass to the glucose polymer, glycogen. Cumulatively, hepatic and skeletal muscle tissue contain about 100 and 300 to 400 g of carbohydrate, respectively. In addition, about 5 to 6 g of carbohydrate circulates freely in the blood in the form of glucose. Thus, the total carbohydrate reserve in a human may be about 500 g or about 2000 kcal.

Catabolism of hepatic glycogen stores and subsequent release of glucose into circulation is a principal euglycemic homeostatic mechanism. During exercise, this mechanism supports muscle activity by maintaining circulatory glucose delivery. In addition to glycogenolysis, hepatocytes also produce glucose from circulating substrates such as lactate, glycerol, and alanine and other amino acids. Muscle glycogen stores also provide a glucose source for the muscle cells in which they are stored. In fact, this energy source is extremely important during training and competition, especially as the intensity of the bout increases. Because muscle cells do not produce glucose 6-phosphatase the fate of glycogen-derived glucose 6-phosphate is to enter glycolysis within that cell.

Lactate produced by the glycolysis increases during exercise relative to intensity. Muscle tissue is the primary tissue responsible for the observed increased in circulating lactate

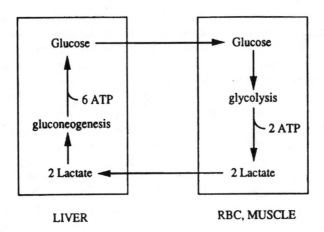

FIGURE 13.5
The Cori cycle.

concentration, while erythrocytes, liver, skin, and adipose tissue may also contribute to some degree. In skeletal muscle, lactate is mostly produced by FT fibers via glucose derived from glycogen stores. Lactate is able to diffuse into the extracellular fluid and potentially circulate to the liver, whereby it is oxidized back to pyruvate, a substrate for gluconeogenesis. The potential for the utilization of this new glucose molecule by skeletal muscle confers a cyclic concept. This cycle has been called the *Cori cycle* or lactic acid cycle (Figure 13.5). However, only a portion of the lactate produced by working skeletal muscle engages in the Cori cycle. Lactate is also available to other skeletal muscle fibers, especially those with greater oxidative capacity, such as ST fibers. In addition, cardiac muscle cells will utilize more and more lactate during exercise. However, the importance of the Cori cycle as a source of circulatory glucose during exercise cannot be overlooked. For instance, 3-mercaptopicolinic acid (MPA) inhibition of phosphenolpyruvate-carboxy kinase (PEPCK), a key gluconeogenic enzyme, can result in hypoglycemia, hyperlactacidemia, and increased muscle glycogenolysis in exercising rats.

In a situation somewhat similar to the Cori cycle, alanine is also involved in a cyclic operation. Alanine derived from the skeletal muscle amino acid pool, as well as from the catabolism of muscle protein and transamination reactions, can diffuse into the blood and circulate to the liver. Once inside hepatocytes, alanine can be converted to pyruvate via transamination and hence become a substrate for gluconeogenesis. This alanine-derived glucose can diffuse into the blood and circulate back to working muscle. This operation has sometimes been referred to as the alanine cycle or the glucose-alanine cycle (Figure 13.6).

During activity, carbohydrate as an energy substrate may come from glycogen stores in muscle cells themselves and circulating glucose. The concentration of glucose in the blood appears to be elevated during higher-intensity exercise in both trained and untrained individuals. Even exercise at 50% VO$_2$max resulted in a maintained increase in circulatory glucose. The rise in plasma glucose concentration is attributable to increased glucose production by the liver, accompanied by a decreased secretion of insulin. Not only will the reduced insulin level decrease glucose uptake in cells such as adipocytes, but it will also allow for greater gluconeogenesis in the liver and glycogenolysis in the liver and muscle. It has been speculated that a drop in circulating insulin levels is a mechanism for conserving blood glucose for obligate tissue such as the brain and RBCs since the increase in RQ reflects more glucose utilization than is created by hepatic glucose production. In the brain and RBCs, the uptake of glucose is concentration driven not insulin driven.

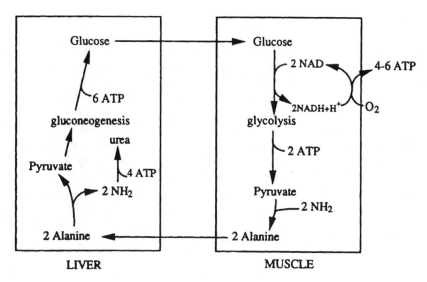

FIGURE 13.6
The alanine cycle.

At rest, skeletal muscle utilizes primarily fatty acids as an energy substrate; however, during exercise the utilization of carbohydrate increases and in relation to the intensity of exercise. Skeletal muscle along with whole body RQ increases during exercise, reflecting the increased carbohydrate utilization. While it is generally assumed that an increased utilization of carbohydrate by skeletal muscle cells was responsible for the increase in RQ, there have been suggestions that extramuscular tissue may actually utilize less carbohydrate during exercise.

Glucose entry into muscle cells is enhanced during exercise. As insulin levels are typically decreased during exercise, the enhanced glucose uptake can not necessarily be explained by insulin-induced translocation of GLUT4 transporters to the sarcolemma. However, some argument can be made that muscle cell contraction amplifies the influence of the insulin that is present. It is likely that the events or properties associated with muscle contraction allow for some insulin-independent glucose transport operation to occur.

The rate of catabolism of skeletal muscle glycogen appears to be related to the intensity of exercise as well as influenced by the duration of the activity. For example, exercising at low intensity for 2 h only reduces muscle glycogen levels by 20%, while higher intensity depletes pre-event stores. More definitively, exercise intensities approximating 50%, 75%, and 100% VO_2max produced glycogenolysis rates of 0.7, 1.4, and 3.4 mmol/kg/min, respectively. Catabolism of muscle glycogen stores is not merely limited to working muscle fibers. Epinephrine-stimulated glycogenolysis occurs in inactive muscle fibers within exercising muscle tissue as well. As epinephrine will not significantly enhance oxygen uptake and utilization in inactive muscle tissue it is not surprising that lactate release by inactive muscle tissue, is enhanced during exercise. Lactate is then available for working muscle cells, primarily ST fibers.

Recently some clarity was rendered to the question as to whether glycogen turnover existed during exercise. Without doubt there is a net breakdown of muscle glycogen during exercise; however, is it because breakdown simply occurs unopposed by synthesis or that breakdown is simply in excess of synthesis? Isotopic labeling of glucose and lactate allowing for the incorporation of the labels in glycogen stores in exercised rats allowed investigators to conclude that some glycogen synthesis occurred during exercise. Similar observations were made in human studies as well.

Clearly, muscle glycogen depletion is closely associated with muscular fatigue during prolonged exercise. However, the physiological mechanisms responsible are less clear. The resulting muscular fatigue can not simply be explained by the inability of other substrates such as blood glucose and FFA along with intramuscular FFA to sustain ATP levels. Individuals whose glycogen levels have been depleted prior to a bout of exercise are still able to engage in a reasonable exercise effort. It may be that the additional carbohydrate supplied by muscle glycogen may provide alternative functions supportive of muscle fiber activity. For instance, it may be important for the replacement of key Krebs cycle intermediates such as α-ketoglutarate and oxaloacetate lost during exercise.

Initial muscle glycogen stores are also very important in allowing an individual to sustain prolonged moderate-to-heavy exercise. For example, an initial glycogen content of 1.75 g/100 g of wet muscle may allow individuals to tolerate a standard workload of 114 min, whereas an initial glycogen content of 0.63 and 3.31 g/100 g wet muscle allow for 57 min and 167 min at that same workload.

Once glycogen is depleted, the timeframe for repletion is quite protracted. Only about 5% of muscle glycogen is replaced per hour. Thus, glycogen repletion may take place over the course of the next day after the exhaustive event. This is an important concept, especially for mutistage endurance athletes such as cyclists (i.e., Tour de France). These and other athletes should eat at least 100 g of carbohydrate within 15 to 30 min after completion of the event, followed by at least 100 g of carbohydrate every 2 to 4 h thereafter.

Pre-Event and Peri-Event Carbohydrate

The status of muscle glycogen stores at the onset of exercise is one of the most significant factors influencing duration of endurance performance. It is generally agreed that a preevent carbohydrate-containing meal will be very beneficial in maximizing those stores. However, the timing of the meal requires some consideration. A high-carbohydrate meal consumed 2½ to 5 h prior to an event will allow glycogen stores to be increased and perhaps maximized at the onset of exercise. Larger meals and/or those containing a significant fat content should be consumed closer to 4 h prior to the event. This recommendation is based upon their effect on the rate of clearance from the stomach and rate of absorption. Smaller meals consisting largely of carbohydrate can be consumed closer to the event (i.e., 1 to 2 h).

Triglyceride and Fatty Acid Metabolism and Exercise

Adipocyte triglyceride stores provide FFA as well as glycerol, both of which can be utilized during exercise. Hormone-sensitive lipase in adipocytes hydrolyzes the ester bonds between glycerol and fatty acids in triglyceride molecules. FFAs liberated from adipocytes are circulated to muscle loosely bound to albumin. Glycerol liberated from adipocytes dissolves into the blood and circulates to the liver, where it can be used for gluconeogenesis.

A 70-kg man with 15% body fat would theoretically have about 10,500 g of triglyceride contributing to his mass. This could be viewed as 94,500 kcal of potential energy. While not all of this triglyceride is readily available, much of it is, and allows an understanding of the great energy potential of stored triglyceride. Most of the triglyceride in the human body is stored in adipocytes, while a relatively minor portion of human body fat is found within muscle tissue. However, skeletal muscle triglyceride is extremely significant as an energy contributor for that tissue, especially during exercise.

Electron microscopy has revealed the presence of tiny triglyceride-rich droplets typically situated near mitochondria. Wet skeletal muscle may contain 7 to 25 μmol of triglyceride per gram of tissue and may collectively contain 150 to 200 g of triglyceride. Training enhances the concentration of lipid droplets in muscle fibers, especially ST fibers. Aerobic training can enhance the triglyceride content of ST fibers by as much as 1.8-fold after a couple months.

Circulating lipoproteins, primarily chylomicrons and VLDL, also provide a source of fatty acids to muscle. In fact, it is believed that fatty acids in the skeletal muscle triglyceride pool are derived primarily from circulating lipoproteins. Since skeletal muscle cells do not make fatty acids, the balance of fatty acids in muscle triglyceride pool is attributable to circulating FFA. Lipoprotein lipase (LPL) is the enzyme complex responsible for the translocation of lipoprotein fatty acids into muscle, which then can be esterified to glycerol to reform triglyceride.

As mentioned above, fatty acids hydrolyzed from adipocyte triglyceride can reenter circulation in the form of FFA. Hormone-sensitive lipase, which is under the stimulus of catabolic hormones such as epinephrine, glucagon, and cortisol, is the enzyme responsible for liberating fatty acids from the adipocyte triglyceride pool. Furthermore, a lipase enzyme has been isolated in muscle which has been suggested to be a molecular precursor to LPL. This enzyme appears to epinephrine to be stimulated in both skeletal and cardiac muscle and is responsible for liberating fatty acids from muscle fiber triglyceride.

Regardless of their source, FFA must first be activated within muscle cells prior to oxidation for energy. Acyl CoA is formed for longer-chain fatty acids in the cytosol, while shorter-chain fatty acids become activated within mitochondria. Once in the mitochondrial matrix, fatty acids undergo β-oxidation, producing NADH and $FADH_2$, which transfer electrons to the electron transport chain for ATP generation. In addition, the end product of most fatty acid oxidation, acetyl CoA, is available to the Krebs cycle. Thus, the energy potential of fatty acid oxidation is great. For instance, when all factors are considered, the oxidation of palmitate (16:0) yields 129 ATP molecules.

Chronic endurance training enhances the fatty acid oxidation potential of trained fibers. Major factors included in this adaptation include an increase in the number and size of mitochondria along with an accompanying enhancement in the activity of β-OH-acyl CoA-dehydrogenase, a principal enzyme in β-oxidation, as well as enzymes in the Krebs cycle. The increase in mitochondria is especially apparent in ST fibers. The increased capillarization allows for increased oxygen and nutrient delivery and a decrease in the diffusion distance for the exchange of substances between muscle fibers and circulation.

As mentioned above, training enhances the concentration of intramuscular triglyceride stores, especially ST fibers vs. FT fibers. For instance, training can produce a 5-fold greater triglyceride content in ST fibers than FT fibers. The fatty acids released from this intramuscular pool appear to be a very important energy source during exercise. Meanwhile, liberated glycerol diffuses into the blood. Muscle biopsies quantifying the actual muscle fiber triglyceride content, as well as measurement of blood glycerol content, are indicative of intramuscular triglyceride utilization during exercise. As discussed below, the relative contribution of intramuscular fat to total energy utilization in muscle fibers depends upon the intensity of the exercise as well as the duration. Intramuscular triglyceride may provide as much as half of the total fat used during an exercise bout and, as mentioned above, endurance training enhances the ability of muscle fibers to utilize intramuscular stores of triglyceride. For example, the contribution of intramuscular triglyceride-derived fatty acids to total fat utilized during a bout of exercise can increase from approximately 35 to 57% in a trained state.

As mentioned above, circulating triglycerides contained within lipoproteins are also a potential fatty acid source for working skeletal muscle, as suggested by reduced concentrations during prolonged exercise. For example, circulating triglycerides were determined to be 30% lower immediately following a 70-km cross-country ski race. Furthermore, plasma triglycerides may also remain lower than preevent levels for 24 to 48 h after the event. Shorter bouts of exercise do not elicit significant reductions in plasma triglyceride levels in normolipemic individuals and those who do not consume a preevent meal. However, reductions in plasma triglycerides can occur in hyperlipidemic individuals or normolipemic individuals who consume a fat-containing preevent meal. For example, a bout of exercise after a fat-containing meal can reduce circulatory triglycerides by 30 to 35% compared to individuals consuming the same meal but not exercising. Furthermore, the reduction in plasma triglycerides is accompanied by an increase in plasma FFA and glycerol.

Bouts of endurance exercise appear to increase the clearance rate of exogenous triglycerides and fasting triglyceride levels for several hours postevent. For example, during the first day following a marathon by elite runners, the clearance rate of diet-derived circulating triglycerides increased by 76% and fasting triglyceride levels were reduced by 26%. Furthermore, as an adaptation to endurance training, the clearance rate of exogenous triglycerides can generally increase by 25 to 50%. It seems that endurance training augments LPL activity in response to fat-containing diet, therefore allowing more fatty acids to be available for skeletal muscle oxidation. For example, 70% more fat was oxidized by elite cyclists after consuming a high-fat diet in comparison to consuming a low-fat diet. Skeletal muscle LPL activity has been shown to be increased 2- to 3-fold as a result of an exercise bout and remains elevated for several hours thereafter. This increased activity, which is most significant in ST fibers, not only allows for greater fatty acid utilization during activity but also repletion of triglyceride stores. Furthermore, endurance training results in higher resting LPL activity in trained muscle. This serves not only to assist in repletion but also to augment triglyceride stores.

Protein and Amino Acid Metabolism and Exercise

Skeletal muscle protein-derived amino acids are a potential energy source during exercise. Consuming protein and/or amino acid-rich foods or sport drinks during training or competition is not as common as carbohydrate-containing resources. Therefore, amino acids utilized during exercise are principally derived from skeletal muscle proteins and amino acid pools, with the latter only amounting to 0.5 to 1.0% of total body amino acids. A 70-kg man with about 40% skeletal muscle would have 12,000 to 13,000 g of body protein in skeletal muscle alone. This is based upon the notion that human skeletal muscle is approximately 22% protein by weight. However, it is generally believed that no more than 3 to 4% of the body's protein is engaged in turnover at any given time, thereby limited the availability of amino acids. While the utilization during weight-training is limited, amino acids typically supply only 5 to 10% of energy turnover during prolonged endurance exercise.

Exercise induces changes in muscle protein turnover. Protein turnover is determined by the balance between protein synthesis and degradation. An imbalance in turnover can be the result of contrasting directional fluctuations in both synthesis and degradation, or, perhaps, an augmentation of either while the other remains the same. Increases in the amino acid pool in both muscle fibers and the plasma are typical of exercise bouts and relative to exercise intensity and duration. However, the nature of the shift towards protein catabolism was not entirely clear. When looking at daily whole-body protein turnover, a positive nitrogen balance is typically associated with both resistance training and endurance training. For instance, 1 h submaximal daily training on bicycle ergometer resulted in positive daily protein turnover. However, since most of the information regarding protein turnover has suggested that protein synthesis decreases during exercise, there is likely an augmentation of protein synthesis after the completion of exercise. This is indeed the case.

Muscle tissue itself is somewhat limited in its ability to completely metabolize amino acids for energy. However, relative to hepatocytes, skeletal muscle cells demonstrate a greater capacity to metabolize the branch-chain amino acids (BCAA) via branch-chain α–keto acid dehydrogenase. Skeletal muscle cells are also able to synthesize glutamine via glutamine synthetase. During exercise of longer duration, alanine and glutamine are released from muscle into circulation in amounts greater than what can be accounted for by the muscle protein concentration of these amino acids. This demonstrates that amino acid metabolism is indeed occurring during exercise. The BCAA transaminase reaction which removes the amino group from valine, leucine, and isoleucine appears to have a relatively high K_m. Therefore, its operative activity is supply driven. It may be that most of the nitrogen used for the transamination of pyruvate in exercising muscle is derived from the BCAA. In conjunction, the availability of pyruvate is dramatically increased during exercise. Pyruvate is derived primarily from intracellular glycogen stores via glycolysis and BCAA which constitute approximately 20% of skeletal muscle protein mass. Pyruvate is available for transamination to alanine. In addition, the carbon skeletons derived from the BCAA are ultimately metabolized to succinyl CoA and acetyl CoA, which help fuel working muscle fibers.

During very brief duration of maximal-intensity exercise the contribution of muscle protein to the production of ATP is negligible. However, as exercise is prolonged or repeated, the catabolism of muscle protein and the contribution of muscle-derived amino acids to energy expenditure increases. This is largely due to associated increases in circulating cortisol. For instance, after 10 to 20 min of exercise at 70% VO_2max the concentration of alanine increases by 60% in muscle cells.

Coordinated Energy Metabolism During Exercise

ATP is the energy currency spent during muscular activity. The hydrolysis of ATP not only fuels muscle fiber contraction but also allows for relaxation, postexercise recovery, and adaptation. Skeletal muscle fibers are endowed with three principal ATP-regenerative mechanisms: (1) ATP-CP (creatine-phosphate) system, (2) anaerobic ATP generation, and (3) aerobic ATP production. The latter two mechanisms are discussed in greater detail in Chapter 11. While detailed discussion of creatine phosphate (Figure 13.2) is provided in Chapter 14, it deserves introduction here first. Certain cell types, chiefly muscle and brain, are endowed with an accessory means of rapid regeneration of ATP called creatine phosphate. Briefly, creatine phosphate is similar to adenosine triphosphate in that the phosphate bond has a high-energy potential. Hydrolysis of the phosphate bond liberates sufficient energy to reattach phosphate to ADP, reforming ATP.

Much of the investigation into integrated energy metabolism during exercise has focused upon aerobic-based or endurance activities such as cycling and running. Furthermore, it has been determined that while protein does contribute some to meeting the energy demands of working skeletal muscle and the human body as a whole, most of the attention has focused upon carbohydrate and fat. Here there are two energy resources for working skeletal muscle, (1) intracellular resources, which are muscle glycogen and triglyceride stores, and (2) extracellular resources, which are circulating glucose and fatty acids, the latter of which may be either independent or via lipoproteins. The contribution of these resources depends upon several factors such as level and duration of the activity, status of the preevent stores, and the level of training and cellular adaptation. For instance, the contribution of these sources at varying levels of intensity is depicted in Figure 13.7. At 25% of VO$_2$max, most of the energy utilized by skeletal muscle in fasting subjects is derived from plasma fatty acids and a little from muscle triglyceride stores. Very little of the energy expended by skeletal muscle is derived from glycogen or circulating glucose. However, as the intensity increases to 65% VO$_2$max, muscle glycogen becomes the predominant energy source followed by plasma fatty acids and muscle triglyceride. Plasma glucose continues to make a small contribution. As intensity is increased even further, to 85% VO$_2$max, muscle glycogen contributes well over half of the energy to working skeletal muscle, again followed by plasma fatty acids and muscle triglycerides. It is important to keep in mind that while the amount of plasma fatty acid utilized decreased when 65% VO$_2$max is compared to 25% VO$_2$max the total amount of fat oxidized was actually greater due to the increased contribution of muscle triglyceride and an increased energy expended by the muscle. The varying contribution of energy sources is largely controlled by hormones. For instance, as the intensity of an exercise bout increases so will the circulatory levels of epinephrine and norepinephrine as well as cortisol. These hormones promote skeletal muscle glycogenolysis and lipolysis.

As mentioned above, the contribution of muscle triglyceride to working skeletal muscle energy expenditure can indeed increase as a training effect (Figure 13.8). This is largely due to an increased storage and thus availability of muscle fatty acids as well as increases in oxidative enzymes involved in fatty acid breakdown. Whether or not the activity of muscle fiber lipase increases is still unclear, but it is likely. The increased ability to utilize fatty acids results in a reduced contribution of carbohydrate and a potential sparing of glycogen and prolongation of an activity.

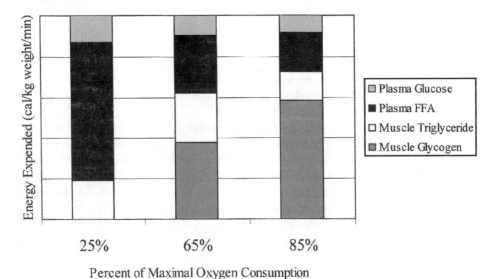

FIGURE 13.7
Relative contributions of energy substrates at differing levels of exercise intensity.

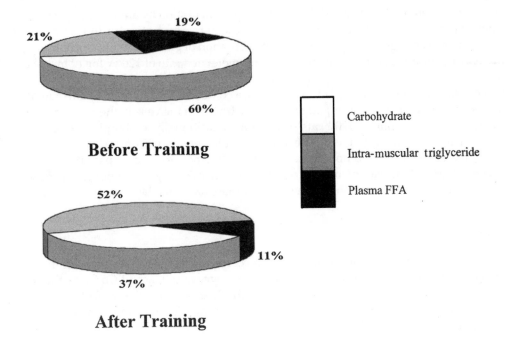

Before Training

After Training

Carbohydrate

Intra-muscular triglyceride

Plasma FFA

FIGURE 13.8
Substrates used during a bout of exercise as influenced by training.

Vitamins, Minerals, and Exercise

The influence of vitamin status upon exercise performance cannot be understated. As described in Chapter 8, several vitamins and minerals are directly involved in the metabolism of energy that fuels both exercise as well as recovery and adaptive processes. Other vitamins and minerals are involved in protein and connective tissue turnover, neurological function, erythrocyte production, and immune and antioxidant functions. Therefore an imbalance in one or more vitamins and/or minerals can markedly impact performance. Furthermore, it is likely that chronic training increases the daily requirement for some of these nutrients. This concept appears to be recognized by athletes. For instance, survey data suggest that 75% of college athletes believed that they needed more vitamins than nonathletes. Furthermore, vitamins are one of the most commonly consumed purported ergogenic aids. Conversely, the intake of some vitamins has been reported to be low for some athletes. These vitamins include B_6, A, C, and B_{12}. This section will attempt to address whether there are increased needs for vitamin during athletic training as well as the impact of supplementation.

Vitamin C

Ascorbic acid is involved in the synthesis and metabolism of several substances important to performance. These include the production of collagen, epinephrine, norepinephrine, carnitine, and the absorption of iron. Body pools of vitamin C become saturated with intakes between 100 to 200 mg/d. Vitamin C supplementation by athletes has been studied extensively. However, despite the wealth of research information in this area, no clear answers have emerged. For example, supplementation of either 1000 mg of vitamin C, or a placebo, by individuals training on a cycle ergometer at a rate of 120 W for 10 min showed that mechanical efficiency rose in the vitamin C group. Further, when athletes were provided 1000 mg of vitamin C for 2 weeks during a continuous training program of moderate intensity, testing on a bicycle ergometer demonstrated an increase in the physical working capacity at a heart rate of 170 beats per minute. Additionally, blood glucose levels were lowered and free fatty acid levels rose during supplementation. Contrarily, supplementing vitamin C at 300 mg/d did not appear to enhance the performance capabilities in a 50-km ski race. Furthermore, supplementation of vitamin C at 300 mg/d did not enhance the running and training time of identical twins in comparison to his/her unsupplemented mate.

Thiamin

Thiamin functions in humans primarily as a coenzyme in several reactions of the energy metabolic pathways, including the conversion of pyruvate to acetyl CoA and the conversion of α-ketoglutarate to succinyl CoA in the Krebs cycle. The RDA is based upon 0.5 mg/1000 kcal consumed, therefore the recommendation for athletes and individuals who train regularly is probably higher than sedentary individuals. Some of the information supporting a greater thiamin intake or supplementation for humans is derived from animal studies. For instance, when race horses were fed a diet supplemented with thiamin, they ran faster. Other studies have also resulted in positive data supporting thiamin as an ergogenic aid. However, human studies are lacking and it is difficult to truly evaluate thiamin in this manner.

Of the human studies performed, thiamin failed to improve arm holding and breath holding in swimmers receiving a thiamin supplement of 5.0 mg daily for a week prior to the test. Elsewhere it was determined that a higher intake of thiamin did not improve strength or alter blood measures (i.e., lactate, pyruvate, glucose). The effect of increased thiamin intake upon exercise performance is still unclear.

Vitamin B$_6$

Vitamin B$_6$ is involved in amino acid metabolism as well as glycogen metabolism in the liver. Preliminary investigations have determined that exercise may significantly alter vitamin B$_6$ metabolism and excretion. Supplemental vitamin B$_6$ at 51 mg daily for 6 months failed to improve endurance performance of trained swimmers. One research team did observe increases in growth hormone levels when vitamin B$_6$ was infused during a bout on a cycle ergometer. Thus, the true significance of vitamin B$_6$ upon exercise performance is also unclear. Activity may indeed increase needs for these individuals, due to altered protein metabolism. However, whether or not larger supplemental doses would increase performance is unknown.

Vitamin B$_{12}$

Vitamin B$_{12}$ supplementation is common among athletes. In fact, some athletes practice megadosing, while others receive vitamin B$_{12}$ injections prior to competition. Despite its widespread use as a purported ergogenic aid, very little scientific literature investigating its efficacy as an ergogenic aid exists. Out of the limited number of studies in this area there does not appear at this time to be any evidence to support its use as a supplement, providing dietary intake is adequate. For example, 10 μg of vitamin B_{12} did not improve leg and grip strength of children. In addition, adolescent males supplemented with 50 μg of vitamin B_{12} daily for 7 weeks showed no improvement in half-mile run times or Harvard Step-Test performances. Lastly, 31 healthy young males receiving vitamin B_{12} injections of 1 mg, 3 times a week, for 6 weeks showed no improvement in pull-ups, leg-lifts, hand-grip strength, standing broad jump, or coordination.

Folic Acid and Biotin

Very limited information is available with regard to folic acid and biotin supplementation and athletic performance. Therefore, it would be difficult to attempt to draw conclusions at this time.

Iron

It seems that long distance runners, especially women, may be at increased risk for reductions in blood hemoglobin concentration. This phenomenon is called *runner's anemia* and is believed to be the result of a few coinciding events. First, women average greater iron loses, in comparison to men, due to menstruation. Second, both men and women runners experience the destruction of RBCs due the high repetition and force of foot impact. Furthermore, many distance runners eat a diet wherein their iron is derived mostly from plant sources, which is less efficiently absorbed. Last, and perhaps less important, small amounts of iron can be lost in sweat. Thus, a distance runner should consider his/her iron status and possible need for a supplement.

Water and Exercise

Plasma volume tends to decrease during a bout of exercise. This is the consequence of increased sweating, as well as a redistribution of water from the vascular compartment to the interstitial spaces. The loss of water, via the former mechanism, during a bout of activity is enhanced by the intensity of the bout and the ambient temperature and humidity. It is estimated that plasma volume decreases by 2.4% for each 1% loss in body weight during the increased sweating associated with training or competition. About 0.58 kcal of heat can be removed from the human body in every ml of water or about 580 kcal/l of sweat.

The shift of water from the vascular to the interstitial space as a response to exercise is initiated within the first minute or so of exercise. This redistribution is attributed to increased blood pressure resulting in increased hydrostatic pressure in capillaries and increased oncotic pressure in the interstitial space. The movement of protein from the capillaries into the interstitial space is responsible for the increased osmotic (oncotic) pressure in that compartment.

Hypohydration of the plasma or hypovolemia can result in significant reductions in athletic performance. For instance, as little as a 2 to 3% loss in body weight, as water, can result in detectable decreases in performance. As more water is lost, the impact upon physiological function and athletic performance intensifies. For instance, every liter of water lost will increase heart rate by as much as 8 beats per minute and cardiac output to decline by about 1 l/ min. One of the most critical homeostatic functions that is compromised by a reduction in plasma volume is the ability to dissipate heat from the body. For every liter of water lost, core temperature can increase by 0.3°C. Increased core temperature, coupled with hampered blood flow to extremities for heat removal, can lead to heat exhaustion at losses of about 5% body weight as water. Furthermore, a 7% reduction can result in hallucinations and dehydration; beyond 9 to 10% is associated with heat stroke, coma and eventually death.

Hydration status prior to a training session or competition can result in significant decreases in performance. For example, when trained runners were dehydrated by 3% of their body weight via a diuretic, running speeds in 5,000- and 10,000-m races declined by 6 to 7%. It is generally recommended that individuals ingest about 500 ml of water or water-based fluid approximately 2 h prior to a bout of activity. This will allow for rehydration, if need be, and excretion of residual water. Furthermore, it has become apparent that ingestion of fluid within an hour of exercise may result in a slightly lower core body temperature and heart rate at the onset and during exercise. This is considered beneficial as it reduces some of the physiological stress associated with exercise.

During training sessions or competition of longer duration than usual, fluid intake becomes more critical with the duration of the effort. It is recommended that for efforts such as a 10,000 meter (10-km) run or longer 100 to 200 ml (3 to 6 oz) be consumed at every aid station. For shorter events, such as those that conclude within 1 h, pure water will provide the most benefit; however, during longer endurance events, water replacement may be most beneficial in the form of a sport drink composite.

Common Nutrition Practices Used in Attempts to Enhance Performance

Athletes continuously look for means to enhance their performance. While many practices certainly have merit, sadly there are many more that do not. Ergogenic practices include glycogen loading, bicarbonate loading, caffeine ingestion, and nutritional supplementation. Many of the more common supplements will be discussed in the ensuing chapter; however, glycogen loading, bicarbonate loading, sport drinks, caffeine, and protein will be discussed here.

Carbohydrate Supercompensation (Glycogen Loading)

Glycogen loading is a means of maximizing muscle glycogen stores and is used to enhance endurance performance of greater than 90 to 120 min. As muscular fatigue is closely associated with depletion of muscle glycogen stores, augmentation of these stores can theoretically allow an individual to perform at a moderate to higher intensity level for a longer period of time before exhaustion. The classic method of glycogen loading involved depleting muscle tissue of its glycogen over a 3-d period of exhaustive exercise and a low carbohydrate diet followed by 3-d of a very high carbohydrate diet (>90% of kilocalories). However, many participants experienced hypoglycemia, irritability, and fatigue during the first half of the protocol and demonstrated poor compliance during the latter half of the protocol.

A more modern approach to glycogen loading appears to be very tolerable and as effective in maximizing glycogen stores. This method entails a tapering down of exercise during the 6 days prior to an event, while at the same time increasing the carbohydrate portion of the diet. Carbohydrate is increased from approximately 350 g to 550 g or 70% of total kcal during the last 3 d. Such a high carbohydrate load typically comes from the consumption of pastas, rice, and breads. The use of synthetic low-residue, high-calorie, maltodextrin-rich drinks to partially substitute for some of the food volume has proven to be as effective in glycogen loading. Carbohydrate consumption culminates 3 to 4 h prior to competition in a preevent meal that contains at least 300 g of carbohydrate. Exercise activities that demonstrate benefit from glycogen loading may include: soccer, marathons, triathlons, ultramarathons, ultraendurance events, cross-country skiing, and long-distance swimming or cycling.

One potential problem associated with glycogen loading is the associated weight gain. For instance, augmenting glycogen stores from 15 g/kg to 40 g/kg in 20 kg of muscle would represent an increase in about 1 lb of glycogen and 3 lb of associated water. An individual must evaluate whether an increase in body weight might effect performance. For instance, a sprinter might find that the extra mass may reduce running speed.

Caffeine and Exercise Performance

Caffeine (1,3,7-trimethylxanthine) is considered illegal by the International Olympic Committee (IOC) when ingested in quantities that produce urinary levels greater than 12 µg/ml following competition. This makes caffeine a somewhat unique substance in that some ingestion during training and prior to an event is not illegal. In fact, most individuals consuming caffeinated beverages prior to an event will not approach the legal limitation following competition.

Caffeine is a methylxanthine compound and occurs naturally in plant sources such as coffee bean, tea leaf, kola nut, and cacao seed. The average cup of coffee contains 50 to 150 mg/cup of caffeine, while tea has about 50 mg/cup, and caffeinated cola drinks about 35 mg/12 oz. While chocolate contains some caffeine, most of its methylxanthine is derived from theobromine. The term "caffeine" will be used in a general sense in this discussion, but will also be inclusive of other methylxanthines (i.e., theobromine, theophylline).

After absorption, caffeine is taken up by most tissues in the body. However, the brain appears to most sensitive to caffeine. Wakefulness or sleep latency are probably two of the most common manifestations. At least some of the stimulatory effects of caffeine are related to its ability to inhibit phosphodiesterase, the enzyme that hydrolyzes the second messenger molecule cyclic monophosphate (cAMP). Thus, caffeine could prolong the influence of ligands utilizing cAMP as a second messenger (i.e., glucagon and epinephrine). However, it does seem that neural stimulation may actually occur prior to caffeine reaching its potency threshold. At this time there is evidence to suggest that caffeine may also inhibit the activity of chloride channels in neural membranes, resulting in stimulation of neuronal activity.

Caffeine also antagonizes adenosine, which can influence CNS activity. Adenosine can inhibit neural activity, both direct action at postsynaptic sites as well inhibiting presynaptic neurotransmitter release. Caffeine and adenosine are structurally similar and therefore will compete for the same binding sites. However, with time more adenosine receptors are produced and more and more caffeine must be consumed to effectively compete. It also appears that if caffeine ingestion is discontinued, the properties of adenosine interaction with receptors go unchallenged and can be more potent because of the augmentation in receptors. This probably accounts for a lot of the side effects associated with caffeine withdrawal. Last, some of the effect of caffeine may also be indirect. For example, caffeine ingestion typically is associated with increases in plasma epinephrine levels.

Theoretically caffeine has the potential to be an ergogenic aid for at least three reasons. First, caffeine and related substances have a CNS stimulatory effect. Second, caffeine may have direct action upon skeletal muscle and increase its performance. It has been speculated from *in vitro* efforts that caffeine may positively influence Ca^{2+} transport and key enzymes in metabolic pathways (i.e., glycogenolysis). Third, caffeine may increase the availability and thus the utilization of fatty acids and potentially decrease carbohydrate utilization and possibly prolong glycogen stores.

Early reports of caffeine-enhancing endurance exercise showed that ingesting 330 mg of caffeine 1 h prior to cycling at 80% VO_2max by trained individuals extended the time till exhaustion from 75 to 96 min. A subsequent study reported that 250 mg of caffeine was associated with an increased work performance of 20% in a 2-h period. Both of these studies suggested that fat utilization was augmented by approximately 30% as a result of caffeine ingestion, and a later study reported glycogen sparing with caffeine ingestion of 5 mg/kg body weight. These studies were indeed preliminary and somewhat suspect in their conclusions due to methodology. However, these preliminary reports did bring great attention to the potential ergogenicity of caffeine.

Over the ensuing decade or so, reports of the effectiveness of caffeine as an ergogenic aid were somewhat equivocal. However, improvements in investigative protocols have recently shed light upon the efficacy of this agent in enhancing athletic performance. Several studies using caffeine doses between 3 to 13 mg/kg in elite and recreationally trained athletes running or cycling at 80 to 90% VO_2max yielded improvements in performance between 20 to 50%. Doses between 3 to 6 mg/kg did not result in urinary caffeine levels exceeding the IOC acceptable limit, and side effects were uncommon. Meanwhile, at doses of 9 mg/kg and higher, a correspondingly higher number of athletes had urinary caffeine levels greater than IOC accepted levels and side effects such as dizziness, insomnia, headache, and gastrointestinal distress were reported. Caffeine ingestion was associated with an increase in plasma epinephrine (resting and exercise) and FFA at rest and during the first 15 min of exercise. It is of interest that the effect of caffeine on these plasma parameters was not significantly affected at the 3 mg/kg dose; however, performance was increased. Furthermore, it is of interest that caffeine ingestion did seem to "spare" muscle glycogen utilization. However, this effect was limited to the first 15 min of the exercise period.

Bicarbonate Loading

Bicarbonate (HCO_3^-) is a naturally occurring buffer in human extracellular fluid. It serves to assist in the neutralization of metabolic acids such as lactic acid and to maintain the optimal pH of the extracellular compartment.

$$HCO_3^- + H^+ \longleftrightarrow H_2CO_3 \longleftrightarrow H_2O + CO_2$$

Ingestion of sodium bicarbonate or similar alkaline salts by athletes is commonly called "bicarbonate loading" and is purported to assist performance by delaying the onset of fatigue related to increased lactic acid generation. Ingestion of sodium bicarbonate at a dosage of 0.3 g/kg body weight in 1 l of water may enhance performance in high-intensity exercise bouts of training or competition lasting 1 to 10 min (i.e., 400 to 3000-meter run/sprint). Bicarbonate loading may also assist in repeated bouts of high-intensity efforts.

The true efficacy of bicarbonate loading as an ergogenic aid is still unresolved. Currently it is not banned by athletic governing bodies. While at this time bicarbonate loading appears relatively safe, individuals may experience gastrointestinal discomfort such as abdominal pain and diarrhea.

Sport Drinks

Sport drinks were pioneered in the 1960s by scientists at the University of Florida, who developed a product designed to provide both fluids, energy, and electrolytes to athletes. The product became known as "Gatorade" named after "The Gators," the University of Florida football team, and a multimillion dollar industry was born. Today there are a number of sport drinks, as well as "spin-off" products (sport gels and bars) commercially available.

As discussed in detail in Chapter 7, sweat is primarily a composite of water and electrolytes. It is secreted by sweat glands in the skin, primarily under autonomic control as well as circulating catecholamines. Sweating is a primary mechanism for removing heat from the human body and, as mentioned above, 1 l of sweat allows for the removal of about 580 kcal of heat energy. Thus, if an activity, such as running for 2 h, generates about 850 to 900 kcal of heat, then theoretically as much as 1½ l of sweat may have evaporated from the skin surface. The primary electrolytes lost from the body in sweat are sodium and chloride. While their concentration in sweat is lower than in the plasma, more copious episodes of sweating will result in significant losses of these electrolytes over time. Also, the more copious the flow of sweat, the more concentrated the sweat solution will be with sodium and chloride, although one beneficial effect of training is a reduction in electrolyte loss during bouts of copious sweating, via more aggressive sweat gland tubule reabsorption. However, it should be realized that even under extreme sweating situations, the concentration of sodium and chloride is still but half that of the plasma. Thus, sweat is dilute compared to blood. Sport drinks provide an avenue of fluid replacement to help maintain blood volume during exercise as well as to provide the replacement of electrolytes lost in sweat. Sport drinks may include other ingredients such as potassium, phosphorus, chromium, calcium, magnesium, iron, caffeine, and certain vitamins.

The energy in sport drinks is provided largely in the form of carbohydrates such as glucose, sucrose, fructose, corn syrup, maltodextrins, and glucose polymers. These carbohydrates usually make up about 4 to 11% of the sport drink. Glucose and fructose are monosaccharides, whereas corn syrup is derived from corn starch, which has been partially digested to short, branching chains of glucose. Maltodextrin is just a few glucose molecules linked together with a branching point. Glucose polymers may just be short chains of glucose. Even Coca-Cola® can be regarded as a sports drink and is popular with many athletes. Coke's carbohydrate source is a high-fructose corn syrup — corn syrup with added fructose.

As mentioned previously, one of the principal factors involved in the onset of exhaustion or fatigue is a depletion of muscle glycogen stores. Glucose, via the carbohydrate source in sport drinks, is available to working muscle. While this carbohydrate may not truly slow the rate of glycogen depletion in muscle during a bout of exercise, the glucose can become a primary energy source late in an endurance event when glycogen stores are becoming exhausted. This may allow the continuation of an effort for a brief, yet competitively significant, period of time after glycogen exhaustion.

For a well-nourished and hydrated weight-training athlete there is probably not a need for a sport drink unless they are training for longer periods of time and/or sweating profusely. Furthermore, the activity should be of at least a moderate intensity, thereby causing glycogen utilization and sweating. It was mentioned above that activity performed at 25% VO_2max utilizes primarily fatty acids for energy and minimal amounts of muscle glycogen. Thus, need for a sport drink for endurance training/competition or several repeated events largely depends on the duration of exercise and its intensity and the environmental conditions. Generally, for single shorter events such as 5K runs and ½-h aerobic sessions, the use of a sport drink is probably not warranted physiologically. However, they may be beneficial psychologically (taste, caffeine) or for comfort (i.e., alleviation of dry mouth). For bouts lasting an hour or slightly longer, water replacement becomes more necessary. At this time, glycogen stores are not nearly depleted, and thus the need for the carbohydrate is not fully substantiated. Furthermore, because the electrolyte content of sweat is less than blood, electrolyte loss may not be detrimental to performance at this point. Eating after the event will replace these substances (glucose and electrolytes). Thus, for activities lasting up to 1 h it would be beneficial to drink some water prior to and during an event to help replace sweat water loss, while the need for electrolytes and carbohydrates is not critical at this point.

For more endurance sessions, such as those lasting up to or greater than 2 h, a sport drink becomes more appropriate. The water helps replace the water lost in sweat, while the carbohydrate helps fuel the athlete late in the event and, hopefully, prolong the onset of exhaustion. Also, the ingestion of electrolytes allows for the replacement of that which is lost in sweat. For an endurance athlete of typical size (68 kg), roughly 30 to 60 g of carbohydrate per hour will probably be sufficient. This amount can be met by ingesting a 4 to 8% carbohydrate-containing solution at about 625 to 1250 ml/h. For smaller or larger endurance athletes, recommendations can be obtained by dividing the body weight in kg by 68 and then multiplying the product by the fluid recommendations for the 68-kg athlete. For instance, recommendations for a 50-kg individual athlete is about 462 to 925 ml of a 4 to 8% carbohydrate-containing beverage per hour of exercise.

With regard to gastric emptying, a solution provided at a cooler temper (5 to 15°C) will traverse the pyloric sphincter more rapidly. Furthermore, the addition of carbohydrates and other solvents (electrolytes, etc.) will slow gastric emptying relative to the energy nutrient content. The primary reason seems to be due to the feedback mechanisms applied (i.e., CCK) as energy nutrients reach the duodenum. It was once thought that increasing the osmolarity of the solution, as related to the carbohydrate content, significantly slowed gastric emptying. However, this is not a significant factor when the carbohydrate concentration is lower (4 to 7%), but may be a factor if the carbohydrate concentration is increased. Furthermore, mild to moderate exercise intensity (up to 70% VO_2max) does not hinder gastric emptying, even when exercise lasts several hours.

Suggested Readings

Granjean, F., Hursh, L.M., Majure, W.C., and Hanley D.F., Nutrition knowledge and practices of college athletes, *Med. Sci. Sports Exercise*, 13, 82, 1981.

Dudley, G.A., Abraham, W.M., and Terjung, R.L., Influence of exercise intensity and duration on biochemical adaptations in skeletal muscle, *J. Appl. Phys.*, 53, 844, 1982.

Percy, E., Ergogenic aids in athletics, *Med. Sci. Sports Exercise*, 10, 298, 1978.

Hoogerwerf, A. and Hoitink, A.W., The influence of vitamin C administration on the mechanical efficiency of the human organism, *Int. Z. Angew. Physiol. Arbeitsphysiol.*, 20, 164, 1963.

Howard, H., Segesser, B., and Korner, W.F., Ascorbic acid and athletic performance, *Ann. N.Y. Acad. Sci.*, 258, 458, 1975.

Jetzler, A. and Haffler, C., Vitamin C-bedarf bei einmaligar sportlicher dauerleistung, Wien. *Med. Wochenschr.*, 89, 332, 1939.

Vinarickij, R., An attempt to improve the efficiency of medium distance runners by large doses of vitamin B1, B2 and C, *Scripta Med.*, 27, 1, 1954.

Wetzel, N.C., Hopwood, H.H., Kuechle, M.E., and Grueninger, R.M., Growth failure in school children: further studies of vitamin B_{12} dietary supplements, *J. Clin. Nutr.*, 1, 17,1952.

Montoye, H.J., Spata, P.J., Pinckney, V., and Barron, L., Effects of vitamin B_{12} supplementation on physical fitness and growth of young boys, *J. Appl. Physiol.*, 7, 589, 1955.

Tin-May-Than, Ma-Win-May, Khin-Sann-Aung, and Mya-Tu, M., The effect of vitamin B_{12} on physical performance capacity, *Br. J. Nutr.*, 40, 269, 1978.

Bouchard C., Shepard, R.J., Stephans, T., Eds., *Physical Activity, Fitness, and Health:* International proceedings and consensus statement, Human Kinetics Publishers, Champaign, IL, 1994.

Wolinsky, I. and Hickson, J.F., *Nutrition in Exercise and Sport,* 2nd ed., CRC Press, Boca Raton, FL, 1994.

14

Nutrition Supplements and Nutraceuticals

It is difficult to say when the first nutrition supplements were utilized. For example, it is legend that in 4000 B.C. the Persian physician Melampus provided iron supplements to Persian sailors to compensate for hemorrhagic losses resulting from battle wounds. While the origin of nutrition supplementation is somewhat vague, the enthusiasm for their application in modern times goes without question. Approximately half of the American population utilizes one or more nutrition supplements daily. This includes 48% of children ages 3 to 5 years of age, 35.8% of Americans ages 20 to 29, 46.2% for ages 50 to 59, and 50.6% for those 80 years older. The nutrition supplement industry has never enjoyed greater sales and has developed into a multibillion dollar industry worldwide. In the U.S. alone, $8.2 billion were spent on nutrition supplements in 1995. More globally, the world as a whole spent $28.2 billion on supplements that year. Thus, the U.S. accounted for about 30% of total supplement sales that year. For sport supplements alone, Americans spent $800 million in 1995, while all of Europe spent only 400 million. Sport supplements are used to improve athletic performance, either training- or competition-related. Their purported benefits include increased power and strength, increased endurance, increased muscularity, and improvement in certain psychological aspects that are relative to athletic performance.

Along a similar line to performance-enhancing supplements, the recognition and consumption of various plants and plant extracts or animal foods to prevent or treat various disease states dates back many centuries as well. For example, in ancient Egypt, Pliny stated that eating cabbage and onions cured over 100 different diseases. In addition, green tea has been consumed in China for over 40 centuries for its purported medicinal properties.

With some exceptions, nutrition supplements are preparations of one or more plant, animal, or microbial components. They are either isolated or extracted from a resource or they are created synthetically in laboratories. Typically, supplements are substances, or analogs of substances, commonly found in foods and/or made in the human body such as amino acids, omega-3 fatty acids, lecithin, creatine, carnitine, and ascorbic acid. Also, supplements can include extractions from more exotic life forms such as shark cartilage, ginseng, Brewer's yeast, and ginkgo. They are generally marketed to individuals trying to fill nutrient voids in their existing diet, trying to enhance athletic or physiological performance, and/or trying to prevent or treat disease and enhance vitality. In the U.S., nutrition supplements are not strongly regulated by the Food and Drug Administration. Therefore, the labels of nutrition supplements can certainly mislead the consumer, while the dosage recommended by the manufacturer may not be appropriate.

As alluded to earlier, the consumption of natural entities for their purported medicinal properties has been recorded throughout history. These natural entities are ingested as components of traditional foods such as broccoli, fish, citrus fruits, or whole grains or somewhat exotic foods such as teas made from bark extracts or herbs. Therefore, while the field of nutraceuticals along with the name itself seems pretty new, food therapy has been around for millennia. Perhaps the simplest definition of a nutraceutical would be a component of foods or other ingestible substances that has potentially beneficial effects on human health and function. In general, they are not viewed as essential nutrients, but as beneficial nutrient. Nutraceuticals include plant-derived factors (phytochemicals or medicinal botanicals) and factors derived from animal sources (i.e., fish oils) as well as potentially microbial sources. The activities of nutraceuticals are broad and include antioxidation, enzyme system activation or inhibition, hormone activity modifiers (i.e., agonists and antagonistics), or perhaps a substances serving as precursors for one or more beneficial molecules. While essential vitamins and minerals have been argued to be nutraceutical substances, their essentiality disallows their inclusion.

Some of the more recognized nutraceuticals include flavonoids, carotenoids, allyl compounds, protease inhibitors, saponins, licorice, fibers, and omega-3 and omega-6 polyunsaturated fatty acids. Many food sources provide several nutraceuticals. For example, citrus fruits may contain in excess of 170 different phytochemical compounds. Soy contains phytates, protease inhibitors, saponins, and flavonoids. Whole grains contain flavonoids, tocotrienols, ellagic acid, fibers, and saponins. Fish, especially cold-water fish, can provide docosahexaenoic acid (DHA) and eicosapentaenoic acid (EPA).

A primary difference in the definition between nutraceuticals and nutritional supplements is that nutraceuticals are ingested in the form of intact foods such as fruits, vegetables, fish, fibers, soy products, and teas. On the contrary, nutrition supplements are mostly substance isolates ingested either independently or in a formula with other supplemented substances. As the list of nutraceuticals and nutrition supplements is indeed immense, this chapter will only serve to discuss several of the more prominent ones at present.

Herbs

Several herbs with known pharmacological potential are available as nutritional supplements. Because of this, the Committee of the American Herbal Products Association (AHPA) has established a classification system applicable to the use of herbs. This classification is based on the associated data for the specific herb in isolation and in the normal quantity consumed for a therapeutic effect. The classification will be listed below for several herbs.

Class 1. Herbs which can be safely consumed when used appropriately.

Class 2. Herbs to which the following restrictions apply:

    a. classified for external use only.

    b. not to be used during pregnancy.

    c. not to be used while nursing.

    d. other restrictions as noted.

Class 3. This class is for those herbs that should be used under the recommendation and supervision of an expert. The labeling of the product must also including proper dosage, contraindications, potential adverse effects, and other information related to safe use of the supplement.

Class 4. Data for this class of herbs are insufficient.

Arginine

Since the recognition that the amino acid arginine has the potential to function as a secretagogue for human growth hormone, its use as a supplement by athletes and other populations has become common. Under basal conditions, ingestion of gram doses of arginine, either independently or in combination with other secretagogues (i.e., lysine, ornithine) can elevate growth hormone levels. However, this effect has not always been reproducible in clinical investigations.

It was also reported that ingestion of arginine (1.5 g in combination with 1.5 g of lysine immediately prior to resistance exercise) failed to raise growth hormone levels above what is typically produced by resistance training alone. Interestingly, one investigation revealed that ingestion of glutamate–arginine actually diminished the elevated growth hormone response to exercise in comparison to a placebo group. Therefore, arginine supplementation may only have practical potential for elevating growth hormone levels under basal situations. Furthermore, it is not clear if any elevations in growth hormone by supplementation of arginine would lead to greater hypertrophic gains than that typically experienced and impact important growth-associated factors such as insulin-like growth factor 1 (IGF-I).

The secretogogue properties of arginine appear to be age related. Elderly individuals may not respond to oral arginine as young people do. Thus, arginine ingestion may not be a viable therapeutic avenue to augment the waning growth hormone and IGF-I levels characteristic of advanced age.

Very little work has been performed in the area of performance capacity and l-arginine supplementation. However, there is evidence that l-arginine supplementation can improve exercise capacity in patients with stable angina pectoris. Researchers have suggested that the positive influence of aginine is related to an improvement in the efficiency of the arginine/nitric oxide system. Arginine is a precursor for nitric acid, which is a potent local vasodilator. Thus arginine supplementation may have improved myocardial perfusion in these individuals by serving as a precursor for nitric oxide.

The mechanism involved for stimulatory influence of arginine upon the anterior pituitary gland remains unclear at present. However, it does seem that arginine and certain other amino acids may exert at least some of their influence directly by interacting with specific cells of the anterior pituitary gland (rat) and evoking an increase in cytosolic calcium concentration. The investigators reported that about 40% of anterior pituitary gland cells were responsive in this manner.

Aspartic Acid

The nonessential amino acid, aspartic acid, is involved in the formation of urea in the liver. Blood ammonia concentrations are known to increase as a result of higher intensity, longer duration training, and this situation is associated with fatigue. Therefore, supplementation of aspartic acid was theorized to potentially increase urea synthesis and alleviate ammonia-related premature fatigue. Very few studies have been performed in this area. The conclusions of one study stated that there was no difference in exhaustion time in young trained males exercising at 75% VO_2max. Other investigators provided 7.2 grams of potassium, magnesium aspartate during a 24-hour period prior to a bout of treadmill walking lasting 90 minutes at 62% VO₂max. They reported no apparent benefit to supplementation as assessed by cardiorespiratory, hematological, and metabolic parameters. Another investigation reported that aspartic acid supplementation also failed to reduce plasma ammonia concentrations during and after high-intensity resistance training. Researchers also reported that supplementation of potassium and magnesium salts of aspartic acid failed to improve metabolic parameters (ATP, phosphocreatine, lactate, and L-aspartate) or force generation in electrically stimulated quadriceps of rats, nor were there changes in submaximal endurance time in humans. On the contrary, some investigators have reported positive benefits associated with aspartic acid supplementation at a higher dosage. One group of investigators reported that time to exhaustion during an endurance bout was extended by 40%.

Boron

Boron supplementation is often purported to increase testosterone release. One study utilizing postmenopausal women taking 3 mg of boron per day while following a low magnesium diet did demonstrate elevations in serum estrogen and testosterone. However, boron supplementation of 2.5 mg daily for 7 weeks in nonsteroid-using male body builders failed to increase lean body mass, strength, or circulating testosterone levels. Other investigations also failed to demonstrate changes in circulating hormone levels as well.

Carnitine

Carnitine (β-hydroxy-γ-trimethylammonium butyrate) is widely distributed in the human body but is particularly concentrated in muscle. It is synthesized from lysine and methionine in the liver and kidneys. Carnitine transport mechanisms are necessary for the translocation of longer-chain-length fatty acids from the cytosol to the mitochondrial matrix, the site of fatty acid oxidation. Shorter-chain-length fatty acids are able to diffuse into the mitochondrial matrix without assistance.

The first step in the translocation of long-chain activated fatty acids from the cytosol to the mitochondrial matrix is conversion of long-chain acyl CoAs to acylcarnitine. Carnitine palmitoyl transferase I (CPTI), present in the outer mitochondrial membrane, performs this task. Acylcarnitine is then able to penetrate the inner mitochondrial membrane by moving through the carnitine acylcarnitine translocase antiport system (Figure 11.12). One acylcarnitine molecule enters the matrix in exchange for one free carnitine molecule moving from the matrix to the mitochondrial intermembrane space. Once inside the matrix, acyl CoA molecules are liberated from carnitine by another carnitine-dependent enzyme complex called carnitine palmitoyl transferase II (CPT II). Acyl CoA molecules are then available for oxidation.

Once the role of carnitine was established, supplementation soon followed with the hopes that it could be an ergogenic aid or even increase normal fat utilization, allowing for weight loss in nonexercising individuals. However, after a couple of decades researchers have generally failed to demonstrate that carnitine supplementation is indeed useful in either of these tasks. In a recent review it was stated that the literature suggests that carnitine supplementation does not enhance fatty acid utilization or spare glycogen, nor does it postpone the onset of fatigue. Furthermore, it was stated that carnitine supplementation does not enhance fat or weight loss nor will it improve exercising VO_2max. In conjunction, carnitine does not appear to enhance recovery from exhaustive efforts as well.

While most of the literature has failed to find a positive effect of carnitine supplementation and athletic performance, there is some evidence that carnitine administration preexercise may have some ergogenic merit. In a study with moderately trained young men, who ingested 2 g of carnitine prior to exercising maximally on a cycle ergometer, the researchers reported that there was increase in both maximal oxygen uptake and power output.

Carnitine supplementation may be beneficial in patients with end-stage renal disease (ESRD), peripheral artery disease (PAD), and perhaps other clinical situations. Endogenous carnitine stasis is negatively impacted by ESRD, as synthesis is decreased and carnitine is lost during dialysis. Individuals on dialysis typically demonstrate decreased skeletal muscle carnitine levels, relative to length of time on dialysis, as well as decreased exercise performance. It has been reported that carnitine supplementation in these individuals is effective in increasing total muscle carnitine levels and increasing VO_2max. Propionyl-L-carnitine (PLC) has been reported to be more effective in improving muscle metabolism in individuals with PAD.

Interestingly, supplementation of carnitine at 90 mg/kg body weight, along with asparagine and aspartate, led to utrastructural anomalies in the soleus muscle of swimming-trained rats. The anomalies include focal degeneration of myofibrils and Z-line streaming and disruption along with mitochondrial disorganization and disruption.

Carotenoids

The carotenoids are perhaps the recognizable form of coloring pigment in plants. As discussed in Chapter 2, most naturally occurring carotenoids are tetraterpenoids. They have a basic structure of 40 carbons with unique modifications. The carotenoid family includes molecules such as α-,β-, and γ-carotene, lutein, zeaxanthin, lycopene, cryptoxanthin, vioaxanthin, bixin (24-carbon food additive), crocin, and persicaxanthin. There may be as many as 450 different carotenoids. Recently, it was reported that supplementation of β-carotene (50 mg/d), the most popular carotenoid supplement, for as long as 5 years did not alter the levels of lycopene, lutein/zeaxanthin, retinol, or α-tocopherol while concomitantly increasing α-carotene and β-carotene levels.

Numerous epidemiological studies have reported an inverse relationship between carotenoid intake and the incidence of heart disease and certain cancers. It is speculated that some of the protection is related to free-radical scavenging. β-Carotene is the predominant carotenoid in the human diet and is the form commonly used in supplements. However, several investigations have failed to demonstrate that β-carotene supplementation is indeed beneficial in preventing or treating heart disease and cancer. In fact, in American and Finnish investigations β-carotene supplementation actually increased the incidence of lung cancer in cigarette smokers. Furthermore, several reviews have stated that β-carotene supplementation is not a recommended protocol for the prevention of heart disease and cancer. They speculate that it is likely that fruits and vegetables contain other factors that

are necessary in combination with or supportive of β-carotene for its prophylactic properties. Thus, it is best to obtain carotenoids from a diet rich in fruits and vegetables rather
than supplements.

Chondroitin Sulfate

Chondroitin sulfate belongs to a class of molecules called glycosaminoglycans (mucopolysaccharides). These molecules consist of chains of complex carbohydrates characterized by their content of amino groups and uronic acids. Upon association with protein
molecules, the resulting compounds are called proteoglycans. Chondroitin sulfate is in
essence a disaccharide composed of β-glucuronic acid bonded to N-acetylgalactosamine
sulfate. The sulfate of N-acetylgalactosamine sulfate is found either at the 4th or 6th carbon.

Chondroitin sulfate is an integral portion of cartilagenous connective tissue such as bone,
tendons, and ligaments, as it associates with structural elements. It appears to be able to
associate with a relatively large number of water molecules, thereby providing cushioning
and lubrication to cartilage connective tissue structures. Chondroitin sulfate is supplemented by many individuals with joint concerns. Supplemental doses have been purported to benefit individuals with osteoarthritis (OA) by enhancing the activity of
chrondrocytes. More investigation is needed in this area.

Chromium

Chromium, deemed essential for life, is a trace mineral found in a variety of foods such as
brewer's yeast, American cheese, mushrooms, and wheat germ. Although no RDA has
been determined, an ESSADDI of 50 to 200 µg has been established by the Food and Nutrition Board.

Chromium supplementation has been purported to aid in weight reduction, increase
lean body mass, and potentiate the actions of insulin. Chromium is marketed mostly in the
form of chromium picolinate, but other forms such as chromium nicotinate and chromium
chloride supplements are also available. The picolinate form has been found to be lipo-
philic, therefore increasing chromium's absorptive efficiency and glucose uptake by skeletal muscle cultures when compared to other available complexes.

Recently, it was determined that chromium is the biologically active component of glucose tolerance factor (GTF) that potentiates insulin activity and aides in normal insulin
function. As it relates to athletes and others with insufficient intake and excessive losses,
supplementation may be effective to promote optimal insulin effectiveness. As it relates to
improving body composition, numerous recent studies have shown that chromium supplementation is ineffective in the parameters of weight loss and increasing lean body mass
or muscular strength. However, one poorly designed study did demonstrate that chromium supplementation increased lean body mass in exercising humans. Using untrained
college students and trained football players, 200 µg/d of chromium picolinate or placebo
was supplemented for 40 to 42 d while subjects participated in a resistive training program.
It was reported that participants receiving chromium supplements gained significantly
more lean body mass compared to the placebo group. However, inadequate assessment

methods were used to determine these findings. Lean body mass was reported to be estimated from circumference measurements. Observed changes were so minimal that human measurement error may have influenced the results.

The following reports will demonstrate the ineffectiveness of chromium in its previously mentioned parameters. In one well-designed double-blind study, after 8 weeks of 3.3 to 3.5 µmoles/d of chromium supplementation vs. placebo during a resistive training program, no positive effects of changes in body in composition or strength gain in men were observed. The researchers found that supplementation did increase both serum chromium concentrations and urinary excretions. Consistent with this finding was another double-blind study whereby football players utilized chromium picolinate (200 µg/d) for 9 weeks during a strength-training program during spring training. Repeated measures testing was performed pre-, mid-, and postsupplementation using underwater weighing, anthropometric measurements, and urinary chromium excretion. No significant findings between placebo and experimental groups were found pertaining to changes in skinfold measurements, percent body fat, lean body mass, or circumference measurements. Urinary chromium excretion was reported to be five times greater than placebo group at mid- and postsupplementation assessments, suggesting adequate chromium stores and additional supplemented chromium were excreted via the urine. In addition, the placebo group urinary chromium excretion was low and undetectable throughout all phases of the trial. It was concluded in this trial that chromium picolinate supplementation was ineffective as a body composition and strength altering agent.

In another investigation, this time using untrained individuals, no significant findings related to changes in body composition, percent body fat, strength, and lean body mass gains after a 12-week supplementation of 200 µg/d of chromium during a resistive-training program. Chromium intake from food diaries was estimated at 36 µg/d. Consistent with other studies, chromium excretion in the experimental group increased after 6 weeks of supplementation and remained elevated at 12 weeks of training. In regard to strength changes, both placebo (33%) and chromium (24%) supplemented groups produced significant gains in total body muscular strength.

Yet another report of chromium's ineffectiveness was recently published. Researchers performed a double-blind study utilizing 37 men and 22 females all of whom were untrained and of college age. No significant differences for men and women were found after 12-week supplementation of 200 µg/d of chromium picolinate pertaining to strength gains. However, males receiving both placebo and chromium and females receiving placebo were found to have small increases in body weight. Females receiving chromium supplement gained 2.5 kg of body weight. In addition, the experiment failed to assess lean body mass and chromium present in the diet.

The accumulation of research has indicated that chromium, in any form, has been found to be ineffective as a supplement to increase lean body mass, significantly alter body composition, or improve strength in both trained and untrained individuals. Assessment of urinary chromium excretion indicates that ingested chromium can reach maximal levels in tissue, therefore allowing for the remainder to be excreted. Although there is limited information pertaining to safety of chromium, a recent case study reveals that exogenous chromium picolinate may become toxic when ingested at 6 to 12 times the recommended dosage over the course of many months. Such ingestion caused renal impairment and required dialysis to restore renal function. At this time, exogenous chromium is considered safe when consumed in recommended quantities. However, although unproven in human subjects, *in vitro* studies have suggested that chromium can accumulate in cultured cells and cause chromosomal damage.

Creatine

Creatine and creatine phosphate (Figure 13.2) are found in muscle, brain, and the blood. Three amino acids (arginine, glycine, methionine) and two organs (kidneys and liver) are needed to manufacture creatine. In the kidneys, the guanidino group from arginine is attached to glycine by arginine-glycine transaminase forming glycocyamine. Glycocyamine (guanidoacetate) circulates to the liver and is converted to creatine by receiving a methyl group from *S*-adenosyl-methinione. Creatine then circulates and accumulates largely in skeletal and cardiac muscle and the brain. ATP phosphorylates creatine to form creatine phosphate within the mitochondria. The enzyme creatine kinase (creatine phosphokinase) catalyzes this reaction. Creatine phosphate provides a small phosphate reserve for regenerating ATP. For example, in skeletal muscle the limited quantity of ATP will be exhausted in less than a second during myocyte contraction. ATP may be rapidly regenerated by transfer of the phosphate group from creatine phosphate to ADP to regenerate ATP, again regulated by creatine kinase. In order for creatine phosphate to perform this function it must have translocated from the mitochondria and associated with contractile proteins of cytosolic myofilaments. This activity, along with the actions of adenylate cyclase, maintain ATP at operational concentrations briefly while energy pathways augment their glycolytic and oxidative ATP-generating activities.

Free creatine is subject to nonenzymatic cyclization to form creatinine, which enters the blood and becomes part of the renal ultrafiltrate and subsequently the urine. About 1.6% of the body's creatine spontaneously cyclizes to form creatinine. Skeletal muscle contains about 3 to 5 g of creatine per kilogram of tissue. Since the quantity of urinary creatinine closely correlates with the quantity of skeletal muscle mass, it can be used as a clinical assessment tool for body protein status. For example, for every gram of urinary creatine present, about 18 kg of skeletal muscle can be assumed.

A typical diet contains 1 to 2 g of creatine. However, individuals who eat more red meat receive more creatine and vegetarians receive less. Men typically tend to eat more creatine than women. Over the last half decade or so, creatine has become one of the more popular nutrition supplements, due to its purported ergogenic properties. It is usually marketed in the form of creatine monohydrate, and manufacturers recommend ingesting "loading doses" as high as 20 g/d for 5 d, followed by "maintenance doses" of 5 to 10 g/d thereafter. The rationale for creatine supplementation is that it will result in larger amounts of muscle creatine and creatine phosphate and thus positively influence the ability to maintain optimal ATP levels in working muscle.

Scientific investigation of muscle creatine loading and the efficacy of creatine as an ergogenic aid is mostly supportive as related to high-intensity bouts of activity. In one investigation, it was determined that total muscle creatine concentration in men increased by 20% after 6 d of supplementing 20 g. Furthermore, the augmented level of muscle creatine was maintained for 30 d when the supplemental dosage was 2 g daily. Muscle creatine levels returned to presupplemented levels after discontinuation of creatine supplements for 30 d. In the same study it was also determined that a similar increase in total muscle creatine can be achieved by supplementing 3 g of creatine for 28 d.

Several studies have demonstrated that creatine supplementation can enhance muscular strength and performance and potentially lead to increases in lean body mass. For example, one study demonstrated that creatine supplementation resulted in a greater knee extension torque production as measured on a Cybex II isokinetic dyanamometer. Another investigation revealed that creatine supplementation experienced a 6% increase in their one repetition maximum (1 RM) free weight bench press. Yet another study demonstrated that creatine-supplemented men were able to complete ten bouts of 6-sec high-intensity exercise on a friction-loaded Cardiotonic Wingate cycle ergometer while placebo-treated men were not able to complete the regimen.

With regard to increases in body mass associated with creatine supplementation, a few investigations have reported an increase of 0.5 to 1.0 kg and as much as 1.7 kg. The investigators in the latter study attributed the increase in body mass to fat-free mass. However, it is not conclusively known as to whether the composition of the fat-free mass was largely water due to increased intracellular osmolality related to the augmented creatine levels in muscle. Some evidence is provided by associated reductions in urinary volume coinciding with augmentations in tissue creatine.

At this time most of the evidence supporting creatine as a credible ergogenic aid are focused on activities of higher intensity. Whether or not creatine supplementation can be applied to some training aspect for more endurance-based activities remains to be conclusively investigated. Other areas of promise for creatine supplementation may be for the managment of skeletal myopathies as well as cardiomyopathies and heart failure. While creatine supplementation is generally regarded as safe by many scientists, the risk of toxicity is largely unknown at this time.

Coenzyme Q10 (Ubiquinone)

Coenzyme Q10 is also known as CoQ10 and ubiquinone; however, they are not entirely synonymous. Ubiquinone is an aromatic ring system with isoprenoid units attached (Figure 14.1). The number of isoprenoid units attached can vary by organism. In mammals, the mitochondrial ubiquinone structure has 10 isoprenoid units, hence Q10. In mitochondria there is more ubiquinone than in other members of the respiratory chain and many scientists believe that ubiquinone functions as a mobile component of the respiratory chain, collecting reducing equivalents from more anchored flavoprotein complexes and passing them on the cytochromes. Skeletal muscle ubiquinone content has been reported to be positively associated with molecular oxygen availability, respiratory activity, and oxidative energy-releasing processes, but not fermentation activity. Therefore, the high content of ubiquinone probably allows for dual function: respiratory chain activity and antioxidation. While some of the earliest attention focused upon supplementation of ubiquinone was probably for ergogenic purposes, clinical applications are now gaining greater attention as well.

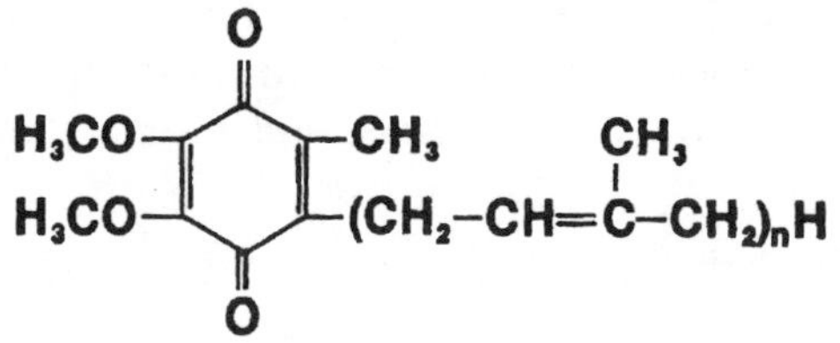

FIGURE 14.1
Ubiquinone (coenzyme Q). The "n" will vary between animals. Humans have ten; hence the common names Q10 or CoQ10.

First, with regard to athletic performance, the ergogenic efficacy of ubiquinone is unclear. In a study using ten male bicyclists provided with 100 mg of ubiquinone per day or placebo for 8 weeks, no significant improvement was observed in cycling performance, VO_2max, submaximal physiological parameters, or lipid peroxidation. In another study, ubiquinone (100 mg) was incorporated into a coenzyme athletic performance system (CAPS) that also included cytochrome c (500 mg), inosine (100 mg), and vitamin E (200 IU), which was ingested 3 times daily by 11 highly trained male triathletes for 4 weeks. This was a double-blind crossover design so the athletes also participated in a placebo trial. The researchers reported no significant improvement in endurance performance nor were there changes in blood glucose, lactate, or free fatty acids (FFA) at exhaustion. Ubiquinone supplementation (120 mg/d) for 6 weeks has also been reported to be ineffective at improving exercise performance or antioxidant capacity in trained young and older men.

In another study, despite improvements in the subjective perception of vigor in the ubiquinone supplemented (150 mg/d for 2 months) group, improvements in VO_2max or lactate threshold were not observed in middle-aged, untrained men. In yet another investigation, investigators failed to find a significant exercise performance benefit associated with ubiquinone supplementation. Here, highly trained cyclists and triathletes utilizing a ubiquinone supplement did not demonstrate significant improvements in oxygen uptake and anaerobic and respiratory compensation thresholds or changes in blood lactate, glucose, and triglyceride kinetics, heart rate, or blood pressure during and after graded cycling to exhaustion.

Contrary to studies reporting no ergogenic benefit, several investigations have found improvements in athletic performance and antioxidant potential with ubiquinone supplementation. One investigation studied the effect of an antioxidant supplement containing 60 mg of ubiquinone in combination with 294 mg vitamin E and 1000 mg vitamin C and found improvements in serum and LDL antioxidant potential in endurance athletes. Meanwhile, another investigation reported that ubiquinone treatment markedly suppressed exercise-induced lipid peroxidation in organs such as liver, heart, and gastrocnemius. Also, utilizing a double-blind crossover design, ubiquinone supplementation (90 mg/d) was reported to improve indexes of physical performance including VO_2max in Finnish top-level cross-country skiers.

In addition to possibly augmenting athletic performance, ubiquinone supplementation has also been purported to have therapeutic application in certain clinical situations. While the results of clinical investigations have not always conclusively demonstrated that ubiquinone supplementation has a beneficial impact as either a primary or adjunctive treatment of chronic congestive heart failure, there is a growing body of evidence that suggests that there may at least be a minimal benefit of 100 mg daily. One metaanalysis of eight controlled clinical trials of ubiquinone treatment of congestive heart failure patients revealed that several cardiac parameters were improved. These parameters included ejection fraction (EF), stroke volume (SV), cardiac output (CO), cardiac index (CI), and end diastolic volume index (EDVI). Without question, further investigative efforts need to occur in order to better understand the potential application of ubiquinone, both independently and as adjunctive therapy for the treatment of chronic cardiac failure.

Choline

Choline (Figure 14.2) or 2-hydroxy-*N,N,N*-trimethyl-ethanaminium is a water and ethanol-soluble and hygroscopic substance widely available in foods (naturally or as an additive),

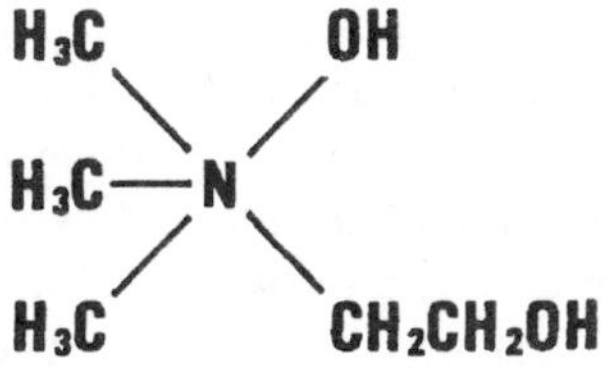

H₃C   OH

H₃C — N

H₃C   CH₂CH₂OH

FIGURE 14.2
Choline.

primarily consumed in the form of the phospholipid phosphatidylcholine. Choline serves as the precursor for the synthesis of actylcholine, which, among other locations, is also the neurotransmitter at neuromuscular junctions. Choline is also a precursor for betaine which serves as a methyl donor in single-carbon operations such as the synthesis of methionine from homocysteine and the formation of creatinine.

Whether or not dietary supplementation under typical situations has merit is still a matter of debate. Human deficiency is rare because of dietary supply and endogenous synthesis via methionine. Choline supplementation has been purported beneficial in the treatment of short-term memory loss in Alzheimer's disease.

DHEA

Dehydroepiandrosterone or DHEA is a steroid hormone synthesized and secreted by the adrenal glands. DHEA and its sulfated form, DHEAS, circulate to peripheral tissue where they are converted into androgens and/or estrogens. The level of circulating DHEA and DHEAS usually peaks during the 20 to 30s and then declines steadily during the aging process, although there appear to be individual variations within age groups as well as variations depending upon gender, race, and health status. Great interest in DHEA has been revitalized in the last decade or so as several investigators have reported inverse relationships between circulating DHEA levels and the incidence of heart disease, various cancers, and several other age-related diseases.

In the human, like other mammals, the cortex region of the adrenal gland has three distinct regions referred to as the zona glomerulosa, the zona fasciculata, and the zona reticularis. It is generally believed that the zona reticularis is the primary DHEA-synthesizing area of the adrenocortical parenchyma. Cholesterol is the precursor for DHEA synthesis and is derived primarily from cholesterol esters present in cytoplasmic lipid droplets. ACTH or cAMP stimulates an esterase to liberate cholesterol which translocates to the mitochondria and undergoes conversion to pregnenolone by the cytochrome P_{450} side chain cleavage enzyme. Cleavage of the cholesterol side chain must first be preceded by hydroxylations at C_{22} and subsequently C_{20}. Removal of the 6-carbon isocaproaldehyde side chain yields a 21-carbon pregnenolone. Pregnenolone can then be hydroxylated at the 17-carbon position to yield 17-hydroxypregnenolone, which can then be converted to dehydroepiandrosterone by C_{17-20} lyase. The enzyme, C_{17-20} lyase, is found primarily in the adrenal cortex and the gonads. Most of the DHEA formed in the adrenal glands is quickly modified by the addition of sulfate to form DHEAS. It should be mentioned that DHEA can also be sulfated in liver parenchyma. While DHEAS is relatively inactive, removal of the sulfate group by peripheral tissue will reactivate the steroid structure.

DHEA circulates in the blood both independently as well as bound loosely to albumin and sex hormone-binding globulin (SHBG). On the other hand, DHEAS circulates in the blood strongly bound to albumin and also undergoes tubular reabsorption. The strong bonding to albumin along with efficient tubular reabsorption contributes to very slow clearance from the blood. However, DHEAS must first undergo sulfate removal, converting DHEAS back to DHEA, to be converted to active steroid molecules in the periphery. In this sense DHEA becomes an intermediate for DHEAS metabolism. With the exception of cholesterol itself, DHEA and its sulfate conjugate dehydroepiandrosterone sulfate (DHEAS) represent the steroid of highest quantity found in the human blood.

Relative to other mammals, humans and other primates produce high levels of DHEA. This allows humans to derive significant quantities of active sex steroids in peripheral tissue from the prohormone DHEA. It has been estimated that greater than 50% of the total androgens in the periphery of adult males is derived from DHEA. In women, the formation of peripheral estrogens from DHEA may be as high as 75% before menopause and 100% after menopause. On the other hand, for lower mammals, such as rodents, reliance is almost entirely upon ovarian and testicular tissue for sex steroids. Perhaps the primary advantage for primates in deriving such a significant proportion of their peripheral active sex steroids from DHEA is that it allows for local control of sex steroid levels as dictated by the needs of specific tissue.

As mentioned above, DHEA and DHEAS circulate to peripheral tissue where they are converted to androstenedione and then to androgens and estrogens. The ability of target peripheral tissue to convert DHEA and DHEAS into androgens and/or estrogens is attributed to the expression of steroidogenic and metabolizing enzyme systems such as 3β-hydroxysteroid dehydrogenase/Δ^5-Δ^4-isomerase (3β-HSD). Because circulating steroid precursors are intracellularly converted to active androgen and estrogen structures in peripheral tissue, this area of endocrinology is often referred to as intracrinology (Figure 14-3).

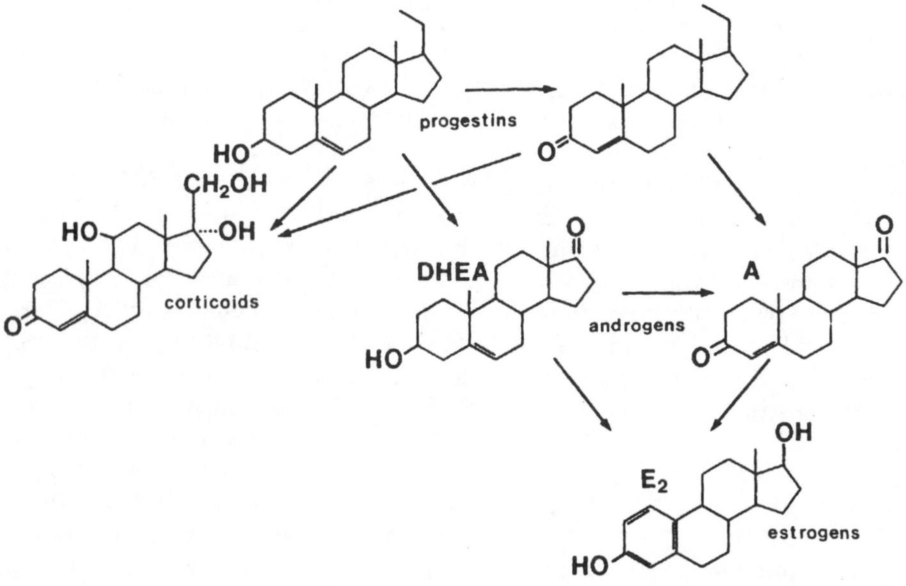

FIGURE 14.3
Interconversion of steroids. "A" denotes androstenedione.

The secretion of DHEA and DHEAS by the adrenal glands increases during adrenarche in children around 6 to 8 years of age, and maximal levels are typically observed between ages 20 to 30. After that time plasma DHEA and DHEAS levels on average decline steadily during the remaining decades of adulthood. Because of this, DHEA supplementation should not be considered prior to the age of 30 and should be physician advised. DHEA supplementation is banned by the International Olympic Committee (IOC). More clinical investigations are warranted in this area before general dose recommendations can be made. In one cross-over DHEA trial, whereby men and women 40 to 70 years of age received either 50 mg of DHEA or a placebo for 6 months, total DHEA and DHEAS levels were elevated to levels resembling younger adults. Also, a twofold increase in androstenedione, testosterone, and dihydrotestosterone was observed in women and only a small rise in androstenedione was observed in men. HDL-cholesterol decreased slightly in the women and insulin sensitivity was unaltered. Insulin-like growth factor 1 (IGF-1) levels increased and IGF binding protein-1 (IGFBP-1) decreased in both genders, suggesting increased IGF-1 availability to target tissue. There was an associated increase in physical and psychological well-being in both genders as well.

In a double-blind investigation of longer duration (1 year), men and women, ages 50 to 65 years of age and with basal DHEA levels below or near the lower end of the range for younger adults, received either 100 mg of DHEA or a placebo. Those participants receiving the DHEA demonstrated an increase in DHEA near or beyond the upper limit of the younger adults. In men, androstenedione levels were doubled; however, in the women a three- to fourfold increase in the levels of androstenedione, testosterone, and dihydrotestosterone were observed. Furthermore, the level of SHBG was halved in the women, perhaps due to a feedback inhibition upon the liver in light of the elevated levels of androgens. One woman developed facial hair by the close of the study.

Echinacea

Echinacea purpurea (L.) Moench is another class 1 herb, commonly referred to as echinacea. Many believe it to be an immunostimulant to strengthen the body against infections. In two studies, acidic arabinogalactan, the purified polysaccharide from plant cell cultures of *Echinacea purpurea*, effectively activated macrophage activity against microorganisms. In these studies, B cells were not activated and T cells were not induced to produce interleukin 2, interferon β2 or interferon γ. However, an increase in T cell proliferation was noted and B lymphocytes demonstrated a small proliferation after an incubation with echinacea.

Echinacea seems to be nontoxic, but it is suggested that it not be used for more than an 8-week period. Currently, it seems to be safe and if effective, its impact is minimal, but caution should be noted with use. Natural human body defense mechanisms are purported to be enhanced with echinachea use.

Flavonoids

Flavonoids are present in plants as coloring agents. They are also called anthoxanthins. These molecules are glycosides with a benzopyrone foundation. There is molecular variation of the members among the subtypes of flavonoids (flavones, flavonols, flavanones, flavanonols, and isoflavones) and there may be as many as 800 total flavonoids in these subtypes. Investigation into the physiological impact of ingesting flavonoids has revealed some potential beneficial function to human health. This class of molecules has been reported to have antioxidant, antiinflammatory, and antitumor properties, along with inhibition of platelet aggregation.

Flavonoids are found in fruits, vegetables, nuts, and grains. Citrus fruits, for example, contain more than 60 flavonoids, including the more reknowned flavonoids *hesperidin* and *quercetin*. Other good sources of flavonoids are soy, which contains a significant amount of isoflavones such as genistein and diadzein. The flavonol quercetin is a major flavonoid in the Western diet and is found in rich amounts in broccoli, red and yellow onions, kale, red grapes, cherries, apples, and cereals. Quercetin has been reported to have anticarcinogenic and antioxidant capabilities.

A study of older men in the Netherlands revealed that flavonoid consumption was inversely related to heart disease mortality and those men with the highest flavonoid intake had 60% less mortality from heart disease than those with the lowest flavonoid consumption. Isoflavones can be found in red wine and grape juice and may serve to protect LDL from oxidation as well as inhibit platelet aggregation, thus reducing atherosclerosis and stenosed coronary vessel thrombosis.

Garlic (*Allium sativum*)

Originally from central Asia, garlic is now grown worldwide. Garlic is purported to have antibiotic, expectorant, and antidiabetic properties, as well as reducing blood pressure and inhibiting blood clotting. Its medicinal components are a volatile oil containing alliin, allinase, and allicin, and scordinins, along with selenium and vitamins A, C, E, and some B vitamins as well. Allinase is an enzyme that converts alliin to allicin when fresh garlic cloves are crushed. Along with fresh garlic crushed or chopped used in food preparation, garlic and processed garlic have become a popular nutrition supplement in the form of pills and tablets.

Garlic is used as a food item in all parts of the world. It belongs to the allium vegetable family along with onions, ginger, scallion, leeks, and chives. Thus, these food items will also have many of the same beneficial compounds as garlic. Research efforts have demonstrated that the allium compounds may induce glutathionine-s-transferase, an enzyme involved in detoxification which is believed to be beneficial in the prevention of heart disease and cancers. The allium compounds may also reduce the amount of nitrates available in the gut and thereby reducing the formation of carcinogenic nitroamines. It is also becoming more clear that garlic supplementation can lower blood cholesterol levels in hypercholesterolemic individuals. Garlic extracts may also inhibit thromboxane synthase, thus decreasing the formation of thromboxane A_2, a vasoconstrictor and platelet aggregation promotor.

Ginger

Zingiber officinale Roscoe, commonly known as ginger, has been gaining much attention in the relief of nausea and vomiting. The fresh root falls under class 1 and interestingly enough the dried root falls under class 2b and 2d. Its classification as 2d restricts those with gallstones from its use as a therapeutic agent.

Medicinally, ginger has been reported to have antiinflammatory properties and has relieved persons with severe nausea and vomiting. It has also been used to improve conditions associated with gastric and duodenal ulcers, but patients were prone to relapse. As an antiinflammatory, ginger has been noted to have equivalent activity to acetylsalicylic acid when studied in the rat. Ginger has also demonstrated antipyretic activity when studied *in vitro*.

Most of the research on ginger points its use as an antiemetic. It has been used to treat severe instances of nausea, vomiting, and motion sickness. Although it has not been approved for use as an agent for relieving vomiting and nausea in pregnancy, a recent investigation to determine its effectiveness found beneficial effects of ginger and pyridoxine in pregnant women. In another study performed to determine the effects of ginger in the treatment of hyperemesis gravidarum, positive effects were found compared to a placebo when ginger was take in 1-g doses over a 4-d period.

The safety of ginger ingestion by pregnant women is inconclusive. Information pertaining to pregnancy outcome and ginger use has yet to be published. However, there has been one instance reported of a spontaneous abortion; therefore, current recommendations by German's Commission E and the American Herbal Product Association declare that ginger not be used during pregnancy.

Ginkgo

Ginkgo biloba is the sole remaining member of the Ginkgoaceae family; the other members, known only in fossilized remains, have long been extinct. The ginkgo tree grows in temperate climates of the northern hemisphere. Seeds of *G. biloba* have long been used in Chinese traditional medicine, and acetone–water extracts from ginkgo leaves are used in several European countries as part of phytotherapy. Ginkgo has been well studied, especially by German investigators, as several hundred papers grace medical literature. Much of the purported effects of ginkgo are in the area of improved memory and concentration. Furthermore, ginkgo has been used prophylactically and in treatment of cardiovascular and cerebrovascular diseases and asthma.

The leaves of *G. biloba* are endowed with several metabolites which may bear pharmaceutical properties including flavonoids (ginkgo flavone glycosides) and terpenoids (ginkgolides and bilobalide). As many as 40 different flavonoid structures have been identified in ginkgo leaves, including catechins, dehydrocatechins, flavones, biflavones, and flavonols. Other constituents of ginkgo leaves include steroid structures (sitosterol, sitosteroid glycoside, stigmasterol), polyprenols, simple organic acids, long-chain benzoic acid derivatives, long-chain phenols, lower aliphatic acids, carbohydrates, cyclitols, straight-chain hydrocarbons, alcohols and ketones, and carotenoids.

Much of gingko purported activity is attributed to the presence of ginkgolides, which are methylmononorditerpene trilactones. These terpene compounds consist of six 5-membered rings in a cage-shaped conformation and ginkgolide forms A, B, C, J, and M have been identified, the last of which may only be present in significant quantities in the root. These forms differ in the number and positioning of their hydroxyl groups. In addition, an active sesquiterpene trilactone molecule, also bearing a cage design, has been identified and named bilabolide. It is found in the leaves as well as in the root. The ginkgolide and bilabolide content of dried ginkgo leaves is approximately 0.005 to 1%.

Preparations from ginkgo leaves and seeds have been used to treat asthma. In Western Europe ginkgo leaf extracts are used to treat cerebral insufficency and peripheral arterial vascular disorders. Cerebrovascular insufficiency symptomology such as forgetfulness, dizziness, depression, anxiety, absentmindedness, and confusion as well as peripheral perceptions of "pins and needles" and coldness have been reported to be relieved by ginkgo. Blood circulation to cerebral and peripheral tissue as well as improvements in blood's rheological properties have been reported. Furthermore, it has been suggested that ginkgo increases tolerance to cerebral hypoxia.

Flavonoid structures in ginkgo preparations presenting antioxidant properties may be beneficial in squelching free radicals, especially during periods of hypoxia, ischemia, or metabolic disturbances. In support of this notion is the report that the flavonoids in ginkgo preparations may protect erythrocytes from hemolysis. Furthermore, the ginkgolides may be potent platelet-activating factor (PAF)-antagonists. It seems that they may displace PAF from its receptor binding sites.

Enriched ginkgo leaf extracts such as GBE, containing 24% ginkgo flavone glycosides and 6% terpene lactones (ginkgolides A, B, C, and J and bilobalide combined) as well as 5 to 10% oligomeric proanthocyanidins, about 9% organic acids, and a limited quantity of ginkgolic acids and ginkgols, have been used extensively in clinical investigation. Most of these investigations did indeed report positive results in improving cerebral insufficiency and intermitent claudication, in doses approximating 120 to 160 mg GBE for several weeks. GBE has also been reported to positively influence dizziness, tinnitus, and learning impairment.

Ginkgo preparations of the above specifications are currently marketed in Germany and France. However, serious reservations for the use of ginkgo preparations have been published, and scientists have suggested that many of the studies reporting positive results with ginkgo preparations were biased. Furthermore, it has been warned that ginkgo preparations should be considered only as a potential treatment protocol and should not be used prophylactically.

Glycerol

Glycerol has also been considered a candidate for supplementation during endurance events. This notion is based upon glycerol's potential to be converted to glucose in hepatocytes and be released into the blood. Theoretically, this could decrease the rate of breakdown of glycogen stores. However, it seems that the torpid rate of conversion of glycerol to glucose seriously decreases its candidacy.

Alternatively, glycerol supplementation in conjunction with water consumption may be of benefit to endurance athletes preparing to perform in warmer environments. It may be that glycerol can enhance water retention prior to an event and thus may allow more sweat to be lost prior to any reductions in performance due to dehydration. It has been reported that glycerol-induced hyperhydration (1 g glycerol per kg body weight + 21.4 ml H_2O per kg body weight) prior to moderate exercise was more effective than water-induced hyperhydration in reducing the thermal stress associated with the heat. Furthermore, researchers reported that ingestion of 1.2 g of glycerol per kg + 25 ml H_2O per kg body weight improved cycling performance to exhaustion at 65% VO_2max in a neutral laboratory environment. Interestingly, the researchers noted a lower heart rate and rectal temperature during the glycerol trial and speculated that some of the benefits may be attributable to an increased plasma volume.

The physiologic impact of glycerol-induced hyperhydration was later confirmed in reports from the U.S. Army Research Institute of Environmental Medicine as researchers provided 1.5 g glycerol + 37 ml H_2O per kg body weight in a test subject. They reported a greater retention of body fluids as glycerol maintained extracellular fluid osmolality at the greater volume. However, the researchers did indeed raise important glycerol dosage issues and the question of potential for tissue damage associated with increased intracellular volume damage.

HMB (β-hydroxy-β-methylbutyrate)

β-Hydroxy-β-methylbutyrate, or more commonly HMB, is a metabolite of the essential amino acid leucine. It is synthesized naturally in humans as well as being available in some foods (i.e., citrus and catfish). Whether HMB has a necessary physiological function or is merely a metabolite remains unclear. However, because HMB is purported to prevent muscle catabolism associated with resistance training, HMB became a popular nutrition supplement among body builders and strength trainers. As is typical with many supplements geared to this population, the marketing exceeds the research.

At this time, there are only a couple of published scientific efforts attempting to gain insight into the efficacy of HMB as a supplement. Investigators have reported that supplemental doses of either 1.5 or 3.0 g HMB per day for 3 weeks during supervised strength-training sessions gained more lean body mass than did the unsupplemented group. The greatest gains were observed in the 3.0-g supplemented group. Furthermore, it was reported that muscle protein catabolism decreased during the first 2 weeks of the trial and there was less evidence of muscle damage as a result of training. As an adjunct to this investigation, the researchers also reported that 3.0 g of HMB per day for 7 weeks while undergoing intense resistance training resulted in an increase in fat-free mass and bench press strength. While these results are indeed promising, more investigation needs to be completed in this area.

Laetrile

Once referred to as vitamin B_{17}, laetrile (Figure 14.4) has experienced periods of popularity since the 1920s after it was theorized that it destroyed cancer cells. Laetrile has been popularized on and off as a potential antitumor factor; however human studies conclusively demonstrating this activity were lacking. One such study reported that laetrile neither caused the shrinkage of tumors nor increased survival time or alleviated symptomology in cancer patients. It was concluded that laetrile was of no clinical value in the treatment of cancer or improving the quality of life in cancer patients. While laetrile has been banned by as many as 30 states in the U.S., it can still be purchased in various countries throughout the world.

Chemically laetrile (amygdalin) can be isolated from the seeds of peaches, apricots, apples, and plums among others. It is cyanogenic, and there are several reports of cyanide

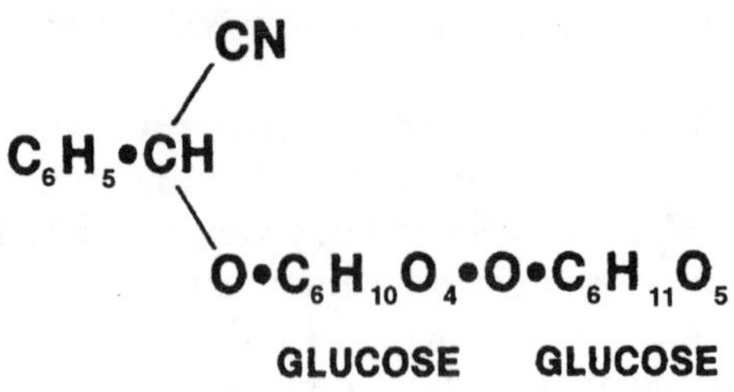

$$\text{C}_6\text{H}_5\bullet\text{CH}\overset{\displaystyle\text{CN}}{\diagdown}$$

$$\text{O}\bullet\text{C}_6\text{H}_{10}\text{O}_4\bullet\text{O}\bullet\text{C}_6\text{H}_{11}\text{O}_5$$

GLUCOSE   GLUCOSE

FIGURE 14.4
Laetrile.

poisoning in the medical literature from ingestion of laetrile in doses suggested by laetrile advocates. Hepatotoxicity and neuromyopathy have been reported with laetrile use. It would appear that oral ingestion of amygdalin leads to its conversion to cyanide by intestinal bacterial β-glucosidase. Therefore, intravenous administration may reduce this risk of toxicity. Currently, laetrile is not accepted as a therapy by the American Medical Association.

Licorice

Licorice, also known as liquorice, glycyrrhiza, sweet wood, liquiritiae radix, and others, comes from the *Glycyrrhiza glabra* plant and consists of the dried unpeeled roots and stolons. Licorice has been extensively studied both for its food and medicinal potential. In the latter half of the 18th century, sugar was added to licorice extract and it quickly became a popular confection. On the other hand, the use of licorice in treating human ailments such as stomach pains and oral cavity ulcers has been recognized for thousands of years. It appears that its most important component is the saponin glycoside, *glycyrrhizin*. Glycyrrhizin, also known as glycyrrhizic and glycyrrhizinic acids, is reponsible for most of licorice's taste and probably much of its medicinal quality. Its concentration, either in the form of calcium or potassium salt, is typically up to 24%.

Upon hydrolysis, glycyrrhizin yields 2 molecules of glucuronic acid and a pentacyclic triterpene agycone, glycyrrhetinic (glycyrrhetic, glycerretic) acid, and other triterpenes. Other components of licorice extract include amines, amino acids, coumarins (glycyrin, herniarin, licopyranocoumarin, etc.), flavonoids and isoflavonoids (glicoricone, liquiritigenin, glisoflavone, licoflavonol, etc.), sugars, gums, lignin, resins, starch, steroids (β-sitosterol, stigmasterol, 22,23-dihydrostigmasterol, etc.), tannins, triterpenes (β-amyrin, glabrolide, 18-β-glycyrrhetinic acid, glycyrrhetol, etc.), and a volatile oil containing substances such as acetylsalicylic acid, salicylic acid, and methylsalicylate.

Licorice has a long list of purported therapeutic uses, including function as an antiplatelet agent; an antihypotensive agent; a antihypercholesterolemic agent, a laxative; an antibacterial, fungicical, and viral agent; an immunostrengthening agent; and an antiallergy, antiinflammatory, and anticarcinogenic agent.

Ornithine

Ornithine and its derivative *ornithine-α-ketoglutarate* (OKG) have received considerable interest from weight-training athletes. While ornithine is an amino acid, it is not found in protein. It exists independently in the human body and is fundamentally involved in the formation of urea. Supplemental ornithine was popularized after scientists reported that when ornithine was infused into blood there was a corresponding increase in growth hormone. In one study, supplementation of 1 g of ornithine, in conjunction with 1 g of arginine, resulted in increases in total strength and lean body mass and lowered urinary hydroxyproline, an indicator of muscle tissue breakdown. However, these investigative efforts need to repeated, and ornithine has to be tested independent of arginine, which is a known growth hormone secretagogue.

OKG has been used clinically for many years, especially in countries abroad. Oral supplementation of 10 to 20 g/d has been shown to be beneficial in patients recovering from burns, malnutrition, various wounds, or surgery. It seems that OKG not only increases circulating growth hormone levels in these patients, but also protein synthesis, while at the same time decreasing protein breakdown.

Phytoestrogens

Phytoestrogens are flavonoids broadly grouped into four main classes: isoflavones, lignans, coumestans, and resorcyclic lactones. Phytoestrogens are available in a vast array of plants typically consumed by humans. *Phyto* refers to plants while *estrogen* alludes to their ability to estrogen have estrogen-like properties, however, much less potent then synthetic estrogens. Phytoestrogen isoflavones are found mostly in legumes such as soybeans, lentils, and beans (i.e., kidney, lima, broad, haricot). Soy products will contain some isoflavones. Lignans are found in many plant foods including cereal grains, fruits, and vegetables. They are found in higher concentration in flaxseed (linseed). Coumestans are found in sprouts and fodder crops such as alfalfa. Last, resorcyclic acid lactones are mycotoxins that develop in stored crops. Therefore, they are not true phytoestrogens.

Most of the attention is focused upon isoflavones and lignans. Epidemiological studies indicate that diets rich in phytoestrogens are inversely associated with cardiovascular disease and certain cancers. Thus, these substances are currently being evaluated for their preventive and treatment potential. See Chapter 17 for a more in depth discussion of phytoestrogens and cancer.

Pyruvate

Pyruvate is a 3-carbon α-keto acid and is a key intermediate of energy metabolism. It is formed in a later step in glycolysis and in mitochondria-endowed cells it can enter these organelles and undergo conversion to acetyl CoA via pyruvate dehydrogenase or oxaloacetate via pyruvate decarboxylase. Acetyl CoA can subsequently condense with oxaloacetate (OAA) to form citrate, a molecule that can undergo the first reaction in the Krebs cycle or exit the mitochondria and be converted back to acetyl CoA and OAA, by citrate lyase. Cytosolic acetyl CoA can then be used for fatty acid synthesis under the influence of insulin. Pyruvate is also available for alanine transaminase (ALT) to create alanine, especially in skeletal muscle during periods of fasting and prolonged activity.

Currently pyruvate is being consumed as a nutrition supplement, primarily as an agent to enhance weight and body fat loss in individuals on hypocaloric diets. It is secondarily utilized to reduce total blood cholesterol and LDL-cholesterol as well as an ergogenic aid. Although limited in number, the results of the studies have led researchers to suggest that pyruvate may have some clinical applications.

Recently, an investigation reported that obese women consuming 30 g of supplemental pyruvate (20 g sodium pyruvate + 16 g calcium pyruvate) in conjunction with a low-energy liquid diet experienced a greater weight and body fat loss than obese women consuming a isocaloric polyglucose placebo in conjunction with the low-energy diet. Nitrogen balance was not different between the two groups. The diets provided approximately 1000 kcal (4.25 MJ/d) and consisted of 68% carbohydrate, 22% protein, and 10% fat. The mechanism for the enhanced weight and fat loss was unclear to the investigators. However, they did speculate that the pyruvate may become involved in a pyruvate–phosphenol pyruvate futile cycle. Differences in activity, thermal effect of food (TEF), and RMR were ruled out as possible explanations.

A subsequent study utilizing a less restrictive hypocaloric diet (0.09 MJ/kg/d or between 1600 to 1800 kcal) and pyruvate substitution for a polyglucose contribution to carbohydrate calories in hyperlipidemic individuals attempted to determine if there was a positive impact on serum lipid levels. Despite greater weight and body fat loss in the pyruvate group, there was not a positive change in serum lipids.

In another follow-up study, pyruvate and dihydroxyacetone were substituted for the polyglucose component (20% of energy) of hypercaloric (1.5X REE) diet fed to obese subjects for 3 weeks after they participated in a hypocaloric (1.3 MJ/d) feeding trial for the previous 3 weeks. The results suggested that substitution of polyglucose with the 3-carbon compounds led to less weight and body fat gain, while nitrogen balance was not different between groups.

The interpretation of these studies is somewhat difficult, especially when it comes to potential application. Is pyruvate really a supplement or a substitute? Its true application may be as a partial substitute for traditional carbohydrates in synthesized diets. Research in dietary pyruvate metabolism is still young, and many questions need to be answered.

Saponins

Saponins are a group of triterpene or steroid glycosides with diverse structures. In general, these molecules are amphiphilic. Their presence has been identified in hundreds of different plant species, but few of them are consistantly consumed by humans. Some foods with respectable saponin levels that are more prevalent in the human diet include alfalfa sprouts, chick pea, soybeans, navy beans, kidney beans, spinach, asparagus, sesame seeds, lentil, green peas, and oats.

Saponins have long been suspected to influence lipid levels in humans. Those reports indicating a hypocholesteric impact demonstrated the greatest reductions in individuals with higher serum cholesterol levels at the onset. At this time, there appears to be two viable explanations or mechanisms for saponin hypocholesterolemic activity. First, some saponins can form insoluble complexes with cholesterol in the gut and limit its absorption. Second, saponins can participate with bile acids in the gut in the formation of micelles. However, the micelles that form are extremely large, having molecular weights in the millions. This has been suggested to block the reabsorption of bile acids in the distal ileum. Bile acids are thus lost in the feces. This hinders enterohepatic circulation and forces the liver to dedicate more cholesterol to the formation of new bile acids, thereby reducing the amount available for VLDL synthesis.

Saw Palmetto

Saw palmetto is the name commonly given to the plant *Serenoa repens* Small. It is a dwarf palm tree of the family Arecaceae found native in the West Indies and southeastern U.S. In addition, it is a class 1 herb as defined by the American Herbal Products Association; therefore it can be safely consumed when used appropriately.

Those supplementing saw palmetto aim to treat benign prostate hyperplasia. There have been numerous trials to determine the efficacy of the use of *Serenoa repens*. In one large study, patients treated with saw palmetto experienced a 50% volume decrease in residual urine, a 37% decrease in urination frequency, and 54% decrease in nocturia. Therefore, it was concluded by this study that saw palmetto is effective in the treatment of symptoms associated with enlarged prostate but will not cure the ailment. These finding are also consistent with another trial performed.

The mechanism of action and active ingredients are unknown at this time. Further studies isolating these substances would be useful in the determination of the mechanistic action of this plant. From the available data, it would seem fair to state that saw palmetto is safe and effective in the treatment of symptoms of benign prostate hyperplasia. In addition, there are many other studies determining the treatment effects of saw palmetto, but these studies have yet to become available in English and could not utilized at present.

Soy Products

Soybeans are endowed with compounds that are associated with anticancer activity and reducing serum cholesterol levels. These compounds include phytates, protease inhibitors, saponins, phytosterols, and isoflavonoids. Epidemiological studies have suggested that consumption of soybeans and soy products is a contributing factor in the low incidence of breast and prostate cancer in Japan. Also, Chinese people who eat soybeans and/or tofu regularly have half the incidence of stomach, colon, rectal, breast, and lung cancer in comparison to a Chinese individuals consuming relatively lower amounts of soy foods. It is speculated that at least some of the anticancer activity attributed to soy is due to the presence of protease inhibitors, isoflavones, genistein, and diadzein.

It has been suggested that one particular component of soybeans, a protease inhibitor called *Bowman-Birk inhibitor (BBI)*, is the most potent anticarcinogenic agent. Researchers have reported 100% suppression of dimethylhydrazine (DMH)-induced colon carcinogenesis in mice whose diet was supplemented with BBI. Other investigators with BBI and carcinogenesis found DMH-induced liver cancer was suppressed by 71% in mice; topically administered 7,12-dimethylbenzanthracene (DMBA)-induced oral cancer was suppressed by 61 to 86% in hamsters; and 3-methylchloranthrene (MCA)-induced lung tumorogenesis was supressed by 48% in mice. Other experiments using a soybean concentrate, called BBI concentrate (BBIC), in which the active ingredient is assumedly BBI, also revealed significant reductions in the amount of DMH, DMBA, MCA, and/or radiation-induced carcinogenesis in various mammalian tissue.

Other compounds in soybeans are believed to have at least some influence in the development of neoplasms. Inositol hexaphophate (IP_6) or phytic acid appears to reduce the number of tumors per animal in both azoxymethane (AOM)-induced colon carcinogenesis in rats and DMH-induced colon and mammary carcinogenesis in mice and rats, respectively. These studies demonstrated that this soy compound can indeed influence carcinogenesis by reducing the number of tumors per animal. However, there are relatively fewer investigations that support the idea that IP_6 can actually suppress carcinogenesis when comparing the number of animals with tumors in the in the IP_6 diet-administered group to the treatment group not receiving IP_6.

Another compound, β-sitrosterol, has also been reported to influence carcinogenesis *in vivo*. When this soy-derived compound was added to the diet of mice, there was a reduction in the number of animals with *N*-methyl-*N*-nitrosurea (NMU)-induced colon tumors. However, when only counting the number of animals with only malignant tumors, there was an increase of 50%. Thus, identifying this compound as an independent anticarcinogenic agent is suspect at this time.

St. John's Wort

Hypericum perforatum L., referred to by many as St. John's Wort, is an extremely popular substance in the treatment of depression. In Germany, hypericum extracts are the most widely prescribed antidepressants. It contains up to 10.0% tannins and is classified as a class 2d herb because it may enhance pharmaceutical MAO inhibitors. It has been proven against placebo to be effective in treating mild to moderate depression.

The major benefit of the use of hypericum is that it does not produce the undesirable side effects shown by conventional antidepressive drugs. Effective treatment by hypericum requires a 10- to 14 d lag time to allow for CNS adaptations. In rats, a 50% increase of 5-HT1 A and 5-HT2 A receptors was found when compared to a control group and affinity of these serotonergic receptors was unchanged.

Occasionally, persons with fair skin may be susceptible to skin irritations, rashes, swelling, and hyperpigmentation with prolonged exposure to sunlight. This photosensitizing reaction is due to a phototoxic reaction occurring from light activation of the plant substance furocoumarins. This reaction results in free radical formation and manifests as severe sunburn or second degree burns.

Vanadium

Vanadium, another trace mineral, is biologically found primarily in the pentavalent state (VO_3^- or $H_2VO_4^-$). It can also be found in the tetravalent state of VO^{+2}. It has gained gross attention in the past decade by weight-training individuals seeking to enhance lean body mass manufacturing. However, despite the attention it has received, very little research has been conducted on its purported use in this area.

At this time, vanadium is considered nonessential as it relates to human life. It is estimated that an intake of 10 µg daily should meet any postulated nutritional demands of humans. Since vanadium has not been determined to be an essential element for humans, no RDA has been established. Supplementation can be obtained in both tablet and liquid forms.

Several roles for vanadium have been purported. One use includes enhancement of amino acid uptake due to an insulin-like role. It is believed that an increased uptake of amino acids will contribute to greater growth of skeletal muscle. It has also been tested as a fasting blood glucose lowering agent in those with noninsulin diabetes mellitus.

Regarding strength-training athletes, one well-designed investigation studied the effects of vanadyl sulfate (0.5 mg/kg/d) on body composition and performance in two groups during a weight training program. In this 12-week double-blind trial comparing vanadyl sulfate to placebo, performance was measured using one and ten repetitions maximum for the leg extension and bench press whereas body composition was assessed by DEXA scans. The study found that strength increased significantly and similarly in both groups. The other parameter, body composition, was unchanged in both groups. Therefore, the researchers concluded that vanadyl sulfate was ineffective as a performance enhancer and anthropometric altering agent.

Toxicity studies of vanadium are also limited. In addition, long-term supplementation has yet to be assessed. Vanadium supplements taken at doses of 13.5 mg/d or 9 mg/d for 6 weeks and 16 months, respectively, were found not to be toxic. However, larger doses have been reported to produce diarrhea, green tongue, gastrointestinal disturbances, and cramps.

Valerian

Valeriana officinalis L. or valerian root is a class 1 plant belonging to the genus *Valeriana*, which contains about 230 species. Valerian root contains two known active substances, valepotriates and sesquiterpenes, that are important to pharmacological interest due to their sedative effects.

The use of valerian dates back to the Greek and Roman physicians who used it as a diuretic, anodyne, and spasmolytic agent. Currently, it is applied as a mild sedative and sleeping agent. The valepotriates are of particular interest due to their cytotoxic effect and use in standardization of valerian.

In a double-blind study using a preparation of mostly sesquiterpenes compared to a placebo, a "good and significant effect on poor sleep" was reported. Of the participants, 40% reported perfect sleep and 89% reported improved sleep from the preparation. In a pilot study comparing valerian to a placebo, it was concluded by using polysomnography that valerian's action increases slow wave sleep and causes a decrease in sleep stage 1 in those individuals who exhibit low baseline values.

To date, there have been no reported adverse reaction in humans. This may be due to the poor gastrointestinal absorption rate of valepotriates and the quick degradation associated with this substance. However, at high doses, valerian may cause CNS disturbances and reduce the excitability of the brain and spinal cord. Reported minor side effects in those habitually using valerian include headache, excitability, and insomnia.

Yohimbine

Yohimbine is an indole alkaloid obtained from the West African tree called Pausinystalia yohimbe tree. Its root name is *Rausinystalia yohimbe* Pierre ex Beille and commonly goes by the name yohimbe as well as johimbe. Yohimbe is a class 2d plant because it may enhance actions of pharmaceutical MAO inhibitors. It is also contraindicated in existing liver and kidney diseases as well as chronic inflammation of sex organs and/or the prostate gland. Its reputation as an aphrodisiac has been reported through testimonies, but no effect on sex drive in humans has been properly demonstrated. For more than 70 years this plant has been used to treat male sexual difficulties.

When taken in recommended doses, the predominant activity in man is antagonism of alpha 2-adrenoceptors. Its purported mechanism is caused by inhibition of central alpha 2-adrenoceptors, thus causing increased epinephrine and norepinephrine turnover and resulting in sympathetic outflow.

The use of yohimbine in erectile disorders has been evaluated in placebo-control studies and does appear to have a modest therapeutic benefit. In a small study using six male subjects with a history of sexual problems, five reported positive results when ingesting yohimbine as necessary. It was also reported that the sixth subject did not comply with the treatment and did not experience any positive results. The researchers purported that yohimbine is an effective agent for sexual disorders caused by serotonin reuptake blockers.

In a larger double-blind crossover trial of yohimbine vs. placebo, 33% of the subjects completing the trial had subjective improvement of erection while taking yohimbine compared to 15% who responded to placebo and 36% who did not respond to either treatment. The remaining 15% responded to both yohimbine and placebo treatments.

Treatment of erectile disorder using yohimbine at this time is inconclusive. Researchers suggest further trials be conducted to determine the safety and effectiveness of yohimbine treatment even though yohimbine does demonstrate a modest effect. Standard doses of yohimbe contain 5 to 6 mg of yohimbine taken 3 to 4 times daily.

Evaluation of safety is essential, due to the many adverse side effects reported, such as excessive sweating, facial flushing, increased heart rate and blood pressure, restlessness, irritability, shakes, and increased anxiety. According to the American Herbal Product Association, this plant is not recommended for long-term use. Also noted, it can stimulate the nervous system and high doses may cause a lowering in blood pressure.

References and Suggested Readings

Arginine

Suminski, R.R. et al., Acute effect of amino acid ingestion and resistance exercise on plasma growth hormone concentration in young men, *Int. J. Sport Med.*, 7(1), 48–60, 1997.

Isidori, A., et al., A study of growth hormone release in man after oral adminstration of amino acids, *Curr. Med. Res. Opin.*, 7(7), 475–481, 1981.

Lambert, M.I., et al., Failure of commercial oral amino acid supplements to increase serum growth hormone concentrations in male body-builders, *Int. J. Sport Nutr.*, 3(3), 298–305, 1993.

Eto, B., et al., Glutamate-arginine salts and hormonal responses to exercise, *Arch. Physiol. Biochem.*, 103(2), 160–164, 1995.

Fogelholm, G.M., Naveri, H.K., Kiilavouri, K.T., and Harkonen, M.H., Low-dose amino acid supplementation: no effects on serum human growth hormone and insulin in male weightlifters, *Int. J. Sport Nutr.*, 3(3), 290–297, 1993.

Corpas, E., Blackman, M.R., Roberson, R., Scholfield, D., and Harman, S.M., Oral arginine-lysine does not increase growth hormone or insulin-like growth factor-I in old men. J. Gerontol., 48(4), M128–M133, 1993.

Ceremuzynski, L., Chamiec, T., and Herbaczynska-Cedro, K., Effect of supplemental oral L-arginine on exercise capacity in patients with stable angina pectoris, *Am. J. Cardiol.*, 80(3), 331–333, 1997.

Villalobas, C. et al., Mechanisms for the stimulation of rat anterior pituary cells by arginine and other amino acids, *J. Physiol. (Lond.)*, 502(Pt. 2), 421–431, 1997.

Aspartic Acid

Maughhan, R.J. et al., The effects of oral supplementation of salts of aspartic acid on the metabolic response to prolonged exhausting exercise in man, *Int. J. Sports Med.*, 4, 119–123, 1983.

Hagan, R.D., Upton, S.J., Duncan, J.J., Cummings, J.M., and Gettman, L.R. Absence of effect of potassium-magnesium aspartate on physiologic responses to prolonged work in aerobically trained men, *Int. J. Sports Med.*, 3(3), 177–181, 1982.

Tuttle, J.L., Potteiger, J.A., Evans, B.W., Ozmun, J.C. Effect of acute potassium-magnesium aspartate supplementation on ammonia concentrations during and after resistance training, *Int. J. Sports Nutr.*, 5(2), 102–109, 1995.

deHaan, A., van Doorn, J.E., and Westra, H.G., Effects of potassium + magnesium asparate on muscle metabolism and force development during short intensive static exercise, *Int. J. Sport Med.*, 6(1), 44–49, 1985.

Wesson, M. et al., Effects of oral administration of aspartic acid salts on the endurance capacity of trained athletes, *Res. Q. Exercise Sport*, 59, 234–239, 1988.

Lancha, A.H., Recco, M.B., Abdalla, D.S. and Curi, R. Effect of aspartate, asparagine, and carnitine supplementation in the diet on metabolism of skeletal muscle during a moderate exercise, *Physiol. Behav.*, 57(2), 367–371, 1995.

Boron

Nielsen, F.H., Hunt, C.D., Mullen, L.M., and Hunt, J.R. Effect of dietary boron on mineral, estrogen, and testosterone metabolism in postmenopausal women, *FASEB J.*, 1, 394–397, 1987.

Green, N.R. and Ferrando, A.A., Plasma boron and the effects of boron supplementation in males. *Environ. Health Perspectives*, 102, 73–77, 1994.

Meacham, S.L., Taper, L.J., and Volpe, S.L. Effects of boron supplementation on bone mineral density and dietary, blood, and urinary calcium, phosphorus, magnesium, and boron in female athletes, *Environ. Health Perspectives*, 102, 79–82, 1994.

Meacham, S.L., Taper, L.J., and Volpe, S.L., Effects of boron supplementation on blood and urinary calcium, magnesium, and phosphorus and urinary boron in athletic and sedentary women, *Am. J. Clin. Nutr.*, 61, 341–345, 1995.

Carnitine

Heinenen, O.J., Carnitine and physical exercise, *Sports Med.*, 22(2), 109–132, 1996.

Colombani, P. et al., Effects of L-carnitine supplementation on physical performance and energy metabolism of endurance-trained athletes: a double-blind crossover field study, *Eur. J. Appl. Physiol.*, 73(5), 434–439, 1996.

Vecchiet, L. et al., Influence of L-carnitine administration on maximal physical exercise, *Eur. J. Appl. Physiol.*, 61(5-6), 486–490, 1990.

Brass, E.P. and Hiatt, W.R., The role of carnitine and carnitine supplementation during exercise in man and in individuals with special needs, *J. Am. Coll. Nutr.*, 17(3), 207–215, 1998.

Fagher, B., Gederblad, G., Erikson, M., Moritz, U., Nillson-Ehle, P., and Thysell, H., 1-Carnitine and hemodialysis: double blind study of muscle function and metabolism and peripheral nerve function, *Scand. J. Clin. Invest.*, 45, 169–178, 1985.

Golper, T.S., Wolfson, M., Ahmad, S., Hirschberg, R., Kurtin, P., and Katz, L.A., Multicenter trial of 1-carnitine in hemodialysis patients. I. Carnitine concentrations and lipid effects, *Kidney Int.*, 38, 904–911, 1990.

Ahmad, S., Robertson, T., Golper, T.A., Wolfson, M., Kurtin, P., Katz, L.A., Hirshberg, R., and Nicora, R., Multicenter trial of 1-carnitine in hemodialysis patients. II. Clinical and biochemical effects, *Kidney Int.*, 38, 912–918, 1990.

Lancha,, A.H., Jr., Supplementation of aspartate, asparagine and carnitine in the diet causes marked changes in the ultrastructure of soleus muscle, *J. Submicrosc. Cytol. Pathol.*, 29(3), 405–408, 1997.

Carotenoids

De Luca, L.M. and Ross, S.A., Beta-carotene increases lung cancer incidence in cigarette smokers, *Nutr. Rev.*, 54(6), 178–180, 1996.

van Poppel, G. and van den Berg, H., Vitamins and cancer, *Cancer Lett.*, 114 (1-2), 195–202, 1997.

Steinbrecher, U.P., Dietary antioxidants and cardioprotection—fact or fallacy?, *Can. J. Physiol. Pharmacol.*, 75(3), 228–233, 1997.

Mayne, S.T. et al., Effect of supplemental β-carotene on plasma concentrations of carotenoids, retinol, and α-tocopherol in humans, *Am. J. Clin. Nutr.*, 68, 642, 1998.

Chondroitin Sulfate

Pipitone, V.R., Chondroprotection with chondroitin sulfate, *Drug Exp. Clin. Res.*, 17(1), 3–7, 1991.

Chromium

Food and Nutrition Board, National Research Council, *Recommended Dietary Allowances*, 10th ed., National Academy Press, Washington, D.C., 1989.

Evans, G.W. and Pouchnik, D.J., Composition and biological activity of chromium-pyridine carboxylate complexes, *J. Inorg. Biochem.*, 49(3), 177–187, 1993.

Lefavi, R.G., Anderson, R.A., Keith, R.E., Wilson, G.D., McMillan, J.L., and Stone, M.H., Efficacy of chromium supplementation in athletes: emphasis on anabolism, *Int. J. Sport Nutr.*, 2 (2), 111–122, 1992.

Lukaski, H.C., Bolonchik, W.W., Siders, W.A., and Milne, D.B., Chromium supplementation and resistance training: effects on body composition, strength, and trace element status of men, *Am. J. Clin. Nutr.*, 63 (6), 954–965, 1996.

Trent, L.K. and Theilding-Cancel, D., Effects of chromium picolinate on body composition, *J. Sports Med. Phys. Fitness*, 35 (4), 273–280., 1995.

Clancy, S.P., Clarkson, P.M., DeCheke, M.E., Nosaka, K., Freedson, P.S., Cunningham, J.J., and Valentine, B., Effects of chromium picolinate supplementation on body composition, strength, and urinary chromium loss in football players, *Int. J. Sport Nutr.*, 4 (2), 142–153, 1994.

Hallmark, M.A., Reynolds, T.H., DeSouza, C.A., Dotson, C.O., Anderson, R.A., and Rogers, M.A., Effects of chromium and resistive training on muscle strength and body composition, *Med. Sci. Sports Exerc.*, 28 (1), 139–144, 1996.

Hasten, D.L., Rome, E.P., Franks, B.D., and Hegsted, M., Effects of chromium picolinate on beginning weight-training students, *Int. J. Sport Nutr.*, 2 (4), 343–350, 1992.

Evans, G.W., The effect of chromium picolinate on insulin controlled parameters in humans, *Int. J. Biosoc. Med. Res.*, 11, 163–180, 1994.

Cerulli, J., Grabe, D.W., Gauthier, I., Malone, M., and McGoldrick, M.D., Chromium picolinate toxicity, *Ann. Pharmacother.*, 32 (4), 428–431, 1998.

Stearns, D.M., Wise-Sr., J.P., Patierno, S., and Wetterhan, K.E., Chromium (III) picolinate produces chromosome damage in Chinese hamster ovary cells, *FASEB J.*, 9, 11643–1649, 1995.

Stearns, D.M., Belbruno, J.J., and Wetterhahn, K.E., A prediction of chromium (III) accumulation in humans from chromium dietary supplements, *FASEB J.*, 9, 1650–1657, 1995.

Creatine

Hultman, E. et al., Muscle creatine loading in men, *J. Appl. Physiol.*, 81(1), 232–237, 1996.

Greenhaff, P.L. et al., Influence of oral creatine supplementation on muscle torque during repeated bouts of maximal voluntary exercise in man, Clin. Sci., 84, 565–571, 1993.

Balsom, P.D. et al., Creatine supplementation and dynamic high-intensity intermittent exercise, *Scand. J. Med. Sci. Sports*, 3, 143–149, 1993.

Birch, R., The influence of dietary creatine supplementation on performance during repeated bouts of maximal isokinetic cycling in man, *Eur. J. Appl. Physiol. Occup. Physiol.*, 69, 268–270, 1994.

Earnest, C.P., The effect of creatine monohydrate ingestion on anaerobic power indices, muscular strength, and body composition, *Acta Physiol. Scand.*, 153, 207–209, 1995.

Greenhaff, P.L., The effect of oral creatine supplementation on skeletal muscle phosphocreatine resynthesis, *Am. J. Physiol.*, 266: (*Endocrinol. Metab. 29*), E725–E730, 1994.

Williams, M.H. and Branch, J.D., Creatine supplementation and exercise performance; An update, *J. Am. Coll. Nutr.*, 17(3), 216–234, 1998.

Coenzyme Q

Karlsson, J., Lin, L., Sylven, C., and Jansson, E., Muscle ubiquinone in healthy physically active males, *Mol. Cell Biochem.*, 156(2), 169–172, 1996.

Braun, B., Clarkson, P.M., Freedson, P.S., and Kohl, R.L., Effects of coenzyme Q10 supplementation on exercise performance, VO2 max, and lipid peroxidation in trained cyclists. *Int. J. Sport. Nutr.*, 1(4), 353–365, 1991.

Snider, I.P., Bazzarre, T.L., Murdoch, S.D., and Goldfarb, A. Effects of coenzyme athletic performance system as an ergogenic aid on endurance performance to exhaustion, *Int. J. Sport Nutr.*, 2(3), 272–286, 1992.

Laaksonen, R., Fogelholm, M., Himberg, J.J., Laakso, J., and Salorinne, Y., Ubiquinone supplementation and exercise capacity in trained young and older men, *Eur. J. Appl. Physiol.*, 72(1-2), 95–100, 1995.

Porter, D.A., Costill, D.L., Zachwieja, J.J., Fink, W.J., Wagner, E., and Folkers, K., The effect of oral coenzyme Q10 on the exercise tolerance of middle-aged, untrained men, *Int. J. Sports. Med.*, 16(7), 421–427, 1995.

Weston, S.B., Zhou, S., Weatherby, R.P., and Robson, S.J., Does exogenous coenzyme Q10 affect aerobic capacity in endurance athletes?, *Int. J. Sport Nutr.*, 7(3), 197–206, 1997.

Vasankari, T.J., Kujala, U.M., Vasankari, T.M., Vuorimaa, T., and Ahotupa, M., Increased serum and low-density-lipoprotein antioxidant potential after antioxidant supplementation in endurance athletes, *Am. J. Clin. Nutr.*, 65(4), 1052–1056, 1997.

Faff J. and Frankiewicz-Jozko, A., Effect of ubiquinone on exercise-induced lipid peroxidation in rat tissue, *Eur. J. Applied Physiol.*, 75(5), 413–417, 1997.

Ylikoski, T., Piirainen, J., Hanninen, O., and Penttinen, J., The effect of coenzyme Q10 on the exercise performance of cross-country skiers, *Mol. Aspects Med.*, 18(Suppl.), S283–S290, 1997.

Sojo, A.M. and Mortensen, S.A., Treatment of chronic cardiac insufficiency with coenzyme Q10, results of meta-analysis in controlled clinical trials, *Ugeskr. Laegr.*, 159(49), 7302, 1997.

Sinatra, S.T., Coenzyme Q10: a vital therapeutic nutrient for the heart with special application in congestive heart failure, *Conn. Med.*, 61(11), 707, 1997

Hofman-Bang, C., Rehnqvist, N., Swedberg, K., Wiklund, I., and Astrom., Coenzyme Q10 as an adjunctive in the treatment of chronic congestive heart failure. The Q10 Study Group, *J. Card. Fail*, 1(2), 101, 1995.

DHEA

Labrie F., Intracrinology. *Moll. Cell. Endocrinol.*, 78, C113–C118, 1991.

Labrie F., DuPont A., and Belanger A., Complete androgen blockage for the treatment of prostate cancer, in *Important Advances in Oncology*, de Vita, V.T., Hellman, S., and Rosenberg, S.A., Eds, J.B. Lippincott, Philadelphia, 1985, 193–217.

Labrie, C., Belanger, A., and Labrie F., Androgenic activity of dehydroepiandrosterone and androsterenedione in the rat ventral prostrate, *Endocrinology*, 123, 1412–1417, 1988.

Migeon, C.J., Keller, A.R., Lawrence, B., and Shepart, T.H., II, Dehydroepiandrosterone and adndrosterone levels in human placenta: effect of age and sex: day-to-day and diurnal variations, *J. Clin. Endocrinol. Metabol.*, 17, 1051–1062, 1957.

Orentreich, N., Brind, J.L., Rizer, R.L., and Vogelman, J.H., Age changes and sex differences in serum dehydroepiandrosterone sulfate concentrations throughout adulthood, *J. Clin. Endocrinol. Metab.*, 59, 551–555, 1984.

Vermeulen, A., Deslypene, J.P., Schelthout, W., Verdonck, L., and Rubens, R., Adrenocortical function in old age: response of acute adrenocorticotropin stimulation, *J. Clin. Endocrinol. Metab.*, 54, 187–191, 1982.

Barrett-Conner, E., Khaw, K.T., and Yen, S.S.C., A prospective study of dehydroepiandrosterone sulfate, mortality and cardiovascular disease, *N. Eng. J. Med.*, 315, 1519–1524, 1986.

Zumff, B., Levin, J., Rosenfeld, R.S., Markham, M., Strain, G.W., and Fukushima, D.K., Abnormal 24-hr mean plasma concentrations of dehydroepiandrosterone and dehydroisoandrosterone sulfate in women with primary operable breast cancer, *Cancer Res.*, 41, 3360–3363, 1981.

Stahl, F., Schnorr, D., Pilz, C., and Dorner, G., Dehydroepiandrosterone (DHEA) levels in patients with prostatic cancer, heart diseases and under surgery stress, *Exp. Clin. Endocrinol.*, 99, 68–70, 1992.

Neville, A.M. and O'Hare M.J., The Human Adrenal Cortex. *Pathology and Biology—An Integrated Approach*, Springer-Verlag, Berlin, 1982.

Murray, R.K., Granner, D.K., Mayes, P.A., and Rodwell, V.W., *Harper's Biochemistry*. Appleton & Lange, San Mateo, CA, 1988.

Dunn, J.F., Nisula B.C., and Rodbard D., Transport of steroid hormones: binding of 21 endogenous steroids to both testosterone-binding globulin and corticosteroid-binding globulin in human plasma, *J. Clin. Endocrinol. Metab.*, 53, 58–68, 1981.

Plager, J.E., The binding of androsterone sulfate, etiocholanolone sulfate, and dehydroisoandrosterone sulfate by human plasma protein, *J. Clin. Invest.*, 44, 1234–1239, 1965.

Wang D. and Bulbrook, R.D., Binding of the sulfate esters of dehydroepiandrosterone, testosterone, 17-acetoxypregnenolone and pregnenolone in the plasma of man, rabbit, and rat, *J. Endocrinol.*, 39, 405–413, 1967.

Kellie, A.E. and Smith, E.R., Renal clearence of 17-oxo steroid conjugates found in human peripheral plasma, *Biochem. J.*, 66, 490–495, 1957.

Belenger, A., Brochu, M., and Clinche J. Levels of plasma steroid glucoronides in intact and castrasted men with prostatic cancer, *J. Clin. Encrinol. Metabol.*, 62, 812–815, 1986.

Labrie, F., Belanger, A., DuPont, A., Luu-The, V., Simard, J., and Labrie, C. Science behind total androgen blockade: fron gene to combination therapy, *Clin. Invest. Med.*, 16, 487–504, 1993.

Moghissi, E., Ablan, F., and Horton, R., Origin of plasma androstanediol glucuronide in men, *J. Clin. Endocrinol. Metab.*, 59, 417–421, 1984.

Orentreich, N., Brind, J.L., Rizer, R.L., and Vogelman, J.H., Age changes and sex differences in serum dehydroepiandrosterone sulfate concentrations throughout adulthood, *J. Clin. Endocrinol. Metab.*, 59, 551–555, 1984.

Vermeulen, A., Deslypene, J.P., Schelthout, W., Verdonck, L., and Rubens, R., Adrenocortical function in old age: response of acute adrenocorticotropin stimulation, *J. Clin. Endocrinol. Metab.*, 54, 187–191, 1982.

Yen, S.S.C., Morales, A.J., and Khorram, O., Replacement of DHEA in aging men and women: Potential remedial effects, *Ann. N.Y. Acad. Sci.*, 774, 128, 1995.

Echinacea

McGuffin, M., Hobbs, C., Upton, R., and Goldberg, A., *American Herbal Products Association's Botanical Safety Handbook*, CRC Press, Boca Raton, FL, 1997.

Leuttig, B., Steimuller, C., Gifford, G.E., Wagner, H., and Lohmann, M.L., Macrophage activation by the polysaccharide arabinogalactan isolated from plant cell cultures of *Echinacea purpurea*, *J. Natl Cancer Inst.*, 81(9), 669–675, 1989.

Stimpel, M., Proksch, A., Wagner, H., and Lohmann, M.L., Macrophage activation and induction of macrophage cytotoxicity by purified polysaccharide fractions from the plant *Echinacea purpurea*, *Infect. Immun.*, 46(3), 845–849, 1984.

Mengs, U., Clare, C.B., and Poiley, J.A., Toxicity of echinacea purpurea. Acute, subacute and geno-toxicity studies, *Arzneimittelforschung*, 41(10), 1076–81 (Abst.), 1991.

Flavonoids

Kanner, J., Frankel, E., and Granit, E., Natural anti-oxidants in grapes and wines, *J. Agric. Food Chem.*, 42, 64–69, 1994.

Hertog, M.G.L., Feskens, E.J.M., Hollman, P.C.H., Katan, M.B., and Kromhout, D., Dietary antioxidant flavonoids and risk of coronary heart disease, *Lancet*, 342, 1007–1011, 1993.

Demrow, H.S., Slane, P.R., and Folts, J.D., Administration of wine and grape juice inhibits in vivo platelet activity and thrombosis in stenosed canine coronary arteries, *Circulation*, 91, 1182–1188, 1995.

Kinsella, J.E., Frankel, E., German, B., and Kanner, J., Possible mechanisms for the protective role of antioxidants in wine and plant foods, *Food Tech.*, 47, 85–89, 1993.

Ginger

McGuffin, M., Hobbs, C., Upton, R., and Goldberg, A., *American Herbal Products Association's Botanical Safety Handbook*, CRC Press, Boca Raton, FL, 1997.

Lindahl, O. and Lindwall, L., Double blind study of a valerian preparation, *Pharmacol. Biochem. Behav.*, 32(4), 1065–1066, 1989.

Bos, R., Woerrdenbag, H.J., DeSmet, P.A.G.M., and Scheffer, J.J.C., *Adverse Effects of Herbal Drugs*, Springer, Berlin, 1997.

Fischer, W., Kjaaer, S.K., Dahl, C., and Asping, U., Ginger treatment of hyperemesis gravidarum, *Eur. J. Obstet. Gynecol. Reprod. Biol.*, 38(1), 19–24, 1991.

Aikins, P., Alternative therapies for nausea and vomiting of pregnancy, *Obstet. Gynecol.*, 91(1), 149–55, 1998.

Gingko

Woerdenbag, H.J. and Van Beek, T.A., *Ginkgo Biloba*, in *Adverse Effects of Herbal Drugs*, DeSmet, P.A.G.M. et al., Eds., Spinger-Verlag, Berlin, 1997.

Hosford, D. et al., Natural antagonists of platelet-activating factor, *Phytother. Res.*, 2, 1–24, 1988.

Braquet, P., The ginkgolides: potent platelet-activating factor antagonists isolated from *Ginkgo biloba* L., chemistry, pharmacology and clinical applications, *Drugs Future*, 12, 643–699, 1987.

Sticher, O., Quality of *Ginkgo* preparations, *Planta Med.*, 59, 2–11, 1992.

Wichtl, M., Pflanzliche Geriatrika, *Dtsch. Apoth. Ztg.*, 132, 1569–76, 1992.

Tang, W. and Eisenbrand, W., *Ginkgo biloba* L., *Chinese Drugs of Plant Origin*, Springer-Verlag, Berlin, 555–565, 1992.

Glycerol

Lyons, T. et al., Effects of glycerol-induced hyperhydration prior to exercise in the heat on sweating and core temperature, *Med. Sci. Sports Exer.*, 22, 477–483, 1990.

Monter, P. et al., Glycerol, hyperhydration and endurance exercise, *Med. Sci. Sports Exer.*, 24, S157, 1992.

Sawka, M. et al., Total body water (TBW), extracellular fluid (ECF), and plasma responses to hyperhydration with aqueous glycerol, *Med. Sci. Sports Exer.*, 25, S:35, 1993.

Hydroxymethyl Butyric Acid (HMB)

Nissen, S., Sharp, R., Ray, M., Rathmacher, J.A., Rice, D., Fuller, J.C., Connelly, A.S., and Abumrad, N., Effect of leucine metabolite β-hydroxy-β-methylbutyrate on muscle metabolism during resistance training, *J. Appl. Phys.*, 81, 2095–2104, 1996.

Laetrile

Moertel, C. et al., A clinical trial of amygdalin (laetrile) in the treatment of human cancer. *N. Eng. J. Med.*, 306, 4201–4206, 1982.

Hall, et al., Cyanide poisoning from laetrile ingestion: role of nitrate therapy, *Pediatrics*, 78(2), 269–72, 1986.

Leor, R. et al., Laetrile intoxication and hepatic necrosis: a possible association, *South. Med J.*, 79(2), 259–60, 1986.

American Cancer Society, Laetrile — The Official View: Unproven remedies, Web site: http://www.livelinks.com/sumeria/canc/anti.html, 1997.

Licorice

Woerdenbag, H.J. and Van Beek, T.A., *Ginkgo Biloba*, in *Adverse Effects of Herbal Drugs*, DeSmet, P.A.G.M., et al., Eds., Springer-Verlag, Berlin, 1997.

Leung, A.Y., *Encyclopedia of Common Natural Ingedients Used in Food, Drugs, and Cosmetics*, Wiley Interscience, Glen Rock, NJ, 1980, 220–223.

Morton, J.F., Major Medicinal Plants: Botany, Culture, and Uses, Charles J. Thomas, Springfield, IL, 1977, 154–158.

Der Marderosian, A.H. and Liberti, L.E., *Natural Product Medicine*, George F. Strickley, Philadelphia, 1998 317–321.

Pyruvate

Stanko, R.T. et al., Body composition, energy utilization, and nitrogen metabolism with a 4.25 MJ/d low-energy diet supplemented with pyruvate, *Am. J. Clin. Nutr.*, 56, 630–5, 1992.

Stanko, R.T. et al., Pyruvate supplementation of a low-cholesterol, low fat diet: effects on plasma lipid concentrations and body composition in hyperlipidemic patients, *Am. J. Clin. Nutr.*, 59, 423–7, 1994.

Stanko, R.T. and Arch J.E., Inhibition of regain in body weight and fat with addition of 3-carbon compounds to the diet with hyperenergetic refeeding after weight reduction, *Int. J. Obes. Related Metab. Disord.*, Oct 20 (10), 925–930, 1996.

Saw Palmetto

DeFelice, S.L., *Nutraceuticals: Developing, Claiming, and Marketing Medical Foods,* Marcel Dekker, New York, 1998.

McGuffin, M., Hobbs, C., Upton, R., and Goldberg, A., *American Herbal Products Association's Botanical Safety Handbook*, CRC Press, Boca Raton, FL, 1997.

Vahlensieck, W. Jr., Volp, A., Lubos, W., and Kuntze, M., Benign prostatic hyperplasia-treatment with sabal fruit extract. A treatment study of 1,334 patients, *Fortschr. Med.*, 111(18), 323–326, Abstr., 1993.

Champault, G., Patel, J.C., and Bonnard, A.M.L., A double blind trial of an extract of the plant *Serona repens* in benign prostatic hyperplasia, Br. J. Clin. Pharmacol., 18, 461–462, 1984.

Soybeans

Messina, M.J., Persky, V., Setchell, K.D., and Barnes, S., Soy intake and cancer risk: a review of the in vitro and in vivo data, *Nutr. Cancer,* 21(2), 113–131, 1994.

Kennedy, A.R., The evidence for soybean products as cancer preventive agents, *J. Nutr.*, (125), 733S–743S, 1995.

St. Clair, W. et al., Suppression of DMH-induced cancinogenesis in mice by dietary addition of the Bowman-Birk protease inhibitor, *Cancer Res.*, 50, 580–586, 1990.

St. John's Wort

McGuffin, M., Hobbs, C., Upton, R., and Goldberg, A., *American Herbal Products Association's Botanical Safety Handbook*, CRC Press, Boca Raton, FL, 1997.

Volz, H.P., Controlled clinical trials of hypericum extracts in depressed patients-an overview, *Pharmacopsychiatry,* 30 (Suppl. 2), 72–76 (Abstr.), 1997.

Teufel, R. and Gleitz, J., Effects of long-term administration of hypericum extracts on the affinity and density of the central serotonergic 5-HT1 A and 5-HT2 A receptors, *Pharmacopsychiatry,* 30 (Suppl. 2), 113–116, 1997.

Ernst, E., St. John's wort as antidepressive therapy, *Fortchr. Med.*, 113(25), 354–355 (Abstr.), 1995.

Linde, K., Ramirez, G., Mulrow, C.D., Pauls, A., Weidenhammer, W., and Melchart, D., St John's wort for depression — an overview and meta-analysis of randomised clinical trials, *B.M.J.*, 313(7052), 253–258, 1996.

Oztruk, Y., Testing the antidepressant effects of Hypericum species on animal models, *Pharmacopsychiatry,* 30 (Suppl. 2), 125–128, 1997.

Schmidt, Y. and Sommer, H., St. John's wort extract in the ambulatory therapy of depression. Attention and reaction ability are preserved, *Fortchr. Med.*, 111(19), 339–342 (Abstr.), 1993.

Vanadium

Nielsen, F.H., Other trace elements, in Ziegler, E.E. and Filer, L.J., Jr., Eds., *Present Knowledge in Nutrition*, 7th ed., International Life Sciences Institute, Washington, D.C., 1996.

Food and Nutrition Board, National Research Council, *Recommended Dietary Allowances*, 10th ed., National Academy Press, Washington, 1989.

Fawcett, J.P., Farquhar, S.J., Walker, R.J., Thou, T., Lowe, G., and Goulding, A., The effect of oral vandyl sulfate on body composition and performance in weight-training athletes, *Int. J. Sport Nutr.*, 6 (4), 382–390, 1996.

Valerian

McGuffin, M., Hobbs, C., Upton, R., and Goldberg, A., *American Herbal Products Association's Botanical Safety Handbook*, CRC Press, Boca Raton, FL, 1997.
Lindahl, O. and Lindwall, L., Double blind study of a valerian preparation, *Pharmacol. Biochem. Behav.*, 32(4), 1065–1066, 1989.
Schultz, H., Stolz, C., and Muller, J., The effect of valerian extract on sleep polygraphy in poor sleepers: a pilot study, *Pharmacopsychiatry*, 27(4), 147–151, 1994.
Bos, R., Woerrdenbag, H.J., DeSmet, P.A.G.M., and Scheffer, J.J.C., *Adverse Effects of Herbal Drugs*, Springer, Berlin, 1997.

Yohimbe

Riley, A.J., Yohimbine in the treatment of erectile disorder, *Br. J. Clin. Pract.*, 48(3), 133–136, 1994.
Hollander, E. and McCarley, A., Yohimbine treatment of sexual side effects induced by serotonin reuptake blockers, *J. Clin. Psychiatry*, 53(6), 207–209, 1992.
Sonda, L.P., Mazo, R., and Chancellor, M.B., The role of yohimbine for the treatment of erectile impotence, *J. Sex Marital Ther.*, 16(1), 15–21, 1990.

15

Nutrition and Human Reproduction

Pregnancy

While the greater part of this text discusses nutrition as it stems from personal consumption, this chapter begins by addressing points in the life-span of humans in which they are directly reliant upon the nutritional status and provision of nutrients by another human. During pregnancy, the developing embryo and fetus is nourished exclusively by way of the fetal circulation, which in essence is a placenta-modified extension of the maternal circulation.

Ovulation culminates with the expulsion of an ovum, along with attached cells into one of the fallopian tubes. Fertilization by sperm must take place shortly thereafter within the fallopian tube. The fertilized ovum, or zygote, then navigates the remainder of the tube and reaches the uterus. This journey takes about 3 days and is characterized by a series of cell divisions. The earlier divisions are centralized, creating the *morula*. The subsequent divisions promote the creation of a central cavity. This stage is now called a blastocyst and the created cavity is called the blastocyst cavity. The blastocyst will then implant itself within the endometrium within roughly 4 to 5 days after conception. Once implanted in the endometrium, the nutritional requirements of the blastocyst are initially met by endometrial secretions. These secretions will continue to help provide nutritional factors for the next 2 to 3 months as the placental and embryonic vasculatures develop.

Proliferating cells from both the implanted blastocyst, now called an embryo, and the endometrium develop into the early placenta. As early as 16 d postconception, circulation begins. This serves as the mechanism of exchange between maternal blood and now embryonic blood in the placenta. An amniotic sac develops to contain the embryo and bath it with amniotic fluid. The primary role of the placenta is to provide a site of exchange between maternal blood and embryonic/fetal blood. Oxygen and nutrients are derived from maternal blood, while urea, CO_2, and other fetal waste products enter the maternal blood. Factors such as amino acids, ascorbic acid, phosphate, and calcium are actively absorbed at the placenta. Some nutrients reaching the fetal circulation are actually derived from storage in the placenta as well. Therefore the placenta is a temporary organ, providing both regulatory and storage functions.

During pregnancy, most women will experience a weight gain of 11 to 16 kg (25 to 35 lb), and the uterus expands 150-fold. Of the weight gain, about 40% is attributable to the fetus, placenta, and amniotic fluid. The remaining 60% is attributable to maternal weight gain, which will include increased fluid volume, protein, and fat deposition. Maternal cardiac and renal mass will increase in conjunction with a 45 to 50% increase in blood volume. Blood components become diluted during pregnancy. Densitometric estimates of body composition changes during pregnancy show that body fat increases 2 to 8%. Physiologically, cardiac output increases 30 to 50% as both heart rate and stroke volume increase. Also, increased tidal volume (volume of gas exchange/breath), increased renal perfusion and glomerular filtration rate, and increased appetite and absorption of nutrients occur during pregnancy.

The embryonic period occurs during the first 8 weeks of pregnancy. Human growth during this time is largely the result of hyperplasia. Organs begin to develop, and at this time the human form is exceptionally sensitive to teratogenic substances. The remaining 7 months of pregnancy are called the fetal period. Hyperplasia continues during this period and will continue in most organs after birth. Hypertrophy of cells compliments hyperplasia, and during this period the need, both quality and quantity, for nutrients is very high. At term a healthy infant will weigh about 3.4 kg (7.5 lb) and be about 51 cm (20 in) long.

Energy

The energetic cost of pregnancy is high. Extra energy is needed not only to fuel the growth and development of maternal and embyo/fetal tissue, but also to fuel the increased maternal physiological work to support fetal growth. Maternal basal metabolism increases by about 25%. The total energy cost during pregnancy can range from 40,000 to 110,000 kcal. The recommendations made by the National Research Council are based upon an estimated 80,000 kcal energy expenditure for a woman experiencing a 12.5 kg (27.5 lb) weight gain giving birth to an infant weighing 3.3 kg (7.5 lb). As normal pregnancy may last approximately 250 d, the average increased energy requirement is approximately 300 kcal/d (80,000 kcal/250 d). There appears to be a relationship between prepregancy (pregravid) body weight and weight gain during pregnancy and mortality during pregnancy. For underweight women who become pregnant, perinatal mortality rates decrease as the women experience greater weight gains. For example, women who are underweight prior to pregnancy and only gain about 4.5 kg (~10 lb) have approximately a 5 times greater associated perinatal mortality rate in comparison to similar women who gain 13 to 14 kg (30 lb). A gain of 9 kg (~20 lb) during pregnancy is associated with double the perinatal mortality rate of the women gaining 13 to 14 kg.

On the other hand, the perinatal mortality rate decreases for women who are overweight (>135% of Metropolitan Life Weight to Height figure) prior to pregnancy and only gain 7 kg of body weight. Greater weight gains during pregnancy for overweight women increases the likelihood of a higher birth weight and of prolonged labor and complications in delivery.

Protein

Protein needs are increased during pregnancy. The extra protein is needed for the development of new maternal tissue such as the placenta and the expansion of the uterus, breasts, and blood volume, as well as the development of fetal tissue. The total protein requirement for a typical pregnancy is approximately 925 g, or an additional 8.5 g of protein per day at peak requirement during pregnancy. To accommodate the extra need, 10 g have been added to the RDA during pregnancy, which then is approximately 56 to 60 g. In the U.S., the average protein intake of women is estimated at 75 to 110 g/d, so it is likely that protein needs are met for most American women without significant dietary changes.

Vitamins

Requirements are augmented for several vitamins during pregnancy; however, there is also some concern for overconsumption of certain vitamins as well. Vitamin A is necessary for embyogenesis and tissue differentiation. There is a significant transfer of vitamin A between the mother and the fetus, and total fetal vitamin A needs can be met by mobilizing as little as 10% of typical stores of a well-nourished mother. However, low maternal status of vitamin A is associated with preterm birth and intrauterine growth retardation.

Ingestion of excessive amounts of vitamin A can have deleterious effects during pregnancy. The resulting toxicity is typically not associated with food choices but with ingestion of excessive amounts of supplemental vitamin A or pharmacological doses of the vitamin A analog *isotretinoin* (Accutane). Ingestion of isotretinoin, which is used in the treatment of cystic acne, in the early months of pregnancy, can lead to spontaneous abortion and major congenital defects. While most tissue is susceptible to toxicity, the CNS and cardiovascular system are extremely sensitive. Facial anomalies, especially in the regions of the ears and palate, are among the most common external signs of fetal isotretinoin toxicity. Similar anomalies have resulted from supplemental doses of vitamin A of 20,000 to 50,000 IU. Vitamin A derived from dietary carotenoids does not seem to carry such a toxic concern.

The RDA level for vitamin D during pregnancy is 10 µg. This is already the RDA for women under the age of 24 and is an increase from 5 µg for women over the age of 24. The biologically active form of vitamin D, 1,25-dihydroxycholecalciferol, is elevated in the maternal circulation during pregnancy and is able to traverse the placenta and enter the fetal circulation. Deficiency of vitamin D during pregnancy raises concerns for both the developing embryo/fetus and the mother. Neonatal hypocalcemia and tetany, infant hypoplasia of tooth enamel, and maternal osteomalacia are potential results.

Interestingly, pregnant women often exhibit lower plasma levels of pyridoxal phosphate (PLP), the primary active form of vitamin B_6. While the placental transport system for PLP remains unclear at present, the fetal circulation typically demonstrates higher concentrations than the maternal circulation. As no measurable indications of a vitamin B_6 deficiency have been reported in maternal and fetal operations, the reduced maternal vitamin B_6 status during pregnancy is not viewed as critical. The RDA for pregnant women is 2.2 mg/d. Supplemental vitamin B_6 is recommended for those women at risk for inadequate intake (i.e., pregnant adolescents, substance abusers, and women bearing twins).

Maternal folate deficiency is associated with several pregnancy-related anomalies including low birth weight infants, abruptio placentae, and developmental neural tube defects. Like vitamin B_6, the concentration of folate in the fetal blood is typically greater than in the maternal blood. Also, like vitamin B_6, the mechanisms involved in placental transfer of folate are unknown. However, several folate binding proteins have been identified in placental tissue and may serve as membrane receptors for folate. Based upon metabolic turnover evaluation, dietary folate needs during pregnancy have been estimated at 280, 660, and 470 µg/d in the 1st, 2nd, and 3rd trimesters, respectively. Folate deficiency-related megaloblastic anemia during pregnancy is fairly common in developing countries, and folate supplementation is associated with a decreased incidence of low birth weight deliveries and neural tube defects. Periconception folate consumption of 400 µg/d is believed to be an effective level to greatly reduce the occurrence of neural tube defect. However, in many countries the folate consumption of women is below these recommendations. For example, the average folate intake of American women of reproductive age is about 200 to 250µg. In efforts to increase the folate intake of women of reproductive age, the U.S. Food and Drug Administration (FDA) has proposed that additional folate be added to enriched grain products.

Minerals

The metabolism of the major element calcium is significantly altered during pregnancy. Maternal calcium absorption and retention are both increased as circulatory levels of active vitamin D are augmented. However, the level of parathyroid hormone (PTH) in the blood generally does not change. Calcium is translocated across the placenta by an energy-dependent mechanism as it is moving against a concentrational gradient. It has been estimated that the embryo/fetus accumulates about 30 g of calcium throughout its development. The RDA for calcium during pregnancy is 1200 mg, which is also the non-pregnant RDA for younger women and 400 mg above the RDA for women over 25 years of age.

The total iron needs during pregnancy have been estimated at 1040 mg. After delivery, about 200 mg are retained by the mother as the blood volume decreases. During pregnancy and delivery about 840 mg are lost in the formation of the placenta, the development of the embryo/fetus, and hemorrhagic loss during delivery. Iron absorption is increased two- to threefold to meet the increased needs during pregnancy. The RDA for women is increased 15 to 30 mg/d.

Iron-deficiency anemia in early pregnancy is associated with prematurity and low birth weight deliveries. Iron deficiency anemia is still one of the most prevalent nutrition-based disorders, even in developed countries such as the U.S. In the U.S. it has been estimated that 4 to 10% of women of reproductive age present iron deficiency anemia. This is especially a concern for low-income women. Data collected by the Pregnancy Nutrition Surveillance of the Centers for Disease Control and Prevention show that 10%, 14%, and 33% of pregnant women are iron-deficiency anemic during their 1st, 2nd, and 3rd trimesters, respectively.

The concentration of zinc in fetal blood is about 1.5 times greater than maternal circulation. Maternal zinc level decreases during pregnancy and is only approximately 35% below the concentration of age-matched nonpregnant women at term. The transfer of zinc increases throughout pregnancy and reaches a rate of approximately 0.6 to 0.8 mg/d. Pregnant women achieve zinc balance by consuming greater than 9 mg/d. Zinc supplements are recommended for women who typically consume inadequate amounts of zinc or who are at greater risk for reproductive anomalies. Women falling into the latter category include heavy tobacco smokers, drug users, and women carrying multiple fetuses. The RDA for zinc is increased from 12 to 15 mg during pregnancy.

Alcohol

Excessive alcohol consumption during pregnancy increases the risk of fetal alcohol syndrome. Fetal alcohol syndrome is a pattern of malformations that include perinatal and postnatal growth retardation, facial anomalies, physical defects at birth, and abnormalities of the CNS. The incidence of fetal alcohol syndrome in women who consume 1.5 to 8 drinks per week and >8 drinks per week is 10% and 30 to 40%, respectively. Here a "drink" is defined as a 355 ml (12 oz) of beer, 148 ml (5 oz) of wine, or 44 ml (1.5 oz) of 80-proof distilled spirits. These quantities of alcohol beverages contain approximately 17 g of alcohol. While infrequent and limited consumption of alcohol during pregnancy is generally believed to be benign, scientists are unsure as to the threshold for deleterious effects, and suspect that it is probably individualized.

Caffeine

While teratogenic effects of caffeine consumption during pregnancy have been demonstrated in animal studies, a similar response has not been found in humans. However, in humans, higher intakes (>300 mg/d) have been associated with low birth weight at delivery. Therefore pregnant women are advised to keep caffeine consumption below 300 mg/d. A typical cup of brewed coffee (240 ml) contains approximately 125 mg, while instant coffee has about 90 mg, cocoa or hot chocolate 25 m, and cola soda about 50 mg.

Lactation

Lactation is a period of time when a woman is producing breast milk. After birth, circulatory levels of estrogen and progesterone are decreased while prolactin levels remain elevated. This results in the release of milk or *lactogenesis*. Female breasts begin to develop during puberty and undergo further growth and development during pregnancy. The initiation of lactogenesis is indeed hormone related; however, stimulation by infant suckling or other means must be provided within the first few days for the continuation of the process.

The composition of breast milk changes not only from the onset of lactogenesis though the days that follow, but also within a single feeding as well. *Colostrum* is the earliest form of breast milk. Colostrum is a yellowish and relatively viscous solution consisting of a variety of dissolved or suspended substances such as electrolytes and immune factors. It is also higher in protein and lower in fat in comparison to breast milk produced after 1 month. The immune factors help protect the neonate against bacterial and viral factors. Colostrum factors facilitate the passage of an infants first stool (meconium) and contains *Lactobacillus bifidus* which promotes the formation of colonic bifidus bacteria which are believed to have protective properties. Over the first 2 weeks of lactation, breast milk gradually loses many of the characteristics of colostrum, thereby making the conversion from colostrum to *mature breast milk*. The protein content remains high for the first 4 weeks or so. The caloric density of colostrum and mature breast milk is approximately 670 and 740 kcal/l, respectively. Mature breast milk contains protein factors such as lactoferrin, lysozyme, lipase, lactalbumin, and casein; carbohydrates such as lactose and polysaccharides; and lipids such as triglycerides, and polyunsaturated fatty acids. It also contains IgM, IgG, and IgA (sigA) which are immunoglobin factors (Table 15.1).

Energy Demands of Lactation

The energy demands during lactation are greater than during preganancy. This is largely attributable to the rapid growth experienced by the infant. For instance, a newborn infant will double its weight within 6 months and it is estimated the breast milk consumed during the first 4 months alone is energetically equivalent to the total energy requirements of pregnancy. While some of the energy in breast milk is derived from maternal stores, primarily developed during pregnancy, this cannot underscore the huge energy demands during lactation. For instance, it is estimated that the percentage increase in energy demands is about 23% during lactation over a nonpregnant, nonlactating woman. Comparatively, pregnancy only increases the total energy demand by about 14%.

TABLE 15.1

Major Components of Human Breast Milk and Their Function and Considerations

Component	Function
Whey	Energy source (α-lactalbumin predominant protein)
Caesein	Energy source (low content relative to cow's milk); carrier of Ca, Fe, Zn, Cu, and phosphate
Polyunsaturated Fatty Acids	Development of tissue
Immunoglobulins (IgA, IgM, IgE, IgG, EgD)	Protection against bacterial and virus infection
Bifidus factor	Promotes formation of healthy bacterial colonization in infant's lower gastrointestinal tract
Lactoferrin	Iron-binding protein that reduces the availability of iron to bacteria in the gastrointestinal tract
Lactoperoxidase	Destroys bacteria
Lysozyme	Kills bacteria by destroying the cell wall
Macrophages	Destroy bacteria by phagocytosis; synthesize lactoferrin and lyzozyme
Vitamin B_{12}-binding protein	Decreases vitamin B_{12} availability for growth of bacteria
Interferon	Interferes with viral replication in host cells
Lymphocytes	Synthesize IgA
Antistaphylococcus factor	Inhibits the growth of staphylococcal bacteria

Variations in Nutrient Content and the Influence of Nutritional Status

Provided that there is some storage of certain micronutrients in infants, it is generally believed that human breast milk is nutritionally adequate for the first 4 to 6 months of an infant's life. However, after this time breast milk becomes inadequate with regard to some nutrients. As mentioned above, the composition of breast milk will vary, not only from woman to woman, but also show variations during the period of lactation (months) as well as within the same day and within the same feeding. The initial milk secreted during a feeding is often referred to as *foremilk*. On the contrary, the milk that is secreted later in a feeding is called *hindmilk*. Hindmilk tends to have a higher fat content than foremilk; thus mothers should encourage longer feeding periods such as 20 to 30 min to allow for the ingestion of the more energy-dense hindmilk.

The diet and nutritional status of the mother can certainly impact the nutrient composition of breast milk (Table 15.2). With regard to the energy nutrients, barring extremes, dietary intake does not have significant impact upon breast milk total energy or energy nutrient ratios. However, it should be recognized that the fatty acid composition of the mother's diet can influence the fatty acid profile of breast milk. On the other hand, the cholesterol, calcium, phosphate, magnesium, sodium, potassium, chloride, iron, and copper content does not seem to vary with a mother's nutritional intake. In contrast, the manganese, selenium, and iodide of breast milk are positively influenced by the mother's intake, while the fluoride content is negatively influenced. All of the vitamins appear to be positively influenced by the mother's nutritional intake and status. As intake is increased well above recommendations, only the level of vitamin B_6 is elevated in breast milk. This is also true for two minerals, selenium and iodine, as well. Oppositely, reduced intake and status of the vitamins will result in reductions in breast milk levels. One exception is folate, as its content in breast milk is maintained somewhat at the expense of maternal stores. This also appears to be true for calcium.

TABLE 15.2
Influence of Maternal Nutritional Intake on Breast Milk Components

Minimal to No Influence	Positively Influenced	Negatively Influenced
Lactose	Protein	Fluoride
Total fat	Fatty acids	
Calcium	Manganese	
Phosphorus	Selenium	
Magnesium	Iodine	
Sodium	Water-soluble vitamins	
Potassium	Fat-soluble vitamins	
Chlorine		
Zinc		
Copper		

Infancy

The period of infancy spans the period from birth to the completion of the first year. During this time, a human will experience an extremely rapid growth spurt-doubling its length and tripling its birth weight. From an anatomical and physiological standpoint, an infant also experiences a tremendous development of their organs. For a newborn infant many of these organs (i.e., lungs, digestive, and urinary tracts) will, more or less, be used for the first time. The RDAs include recommendations for infants at 0 to 6 months and for 6 to 12 months of age. With the exception of zinc and vitamin A, all recommendations are increased during the latter 6-month period.

Physical Growth

In North America, typical birth weights tend to range between 3.0 to 3.4 kg (7.0 to 7.5 lb) and the average length is about 50 cm (20 in.). A newborn infant's head may actually account for about one third of the total length. The circumference of a newborn infant's head is on average 33 to 35 cm (13 to 15 in.). Male newborns tend to be slightly heavier, longer, and have a larger head circumference than newborn females. As mentioned above, the period of infancy is characterized by extreme growth. In addition to the doubling of their length and tripling of their birth weights, infants will experience a 30% increase in their head circumference by the close of their first year of life. Figure 15.1 displays a technique for measuring an infant's length (height).

Monitoring the rate of change of these anthropometric parameters provides important information about an infant's nutritional state and overall ability to thrive. Growth charts are provided by the National Center for Health Statistics (NCHS), a federal organization. The growth charts include information for weight, length/height, and head circumference for the first 3 years of life. These charts help identify infants of low or high body weight or stature, and body weight for a given length can be used as an indicator of the development of energy stores (adipose tissue). Head circumference is used as an indicator of the development of the brain. Growth charts are provided in Appendix B.

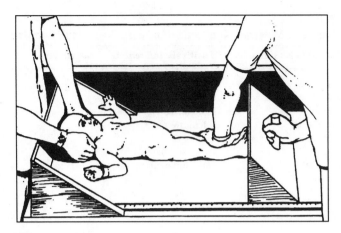

FIGURE 15.1
Measurement of an infant's length.

Energy Needs and Energy Nutrients

At no other point in human existence is the need for energy higher when expressed per unit body weight. A newborn infant may require 3 to 4 times the amount of energy per kilogram body weight in comparison to an adult. The high demand for energy is necessary to support the extreme rate growth and development. For example, a newborn infant may require 90 to 120 kcal/kg body weight, whereas an adult may only require about 30 to 40 kcal/kg for weight maintenance.

An infant's energy requirements are based upon basal metabolism, thermal effect of food, physical activity, maintenance, growth, and energy losses in the urine and feces. Basal metabolism accounts for the greatest proportion of an infant's total energy expenditure and has been estimated at 48 to 55 kcal/kg body weight per day. While the total energy expenditure (TEE) will increase during the period of infancy relative to growth, TEE when expressed per kilogram of body weight will actually decrease. Growth is perhaps the second largest energy expenditure during infancy, especially early infancy. About 4 to 6 kcal is expended per gram of tissue gained. The thermal effect of food is similar to that of adults at 5 to 10% of energy intake or about 4 to 5 kcal/kg body weight per day. While still relatively minor, the energy lost by urinary and fecal excretion is still greater than for adults.

Protein

During the first month of infant's life, the requirement for protein is higher than at any other point in the life span. It has been estimated that about 1.98 g of protein is required per kilogram body weight to allow for proper growth as well as to replace nitrogen lost in urine and feces. This requirement decreases rapidly to about 1.18 g per kilogram body weight by about 5 months of age and continues at this level till the end of infancy. The average protein intake of breast fed infants in developed countries provides about 2.04 g of protein per kilogram body weight. The RDA for infants is 2.2 g/kg body weight for the first 6 months, and then is reduced slightly to 2.0 g/kg body weight for the second 6 months of infancy. An infant's diet providing at least 6.5% of its energy from protein, primarily breast milk, will meet its protein needs for normal growth and development. Furthermore, consumption of protein in higher amounts will not enhance growth. An infant requires nine essential amino acids (Table 6.1). In addition, three other amino acids, namely, tyrosine, taurine, and cysteine, have been suggested to be conditionally essential. In early infancy the conversions of phenylalanine to tyrosine as well as methionine to cysteine are not developed. The latter process, catalyzed by the enzyme cystathionase, does not fully develop until about 4 months of age. Conversely, the conversion of phenylalanine to tyrosine via phenylalanine hydroxylase pathway is mature at the onset of infancy. Therefore, it is still not clear as to why the need for tyrosine is increased during early infancy.

Carbohydrate

Carbohydrate is a major energy contributor during infancy. Breast feeding and the consumption of cow's milk-based formula assures that lactose will be the primary carbohydrate in the diet, at least in the first half of infancy. As infants begin to eat more solid foods, such as infant cereals, vegetables, and fruits, the percentage of energy derived from carbohydrates can increase while the contribution from fat will decrease. It is estimated that at least 5 g of carbohydrate per kilogram body weight is necessary to prevent ketosis in an infant.

Fat and Fatty Acids

Whether it is more beneficial or healthier to provide the energy primarily in the form of carbohydrate or fat is still a matter of debate. The general recommendations for energy nutrients begin after the age of 2. These recommendations, as stated by the American Heart Association and the American Dietetics Association, are to reduce total fat to less than 30% of total energy. It seems that as little as 0.5 to 1.0 g of linoleic acid per kilogram body weight (and a smaller amount of linolenic acid) is needed to prevent essential fatty acid deficiency. While more than one half of the energy in breast milk is derived from fat, human milk in comparison to cow's milk is a better source of both ω-3 and ω-6 polyunsaturated fatty acids. Combined, these essential fatty acids account for about 5 to 6% of the energy in breast milk.

Vitamins and Minerals

The consumption of 700 to 800 ml of breast milk provides an infant with about twice the RDA for vitamin A along with a compliment of carotenoids. On the other hand, consuming the same quantity of breast milk will not allow the acquisition of the RDA for vitamin D. Thus, the American Academy of Pediatrics recommends a vitamin D supplement for infants fed breast milk exclusively. Also, breast milk is not a good source of vitamin K and it will require a couple of months to develop a healthy microbial population in an infant's colon as the digestive tract is sterile at birth. With these facts in mind, an intramuscular injection of vitamin K is routinely provided as a prophylactic measure for newborns. Folate and vitamin B_{12} are extremely important during the first year of life. While an infant's folate stores are somewhat limited at birth, adequate consumption of breast milk, as well as cow's milk-based formulas, will provide at least the minimum requirements for folate, as well as vitamin B_{12}.

It is thought that a human fetus has the potential to acquire sufficient iron stores in the last weeks of gestation to help support the limited supply of iron in breast milk in meeting an infant's needs during the first 4 to 6 months after birth. However, as iron storage status can certainly vary among infants, and intestinal iron absorption is also variable, iron deficiency remains as one of the most common nutrition problems in this population. As the iron content of breast milk is relatively low, iron fortification of infant formulas and foods is very common at present. Zinc stores are moderate in the newborn infant. Therefore, adequate zinc provision for a breast-fed infant, for at the least the first half of infancy, is a combination of breast milk zinc and acquisition from stores.

Progression to Solid Foods

The transition to solid foods should begin when the infant is ready, not necessarily when the feeder is ready. Infants present physical signs when they are prepared for solid foods. One of these signs is a relaxation of the *gag reflex*. The gag reflex propels undesirable items forward and out of the mouth. This reflex is strongest in infants and is still maintained to some degree throughout life. Relaxation of the gag reflex allows an infant to swallow foods of a more solid consistency, such as cereals and purees. The ability of an infant to form his or her mouth around a spoon is another sign that solid foods are becoming more appropriate.

Early in the transition to solid foods, infants do not have the hand dexterity and hand-to-mouth coordination to feed themselves. However, within the ensuing months they develop these capabilities. Also during this time, teeth begin to appear and an infant may begin to take small sips from a cup. Usually by 9 months, an infant is able to participate in a meal and may play with plates, cups, and perhaps help support a cup during a drink. By 10 months, an infant may be eating finger foods and drinking from a cup.

A typical progression of solid food introduction is as follows:

0–4 months:	Breast milk or formula
4–6 months:	Iron-fortified cereals when infant is ready while still breast or formula feeding
6–9 months:	Strained vegetables, fruits, and meats are added to cereals while still breast or formula feeding
9–12 months:	Gradual introduction to cut and mashed table foods; meats should be well cooked to minimize chewing; juice by a small cup becomes appropriate; breast or formula feeding continues.

Adverse Food Reactions

Adverse food reactions include both *food allergies* and *food intolerances*. Food allergies involve an immunologically mediated reaction to food or more specifically a component of the food. An intolerance is a physiologicial, not immunological, response to a component of a food. The most universal food intolerance is lactose intolerance, affecting most people at least to a minor degree. On the contrary, adverse food reactions of the allergic type probably occur in less than 5% of the general population.

The development of many food allergies is believed to originate during infancy or shortly thereafter. Although the digestive tract is rapidly developing during the first few months of infancy, there remains the potential for complete or semicomplete food substances, such as proteins, to be absorbed. When this occurs, the immune system recognizes the substance as foreign or an *antigen*. At the same time *immune memory* of that substance is developed for future reference. Antibodies are produced routinely specific for the antigen.

Antigens can gain access to circulation along the length of the digestive tract. In response, antibodies from all classes, especially IgA, are produced. Antibodies such as IgG will bind to receptors on mast cells, macrophages, monocytes, lymphocytes, eosinophils, and platelets. The subsequent interaction of the antigen to the bound antibody results in activity within that cell. Activities include the release of chemical mediators such as histamine, lekotrienes, and prostaglandins, and the response include vasodilation, mucus secretion, and other events of an immune response (Figure 15.2).

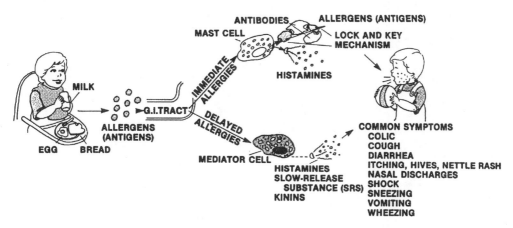

FIGURE 15.2
Events characteristic of an allergic reaction to a food component.

Typically, food allergens are water-soluble glycoproteins with a molecular weight less than 70,000 and are relatively resistant to human digestive processes. Foods that have been identified as containing allergens, thus involved in many food allergies, include peanuts, milk, soy, wheat, fish, tree nuts, and shell fish (i.e., clams, oysters, scallops, crabs, lobster, shrimp). Fish allergy is more common in adults than children. A common allergen in fish such as codfish, is *Gad c* I, which is a calcium-binding glycoprotein found in their muscle tissue. Shrimp contain an allergen functioning similarly to tropomyosin, called *Pen a* I. Chicken egg allergies, which are more common in children, may be the result of ovalabumin, ovomucoid, or ovotransferrin. Both whey and casein components of cow's milk may become allergens.

Suggested Readings

Mitchell, M.K., *Nutrition Across the Life Span*, W.B. Saunders, Philadephia, PA, 1997.

Heird, W.C., Nutrition requirments during infancy, in *Present Knowledge in Nutrition*, 7th ed., Ziegler, E.E., Ed., ILSI Press, Washington, D.C., 1996.

Picciano, M.F., Preganancy and lactation, in *Present Knowledge in Nutrition*, 7th edition,. Ziegler, E.E., Ed., ILSI Press, Washington, D.C., 1996.

16

Cardiovascular Disease and Nutrition

Despite the decline in cardiovascular disease in the U.S. and other western countries in the last 20 years, mortality from cardiovascular disease still remains the number one cause of death. The high incidence of cardiovascular disease in these societies has been blamed on the Western lifestyle, with a diet often cited as one of the most impacting factors. However, it is important to keep in mind that there are numerous types of cardiovascular disease that afflict humans and the influence of nutrition will vary in the development and treatment of these various disorders. The type of cardiovascular disease most often associated with diet is atherosclerosis, which is the build-up of lipid deposits, connective tissue proteins, and mineral complexes within the wall of coronary arteries. This build-up is often referred to as plaque and the initiation of its development can begin very early in life and progress for decades. For instance, while the complications associated with advanced atherosclerosis may not be observed until the waning decades of the human life-span, autopsies on 10- to 14-year-old children have revealed fatty streaks, which are the earliest appreciable sign of developing atherosclerosis. Thus, atherosclerosis should be viewed as a progress rather than a more acute condition.

As plaque grows in size, its thickness causes the vessel wall to expand further and further into the arterial lumen. Eventually blood flow to cardiac tissue "downstream" from the lesion is compromised, resulting in *ischemia* and potential *infarction* (tissue death). Infarction to myocardial tissue or a *myocardial infarction (MI)* is manifested in the form of a heart attack. Cerebrovascular disease may also share similar etiologies with ischemic heart disease. Here the end result would be a stroke.

Without question, the initiation and progression of an atherosclerotic lesion is strongly influenced by genetic, dietary, and behavior factors. As atherosclerotic-related cardiovascular disease is by far the most common clinical cardiac problem, it is often simply referred to as *heart disease*. Other forms of cardiovascular disease, such as hypertension, may certainly be influenced by diet. Hypertension may lead to cardiac hypertrophy and cardiac failure as well as be a significant factor in the initiation and progression of the atherosclerosis. Cardiac mitochondrial and valvular disorders also lead to cardiovascular disease; however, most of these have a genetic basis.

With respect to nutrition, the items most commonly discussed with relation to the etiology of heart disease are cholesterol, total dietary fat and fatty acid types, obesity, and salt intake. Recently, scientists have also shed light on the potential for other nutritional factors, which, when present in either excessive or deficient amounts, can deleteriously impact the cardiovascular system. These factors include iron, homocysteine, calcium, potassium and copper, as well as certain water-soluble vitamins, namely, folic acids and vitamin B_{12}.

Perhaps foremost among the considerations of risk factors for heart disease is the notion of genetics. The fact that there is a familial basis for atherosclerosis and other cardiovascular anomalies certainly needs to recognized. Quite simply, certain individuals are more prone than others to cardiovascular disease, by inherited "bad genes."

General Energy Metabolism in Myocardial Tissue

Cardiac myocytes require a tremendous amount of energy and on a continual basis. Energy, in the form of high-energy phosphate compounds, must be available to power electromechanical activity, ion pumping, and cellular maintenance. ATP and creatine phosphate are the major high energy phosphates derived from the catabolism of fatty acids, glucose, lactate, pyruvate, acetate, ketone bodies, and to a lesser degree, amino acids.

The rate at which cardiac myocytes utilize different energy substrates is directly related to their relative concentrations in the vascular and interstitial compartments, the mechanical activity of the heart, and the presence of various hormones, either released locally or circulating. Early studies overestimated the contribution of fatty acid oxidation to cardiac ATP production to be as high as 70 to 100%. Later studies suggested that the contribution of fatty acids to oxidative metabolism in on the order of 50 to 70%. The carbohydrate substrates glucose and lactate account for the majority of the remaining oxidative metabolism, with relatively minor contributions from pyruvate, β-hydroxybutyrate, and acetoacetate.

Since myocardial activity can only be sustained by anaerobic metabolism for a brief period of time, cardiac myocytes are endowed with relatively large compartments of mitochondria and a rich supply of myoglobin. In fact, mitochondria may make up almost 40% of the myocyte volume. The inner membrane of mitochondria, the site of oxidative phosphorylation, is approximately 30 times the surface area of the sarcolemma. Further attesting to the fundamental oxidative nature of myocardium is the rich capillary distribution, as a 1 mm^3 region of the left ventricular myocardium of a dog contains approximately 3500 capillaries.

As oxidative metabolic generation of ATP prevails in cardiac tissue, the primary substrates will include fatty acid-derived acetyl CoA, via mitochondrial and peroxisomal β-oxidation, and pyruvate derived from glucose and lactate catabolism. Only under extreme conditions, such as ischemia, will anaerobic glycolytic mechanisms increase, resulting in dramatic changes in substrate utilization.

Endogenous stores of carbohydrate and fatty acids are normally limited in cardiac myocytes. Carbohydrate contribution to total cardiac mass is less than 0.7%, which would also include carbohydrate moieties beyond glycogen stores. Canine cardiac tissue contains approximately 50 μmol fatty acid moieties per gram of wet tissue with the majority (85 to 90%) of the fatty acid being incorporated in the phospholipid pool, and the remaining fatty acids comprising the triglyceride pool (12%) and cholesterol esters (0.5%). A small quantity of fatty acids in cardiac tissue are of the unesterified nature (<0.1%), as the normal dog will contain on the order of 30 nmol/g wet weight. However, once the fatty acid in the extracellular compartment have been considered, the quantity of unesterified fatty acids in the cytosolic compartment has been estimated at <10 μmol/l. As the amount of cytosolic unesterified fatty acids is small and because it is uncertain whether fatty acids associated with membrane phospholipids are available for oxidation and high-energy phosphate production, it seems more likely that the endogenous source of fatty acids as a substrate for β-oxidation is almost entirely reserved for the triglyceride pool.

Beyond endogenous stores, triglyceride is also localized at various sites throughout the heart. Cardiac adipocytes are visually obvious without magnification in the vicinity of superficial epicardial coronary arteries in dogs and rats, while in humans, adipocytes are abundant in the epicardium. Additionally, some triglyceride deposition can be observed in the interstitial space as well as a limited amount in endothelial cells.

Since cardiac myocytes are limited in their ability to store energy substrates in appreciable quantities, they will require a constant perfusion of these molecules by way of coronary circulation. Glucose and lactate circulate independently, while fatty acids are found in the blood either complexed to albumin or esterified in lipoprotein triglyceride. The uptake of circulating unesterified fatty acids by cardiac tissue is very efficient, with extraction estimated as high as 70% on a single transit of blood. The uptake of lactate on a single capillary passage is about 50%, while only a minor proportion of glucose is taken up on a single passage. The uptake of glucose at a normal workload appears to be regulated by insulin. At higher workloads, glucose uptake by cardiac myocytes increases in an insulin-independent manner. Conversely, the extraction of lactate by cardiac myocytes appears to be governed by its concentration in the extracellular compartment.

Fatty acids that circulate esterified to glycerol as part of triglyceride assembled in lipoproteins, are liberated by the catalytic activity of lipoprotein lipase. Phospholipase A_1 activity also exerted by lipoprotein lipase assures exposure of the triacylglycerol-abundant core of chylomicrons and very-low-density lipoproteins. Fatty acids and monoglycerides are the primary products of cardiac lipoprotein lipase activity which are taken up by endothelial and myocardial cells and used for both anabolic and catabolic processes.

The utilization of glucose as an oxidative metabolic substrate in cardiac myocytes begins with glycolysis. Glycolysis is regulated at various steps, the most important of which include hexokinase, phosphofructokinase (PFK), glyceraldehyde 3-phosphate dehydrogenase, and pyruvate dehydrogenase. The latter of these enzyme systems would yield acetyl CoA in the mitochondrial compartment. Glucose entry into cardiac myocytes appears to be a carrier-mediated, nonenergy-dependent process that can be augmented by increased cardiac work, the presence of elevated levels of insulin, epinephrine, and growth hormone, and decreased oxidative metabolism such as during anoxia. Conversely, efficient fatty acid oxidation will lessen glucose transport into cardiac myocytes. Hexokinase is inhibited by its product, glucose 6-phosphate, which, after reversible conversion to fructose 6-phosphate by phosphoglucose isomerase, is a substrate for PFK. PFK is a major regulator for glycolysis and is impacted by cytosolic pH and allosteric factors. Its activity is stimulated by low-energy phosphates such as AMP, ADP, and inorganic phosphate, and decreased by ATP and citrate. The factors that decrease PFK activity are indeed products of fatty acid oxidation. The mitochondrial enzyme complex pyruvate kinase is not only regulated by phosphorylation/dephosphorylation, but is allosterically inhibited by the products of fatty acid oxidation (i.e., NADH and acetyl CoA) and oxidative phosphorylation (ATP).

Fatty acids, derived either from exogenous or endogenous sources, interact with a tissue-specific isoform of fatty acid-binding protein (FABP). The heart-type FABP has been reported to be a relatively small protein (15 kDa), however, it makes a significant contribution to cardiac protein mass. Some early estimates of the contribution of cardiac-type FABP to the cytosolic protein mass were as high as 5 to 6%, although more recent estimates are about one half of the earlier reports. The primary responsibility of cardiac-type FABP appears to be to facilitate the transport of fatty acids to intracellular sites of metabolic conversion.

Before fatty acids can be utilized in oxidative pathways for ATP production, their carboxylic head group must be converted to a reactive thioester in a process referred to as *fatty acid activation*. Fatty acid activation is catalyzed by long-chain, medium-chain, and short-chain acyl CoA synthetases. Activated fatty acids are then available for mitochondrial and peroxisomal β-oxidation. Activated long chain fatty acids must first be transported into the mitochondrial matrix, via a carnitine-dependent shuttle mechanism, prior to engaging in β-oxidation. Acyl CoA esters are first converted into acylcarnitine, by the action of carnitine acyltransferase I located at the inner surface of the mitochondrial inner membrane, and then transported across the inner membrane by carnitine-acylcarnitine translocase. Once inside the matrix, acylcarnitine is reconverted to acyl CoA by carnitine acyltransferase II. β-Oxidation of acyl CoA in the mitochondrial matrix yields acetyl CoA, NADH, and $FADH_2$, and integration of acetyl CoA into the tricarboxylic acid cycle yields more NADH and $FADH_2$. The reduced electron transfer complexes ($NAD^+ \rightarrow$ NADH and FAD $\rightarrow$ $FADH_2$) deliver electrons to the respiratory chain located within the mitochondrial inner membrane to support ATP synthesis.

The peroxisomes of cardiac myocytes also possess the ability to oxidize fatty acids; however, their oxidative capacities are limited to long-chain acyl CoA. Furthermore, peroxisomal β-oxidation is somewhat incomplete in that long-chain acyl CoA are catabolized to acetyl CoA and short-chain acyl CoA moieties that need to be further degraded in mitochondria.

Cardiac Energy Metabolism During Reduced O$_2$ Delivery (Ischemia)

The hallmarks of alterations in normal cardiac function, structure, or perfusion include modifications in energy substrate metabolism. For example, in low-flow ischemic hearts there is a resultant accumulation of cytosolic fatty acids. Furthermore, hypoxic and ischemic conditions in humans and experimental animals result in the accumulation of lipid droplets. The appearance of lipid droplets is similar to other heart conditions where there are genetic fatty acid defects in metabolism. During adaptive cardiac hypertrophy there is often a trend towards the utilization of less fatty acid and more glucose for oxidative ATP generation.

Ischemia resulting in oxygen deficiency in cardiac myocytes causes a significant reduction in oxidative metabolism. However, it still persists as the primary means of residual ATP generation. All parameters of mitochondrial function become depressed with ischemia, and in contrast to normal aerobic metabolism, glucose becomes the primary contributor of substrates for the tricarboxylic acid cycle. During decreased oxygen delivery to myocardium there is increased glycogenolysis to provide more glucose. Furthermore, under conditions of extreme anoxia, cardiac glycogen stores may become essentially depleted within 4 min. Glucose transport into cardiac myocytes as well as the activity of hexokinase and PFK are increased during decreased oxygen delivery. However, in severe anoxia resulting from ischemia, glycolysis is ultimately reduced, primarily due to the inhibitory effect of lactate, both directly upon glyceraldehyde 3-phosphate dehydrogenase, and indirectly by its regulation of the sole remaining means for oxygen-deficient cardiac myocytes to reoxidize NADH through lactate dehydrogenase.

During myocardial ischemia, many events take place that depress fatty acid oxidation. The resulting decrease in respiratory chain flux in mitochondria increases the NADH:NAD$^+$ ratios in mitochondria and the cytosol and acts to suppress β-oxidation, especially the oxidation of β-hydroxy acyl CoA, which requires NAD$^+$. Mitochondrial accumulations of long-chain acyl CoA has been reported as well during ischemic states. In fact, accumulation of lipid droplets in hypoxic and ischemic cardiac tissue has been well established in both humans and laboratory animals.

Cardiac Energy Metabolism During Hypertrophy

In the adaptive hypertrophic state, energy substrate metabolism also appears to be altered. There appears to be a decrease in fatty acid oxidation in the hypertrophic heart, expressed either per gram of cardiac tissue or per unit of cardiac work. Investigations to assess energy substrate utilization have been done using rat hearts subjected to a volume-overload scenario that resulted in cardiac enlargement. The overloaded hearts demonstrated decreased mechanical performance and O_2 consumption. The production of $^{14}CO_2$ from [U-^{14}C]palmitate was also decreased. However, when the hearts were perfused with octanoate (8:0), the mechanical performance and O_2 consumption were normalized in the overloaded hearts. This suggests that a decrease in oxidative metabolism of fatty acids may not necessarily be the root of the problem.

Despite normal levels of carnitine in the blood, carnitine levels were depressed in the overloaded rat hearts. CoA levels were not altered in the overloaded rat hearts. Therefore, the reduction in long-chain fatty acid oxidation in mitochondria in the overloaded rat hearts may be related to a reduced ability to translocate activated long-chain fatty acids into the mitochondria for subsequent β-oxidation. Furthermore, it has been speculated that a decreased translocation of activated fatty acids in the cytosolic compartment into mitochondria can lead to increased triglyceride synthesis and incorporation into the triglyceride pool within those cardiac myocytes. The existence of an impaired long-chain fatty acid utilization in mechanically overloaded rat hearts mentioned above confirms the reports of other investigators using different models of experimental cardiac overload. A primary underlining aspect of the decreased long-chain fatty acid utilization observed in mechanically overloaded hearts may be related to altered function of a mitochondrial carnitine palmityl transferase (CPT$_o$). This would certainly impair the penetration of long-chain fatty acids into mitochondria and thus limit their contribution to cardiac energy production.

As glucose utilization, as an oxidative substrate, increases relative to the reduction in fatty acid oxidation in adaptive cardiac hypertrophy, the question is whether mechanisms associated with glucose utilization are enhanced? It has been demonstrated that certain features of glucose metabolism are indeed enhanced in dogs with experimental cardiac hypertrophy and congestive heart failure. Progressive pulmonary stenosis was produced resulting in right ventricular hypertrophy in one experimental group, while right ventricular hypertrophy and congestive heart failure was produced in another experimental group secondary to infestation with the canine heartworm *Dirofilaria immitis*. There was a significant shift from heart-type lactate dehydrogenase (H-LDH) towards muscle-type lactate dehydrogenase (M-LDH) isozyme. M-LDH is more associated with tissue more accustomed to anaerobic metabolism, such as white skeletal muscle fibers. Lactate production is significantly increased above control levels, in the hypertrophied right ventricles after 30-min anaerobic incubation, further suggesting an increased ability to metabolize glucose in hypertrophied cardiac tissue.

Cardiac Hypertrophy

Cardiac hypertrophy is heart enlargement that occurs in response to a pathological, or in some cases physiological, stress. There are two basic patterns of cardiac hypertrophy which both display an overall increase in cardiac mass, termed (1) concentric, and (2) eccentric hypertrophy. Concentric hypertrophy is characterized by thickened ventricular walls and ventricular chambers that are diminished in volume. Eccentric hypertrophy is character-ized by thinner ventricular walls along with a greatly increased chamber volume. A heart in a state of eccentric hypertrophy is commonly referred to as being dilated and is common among heart failure patients. Iron-deficiency anemia, beriberi, and chronic abusive alcohol consumption are all associated with eccentric hypertrophy. Hypertension, due to genetic causes or secondary causes, is one of the most often cited factors related to cardiac hyper-trophy. Here the cardiac hypertrophy is more concentric in nature.

The development of cardiac hypertrophy and congestive heart failure is a continuum that begins with an underlying pathological stress. The primary pathological stress in this case is hypertension, which results in an increase the ventricular wall stress in the heart. Complex biochemical mechanisms sense the increase in global wall stress; signal transduc-tion mechanisms involving angiotensin II, endothelin I and G-protein-coupled receptors have been implicated in initiating the biochemical signals to activate various genes that modulate the hypertrophic response. More myofibrils are synthesized and laid in a parallel fashion, resulting in the thickening of the myocyte itself. The ventricular walls (predomi-nantly the left ventricle and intraventricular septum) will grow thicker in a concentric pat-tern of hypertrophy until they reach a dimension in which the wall stress imposed by the underlying hypertension is normalized. During this time of compensation, the heart is characterized by concentric hypertrophy, normal hemodynamic function, and contractility at the whole heart and myocyte level. Normal developed pressure and ejection fraction (fraction of ventricular volume ejected with each beat of the left ventricle) are maintained as well. This condition is referred to as *compensated cardiac hypertrophy* since the heart has compensated for the initial stress laid upon it.

Compensation, however, does not come without a serious price. One must remember that the adult cardiac myocyte is a terminally differentiated cell type that is not designed to significantly alter in size and shape. If the underlying pathological stress is not con-trolled or diminished, the heart will try to continue to remodel and adapt to the ever-changed stress imposed upon it, but will reach a point where it is unable to continue to cope and maintain normal function. During this transition, where the heart begins to lose its functional ability, there are complex physiological and biochemical changes that occur. The ventricles grow dilated and the ventricular walls become thinner. Overall the heart assumes a pattern of eccentric hypertrophy. The heart begins to fail as a mechanical pump and is unable to maintain normal developed pressure and ejection fraction. Consequently, blood is not adequately pumped through the circulation and tends to pool in the extremi-ties and the lungs. Fluid retention in the lungs and edema are classic symptoms of heart failure, and patients manifesting these symptoms are said to be in congestive heart failure.

Currently the molecular events that mediate cardiac hypertrophy in response to hyper-tension or volume overload due to inadequate kidney function are under intense investi-gation. The goal of many cardiovascular researchers is to map out the various pathways that participate in the hypertrophic event so that possible new targets for novel drug ther-apy can be identified that would attenuate or inhibit the hypertrophic process. Until the myriad of biochemical pathways can be sorted out, however, effective preventative mea-sures must be promoted to reduce the risk of hypertrophic heart disease such as controlling weight and blood pressure.

Another type of cardiac hypertrophy that can be observed in athletic individuals is phys-iological hypertrophy. Intense exercise can lead to a rise in blood pressure (seen in weight lifters) or a rise in blood volume (seen in runners). These stimuli act to cause a mild hyper-trophy of the left ventricle. The same principles discussed earlier stimulate the hypertrophy;

an increase in wall stress due to the pressure and/or volume overload leads to a thickening of the left ventricle as a compensatory mechanism. In the case of physiological hypertrophy the hypertrophic response is more mild and should not be confused with cardiac hypertrophy derived from pathological mechanisms. The major difference is in the intensity of the stimuli. Even a world class athlete during a period of intense training imposes an increased workload upon the heart for only a several hours a day. In contrast, an individual with hypertension imposes an increased workload upon the heart continuously, 24 h a day, 7 d a week. Hence the hypertrophic response from pathological stimuli is results in a much more severe hypertrophic response.

Risk Factors for Heart Disease

There are several confirmed risk factors for heart disease. Males are at increased risk as compared to females. As one grows older or ages, the likelihood that they may develop ischemic heart disease increases. Hypertension, renal disease, and diabetes are commonly cited as well. Obesity and the propensity to overweight conditions often have a direct correlation to other diseases or physiological events that increase the risk of heart disease as well. Obesity can result in hyperinsulinemia and syndrome X, which are correlated with heart disease.

Heart disease does tend to run in families and thus genetic predisposition is certainly a major consideration. Hypercholesterolemia is a risk factor for heart disease as it accelerates plaque formation. Cigarette smoking has also long been identified as a heart disease risk factor. Some of these factors, such as gender and age, are seemingly uncontrollable. At this time there is not much that can be done about having the "wrong" genes to eliminate the associated increased risk. However, minimizing the other so called "controllable" risk factors" becomes more important in a practical sense. While obesity may, too, have a strong genetic basis, exercise and caloric restriction may prevent and treat this disorder. Hypertension may be treated with medication and/or diet to reduce this factor as a risk. Hypercholesterolemia may have a genetic basis, particularly if LDL cholesterol is elevated and there are decreased LDL receptors on hepatocytes. Not smoking or cessation of smoking can control one of the most powerful risk factors.

Hypertension

Hypertension is a major risk factor for developing heart disease that results in cardiac hypertrophy, and eventually, if left untreated, it leads to congestive heart failure. In adults, high blood pressure or hypertension, can be defined as a systolic blood pressure greater than 160 mmHg and/or a diastolic greater than 95 mmHg. Previously, 140 mmHg and/or 90 mmHg was considered borderline hypertensive. However, many clinicians and researchers have also defined this as hypertension. In adolescents, the latter readings would be considered definite hypertension. In children, 130 mmHg systolic and 85 mmHg diastolic would be considered high.

Hypertension itself has many etiologies and is broadly defined in two catagories: primary (essential) hypertension and secondary hypertension. Primary hypertension, by far the most common type of hypertension seen in clinical settings, has an unknown etiology and is believed to result from genetic predisposition characterized by poor blood pressure regulation. Secondary hypertension is often the result of another disease process which produces elevated blood pressure as a symptom or side effect. Common causes for secondary hypertension are kidney diseases, which can lead to malfunctioning kidneys and result in poor regulation of blood pressure. Atherosclerotic plaques that develop in the renal arteries cause renal stenosis, which will lead to an increase in blood pressure. Diabetes can also lead to kidney dysfunction due to the destructive effect on the glomeruli encountered during this disease. This kidney dysfunction in turn results in high blood pressure. Other factors that influence both primary and secondary hypertension are cigarette smoking, diet, sedentary behavior, and obesity. These factors are also interrelated to some degree, as it is typical to see individuals who do not exercise, who are overweight, smoke, and consume a high fat/high sodium diet and posses high blood pressure. There are also racial differences, with adult African-Americans having a higher incidence than caucasians. In the U.S., the southern portion, where there are many African-Americans in the population, has the greatest incidence of hypertension and is sometimes referred to as the "stroke belt." From a nutritional aspect, dietary sodium has received the most attention. Survey studies have long demonstrated that the typical Western diet after contains 10 to 15 g of sodium chloride per day in the diet. This amounts to about 5 to 7 g of sodium. This level is far in excess of the amount needed, about 3 to 5 g of sodium chloride. With excess sodium in the diet, the current thinking is that the body responds by attempting to rid itself of the excess sodium. Such mechanisms that come into play involve both the renal and cardiovascular systems and accompanying hormonal control systems. The hormone aldosterone is secreted by the adrenal glands and serves to facilitate sodium reabsorption by the kidney tubules. However, with excess sodium, the synthesis of this hormone is reduced. Antidiuretic hormone produced by the pituitary gland is significant in that it will facilitate the reabsorption of water in the kidney tubules, particularly when excess sodium is consumed, in order to maintain a proper level of sodium blood levels. This often results in greater fluid retention and may contribute to extra blood volume and pressure. However, the cardiovascular system also reacts, in that the cardiac output increases so that there is increased blood flow to the kidneys in order to rid the body of the extra sodium. However, this extra workload by the heart is not energy efficient and can lead to deleterious changes in the myocardium. One thought is that increased peripheral resistance via vasoconstriction will also allow for greater blood flow to the kidneys and allow cardiac output to return to "normal," thus sparing the heart of this extra effort. In essence, the increased peripheral resistance is the lesser of the two evils in terms of the entire organism. Increased renin by the kidney and therefore increased angiotensin I and II is a mechanism by which the vasoconstriction may occur. The kidney is able to monitor the plasma and urine concentration of solutes, and a group of cells in the juxtaglomerular apparatus of the kidney releases renin. These are cells located in the walls of the afferent arterioles proximal to the glomeruli. This enzyme converts the plasma protein angiotensinogen to angiotensin I by releasing a decapeptide. This decapeptide or angiotensin I will be acted upon by angiotensin converting enzyme (ACE) in the small vessels of the lung and will split off a dipeptide from this precursor to produce the active angiotensin II, the vasoconstrictor. This compound has a direct effect upon the kidney to cause decreased excretion of water and sodium, as well as stimulating the release of aldosterone from the adrenal cortex in order to decrease the renal excretion of salt and water. When this system is operating efficiently, it should allow for the ingestion of low to high amounts of salt and, at the same time, the maintenance of normal blood pressure. However, some individuals may not be able to respond adequately to extreme levels of salt in their diet. The kidneys in some individuals may produce excess renin in an attempt to rid the body of the excess sodium.

The usual approach in controlling blood pressure is through pharmacological means. The first class of drugs used were the diuretics, which allowed for the enhanced excretion of water and sodium. Some of the early diuretics used also were troublesome in that excess potassium was lost. The potassium-sparing diuretics were soon developed. A newer type of drugs that became popular was the ACE inhibitors, which lowered the levels of circulating angiotensin II. These drugs proved very effective. Whether or not pharmacological approaches are used, the amount of sodium in the blood should be controlled by the diet. The greatest source of sodium is via the salt shaker, either by addition at the table or while cooking. The taste for salt in Western societies is well known and is thought to be a fundamental concern as it relates to hypertension. Eliminating salt from cooking and at the table can in effect readily decrease the daily sodium intake. Canned and processed foods have a significant amount of sodium added in their preparation. Cured meats such as ham, bacon, and sausages are also high in sodium. A basic difficulty is that many individuals who try to consume a lower salt diet find them bland and flavorless; thus compliance is a problem. Salt substitutes, using herbs that have not been dehydrated with salt, lemon, and other flavoring agents have become popular.

Another concern is simply not the amount of sodium intake, but that of potassium. Another school of thought is that the ratio of sodium to potassium consumed is more significant than the overall sodium intake. Potassium is found in foods such as fruits and vegetables, and can cause vasodilation. Normally, the Western diet is low in fruits and vegetables and consequently so is potassium. Several health agencies have advocated not only careful salt restriction, but increased potassium consumption via more fruits and vegetables in the diet.

Calcium intake is another dietary factor thought to play a role in blood pressure regulation, although the mechanism by which this occurs is less certain. Initially, much of this work was observed in pregnant females who suffered from toxemia of pregnancy. Among the symptoms of this disorder are hypertension and fluid retention. It was discovered that calcium supplements could lower blood pressure in these females, and also prevent the severity of the condition in high-risk patients. Subsequent studies have demonstrated that hypertensive individuals given either calcium supplements or a diet higher in calcium can exhibit reduced blood pressure as well. Once potential mechanism by which calcium may lower blood pressure is by blocking the reabsorption of sodium by the kidney tubules and enhancing sodium excretion. Even previous to such observations, epidemiological studies revealed that populations living in areas characterized by hard water, which are high in calcium and magnesium, had lower incidences of cardiovascular disease, such as stroke and coronary heart disease. British studies revealed that towns where water over the years had become harder also had a decline in incidence of cardiovascular disease, whereas those areas in which water supplies had become more soft, did not have as favorable an outcome. One aspect of water hardness of commercial significance is the use of water softeners. These appliances not only remove calcium and magnesium from the water supply, but through an ion exchange principle, add sodium to the water. If water softeners are to be used, it may be appropriate to use them only for purposes other than drinking water.

Perhaps the easiest method for reducing blood pressure in hypertensive individuals is to encourage weight loss, as so many are overweight — easy in the sense that drugs are not involved. A loss of only a few pounds can have meaningful clinical decreases in blood pressure in many individuals. Of course, lifestyle modification such as increased physical activity and smoking cessation are commonsense interventions.

Cholesterol

Total Fat and Fatty Acid Type

Blood cholesterol levels in general increase with age. However, as a clinician, several things can be done to reduce the risk of ischemic heart disease characterized by atherosclerosis. First, knowing the genetic history of the individual would be helpful, since this is perhaps the strongest risk factor. The weight of the individual is important, since losing pounds can significantly reduce both the overall risk directly or even lower blood cholesterol. Total calories in the form of fat should be examined, followed by fat composition in terms of degree of monounsaturated and polyunsaturated fatty acids relative to saturated fat. Monounsaturated and polyunsaturated fat are well known to reduce blood cholesterol levels, whereas saturated fat has the reverse effect. For instance, it has been estimated that for every 1% increase in total energy from saturated fat, an increase of 2.7 mg/100 ml of blood cholesterol can be predicted. Palmitic acid (16:0), myristic acid (14:0), and lauric acid (12:0) are the only true hypercholesterolemic saturated fatty acids. Palmitic acid represents as much as 60% of the total saturated fatty acid in the American diet with almost all of it derived from animal foods. Palm oil is also rich in palmitic acid, contributing as much as 44% of all fatty acids. Myristic acid is found mostly in butter fat and palm-kernel and coconut oils. Lauric acid is also found in palm-kernal oil and coconut oils. Thus the most hypercholesterolemic fat sources in the American diet are butter, meats, and palm, palm-kernel and coconut oils.

Trans Fatty Acids

The typical American diet, where partially hydrogenated vegetable oils are abundant through food processing, may contain 15 g of *trans* fatty acids or 5% of total calories daily. However, others contend lower values of 8 g/d or 3% of total calories more accurately reflect the American diet. For years, concern with *trans* fatty acids was apparent; yet, supportive scientific evidence was lacking. However, soon after studies suggested that *trans* fatty acids when fed at levels consumed by the typical American diet increased plasma LDL-cholesterol and reduced HDL-cholesterol. Some studies suggest that intake of *trans* fatty acids increases the risk of coronary heart disease. In the Nurses Health Study, a decrease of 2% of calories from *trans* fatty acids reduced the risk of coronary heart disease by 53%.

Dietary Cholesterol

Dietary cholesterol has minimal effects upon blood cholesterol levels, but can be restricted if blood cholesterol levels are very high and limited pharmacological intervention is attempted or the patient does not respond to drug treatment. For instance, for every 25 mg increase in dietary cholesterol, total blood cholesterol is only increased by about 1 mg/100 ml. Furthermore, as cholesterol in foods in highly associated with hypercholesterolemic saturated fat sources, emphasis on reducing these foods would also reduce cholesterol intake without further consideration. Last, cigarette smoking has been long known to reduce HDL-cholesterol levels by as much as 5 to 8 mg/100 ml while also increasing VLDL-cholesterol and glucose levels.

Atherosclerosis

The process of atherosclerosis, which occurs in the intima layer of primarily smaller arterial walls, is rather well known. A key initiating factor is damage to the endothelial layer of blood vessels (Figure 16.1). Free radical-induced oxidized LDL-cholesterol is one such agent as well as direct endothelial contact with free radicals. LDL-cholesterol and platelets can penetrate the damaged endothelium and cause the release of platelet-derived growth factor (PDGF) to stimulate smooth muscle division in the blood vessel wall. Monocytes invade the area and become phagocytic and are termed "macrophages." These cells take up LDL-cholesterol and form foam cells. The deposition of circulating calcium in a vessel wall causes a hardening of the developing plaque. All of these factors result in a growing plaque mass that can narrow a blood vessel to the point of total occlusion, either directly or via thrombosis (Figure 16.2). The occluded vessel results in ischemia in tissue "downstream" resulting in infarction (Figure 16.3).

Pathogenesis of Atherosclerosis

The areas which are targets of this process are not random, but are specific lesion-prone sites. These sites are often permeable to a number of plasma proteins. Endothelial cell

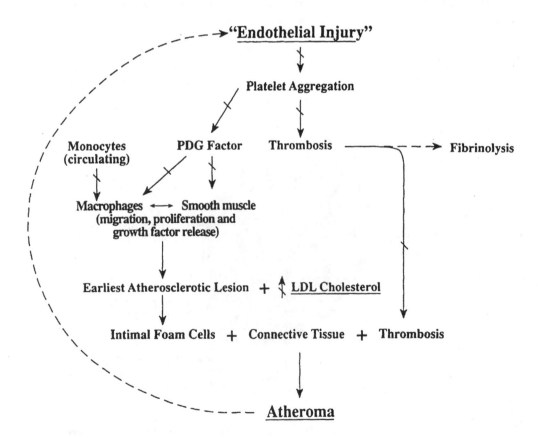

FIGURE 16.1
Sequence of events involved in the formation of an atheroma.

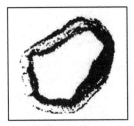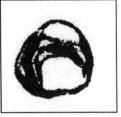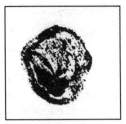

NORMAL ARTERY   FATTY DEPOSITS IN   PLUGGED ARTERY
      VESSEL WALL   WITH FATTY DEPOSITS
      AND CLOT

FIGURE 16.2
Development of atherosclerosis in an artery.

turnover is increased and the glycocalyx decreased in thickness. Monocytes are recruited to these areas initially at the onset of the disease. These monocytes then become activated and are transformed into macrophages, which can generate free radicals as products. Monocytes adhere to the blood vessel wall by secretion of endothelial leukocyte adhesion molecules and several adhesion cytokines, (i.e., interleukin 1β). Oxidized LDL may also facilitate monocyte recruitment and adhesion to lesion sites.

Oxidized LDL, and even glycated LDL such as may occur in diabetics, are not recognized by normal LDL receptors, but are recognized by the macrophage scavenger receptor. This receptor is not down-regulated by the intracellular accumulation of cholesterol and is the normal LDL receptor one would find on hepatocytes. Thus, there is continual uptake of the oxidized LDL by the macrophages, resulting in the formation of foam cells. Another small, dense LDL particle, Lp(a), is subject to oxidation and modification and participates in foam cell formation. The foam cells eventually become necrotic, perhaps due to the oxidized LDL. This is an important event in the transition from the reversible to the less reversible

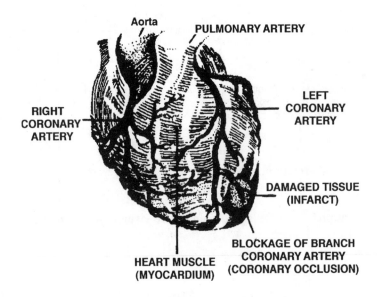

FIGURE 16.3
Some characteristic features of a heart attack. Interference with the flow of blood to the heart muscle results in infarction.

lesion. At this point, smooth muscle cell migration and proliferation in the intima occurs. This event is mediated by platelet-derived growth factor as a chemoattractant. Muscle cell proliferation is thought to be due to fibroblast growth factor. The plaque that develops may rupture due to the activity of certain types of proteolytic metalloenzymes, resulting in thrombosis. Proliferating smooth muscle cells are different in nature than their predecessors, which were more specialized for contraction. These proliferated smooth muscle cells are capable of synthesizing and secreting connective tissue proteins (i.e., type I collagen) that contribute to the formation of the complicated atherosclerotic plaque.

Plasma cholesterol level, in particular oxidized LDL-cholesterol levels, are important in realizing the percent of area covered by lesions. There appears to be a curvilinear relationship between the level of blood cholesterol and coronary heart disease risk. However, the percent area covered by raised lesions is linear. What causes the curvilinear relationship with the disease incidence and cholesterol level is that when 60% of the surface area of a blood vessel is covered with raised lesions, then clinical signs of coronary heart disease do become apparent. Furthermore, the percent area covered is dependent not only on the plasma cholesterol level, but on the presence of other risk factors. For instance, an individual with 200 mg/100 ml cholesterol would be 70 years of age before the 60% level would be reached. However, if the individual is a tobacco smoker and was hypertensive, the same cholesterol level in tandem with these other risk factors would cause that patient to reach the 60% level in the late 40's.

Recently, elevated homocysteine levels have been implicated as a risk factor for heart disease. A deficiency of folate, vitamin B_6, or vitamin B_{12} can interfere with the enzymatic conversion of homocysteine to methionine, and even moderate elevations in blood homocysteine levels are associated with increased risk of heart disease. For example, an increase of 5 μmol/l in plasma homocysteine levels is estimated to increase heart disease risk by 70%. This is equivalent to an increase in risk when serum cholesterol levels increase by 0.5 μmol/l. An increased intake of folic acid by 200 μg/d reduces homocysteine levels by about 4 μmol/l. Homocysteine levels can be regulated by both genetic and environmental (nutritional) factors. Genetic defects in the enzymes cystathione β-synthase, methionine synthase, and methylenetetrahydrofolate reductase can all lead to an augmentation of homocysteine levels. However, folic acid, riboflavin, methionine, choline, and vitamins B_6 and B_{12} may all affect homocysteine metabolism. Elevated serum homocysteine has been suggested to cause oxidative damage, in particular that of LDL. However, it may also interfere with the blood coagulation process, in particular those events associated with dissolution of the fibrin clot.

Clinical Intervention

Clinically, strategies have been developed in order to provide direction for treatment of individuals at risk for heart attack. Much of the strategy is based on reducing total cholesterol levels in the blood and LDL-cholesterol, in conjunction with controlling other risk factors. This strategy allows a clinician to suggest when an intervention is warranted as well as the type of intervention involved, whether it be diet and behavioral modifications with or without pharmacological support. This approach is summarized in Tables 16.1 and 16.2. In Table 16.1, the classification of an adult subject in terms of desirable, borderline, and high blood cholesterol levels is defined. Based on the classification, a recommended follow-up

TABLE 16.1
Initial Classification and Recommended Follow-up Based on Total Cholesterol[a,b]

Classification (mg/100 ml)

<200	Desirable blood cholesterol
200–239	Borderline-high blood cholesterol
≥240	High blood cholesterol

Recommended Follow-Up

Total cholesterol, <200 mg/100 ml	Repeat within 5 years
Total cholesterol, 200 to 239 mg/100 ml without definite CHD or two other CHD risk factors (one which may be male gender)	Dietary information and recheck annually
With definite CHD or two other CHD risk factors (one of which may be male gender)	Lipoprotein analysis: further action based on LDL-cholesterol level

[a] CHD, coronary heart disease; LDL, low-density-lipoprotein.
[b] Patients have a lower level and goal if they are at high risk because they already have definite CHD, or because they have any two of the following risk factors: male gender, family history of premature CHD, cigarette smoking, hypertension, low high-density lipoprotein (HDL)-cholesterol, diabetes mellitus, definite cerebrovascular or peripheral vascular disease, or severe obesity.

TABLE 16.2
Classification and Treatment Decisions Based on LDL-Cholesterol[a,b]

Classification (mg/ 100 ml)

<130	Desirable LDL-cholesterol
130–159	Borderline high-risk LDL-cholesterol
≥160	High-risk LDL-cholesterol

Recommended Follow-Up

	Initiation Level (mg/100 ml)	Minimal Goal (mg/100 ml)
Dietary treatment		
Without CHD or two other risk factors	≥160	<160[c]
With CHD or two other risk factors	≥130	<130[d]
Drug treatment	≥190	<160
Without CHD or two other risk factors		
With CHD or two other risk factors	≥160	<130

[a] CHD, coronary heart disease; LDL, low-density-lipoprotein.
[b] Patients have a lower level and goal if they are at high risk because they already have definite CHD, or because they have any two of the following risk factors: male gender, family history of premature CHD, cigarette smoking, hypertension, low high-density lipoprotein (HDL)-cholesterol, diabetes mellitus, definite cerebrovascular or peripheral vascular disease, or severe obesity.
[c] Roughly equivalent to total cholesterol level of <240 mg/100 ml or <200 mg/100 ml.
[d] As goals for monitoring dietary treatment.

is outlined. For instance, if a subject has between 200 and 239 mg/100 ml for cholesterol, and does not have any risk factors, diet information is provided and an annual recheck of the cholesterol level is recommended. However, if two other risk factors are present, then a lipoprotein analysis is suggested. If the blood cholesterol is greater than 240 mg/100 ml, then a further analysis is recommended, regardless of the presence of other risk factors. It is important to recognize the risk factors in this strategy: male gender, family history of premature coronary heart disease, tobacco smoking, hypertension, low HDL-cholesterol levels, diabetes mellitus, definite cerebrovascular or peripheral vascular disease, or severe obesity. An analysis of the LDL-cholesterol level serves as a guide for further treatment (Table 16.2). A level of 130 mg/100 ml or less is desirable. Borderline elevated LDL-cholesterol levels are 130 to 159 mg/100 ml, and a "high" level is that which is greater than 160 mg/100 ml or greater.

Diet vs. drug intervention is guided by the initial level of the LDL-cholesterol and the presence or absence of two other risk factors (Table 16.2). A minimal goal to achieve is also provided. For instance, if a male patient who is a tobacco smoker has an LDL-cholesterol level of 150 mg/100 ml, then only diet treatment is recommended, with a goal of achieving less than 130 mg/100 ml. However, if the same patient had an LDL-cholesterol level of 170 mg/100 ml, then pharmacological treatment (in addition to diet) would be advised, with a goal to get the cholesterol level down to 130 mg/100 ml or less.

The type of pharmacological treatment advocated is under constant debate. Bile-sequestering resins, such as cholestyramine, fibric acid derivatives (gemfibrozil), probucol, and niacin, are examples of some drugs initially advocated. However, inhibitors of HMG-CoA reductase (lovastatin, pravastatin, simvastatin) are being more commonly used and produce a dramatic lowering of total cholesterol by up to one third in many cases. Combination of various drug categories may be used, as should dietary treatment, whenever drug intervention is in use.

Dietary Guidance

Clinicians may wish to follow the guidelines of the National Cholesterol Education Program's Step 1 and Step 2 diets, when dealing with clients with hyperlipidemias. The basic aim of these diets is to reduce elevated cholesterol levels while maintaining a nutritionally adequate diet. As the designation suggests, the diet should be implemented in two stages with monitoring. The diets are designed to reduce the intake of saturated fatty acids and cholesterol, to promote weight reduction in overweight individuals by reducing excess caloric intake. The Step 1 diet advocates an intake of less than 30% of calories as fat, saturated fats at 10% or less, and cholesterol less than 300 mg/d. The Step 2 diet is often prescribed if the Step 1 diet does not bring about a desired lowering of blood cholesterol. The Step 2 diet requires a further reduction of saturated fat to 7% of the caloric intake in tandem with a reduction of dietary cholesterol intake to 200 mg/d or less. In practice, the Step 1 diet should be followed for up to 3 to 4 months to demonstrate any effective results. Not only should total cholesterol level be monitored, but LDL-cholesterol as well. If the Step 2 diet does not bring about significant cholesterol lowering after 6 months of intensive dietary intervention, then pharmacological interventions should be considered.

With respect to polyunsaturated fatty acids (PUFAs) and monounsaturated fatty acids (MUFAs), both steps of the diet allow for up to 10% of total calories from PUFAs and 10 to

15% of total calories from MUFAs. Carbohydrate should comprise 50 to 60% of total calories and protein 10 to 20% of total calories. The typical American diet by comparison has 37 to 43% of calories from fat, PUFA:SFA of 0.2:1 to 0.6:1, and about 450 mg cholesterol/day. While a low-fat diet of slightly less than 30% of the calories from fat may reduce HDL-cholesterol, more significantly, the LDL:HDL ratio is probably improved. While MUFAs may lower blood cholesterol level, such as provided by olive oil, it is uncertain if MUFAs are more beneficial than PUFAs in cholesterol lowering. The preponderance of evidence suggests that one has no advantage over the other, but that both are equally effective at lowering total cholesterol, particularly LDL-cholesterol. Saturated fats are about twice as effective at increasing serum cholesterol levels as polyunsaturated fats are at lowering them.

Fiber

Dietary fiber may reduce blood cholesterol levels by its interactions and metabolism within the gut, as well by the absorption of its metabolites. Fibers can bind intestinal material including bile acids and cholesterol and toxic compounds. For instance, lignin seems to be very efficient in binding bile acids present in the digestive tract. Pectin and other acidic polysaccharides also appear to bind bile acids. However, cellulose has little ability to bind bile acids. The ability of soluble fibers and lignin to bind bile acids is believed to be responsible for some of the hypocholesterolemic effect of dietary fiber. When more bile acids are complexed to fiber components, less bile acids is reabsorbed by the intestine. Thus, the enterohepatic circulation of bile acids is decreased and more bile acids are excreted in the feces. This is believed to result in the dedication of more hepatic cholesterol to the synthesis of new bile acids. Thus less cholesterol may be available for incorporation into VLDL and export into circulation. As VLDL become LDL, the effect is a reduction in total cholesterol and LDL cholesterol levels.

A second mechanism has been proposed for the hypercholestoremic effects of fibers. Bacterial fermentation of fibrous molecules results in the production of short-chain fatty acids, namely, acetic acid, propionic acid, and butyric acid. While these fatty acids can serve as an energy source for colonic mucosal cells, they can also be absorbed and circulate to the liver via the hepatic portal vein. Once diffused into hepatocytes, that may cause a reduction in cholesterol synthesis.

Soy

Plant sterols in rather large doses may also decrease cholesterol. Sitosterol and campesterol are two of the sterols that may interfere with the reabsorption of cholesterol and bile acids from the gut for recirculation to the liver. Sterols from marine organisms such as oysters and clams have also been advocated. Certain soy proteins may also play a role in lowering blood cholesterol. In humans, the reduction in LDL-cholesterol related to soy intake occurs with either an increase or no change in HDL-cholesterol. Some researchers have also reported a decrease in serum triglycerides. This effect may not only be due to the fiber from soybeans, but to other factors as well. For instance, the rate of removal of circulating LDL-cholesterol from the blood circulation is greater in animal studies when soy protein is part of the diet. Increases in the apo B/E receptor have also been reported in animal studies.

The amino acid pattern of soy protein may also help explain the decreases in total cholesterol; however, the exact mechanism has not been defined. Feeding animals with amino acids patterned after soy protein significantly reduces blood cholesterol levels compared with a casein amino acid pattern. A high molecular weight fraction of soy protein has been isolated that is potent in lowering cholesterol levels. Another suggestion is that the isoflavone content of soy may be responsible for cholesterol lowering due to the similarity in biochemical structure to estrogens, which lower cholesterol levels. Besides cholesterol levels, one isoflavone in soy protein, genistein, is responsible for improved vascular vasodilatory reactivity. Genistein may also inhibit thrombus formation by inhibiting tyrosine kinase, which, when active, leads to thrombus formation and enhanced atherosclerotic lesions.

Fish Oils

Fish are not only a good source of PUFA, but cold-water species are particularly good sources of omega-3 fatty acids. The Physician Health Study did suggest that consumption of fish is helpful in reducing sudden cardiac death as opposed to coronary heart disease as an aggregate condition. This study, performed in the 1980s, was composed of 20,551 men and included an examination of fish consumption behavior of male physicians between 40 to 84 years of age. The intake of fish was followed yearly over a 10-year period and self-reported cardiovascular events were monitored. The results revealed that about 11% consumed fish 5 times per week and 80% 1 to 4 times/week, with an average of 2.5 meals per week containing fish. Men who consumed fish tended to have more cardiovascular disease risk factors, such as hypertension, family history, and high blood cholesterol levels. They also tended to exercise more and use antioxidant supplements more frequently. Data analysis suggested that when considering adjusting for other factors as aspirin intake, age, and β-carotene intake, fish consumption was inversely related to the risk of sudden cardiac death. The trend between fish consumption and a lowering of sudden cardiac death reached statistical significance at one to two servings of fish per week. The results failed to find any association with other food groups, such as red meat, chicken, vegetables, fruits, dairy foods, or fried foods. There was no relationship, however, with fish consumption and myocardial infarction.

Serum triglycerides until recently were not considered important risk factors for heart disease. One thought is that serum triglycerides are a risk factor for atherosclerosis and coronary artery disease if LDL-cholesterol is elevated and HDL-cholesterol is decreased. In particular, if the LDL-cholesterol to HDL-cholesterol ratio is 5 or greater, elevated serum triglycerides may be a powerful additional risk factor. Others believe that elevated serum triglyceride levels as a risk factor are independent of serum cholesterol factors. While the consensus has not clearly formed on the topic, dietary compounds may lower serum levels of triglycerides. The most studied of these have been fish oils, rich in omega-3 PUFA. Such fatty acids as EPA and DHA effectively reduce elevated plasma triglyceride concentrations. These two omega-3 fatty acids may inhibit hepatic fatty acid synthesis and triglyceride synthesis, including VLDL assembly and secretion. Blood pressure has been shown to be reduced with fish oil supplements.

Olive Oil, Oleic Acid, and Phenolic Compounds

As already considered, the Mediterranean diet lowers the risk of heart disease. Such a lowering is often thought to be due to the high levels of monounsaturates, such as oleic acid (18:1). However, this may not be the only factor, and in fact may only partly explain this observation. The Mediterranean diet also contains polyphenolic compounds, which are high in olive oil. The level of these compounds is rather variable, with 50 to 800 mg/kg olive oil being reported. The level of these compounds in olive oil is dependent on soil, degree of ripeness, and cultivar (olive variety). The simple phenolic compounds are *hydroxytyrosol* (3,4-dihydroxyphenylethanol), *tyrosol*, and phenolic acids, such as *vanillic acid* and *caffeic acid*. Complex compounds are tyrosol and hydroxytyrosol esters, oleuropein, and aglycone.

Incubation of LDL with olive oil phenolics (oleuropein or hydroxytyrosol) reduced the fall in vitamin E levels. Normally, virtually all of the vitamin E would have disappeared in 30 min, but 80% remained in the presence of the phenols. Less compounds as isoprostanes, malonaldehyde and lipid peroxides were present. The presence of these substances is relatively indicative of free radical activity. Also, both phenolic compounds prevented the oxidation of linoleic and docosahexaenoic compounds in the LDL phospholipids. Phenols can also inhibit platelet aggregation and increase nitric oxide production. Reduced TXB_2 and LTB_4 production by activated leukocytes is a known effect of olive phenolics.

Vitamin E

As mentioned already, antioxidants have protective properties that blunt the progression of cardiovascular disease. One of the most significant mechanisms is the prevention of key phospholipids and apoproteins associated with LDL from becoming oxidized and therefore becoming less atherogenic. Vitamin E will enhance the ability of LDL to withstand oxidative challenge. Also, vitamin E supplementation has been associated with decreased platelet adhesiveness and thrombosis. In a clinical trial of middle-aged men, vitamin E supplements reduced coronary artery lesion progression. A high level of blood vitamin E as well as diet intake have been found to be associated with reduced risk of atherogenesis, cardiovascular disease, including stroke, in epidemiological survey studies. Prospective studies revealed a 77% decrease in risk of nonfatal heart attacks with vitamin E supplementation. This occurred when 400 to 800 IU units was administered over 18 months. Women tend to be able to have a reduction in risk with as little as 10 IU vitamin E per day.

Other schools of thought of means by which vitamin E may prevent atherosclerosis may be related to modulation of protein kinases and transcription factors. Human aortic endothelial cells that are enriched with vitamin E have significantly reduced adherence of monocytes to these cells. Vitamin E enrichment can reduce the concentrations of LDL in the monocytes as well. Inracellular adhesion molecule-1 production is decreased with vitamin E enrichment. Enrichment of endothelial cells with vitamin E decreased cytokine-stimulated expression of adhesion molecules in a dose-dependent fashion. Interleukin 6 and interleukin 8 were reduced in endothelial cells when stimulated by interleukin 1β with vitamin E enrichment. Vitamin E also appears to be able to enhance prostacyclin, which promotes vasodilatory and antiaggregation properties. Thus it appears that the role of vitamin E as a protective component against heart disease is due to factors other than its role as an antioxidant.

Vitamin C

Vitamin C deficiency in guinea pigs promotes atherosclerotic lesions, and administration of vitamin C can lead to regression of early atherosclerotic lesions. In humans, however, the role of vitamin C is less clear. Recent studies have suggested that if vitamin C supplementation is to be effective in lowering the risk of heart disease, it is perhaps due to supplementation in tandem with vitamin E. Vitamin C may have a sparing effect upon vitamin E; another possibility is that it could reduce vitamin E so as to recycle vitamin E as an antioxidant defense in more lipid-rich particles or cell organelles.

β-Carotene

β-Carotene may also exert an antioxidant effect that helps minimize the events associated with the progression of atherosclerosis. In one study, women fed low β-carotene diets showed an increase in carbonyl content (an indicator of oxidation) in LDL. The subsequent addition of β-carotene supplement decreased the carbonyl content of LDL to levels below baseline. Epidemiological studies have suggested a lower risk of heart disease with a higher plasma concentration of β-carotene. Another study with individuals with cystic fibrosis who were deficient in β-carotene revealed greater lipid peroxidation. These levels were reduced when β-carotene supplements were administered.

Garlic

Garlic supplementation may significantly reduce total cholesterol concentrations without affecting HDL-cholesterol levels. The effect of garlic upon decreased serum cholesterol concentrations is thought to be largely due to a decrease in the LDL-cholesterol fraction. This could be due to an inhibition of hepatic cholesterol biosynthesis, possibly by inhibition of HMG-CoA reductase by allicin and/or other component(s) of garlic. Blood pressure may also be moderately reduced by garlic. This effect could be due to increased nitric oxide production that yields a more vasodilatory state.

Other Nutritional Factors and Cardiovascular Disease

Other nutrients may play a role in cardiovascular disease. One classic example is the lack of thiamin which leads to the syndrome, beriberi. Thiamin is critical in energy metabolism as well as in proper neurological function. Besides the nervous system effects that manifest from a thiamin deficiency, cardiac hypertrophy is a pronounced sign of so-called "wet" beriberi. Supplementation with thiamine can reduce the heart size to its normal size.

Dietary copper deficiency leads to cardiac hypertrophy rather rapidly in growing rats, and the animals can die from cardiac failure, but most likely from aneurysms due to impaired lysyl oxidase activity and subsequent cross-linking of collagen. Individuals with Menke's disease, who are unable to absorb copper, and infants either born with low copper stores or fed diets almost devoid of copper can have such cardiac abnormalities. Fortunately, the number of cases of people consuming diets deficient in copper is very low. The issue of marginal copper intake and any subsequent effects upon the heart remains the subject of much debate. Last, the impact of iron toxicity and selenium deficiency were discussed in greater detail in Chapter 10.

Alcohol-Induced Cardiomyopathy

Ethanol-induced cardiomyopathy has long been confused with beriberi-associated cardiomyopathy. Common features to both cardiomypathies include venticular chamber dilation, tachycardia, elevated venous pressure, and peripheral edema. Contrarily, ethanol-induced cardiomyopathy results in a depressed cardiac output and ventricular hypocontractility. Cardiac output may actually be increased in thiamin deficiency.

Echocardiography can be used to help identify the extent of the pathology, an increased heart-mass-to-body-weight ratio, primarily the result of increased left venticular mass and dimensions (chamber dilation) along with increased thickness of the interventricular septal wall. Some of the pathological remodeling of the heart may be attributed to associated hypertension. The consumption of more than three drinks daily is associated with an increase in systolic blood pressure. A increased renal retention of sodium, which can increase blood volume by osmotic means, is probably responsible for some of the hypertension. Dynamic alterations are associated with alterations in cardiac anatomy. For instance, decreased left ventricular diastolic function is commonly observed. An inhibition of Na^+/K^+ ATPase activity partially explained by reduced mitochondrial oxidative phosphorylation results in poor ion pumping and disturbances in the electrical properties of the myocardium.

On average it requires about 10 years of chronic, excessive ethanol abuse by adults to result in overt signs of cardiac pathology. As the severity of the cardiomyopathy heightens, manifestations of overt failure of both right and left sides of the heart become increasingly apparent. In addition to cardiac complications, noncirrotic damage to the liver may occur. This damage is largely the result of hepatic vascular congestion due to reduced cardiac performance. Blood becomes "backed-up" in the hepatic vessels as venous blood flow is slowed by poor right ventricular performance. While impossible to use diagnostically in humans, postmortem examinations of the myocardium present myofibrillar degeneration, mitochondrial swelling, and cellular edema.

At this time there does not seem to be a clear mechanism responsible for the development of cardiomyopathy related to chronic, excessive ethanol consumption. Cardiac myocytes do not produce alcohol dehydrogenase; thus, ethanol is not metabolized in cardiac tissue. However, long-term ethanol abuse leads to biochemical and clinical changes in myocardium. It is possible that ethanol itself has a direct toxicity effect, or ethanol metabolites created in other tissue may have a deleterious impact. Because ethanol-containing beverages are nonenergy nutrient void, malnutrition can also confound the situation.

The incidence of etahnol-induced cardiomyopathy is greater in men. This is largely attributed to the fact that more alcholics are male. However, women may indeed be more susceptible because of a decreased gastric alcohol dehydrogenase as well as a smaller blood volume. Historically, ethanol consumption has been linked to several toxicity syndromes. For instance, during the mid 1960s, numerous beer drinkers died of acute cardiomypathy resulting from cobalt toxicity. In sub-Saharan populations, iron-overload cardiomyopathy resulted from the brewing of beer in large iron kettles. Wine drinkers were noted to develop cardiomyopathy related to arsenic toxicity. Last, lead toxicity has been reported in individuals who regularly drink "moonshine."

Electrolyte imbalances are often observed in individuals who chronically abuse ethanol. These imbalances include hypokalemia, hypophosphatemia, and reduced extracellular magnesium levels. The level of involvement of these imbalances in the development of cardiomyopathy is undetermined.

References

Alder, A.J. and Holub B.J., Effect of garlic and fish-oil supplementation, on serum lipid and lipo-protein concentration in hypercholesterolemic man, *Am J. Clin. Nutr.*, 65, 445, 1997.

Anderson J.W., Johnstone B.M., and Cook-Newell M.E. Meta-analysis of the effects of soy protein intake on serum lipids, *N. Engl. J. Med.*, 333, 276, 1995.

Applewhite, T.H., Trans-isomers, serum lipids, and cardiovascular disease: another point of view, *Nutr. Res.*, 51, 344, 1993.

Boushey C.J., Beresford S.A.A., Omen G.S., and Motulsky A.G., A qualitative assessment of plasma homocysteine as a risk factor for vascular disease, *JAMA*, 74, 1049, 1995.

Burring, J.E. and Hennekens, C.H., Antioxidant vitamin and cardiovascular disease, 55, S53, 1997.

Das, I., Kha,n N.S., and Sooranna, S.R., Nitric acid synthase activity is a unique mechanism of garlic action, *Biochem. Soc. Trans.*, 23, 1365, 1995.

Gazano, J.M., Antioxidants in cardiovascular disease: randomized trials, *Nutr. Rev.*, 54, 75, 1996.

Gebhardt, R., Multiple inhibitory effects of garlic extracts on cholesterol biosynthesis in hepatocytes, *Lipids*, 28, 613, 1993.

Graham, I.M., Daly, L.E., and Refsum H.M. et al., Plasma homocysteine as a risk factor for vascular disease, *JAMA*, 222, 1775, 1997.

Harats, D., Chevion, S., Nahir, M., Norman, Y., Sagee, O., and Berry, E.M. Citrus fruit supplementation reduces lipoprotein oxidation in young men ingesting a diet high in saturated fat: presumptive evidence for an interaction between vitamins C and E in vivo, *Am. J. Clin. Nutr.*, 67, 240, 1998.

Huff, M.W. and Carroll, K.K. Effects of dietary proteins and amino acid mixtures on plasma cholesterol levels in rabbits, *J. Nutr.*, 110, 1676, 1980.

Jacob, R.A., Individual variability in homocysteine response to folate depletion: an unusual case, *Nutr. Rev.*, 56, 212, 1998.

Khosla, P., Samman, S., and Carroll, K.K., Decreased receptor mediated LDL catabolism in casein-fed rabbits precedes the increase in plasma cholesterol, *J. Nutr. Biochem.*, 2, 203, 1991.

Kromhout, D., Menotti, A., Bloemberg, B. et al., Dietary saturated and trans fatty acids and cholesterol and 25-year mortality from coronary heart disease: the Seven Countries study, *Prev. Med.*, 24, 308, 1995.

Medeiros, D.M. and Wildman, R., New findings on a unified perspective of copper restriction and cardiomyopathy, *Proc. Soc. Exp. Biol. Med.*, 215: 299, 1997.

Meydani, M., Nutrition, immune cells and atherosclerosis, 56, S177, 1998.

Nelson, G.J., Dietary fat, trans fatty acids and risk of coronary heart disease, *Nutr. Rev.*, 56, 250, 1998.

Potter, S.M., Soy protein and cardiovascular disease: the impact of bioactive components of soy, *Nutr. Rev.*, 56, 231, 1998.

Silag, C. and Neil A., Garlic as a lipid lowering agent—a meta analysis, *J. R. Coll. Phys.*, 28, 39, 1994.

Silgy, C.A. and Neil, A.W., A meta-analysis of the effect of garlic on blood pressure, *J. Hyperten.*, 12, 4638, 1994.

Sitori, C.R., Galli, G., Lovati, M.R. et al., Effects of dietary proteins on regulation of liver lipoprotein receptors in rats, *J. Nutr.*, 114, 1493, 1984.

Visioli, F., Bellosa, S., and Galli, C., Oleuropein, the bitter principals of olives, enhances nitric oxide production by mouse macrophage, *Life Sci.*, 62, 541, 1998.

Visioli, F. and Galli, C., The effect of minor constituents of olive oil on cardiovascular disease: new findings, *Nutr. Rev.*, 56, 141, 1998.

Warshatsky, S., Kramer, R.S., and Sivak, S.Z., Effect of garlic on total serum cholesterol—a meta-analysis, *Ann. Int. Med.*, 119, 599, 1993.

Willett, W.C., Stampfer, M.J., Manson, J.E. et al., Trans fatty acid intake in relation to risk of coronary heart disease among women, *Lancet*, 341, 581, 1993.

17

Cancer and Nutrition

Despite massive research and educational efforts cancer, still remains one of the most deadly diseases known to man. In the U.S. all cancers combined are the second leading cause of death. In 1996, cancer probably took the lives about 600,000 individuals. Worldwide, cancer is responsible for the death of some 6 million people annually. While great strides have been made to better understand the mechanisms of cancer and to decrease the rate of incidence of many cancers such as breast cancers, laryngeal cancers, leukemias, ovarian cancer, colorectal cancer, testicular cancer, stomach cancer, and Hodgkin's disease, the death rate of all cancers in America has actually increased by approximately 6% from the early 1970s to the early 1990s. A recent American survey found that 6 out of 10 people believed they would develop cancer in their lifetime. In reality, about 40% will actually develop cancer. Figure 17.1 presents the leading cancer sites and related deaths in men and women in the U.S. in 1991.

Tumors and Cancer

Tumors or *neoplasms* are an uncontrolled proliferation of cells. All tumors arise from one, or possibly more cells, that loose their tight control of reproduction and begin to reproduce uncontrollably. This results in *hyperplasia* of tissue. Tumors can be divided into two subgroups: *benign* tumors and *malignant* tumors or cancer. Benign tumors are different from cancerous tumors in that the involved cells greatly resemble the original cell(s). Furthermore, as the benign neoplasm develops it expands uniformly in all directions and is typically encased within a fibrous sac. These characteristics allow for the successful (complete) surgical removal of many benign tumors without reccurrence. In addition, these tumors are usually poorly vascularized (Table 17.1).

Cancerous neoplasms are different in that the involved cells often do not resemble the original cell(s). Further, the growing mass typically does not present uniform boundaries of expansion and is not encased in a fibrous sac. This makes complete surgical removal complicated and increases the potential for reccurrence. Furthermore, cancerous tissue develops a rich vascular system and perhaps most distressingly, cancerous cells can enter circulation and relocate to other regions of the body and proliferate. This allows for the establishment of new sites of cancerous neoplasm. The ability of cancer to spread is called *metastasis*. Thus, cancer may be defined as a malignant and invasive growth or tumor that tends to recur after excision and to metastasize to other sites.

"Cancer" is a universal term that encompasses anywhere from 100 to 150 different forms of the disease. Theoretically, all nucleated cells have the potential to become tumorous. Therefore, every type of tissue in human body has the potential for developing cancer, and some tissue can even yield several types of cancer. Normal cell activity includes tightly controlled reproduction. However, tumorous cells loose that tight regulation and reproduce uncontrollably.

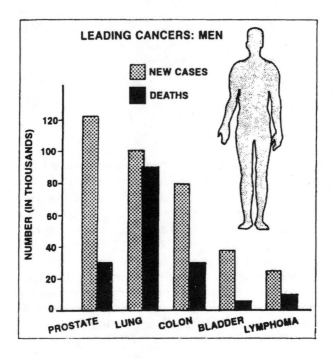

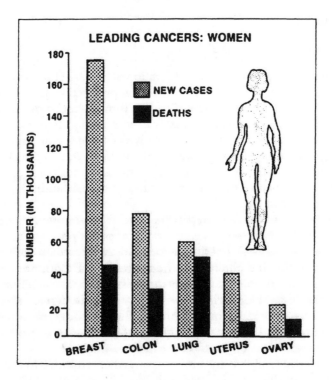

FIGURE 17.1
Leading cancer sites in (a) men and (b) women, with new cases and deaths of each. (Source: *American Cancer Society Facts and Figures*, 1991).

TABLE 17.1
General Characteristics of Benign and Malignant Tumors

Benign Tumor	Malignant Tumor (Cancer)
Neoplasm cells resemble origin cell type	Neoplasm cells do not resemble origin cell type
Neoplasm has uniform boundaries of expansion	Neoplasm does not have uniform boundaries of expansion
Encapsulated in fibrous sack	Nonencapsulated
Remains localized	Spreads to other tissue (metastasis)
	Develops vascular system

Genetic Alterations Causing Cancer

What causes an otherwise "good" cell to begin to proliferate uncontrollably and thus go "bad," potentially giving rise to cancers? There are two primary classes of genes that regulate cell reproduction. These are called *protooncogenes* and *tumor-suppressor genes*. Together the products of these two gene classes choreograph the events of the cell cycle. Or, said another way, they control and regulate those events involved in cell enlargement and division. They are antagonistic in that protooncogenes are supportive of cell proliferation, while tumor suppressor genes provide an inhibitory influence. When mutations occur in these genes, the fine regulation of proliferation for that cell can go awry.

Cells are constantly receiving information, either from circulation or from surrounding cells. Many of these signaling substances promote cell proliferation, while others are inhibitory. Many of signals specifically interact with receptors on the plasma membrane of cells. Once these signals bind with plasma membrane receptors, their information is relayed to the inside of the cell. Many protooncogenes code for proteins that are involved in so-called "molecular bucket-brigades" that relay the growth-stimulating signals from outside the cell to the nucleus. There, the result is an expression of genes that code for proteins that help usher a cell through the cell cycle. Mutations in protooncogenes, resulting in *oncogenes*, can result in the production of proteins at key points in the bucket-brigade. This may allow the bucket brigade to remain active despite the removal of the external signal. For instance, the proteins coded for by mutant *ras* genes maintain an active bucket brigade despite a lack of a signal. Hyperactive *ras* proteins are found in as many as 25% of human tumors, especially those of epithelial tissue.

Some oncogenes result in the overproduction of powerful growth factors such as *platelet-derived growth factor* (PDGF) and *transforming growth factor α*. These and other growth factors can be released from the cell and stimulate the proliferation of surrounding cells, but more importantly, the proliferation of the releasing cell containing the oncogenes or bad genes. Other oncogenes, such as *RET*, *erb-B*, and *erb-B2* code for receptor proteins that, in their aberrant state, produce proliferative signals within a cell despite the absence of the receptor-specific growth factor. The *erb* genes are common to breast cancer. Furthermore, other oncogenes, such as *myc* genes, code for proteins that function as transcription factors increasing the expression of key proteins that increase cell reproduction. Typically *myc* and other transcription factors are produced under the influence of external signals; however, in several forms of cancer *myc* levels remain high.

It is generally agreed that for a cell to become cancerous it must not only over-activate its growth-stimulating efforts but also ignore or dampen the influence of external inhibitory signals. In a manner similar to stimulatory signals, many inhibitory signals are also relayed from receptors on the plasma membrane receptors to the nucleus via a bucket brigade. For example, in some forms of cancer, such as colon cancer, cells do not produce a receptor for transforming growth factor beta (TGF-β). TGF-β is a potent growth inhibiting substance. In another instance, the *NF-1* gene, which inhibits the activity of *ras*, becomes ineffective after its gene has been mutated.

Inheritance

Cancer is not caused by an isolated mutation of a gene that codes for a protein involved in cell reproduction. In actuality, it probably takes a half dozen or more mutated genes, involved in both cell productive and inhibitory operations, to give rise to cancer. Thus, the time frame required to develop mutations in the associated genes that give rise to a cancerous cell can be decades to a lifetime. However, in some cases, the time frame is greatly reduced. Much of this is explained by heredity or the acquisition of one or more mutated cancer-associated genes from a parent. Then, as the zygote begins to proliferate, the mutant gene will be ubiquitous throughout all nucleated cells. In essence, carcinogenesis has hurdled over an early step, the initiation of the first one or two mutations. As a result, cancer can develop in half the time. For example, in individuals presenting an early-onset of colon tumors, this may be the result of the "passing along" of a defective tumor suppressor gene called *APC*. These individuals present hundreds of polyps in their colon, usually before they are 30 to 40 years old. In other examples, the mutant *p53 tumor suppressor gene* is present in many forms of cancer, while mutations in the *BRCA1* and *BRCA2* tumor suppressor genes are involved in the majority of familial breast cancer.

There is another genetic mechanism that may result in the earlier development of cancer. Here again it is caused by molecular mutation to DNA, but in this situation the mutation has occurred to genes that code for proteins that repair DNA, not proteins involved in cell replication. Every day the human genome is under attack by carcinogenic substances. These substances, such as free radicals and toxins, can cause point mutations in DNA. These repair proteins, present in all nucleated cells, endeavor to identify anomalies in our DNA and then repair them. This includes mutations in regions coding for protooncogenes and tumor suppressor genes. Thus, key mutations in the genes coding for these *DNA-proofreading* proteins would increase the likelihood of a cancer-associated mutation becoming a permanent part of that cell's genome. One example of this is presented in individuals afflicted by a familial cancer syndrome called xeroderma pigmentosum. These individuals have a defective copy of gene that directs the repair of DNA damage caused by ultraviolet radiation. As a result, these individuals are prone to several types of sunlight-induced skin cancer.

Stages of Cancer Formation

As discussed above, the stages of tumor formation begin with genetic alterations in cell proliferation-controlling genes. A cell then begins to divide without regulation. With time, descendants of this cell accumulate, causing hyperplasia. With more time, perhaps years, one or more descendent cells can experience another mutation which further decreases their control of proliferation. The cell and its descendants begin to reproduce even more excessively. As hyperplasia continues, cells can undergo even more mutations, some further accelerating proliferation rate while also altering other cell characteristics and function. Still precancerous, "dysplasia" refers to abnormal cell structure and organization of tissue.

There are two possible pathways that dysplastic cells can take. They can progress to *in situ* cancer or spontaneously reverse to hyperplasia. *In situ* cancer exists when cancer cells are present but remain isolated at the site of formation and can remain contained there indefinitely. As mentioned above, tumors that do not have the ability to spread are considered benign or noncancerous. However, cells within these tumors which undergo further mutation in specific genes can begin to invade surrounding areas or metastasize. This last stage or invasive cancer is considered malignant, as cells invade underlying tissue or shed cells into the blood or lymph to initiate the development of secondary tumors.

Cancer Treatment

The treatment of a growing tumorous mass takes into account many considerations. Whether or not the mass is benign or malignant, as well as the stage of development of a malignancy are among the more important considerations. For individuals presenting intermediate-stage cancer development, physicians may apply *combined modality therapy*. Here the most classical sequence of therapy is surgical excision of a mass or radiation therapy, followed by chemotherapy to eliminate any microscopic tumor deposits or rogue cancerous cells not at the site or unaffected by surgery or radiation. Within more recent years, a newer protocol for combined modality therapy employs chemotherapy first and then surgery or radiation treatment. Beyond more established treatments are newer mechanisms being developed and tested to fight cancer. Leading the way among novel approaches to treat cancer is immunotherapy, molecular therapy utilizing viruses, and attacking a cancer's blood supply. All of these will probably be common therapies adding to the cancer treatment arsenal in the 21st century.

Surgery

Today most individuals with skin cancer and as many as one half of the individuals diagnosed with an internal cancer are successfully treated and freed of cancer. The earliest form of treatment was surgical excision of a tumorous mass. This mode of treatment is still the most widely used approach. Surgery is both quick and informative. The excised tissue can be examined by a pathologist who, by looking for a layer of unaltered cells surrounding the neoplasm, can determine if the excision was complete. One drawback to surgical removal is that a surgeon will be unable to remove all the microscopic cancer extensions. Or, in efforts to be more confident, in successful surgery a surgeon may remove excessive healthy tissue. Cancer that has metastasized throughout a body is nearly impossible to treat by surgery alone.

Radiation Therapy

In radiation therapy, an external high-energy *X-ray* or *gamma-ray* beam is focused upon cancerous tissue. Proton and neutron beams are also applied with protons targeting tumor-bearing sites better than X-rays and neutrons being more potent against some cancers. The desired outcome is that cancerous cells will be destroyed and a cancerous mass will be reduced in size. While radiation therapy has been utilized throughout the 20th century, it wasn't until just a few decades ago that the benefits began to outweigh the hazards. The hazards of radiation therapy lie within the overexposure and excessive damage to healthy tissue. Today, sophisticated imaging tools such as magnetic resonance imaging (MRI) and computed tomography (CT) scans allow radiologists to pinpoint the location of cancer and accurately direct the therapy. Furthermore, today powerful megavolt radiation is able to penetrate even the most dense human tissue. In a relatively new technique, called internal radiation treatment (IRT), a radioactive substance is implanted in close proximity to a tumor, thereby tightly localizing the radiation treatment.

Incredible strides have occurred in the last couple decades in improving the successfulness of radiation therapy as well as protecting healthy tissue. For instance, *conformal radiotherapy* begins with a digitally recorded image of the 3-dimensional configuration of the tumor, via CT scans or MRI. This information allows for the basis of a detailed radiation treatment that incorporates an appropriate manipulation of the direction and shape of the beam as well as dictating the intensity and duration of irradiation. Again, the primary advantage to this type of therapy is the maximization of radiation absorbed in the tumorous tissue and a minimization of exposure to surrounding healthy tissue.

Chemotherapy

The first chemotherapeutic agents became available in the 1940s. While promising, they quickly proved inadequate as administered independently or in a sequence. In the 1960s, physicians began to experiment with combining chemotherapeutic agents and some malignancies associated with younger individuals were successfully treated. These included leukemias, lymphomas, and testicular cancer. However, it soon became apparent that the bulk of other cancers could not be treated by chemotherapy alone. Frequently, the efficacy of chemotherapeutic agents is determined by the threshold of tolerance exhibited by the recipient. Anemia, infections, and a propensity for internal bleeding are common side effects. Other side effects of chemotherapy include hair loss, nausea, vomiting, and diarrhea. There are at least four large families of chemotherapeutic agents distinguishable by the mode of anticancer activity.

- *Antimetabolites* act as false substances in biochemical reactions. For instance, the folic acid analog *methotrexate* (4-amino-N^{10}-methyl folic acid) inhibits dihydrofolate reductase and thus decreases the availability of tetrahydrofolate (THF) for use in the formation of nucleic acid bases. Cancer cells can not reproduce, due to limitations in DNA replication. Fluorouracil and gemcitabine are also examples of antimetabolites.

- *Topoisomerase inhibitors* inhibit topoisomerase, which is a key enzyme involved in separating DNA complementary strands for replication. Examples include doxorubicin and CPT-11.

- *Alkalating agents* are able to form chemical bonds with DNA nucleotides, thereby resulting in spatial and other alterations in DNA structure. Examples include cyclophosphamide and chlorambucil.

- *Plant Alkaloids* prevent cell division by interacting and binding to *tubulin*, which is the protein basis of the formation of microtubular fibers that help orchestrate cellular division. Examples include vinblastine, vinorelbine, paclitaxel, and docetaxel.

Bone Marrow Transplantation

Bone marrow transplation today indicates the transplantion of *stem cells*, not necessarily the marrow. Transplantation usually is performed when the marrow itself is diseased or to compensate for the toxic effects of intense chemotherapy. Marrow transplants may most often be employed for treating breast cancer, but the efficacy is questioned. For instance, as many as 2500 American women received marrow transplants in 1994 alone. In cancers of the blood or lymph, transplantation is not controversial and is known to be beneficial. These cancers include non-Hodgkin's lymphoma and other leukemias.

The most common form of transplantation performed today is the autologous transplant whereby stem cells come from the patient. The stem cells are withdrawn prior to chemotherapy. In this procedure there is not the associated risk of GVHD (graft vs. host defense) complication. GVHD occurs when the new tissues (stem cells) derived from a donor produce immune cells that attack the host.

Cancer Risk Factors

The three main contributors of cancer development can be classified as genetic, lifestyle, and/or environmental factors. Although most cancers are related to lifestyle and environmental factors, it is generally accepted that an inherited genetic susceptibility increases the vulnerability to such factors. Reports have shown that the actual genetic risk associated with developing various types of cancers is less than 10% of incidence. Although the genetic component is a small contributor, there are more than 200 hereditary cancer patterns that predispose family members to certain cancers. For example, a woman who has a sister or a mother diagnosed with breast cancer has double the chance of being diagnosed herself. It is important to note that a family pattern could also be a result of sharing an adverse environmental or similar lifestyle patterns.

Other stimuli that have been shown to increase an individual's risk of cancer are smoking, alcohol/drug abuse, obesity, exposure to pollution, a diet low in fruits and vegetables, and prolonged overexposure to the sun. There is probably not a direct cause and effect relationship between consumption of certain natural foods and development of specific cancers, but there does seem to be trends. Listed below are some of the risk factors associated with certain cancers published in the American Cancer Society 1996 Dietary Guidelines.

Breast cancer — influenced by consumption of alcoholic beverages, even in moderate amounts; some studies suggest diets high in fruits and vegetables decrease risk; physical activity also decreases risk; obesity makes risk.

Colorectal cancer — diets high in plant foods (especially those high in fiber) have been shown to decrease risk; diets high in fat and red meat have been shown to increase risk; obesity and physical inactivity appear to increase risk.

Endometrial cancer — being overweight has been shown to increase risk, so physical activity and healthy food choices are important.

Lung cancer — greater than four fifths of all lung cancer cases result from smoking. Those who do smoke, but consume more than 5 servings of fruits and vegetables daily have been found to have lower incidence of lung cancer.

Oral and esophageal cancers — the use of tobacco and alcohol increase the risk of mouth and esophageal cancer. Fruit and vegetable consumption appears to have a positive effect on those that consume these products.

Prostate cancer — intake of animal fat, red meat, and dairy products appears to increase risk for this cancer. Researchers question the role of saturated fat and male hormones in the initiation of prostate cancer.

Stomach cancer — stomach cancer risk has decreased since the availability of refrigeration, fresh foods and food preservation methods. Infection with *Helicobacter pylori* may increase risk. Research has found that increased consumption of fruits and vegetables may decrease risk.

Chemoprevention

Opposite to chemotherapy which is applied in the treatment of cancer, the *chemoprevention* is an attempt to use natural and/or synthetic compounds to prevent the initiation of tumor cell or to intervene in early precancerous stages, before metastasis occurs. While this concept is readily apparent today, it actually began several decades ago. Chemoprevention researchers endeavor to identify and comprehend to the mechanisms of food components or pharmaceuticals that prevent or halt carcinogenesis. Many of the food-endowed, and nontraditional food chemicals include certain vitamins and their metabolites, certain minerals, indoles, isoflavones, flavonoids, isothiocyanates, lignans, liminoids, lycopene, terpenes, ω-3 polyunsaturated fatty acids, phenolic compounds, plant sterols, polyacetylene, protease inhibitors, allium compounds, and quinones. Along with these biological factors, chemoprevention pharmaceuticals including Taxomifen, Oltipraz, and Difluoromethylornithine (DFMO) are just beginning to be tested and better understood.

Dietary and Behavioral Influences on Cancer

Smoking

Perhaps the greatest risk factor for cancer development is tobacco smoke. As many as 30% of the cancer deaths in the U.S. can be attributed to tobacco smoke. Smoking, primarily cigarettes, causes cancers of lung tissue, upper respiratory tract, esophagus, bladder, and pancreas. It also probably causes cancer of the stomach, liver, and kidney. It is also probably involved in myelocytic leukemia and also colorectal cancer. Therefore smoking is considered the single most lethal carcinogen, at least in the U.S. For example, smokers are twice as likely to develop bladder cancer and eight times as likely to develop lung cancer. More specifically, if an individual smokes nine to ten cigarettes daily, he/she increases the risk of lung cancer fourfold and those who smoke a pack of cigarettes daily they increase their risk tenfold. The potency of smoking as a risk factor varies with the number of cigarettes smoked daily. Furthermore, the tar content and the duration of smoking are also strong influencing factors, while the latter is the strongest. Sadly, thousands of other individuals die each year from secondhand smoke or passive smoking.

Energy Intake

The investigation of the relationship between individual macronutrients and carcinogenesis has received far more research money and time than the investigation into the role of energy alone. Investigation of individual macronutrients in human studies, vs. animal studies, are very difficult because humans eat a mixed diet, which cannot be controlled as tightly as a diet fed to laboratory animals. Scientists do agree, however, that obesity is very detrimental in carcinogenesis. Furthermore many researchers believe that simple caloric restriction is one of the most effective dietary means for decreasing cancer risk. The suppression of neuroendocrine hormones and the regulation of growth factors via calorie-restricted diets are thought to be the mechanism by which cancer growth is reduced.

A lack of energy is thought to have many possible roles in the prevention of cancer. This lack is thought to provide an inadequate amount of energy needed to help activate cancer cells or to allow energy for growth. Also, a lack of calories is thought to increase the rate of carcinogen detoxification. In addition, there is strong evidence suggesting that hormonal imbalances related to eating without restriction and the development of obesity are suspect. Hormones of particular suspicion include prolactin, which promotes mammary cancer, and insulin, which probably serves as a tumor growth factor. Reduced glucocorticoid activity associated with *ad libitum* feeding, which inhibits several cancers, is also suggested to play a role. However, caloric restriction appears to be useful only in the primary prevention of cancer. Once established, cancer growth is probably not affected by a lack of calories in the same way and growth will continue at the expense of the individual, even if they are starving.

Even though some researchers have found little or no effect of obesity on breast cancer, the body of evidence does point towards a positive association. Therefore, it is generally accepted that obesity will increase the risk for breast cancer. On the other hand, there seems to be much more ambiguity regarding obesity and colon cancer. Some studies report no effect, while others report a promoting effect in animal models. However, researchers have shown that obesity has a promoting influence in the development of endometrial, renal, and prostate cancers, as well as tumors of the lung.

Dietary Fat

The investigation into the association between dietary fat and cancer has utilized more research dollars than any other single nutrient. Up to this point, findings have not been definitive, but the trends are suggestive of an increased risk for those people consuming diets high in fat. At this time there appears to be strong epidemiologic evidence to support the recommendations for a low-fat diet that limits the amount of red meat, high-fat dairy products and other high-fat foods to <30% of an individual's total fat kilocalories. Countries that consume lower intakes of fat present a lower incidence of a variety of cancers, whereas a greater consumption of animal fat (saturated) and red meat is associated with cancer of the colon, rectum, and prostate.

The exact mechanism involving fat is still unclear, but there are several proposed theories regarding the mechanism. One theory is that dietary fat alters the production of certain hormones, such as estrogen and prolactin, which could be responsible for the promotion of certain cancers. Another theory takes into consideration the type of fat and its negative effect on cell membranes and prostaglandin synthesis, thereby indirectly involving the immune system. Diets high in linoleic acid and other ω-6 PUFAs have been shown to decrease the immune response in animal models, while ω-3 fatty acids have been shown to exhibit a protective effect against cancer formation. However, researchers are unsure whether this protection comes from the presence of ω-3 fatty acids or the absence of ω-6 fatty acids, or both. Some evidence may be derived from rodent studies that demonstrated that when linoleic acid is increased to 5% of the energy intake there is an enhancement of carcinogen-induced mammary, pancreatic, and maybe colon cancer.

In animal studies, it has been demonstrated that dietary fat was positively related to carcinogen-induced breast cancer. However, recent research efforts have found little correlation between diets high in fat and the incidence of human breast cancer. Rather, it is thought that levels of hormones at certain times in a woman's life are more related to a future risk of breast cancer. Young age at first menstruation, number of pregnancies, breast feeding, late menopause, and late age at first pregnancy are all risk factors for breast cancer.

At this time there is no complete agreement as to what dietary factors protect against or promote the development of colorectal cancer. This type of cancer is among the leading causes of cancer death among Americans. Different types of fats (fish oil and ω-3 fatty acids) and varying amounts of fat have been investigated with regard to colon cancer. Researchers have reported that fish oils, ω-3 fatty acids and low-fat diets may indeed be protective against colon cancer in some instances.

There are many hypotheses explaining the mechanism of cancer initiation in the colon. These include the thoughts that increased levels of bile salts can damage the mucosal lining of the colon, initiating cell proliferation resulting in cancer growth; that by-products of fat breakdown will also damage the lining of the colon; or that excess fat in the colon will promote growth of cancer-promoting bacteria. However, what needs to be taken into consideration is that, although the findings are not totally consistent. The NRC Committee on Diet and Health has concluded that the weight of the evidence points to an association between colorectal cancer and a pattern of high dietary fat intake. For instance, one large study performed by Harvard University following the dietary patterns and health of more than 88,000 nurses, demonstrated a clear statistical relationship between animal fat and colon cancer. Those nurses who ate red meat daily were found to be 2 to 3 times more likely to develop colon cancer than those who ate it less than once a month. Furthermore, eating vegetable fat or diary foods did not appear to have an association at all.

To date, most studies have found a positive correlation between total fat, animal fat and saturated fat intake, and prostate cancer. Also, investigative evidence suggests that fat intake is also related to the development of cancers of the pancreas and endometrium.

Conjugated Dienoic Derivatives of Linoleic Acid (CLA)

One somewhat unique fatty acid class that may have an anticarcinogenic property is *conjugated dienoic derivatives of linoleic acid* (CLA). As little as 0.5% CLA in the diet of rats may be enough to significantly reduce carcinogen-induced mammary neoplasm development. It is not yet determined how CLA may act to thwart the development of certain cancers; however, it has been speculated that the *cis*-9, *trans*-11 CLA isomer thwarts cancer development by integrating into cell membranes and acting as an antioxidant. CLAs are produced by microbes in the rumen of cows, and beef and dairy foods are the primary providers. Human studies await for application CLA in human chemoprevention.

Physical Activity

Physical activity appears to decrease cancer risk by reducing the prevalence of obesity and possibly improving immune system functioning. While there is some question as to the true effect of varying levels and durations of activity upon immunological status, there is some evidence to suggest that after a moderate bout of exercise, individuals have higher circulating levels of natural killer cells. Research has shown an inverse relationship between exercise and cancer risk. Because of the strong relationship between increased exercise and decreased obesity, some researchers are not willing to attribute the decreased risk to activity alone. However, some hypothesized mechanisms in support of the relationship between physical activity and certain cancers are that physical activity decreases secretion of testosterone and estrogen, decreasing the likelihood of developing prostate and breast cancer, respectively.

Fiber

While there is some research evidence suggesting that dietary fiber does not reduce the incidence of cancers, the body of encouraging evidence suggesting a prophylactic role of fiber is indeed compelling and is supportive of recommendation for a diet rich in fiber. First, from an indirect role direction, fiber-endowed foods include fruits, vegetables, cereal grains, and other plant-based foods. These foods are generally lower in fat and in addition contain numerous other compounds (phytochemicals) that are protective against cancer. Also, fiber-containing foods are generally lower in energy density and will provide bulk to a meal which may support volume-associated satiety during a meal. This could reduce excessive energy consumption and, potentially, the development or propagation of obesity.

The majority of investigative evidence supports the notion that a higher fiber diet reduces the risk of colon cancers. There are several proposed mechanisms by which fiber protects against colon cancer. The first hypothesis is that fiber increases bulk and in turn dilutes fecal bile acids, which are thought to promote cancer of the colon via the conversion of benign to malignant polyps. Second, dietary fiber may reduce the action of certain colonic bacteria which are responsible for the transformation of primary bile acids (i.e., cholic and chenodeoxycholic) into secondary bile acids (i.e., lithocholic and deoxycholic). These secondary bile acids are thought to promote tumorigenesis in the colon. A third mechanism is that increased dietary fiber is thought to dilute the contents in the lumen of the colon, which will decrease the exposure of mucosal tissue to potential carcinogens. Other researchers have also suggested that dietary fiber will bind to bile acids and speed up their elimination.

The mechanism by which fiber is thought to decrease the risk of breast cancer is less complex. When breast cancer cannot be attributed to genetic predisposition, increased levels of circulating estrogen are suspect. Dietary fiber is speculated to bind with estrogen excreted into the digestive tract and block its reabsorption. Also, compounds such as phytoestrogens found in fiber-containing foods may compete with estradiol for estrogen receptors in breast tissue and in this manner beneficially affect breast cancer risk. Another proposed mechanism is that fiber may positively influence the formation of mammalian lignans, which are protective against breast cancer tumors.

Fruits and Vegetables

As early as 1979, researchers found an inverse correlation between death rates from colon cancer and the consumption of vegetables in different regions of Great Britain. It was speculated that fruits and vegetables that are high in beta-carotene may reduce human cancer rates. In the early 1980s vitamins C and E emerged as antioxidants or free radical scavengers hypothesized to prevent oxidative damage, which may be responsible for the initiation of cancer.

It is generally agreed that a diet high in fruits and vegetables is protective against formation of cancer. The National Cancer Institute in the U.S. estimates that if the following recommendations were widely followed, death from colorectal cancer could be cut in half within 10 years. It is recommended that Americans eat adequate amounts of these foods:

- All kinds of fruits
- Vegetables, especially cruciferous vegetables such as broccoli, cabbage, and brussels sprouts
- Legumes (beans, peas, lentils)
- Whole grain cereals, breads and pastas
- Low-fat, high-fiber snacks such as popcorn, whole grain crackers, and flat breads.

Because of the wide variety of compounds found in fruits and vegetables (i.e., fiber, vitamins, minerals, phytochemicals) and the fact that they are almost all low in fat, it is difficult to pinpoint the exact factor responsible for protecting us against cancer. Researchers began by focusing on single, "traditional" nutrients, especially vitamins C and E. Today, nontraditional nutrients such as carotenoids, terpenoids, and flavonoids including phytoestrogens, are being individually studied to a great extent as well as being studied in concert.

Vitamin C

Over 80% of the vitamin C in our diets comes from vegetables and citrus fruits. There are several theories on how vitamin C acts to reduce cancer risk. The most popular theory is that vitamin C scavenges free radicals and decreases DNA oxidation and alteration. Theoretically, this could prevent some mutations occurring in genes involved in cellular turnover. Vitamin C functions synergistically with other antioxidants as well, namely, vitamin E and glutathione. Also, vitamin C is necessary for hydroxylations carried out by the cytochrome P_{450}-dependent mixed function oxidase system. Further still, vitamin C is purported to have a prophylactic effect by improving immunocompetence, thereby increasing the ability to detoxify carcinogens, such as pesticides and industrial pollutants, and/or block carcinogenic processes. It is important to remember that tobacco smoking enhances the metabolism of vitamin C. This is easily understood when it is realized that it requires approximately twice as much dietary vitamin C to achieve serum levels similar to nonsmokers.

There is a body of epidemiological evidence suggesting that vitamin C intake is inversely associated to cancers of the bladder and larynx as well as cancer of the oral cavity, rectum, lungs, esophagus, and uterine cervix. Furthermore, some clinical trials have reported that large doses of vitamin C can increase survival time in individuals being treated for terminal cancers. Conversely, vitamin C has been reported to be ineffective in other similar investigations. Vitamin C can reduce the formation of nitrosamines in the intestinal tract and potentially reduce the incidence of stomach and esophageal cancers. Several foods contain nitrates. Interestingly, the natural foods containing nitrates, such as cabbage and green leafy vegetables, are also a source of vitamin C as well. Nitrates and nitrites are also found in meats that have been processed, such as during smoking or curing. Nitrosamine formation begins with the conversion of nitrates to nitrites. Vitamin C can inhibit this step. Then nitrosamines are formed when nitrites interact with amines and amides found in protein in the gut. Vitamin C can inhibit this step as well.

It is more than likely that vitamin C has some prophylactic properties relating to the carcinogenesis; however, it is not the panacea it was once touted to be. It is more realistic that vitamin C is just one of many beneficial factors in fruits and vegetables supporting a greater synergistic effect of fruits and vegetables in chemoprevention.

Vitamin E

While vitamin E appears to exert a protective effect against cardiovascular disease, its potential merit as adjunctive therapy in the prevention of some cancers remains unclear, but may hold promise as well. For instance, in a large Finnish study involving 23,000 male smokers, those that received α-tocopherol and β-carotene demonstrated a 34% decrease in prostate cancer. It should also be mentioned that a small, but statistically insignificant, decrease in colorectal cancer was reported as well. In another example, one research investigation found vitamin E to be beneficial in reducing breast cancer in women with family history of breast cancer. More research is indeed warranted with respect to the potential chemoprevention application of vitamin E.

β-Carotene

β-Carotene is the principal carotenoid (carotenes and xanthophylls) in the human diet. Like many other carotenoids, β-carotene functions as an antioxidant. Earlier epidemiological evidence strongly suggested that presence of β-carotene was inversely correlated with certain cancers, including lung cancer. Then in the 1980s large chemoprevention trials were initiated to determine the efficacy of β-carotene and other dietary antioxidants such as α-tocopherol in the prevention of certain cancers in high risk situations. Much to the surprise of the investigators, as well as the scientific community at large, male smokers receiving a β-carotene supplement actually presented a higher incidence (18%) of lung cancer compared with smokers not receiving a supplement.

Researchers speculated that it is likely that fruits and vegetables contain other factors that are necessary in combination with or supportive of β-carotene for its prophylactic properties. Thus, it is best to obtain carotenoids from a diet rich in fruits and vegetables rather than supplements.

Selenium

Some of the earliest reports of a purported anticarcinogenic effect of selenium appeared in the 1940s. It was reported that a relatively higher dietary intake of selenium could protect against azo dye (dimethylaminoazobenzene)-induced hepatic tumors in rats. Later, several reports also indicated that cancer incidence was inversely related to either dietary selenium content or geographic distribution of selenium. For instance, one report in the 1970s revealed that mortality due to lymphomas and cancers of the gastrointestinal tract, peritoneum, lung, and breast were lower for both American men and women residing in areas of greater selenium content in their crops. In another epidemiological effort, blood selenium content of the inhabitants of 24 regions of mainland China was negatively correlated to cancer mortality rates.

It has also been determined by cross-sectional investigation that many cancer patients have lower tissue levels of selenium. However, one concern about a cross-sectional assessment of this nature is that it is difficult to be sure that the subjects were drawn from the same population. For instance, it is possible that the process of cancer formation and progression affected selenium metabolism and status or that individuals might have altered dietary intakes that influenced their selenium status. Several studies of this nature confirmed that a reduction in selenium status was associated with various cancers; however, others did not.

Numerous animal studies have indicated that selenium, provided above the nutritional range, can have an antitumorigenic effect. The models were mostly rodent and the cancer was chemically induced at numerous tissue sites including colon, esophagus, kidney, liver, lung and mammary glands. Here, it may be important for humans to provide selenium in their diet to optimize their status, but not to surpass the threshold for toxicity.

Calcium

Calcium may play a role in preventing colon cancer. It has been suggested that calcium binds to bile acids in the intestinal lumen, thereby decreasing their metabolism by microbes and pathological interaction with colon mucosa. Furthermore, calcium is speculated to decrease the proliferation rate of abnormal mucosal cells. Investigators have reported that men who drank several glasses of milk daily had a significantly decreased incidence of colon cancer.

Dithiolthiones

Dithiolthiones are found in cruciferous vegetables (cabbage family) such as cauliflower, broccoli, cabbage, brussel sprouts, kale, kohlrabi, bok choy, collards, rutabaga, and mustard greens. *Oltipraz* is a synthesized version of diothiothiones, and investigative efforts to present have suggested that it may inhibit the development of neoplasma in lung, colon, and mammary and bladder tissue. All of these reports were the result of animal experimentation. It is believed that Oltipraz induces increased activity of hepatic detoxification systems.

Flavonoids and Phytoestrogens

The *flavonoids* are a large group of naturally occurring compounds found in vascular plants. The Western diet contains about 1 g/d. Multiple beneficial effects of flavonoid consumption have been purported, including anticarcinogenic properties. Certain flavonoids appear to be able to increase the activity of *glutathione-S-transferase* (GST). In preliminary cancer studies, rats consuming a 5% *quercetin* diet developed half as many DMBA-induced mammary tumors. Also, rats consuming a 2% quercetin diet developed one fourth as many tumors.

Isoflavonoids and diphenolic lignans can potentially decrease the development of endocrine-associated cancers, especially breast cancer. These compounds are present in numerous plants and are nonsteroidal. Since these substances possess the potential to bind to estrogen receptors, they were named estrogenic substances. Historically, the compound *mirosterol* was isolated from tuberous roots of a leguminous plant in Thailand. The plant was legendary for its "rejuvenation" properties. One early study of the estrogen potency of mirosterol found it to be as effective as 17β-estradiol in inducing the maturation of young female mouse's reproductive tract. Also, subcutaneous administration of mirosterol was 70% as active as 17β-estradiol in the promotion of mammary duct growth in the rat. Thus, mirosterol was one of the earliest examples of a plant component having properties similar to estrogen. Again, phytoestrogens are not true steroid molecules, but the spacial geometry of their molecular form allows for similarities with mammalian estrogen.

The most common phytoestrogens in the human diet are isoflavones and lignans. Isoflavones are mostly found in soybeans and other legumes while lignans are found in a variety of plant foods such as whole grains, fruits, and vegetables. The most estrogenic isoflavones are *genistein* and *diazdein* and the most estrogenic lignans are *enterodiol* and *enterolactone*. They are consumed in a precursor form that is converted to the active heterocyclic phenols by gut microbes. Phytoestrogens are able to weakly associate to estrogen binding sites; thus they have the properites of estrogen, yet are far less potent. They are about 10^{-3}–10^{-5} times as potent as synthetic estrogen, to be more exact. In addition, they appear to inhibit tyrosine kinase and epidermal growth factor, as well as seem to impede malignant cell proliferation and angiogenesis. This makes them ideal candidates for natural prophylactic compounds against cancer.

True human trials regarding phytoestrogen consumption and cancer incidence are lacking. However, there is encouraging evidence from both epidemiological and animal studies as well as from human cancer cell lines. For instance, the incidence of hormone-dependent tumors (i.e., breast) is lower in Asia and Eastern Europe where the phytoestrogen content of the diet is lower than in Western societies. In animal studies, isoflavone-rich diet decreased mammary tumor numbers and metastasis in experimentally induced cancer. *In vitro* studies of human breast and prostate cancer cell lines are indeed compelling. Breast cell lines saturated with isoflavone demonstrated dose-dependent agonistic activity. Also, prostate cancer cell lines appear to be inhibited with higher doses of genestein; however, the level was higher than could naturally be achieved in the human diet. Also, in a reported case study, an adenocarcinoma specimen, taken from a man utilizing 160 mg of phytoestrogen for 1 week, presented an increased level of *apoptosis* of cancer cells. Apotosis is a cell event whereby a cell in essence commits suicide. Certainly much more information needs to be generated from controlled clinical trials to determine the true efficacy of phytoestrogen in the prevention and treatment of cancer.

Allylic Sulfides

Allylic sulfides are *organosulfur compounds* (OSC) and are components of garlic and onions. Some scientists believe that the regular consumption of these foods can reduce the incidence of cancer, and there is indeed promising evidence to support their claims. Epidemiological evidence is provided by a case-controlled study in northern China by which it was determined that stomach cancer was inversely associated with the intake of OSC-containing vegetables (i.e., onions, garlic, scallions, and Chinese chives).

There are several water-soluble and lipid-soluble OSCs in garlic and onions including *diallyl sulfide* (DAS) and S-*allyl cysteine*. In general, garlic contain OSCs with allyl groups while onions contain OSCs with propyl groups. Garlic is believed to be more potent than OSCs from onions in chemoprevention. A proposed mechanism for OSCs chemoprevention activity is that they increase the activity of glutathione-*S*-transferase which is involved in the detoxification of many carcinogenic substances. Certainly OSCs hold promise of being recognized as a potent chemopreventative agent, and further epidemiological and clinical trials await.

Terpenoids

Terpenoids include d-*limonene*, *limolin*, and *nomilin*, and their derivatives. The monoterpene *d*-limonene is synthesized only in plants beginning with the formation of HMG CoA from acetyl CoA. HMG CoA is then converted to mevalonate by HMG-CoA reductase. Mevalonate is necessary for cell growth. D-Limonene appears to inhibit the activity of HMG-CoA reductase, and thus mevalonate production. The mechanism by which terpenoids reduce cancer formation probably goes beyond the simple reduction of synthesis of cholesterol and ubiquinone and other basic mevalonate derivatives that are necessary for cell proliferation. It is speculated that mevalonate is probably involved in the posttranslational modification of proteins involved in cell turnover.

The limonoids are a class of highly oxidized triterpenes containing a furan ring. Limonin is the triterpene that provides much of the bitter taste to citrus fruits. In carcinogen-induced oral cancer studies, limolin decreased the average tumor burden in DMBA-induced oral carcinogenesis by 60%; nomilin also decreased oral carcinogenesis, but to a much lower, nonsignificant percentage (15%). It may be that these triterpenes increase glutathionine *S*-transferase (GST) activity in select cells. Despite its promising beneficial effects, limolin is too bitter to use as an additive or supplement. Limolin and nomilin also serve as precursors for glucosides.

Limonoid glucosides are formed by the simple addition of a glucose molecule to limonoids. These molecules include limonin 17-β-D-glucopyranoside (LG), nomolinic acid 17-β-D-glucopyranoside (NAG), and nomolin 17-β-D-glucopyranoside (NG). Liminoid glucosides are more concentrated in citrus cultivars, found at 80 to 320 ppm vs. 1 to 2 ppm for limonin and nomilin. Liminoid glucosides are more water soluble and less bitter as well. In preliminary oral carcinogen-induced cancer trials with rats, LG reduced DMBA-induced oral tumor burden by 55%. NG and NAG reduced DMBA-induced oral tumor burden by 20% and 5%, respectively; however, these were statistically nonsignificant trends.

Limonin carboxymethoxime and deoxylimonic acid are produced from limonin via simple reaction or bacterial conversion. In oral cancer studies similar to those mentioned above, limonin carboxymethoxine reduced DMBA-induced oral tumor burden by 55%, while deoxylimonic acid was ineffective. A lot more research is warranted in the area of the terpenoids because their presence within certain plants, especially citrus, may help explain the prophylatic effect of diets rich in fruits and vegetables.

Coffee

Research linking coffee to cancer of the bladder, breast, colon, lung, pancreas, and prostate are inconclusive. The link between coffee and breast cancer may stem from the antagonistic impact that caffeine has on fibrocystic breast lumps; however, many studies have found no relationship between the caffeine and breast cancer. Even in animal studies, the results are not compelling. For instance, when rats were fed the equivalent of 85 cups of coffee per day for 2 years, no bladder tumors appeared. Conversely, some scientists suggest that coffee has a potential co-carcinogenic activity and noted that readily oxidized phenolic compounds, known components of coffee, catalyzed nitrosamine formation. Many researchers agree that small amounts of coffee may help prevent cancer, while large amounts may have a negative impact on cancer formation. Furthermore, if coffee is to be held suspect it is unclear if the caffeine in coffee is to blame for an initiation of cancer, or whether it is other known mutagens in coffee, such as chlorogenic acid, atractylocides, and methylglyoxal.

Alcohol

Cancer risk increases with the amount of alcohol consumed and may start to rise with intake of as few as two drinks per day. Alcohol has been attributed to as many as 3% of all cancer deaths and is most common in oral cavity, esophageal, and laryngeal cancers. The mechanisms involved in cancer production from consumption of alcohol may include promotion of cell division (causing cellular damage), activation of chemical carcinogens; promotion of malnutrition and depletion of vitamin stores, impairment of the immune system, damage to the mucosa of various organs, and possibly exposure to carcinogens in alcoholic beverages (i.e., nitrosamines in beer, urethane in bourbon and sherry).

However, there are multiple problems inherent in identifying alcohol as a cancer-causing agent. Some of these include inability to accurately quantify alcohol intake, confounding interactions between alcohol and smoking, malnutrition status of heavy drinkers, possible cancer-causing substances found in these beverages. For example, the Advisory Committee of the American Cancer Society reports the combined use of alcohol and tobacco leads to greatly increased risk of oral and esophageal cancers; the effect of alcohol and tobacco combined is greater than the sum of their individual effects.

The studies involving breast cancer and alcohol seem less defined. The mechanism is unknown, but is thought to be due to carcinogenic actions of alcohol or its metabolites, to alcohol-induced changes in levels of hormones such as estrogens, or to some other process. Additionally, those who are consuming large amounts of alcohol, regardless of the type, may not be eating foods that are nutrient rich, and therefore chemopreventive. It is also recommended that women with an unusually high risk for breast cancer abstain from drinking any type of alcohol. However, research in this area does seems to be ambiguous. Some research indicates a negative impact of certain types of alcohol on breast cancer, while other research has found little or no relationship.

Unproven Oral Treatment Options

Whenever there is a disease for which science has not found a cure, quackery is bound to flourish. The prevalence of use of questionable treatments has been found to be associated with people who have achieved higher levels of education (i.e., graduate or professional school), higher income (i.e., more than $50,000 annually), and those who have prolonged illnesses.

Krebiozen, popular in the 1950s, was a drug claimed to be manufactured from the serum of Argentinian horses that had been inoculated with a mold (*Actinomyces bovis*) that causes equine lumpy jaw. By stimulating the body's inherent anticancer substances, this drug was purported to halt cancer growth. Upon further investigation, the FDA determined that this was actually creatine monohydrate.

Amygdalin, commonly referred to as laetrile, is found in the pits of fruits such as apricots, peaches, plums, and apples and the active ingredient in this product is cyanide. In the 1970s, 27 states legalized its use for cancer treatment on the basis of two theories. The first theory states that the cancer cells contain an enzyme that initiates the release of cyanide from laetrile, thus killing the cancer cells. The second theory is that cancer is a disease of vitamin deficiency, and laetrile cures this deficiency by acting as the missing vitamin, which is termed vitamin B_{17}. However, even with their popularity, there is no scientific evidence to support any of these claims.

Nutritional Concerns of Conventional Therapies

As stated above, the main treatment options for people diagnosed with cancer include chemotherapy, radiation, surgery, bone marrow transplants, or a combination of these four. Some of the nutritional complications of the treatment process are unique to each therapy are provided in Table 17.2.

TABLE 17.2
Nutritional Concerns Associated with Common Cancer Treatment Therapies

Therapy	Site	Nutritional Complication
Surgery	Head and neck	Problems with chewing, swallowing, and may need prolonged tube feedings
	Abdominal	Malabsorption, diarrhea, flatulence, lack of HCL, intrinsic factor, fluid and electrolyte imbalances
	Pancreatic	Malabsorption, diabetes
Radiation	Head and neck	Loss of sense of taste, alterations in sense of smell, xerostomia, loss of teeth, dental caries (decreased saliva, IgA in saliva, change in flora), mucositis, sore throat, dysphagia, fibrosis, nausea, vomiting, anorexia
	Abdominal	Bowel damage (acute or chronic) diarrhea, flatulence, malabsorption, obstruction, fistula formation, ulceration, colitis, anorexia, nausea, vomiting, fluid and electrolyte imbalances
Chemotherapy		Anorexia, nausea, vomiting

Suggested Readings

Archer, M.C., Cancer and the diet, in *Present Knowledge in Nutrition*, Ziegler, E.E., Ed., ILSI Press, Washington, D.C., 1996.

Griffiths, K., Adlercreutz, H., Boyle, P., Denis, L., Nicholson, R.I., and Morton, M.S., *Nutrition and Cancer*, Isis Medical Media, Oxford, U.K., 1996.

National Research Council, *Carcinogenesis and Anticarcinogenesis in the Human Diet*, National Academy Press, Washington, D.C., 1996.

Craig, W.J., Phytochemicals: guardians of our health. J. Am. Diet. Assoc., 97(Suppl. 2), S199–S204.

Scientific American, What you need to know about cancer, September 1996.

18

Diabetes and Nutrition

Diabetes is a major chronic metabolic disorder afflicting as much as 2% of the population worldwide. In the U.S. alone, approximately 5 to 6% of the population or about 14 million people have currently been diagnosed with diabetes mellitus, the leading cause of blindness, amputation, renal failure, and a significant contributor to the development of heart disease and stroke. Nutrition therapy is a central focus of treatment.

Historically, diabetes mellitus was recognized as early as 3000 years ago. Writings on papyrus describe a condition whereby individuals would urinate frequently and in atypical quantities. Later, Ayurvedic medicine described the sweet nature of the urine of individuals with diabetes mellitus and how ants were attracted to the urine. It also described the general weakness of those individuals as well as the occurrence of emaciation. The 1st-century Greek physician, Aretaeus, is actually credited with the naming of the disorder and described a general "melting down" of the flesh and limbs into the urine. Lipemia was identified in individuals with diabetes mellitus around the turn of the 17th century. In the early 20th century, Banting and Best were able to purify canine islet cell tissue and demonstrate a hypoglycemic effect when it was injected into diabetic animals. After those monumental efforts, the prognosis for individuals diagnosed with diabetes mellitus improved drastically.

Definition, Etiology, and Classification

Diabetes mellitus is not a single disease per se, but rather a group of metabolic disorders characterized by chronic hyperglycemia resulting from defects in insulin secretion, insulin action, or both. If uncontrolled, the chronic hyperglycemia is associated with a variety of organ anomalies. There are two primary types of diabetes as well as other specific types of anomalies resulting in diabetes mellitus-related symptomology. In the past there has been some variation in the naming of the two main types of diabetes mellitus. Recently however, the Expert Committee on the Diagnosis and Classification of Diabetes Mellitus, an international committee of experts working in concert with the American Diabetes Association, published criteria for the diagnosis and classification of individuals with diabetes mellitus. They asserted that it was particularly important to move away from the system that classified diabetes mellitus based upon pharmacological treatment and to base the classification system more upon the etiology of the disease. Their proposal modifies the classification system as stated by the National Diabetes Data Group (NDDG) published in 1979 and endorsed by the World Health Organization (WHO) Expert Committee on Diabetes in 1980. These organizations had classified diabetes mellitus into insulin-dependent diabetes mellitus (IDDM, type I diabetes) and noninsulin-dependent diabetes mellitus (NIDDM type II diabetes). The newer classification system utilizes "type 1" ands "type 2," wherein Arabic numbers replace Roman numerals.

Type 1 Diabetes Mellitus

Type 1 represents approximately 5 to 10% of all known cases of diabetes mellitus in the U.S. Type 1 diabetes mellitus is typically diagnosed before the age of 20, but it may occur at any age. The peak incidence is at about 12 years of age in girls and between 12 to 14 years of age in boys. It has been estimated that as many as 120,000 children in the U.S. alone have been diagnosed with type 1 diabetes mellitus. At diagnosis, individuals are typically lean, and symptoms include polyuria (frequent urination), polydipsia (increased thirst), hyperphagia (increased appetite), and weight loss. Other aberrations include ketosis, electrolyte imbalances, and dehydration.

Type 1 diabetes mellitus encompasses the vast majority of clinical cases that are primarily the result of autoimmune destruction of pancreatic islet β cells. This diabetes type does not include clinical cases where there is nonautoimmune destruction of β cells such as can occur in cystic fibrosis. This form of diabetes has long been referred to as "insulin-dependent diabetes mellitus" (IDDM) or "juvenile-onset diabetes mellitus." In roughly 85 to 90% of type 1 diabetes mellitus diagnostic cases, there are the presence of autoantibody markers such as islet cell autoantibodies (ICAs), insulin autoantibodies (IAAs), glutamic acid decarboxylase autoantibodies (GAD_{65}) as well as autoantibodies to tyrosine phosphatases IA-2 and IA-2β. For the remaining 10 to 15% of individuals with type 1 diabetes, the etiology is unknown. Interestingly, most of those falling into this etiological minority are of African or Asian descent.

Without question, there is a strong hereditary component to the diagnosis of type 1 diabetes mellitus, and a genetic marker has been located. It appears that at least one of the genetic anomalies rendering an individual more susceptible to type 1 diabetes mellitus is located on the histocompatibility region of chromosome 6. Human leukocyte antigen (HLA) genes are divided into three classes: class I, with A,B,C gene subgroups; class II, representing the DP, DQ, and DR loci; and class III genes, which are clustered between the class I and class II genes. The HLA genes code for transmembrane proteins and proteins of the complement system. They are critical for the process of recognizing the difference between host cells and foreign cells, as well as potentiating the immune complement system.

Type 1 diabetes mellitus has a strong HLA association, with linkages to the DQ, A, and B genes, and it is influenced by the DRB genes. The HLA-DR/DQ alleles appear to be either predisposing to or protective against the development of diabetes mellitus. Data suggest that approximately 4 out of 5 individuals diagnosed with type 1 diabetes mellitus are HLA positive.

In addition to a strong genetic component to type 1 diabetes mellitus, there does appear to be poorly understood environmental factors involved as well. Obesity does not seem to be a strong influential factor, as it is in type 2 diabetes mellitus. The consumption of cow's milk during infancy and among young children was speculated to be an influencing factor; however, not enough evidence exists at this time to assign causality to cow's milk. Other factors, such as congenital rubella, mumps, sugar consumption, and infant feeding practices, have also been implemented as causative agents. Many scientists also contend that exposure to viral entities, toxic substances, or diseases such as those just mentioned triggers an autoimmune reaction. One large Swedish study reported that prenatal growth may influence the risk for developing type 1 diabetes mellitus whereby those children with greater birth weights for their gestational age were at a higher risk. Individuals with type 1 diabetes mellitus are also more prone to other autoimmune disorders such as Grave's disease, Hashimoto's thyroiditis, and Addison's disease.

Interestingly the rate of β cell destruction is individualized, leading to a varied onset of signs and symptoms. Therefore, diagnosis may occur as early as infancy or childhood or as late as early adulthood. Some cases have even been reported in individuals in theirs 80s and 90s. However, most of the diagnosis occurs during youth. Early manifestations include ketoacidosis, especially in younger people. For others, a moderate fasting hyperglycemia can progress to a severe state of hyperglycemia and ketoacidosis in the presence of infection or other physiological stress. For many not diagnosed until later in life, residual β cell activity is sufficient to hinder the development of ketoacidosis. Treatment of type 1 diabetes mellitus requires insulin therapy as will be discussed below.

Type 2 Diabetes

This form is the most prevalent form of diabetes and in the past has been referred to as non-insulin-dependent diabetes mellitus (NIDDM) or adult-onset diabetes mellitus. About 85 to 90% of all diabetes mellitus diagnoses in the U.S. are of the type 2 nature. This type of diabetes includes those individuals who present insulin resistance and usually demonstrate a relative insulin deficiency, rather than an absolute deficiency, as in type 1 diabetes mellitus. At the time of diagnosis, as well as often throughout treatment, individuals with type 2 diabetes mellitus do not require insulin therapy. However, periodic or protracted insulin therapy is sometimes adjunctive therapy.

The etiology for this type of diabetes is speculated to be very broad and remains somewhat vague. Rarely are circulating pancreatic islet antibodies observed; therefore β cell destruction has not occurred. Obesity is perhaps one of the factors with the strongest association to type 2 diabetes mellitus, and there is now mounting evidence that obesity may directly result in the development of insulin resistance. Approximately 80% of individuals diagnosed with type 2 diabetes are obese. Furthermore, individuals with centralized or abdominal obesity appear to be more prone to type 2 diabetes than individuals with body fat stores below the waist. In addition, children who have a higher percentage of body fat may be more inclined to develop type 2 diabetes mellitus later in life.

Ethnicity may be a predisposing factor for type 2 diabetes mellitus as well. African-Americans and Hispanic-Americans have a 2 to 3 times greater chance of developing type 2 diabetes mellitus than white Americans. According to the American-based National Health and Nutrition Examination Survey (NHANES) data collected between 1982 and 1984, approximately 10% of Hispanic-American adults, 26% of Puerto Ricans, and 24% of Mexican-Americans were diagnosed with type 2 diabetes mellitus at that time.

Type 2 diabetes mellitus can go undiagnosed for extended periods of time, as the classic signs and symptoms of type 1 diabetes mellitus may not be presented. Individuals with type 2 diabetes mellitus are not as prone to ketoacidosis as type 1 individuals. However, bouts can occur during periods of physiological stress such as infection. The characteristic hyperglycemia develops slowly, and often the initial awareness of the condition by a physician is accidental. Protracted hyperglycemia can result in macrovascular and microvascular anomalies as discussed below.

Upon first examination, individuals with type 2 diabetes mellitus might appear to have normal or even slightly elevated plasma insulin levels. However, with respect to the hyperglycemia, the insulin response is inadequate. Therefore, insulin secretion is defective, concomitant to the reduced sensitivity to the presence of insulin. While exogenous insulin therapy is not required by most individuals with type 2 diabetes mellitus, as much as 40% of these individuals may utilize insulin, either periodically or long term.

Insulin Resistance

The causes of insulin resistance have not been completely revealed. Insulin binds to its receptor on the plasma membrane of cells such as skeletal muscle and adipocytes. It exerts its intracellular effects via a complex phosphorylation chain. The ultimate result is an augmentation of glucose transporter (GLUT4) translocation to plasma membranes, thus allowing for a greater glucose influx into those cells. For a long time, insulin resistance was thought to have its origin with the GLUT4 transporters or insulin receptors. At this time, there is some evidence to suggest that a genetic mutation in the GLUT4 transporter may indeed play a role in the development of insulin resistance. However, its exact involvement, as well as other recognized genetic anomalies (i.e., insulin receptor and islet amyloid polypeptide (IAPP)), is still unclear. It is likely that genetic factors may have a supportive or potentiating effect, along with other factors, in the development of insulin resistance. Increased plasma insulin levels are known to down-regulate the expression of insulin receptors so there can be a quantitative influence as well. However, the change in the number of receptors does not necessarily correlate with insulin sensitivity.

Researchers have reported that insulin-resistant individuals have impaired skeletal muscle glycogen synthesis. At least some of this impairment may be due to the increased level of free fatty acids (FFA) found in the plasma of insulin-resistant individuals. Increased FFA oxidation in skeletal muscle may impair glycogen synthesis and glucose oxidation. The oxidation of FFA may have this effect by altering the redox potential within the cell and influencing key enzymatic steps in the glycolytic pathway. It has also been suggested that increased levels of phosphorylated glucose in insulin-resistant cells, such as may occur when glycolysis is impaired, may lead to a greater flux through the glucosamine pathway. This pathway is normally important for the production of glycoproteins. In rats, infused FFA does indeed increase the quantity of metabolites produced by the glucosamine pathway. This pathway may function as a sensor that reacts to increased intracellular nutrient levels by decreasing the entry of glucose into cells.

The secretion of peptides from enlarged adipocytes has also been suggested as at least a contributing factor to the development of insulin resistance. For example, tumor necrosis factor-α, which has been reported to be released from adipocytes, has been shown to impair insulin receptor autophosphorylation. Further, the hormone leptin has been suggested as having involvement as well. Chapter 12 provides a more detailed description of adipocyte activities as a result of hypertrophy of those cells.

Perhaps some of the benefits of exercise with relation to insulin resistance can be explained by its effect on exercising and resting lipoprotein lipase activity. One of the effects of regular aerobic exercise is an increased ability to transport circulating fat into muscle cells and an enhanced ability to oxidize fat both during exercise and at rest. The net result may be a reduction in fat deposited in adipocytes, thereby allowing for some atrophy of the swollen adipocytes. Theoretically, this would then reduce the release of the signaling molecules alluded to above and potentially ameliorate some of the insulin resistance. Also, exercise promotes the uptake of glucose into working muscle in an insulin-dependent manner.

Insulin resistance, or even marginal insulin resistance, is perhaps more common than once thought. For example, as much as 20 to 25% of healthy American individuals may show signs of insulin resistance as determined by insulin-stimulated glucose uptake. Furthermore, in one investigation, about 13% of normotensive, nonobese individuals with normal fasting glucose had fasting insulin levels measured at 2 SDs above the mean. These individuals also had a greater insulin response to glucose challenge as well.

Pathophysiology of Insulin Resistance

Provided that the β cells are able to produce more and more insulin during insulin resistance, normal glucose tolerance can be maintained. However, once *compensatory hyperinsulinemia* is not sustained, glucose intolerance is developed. The compensatory hyperinsulinemia is indeed a paradox. While the hyperinsulinemia can help control glucose tolerance, it is also associated with varieties of physiological anomalies. Hyperinsulinemia is associated with elevations in plasma triglycerides and lower HDL-cholesterol. Smaller and more dense LDL particles become more prominent in the blood, while lipemia after a meal is elevated and hypertension is common. The presence of these risk factors has been termed "syndrome X" and the hyperinsulinemic individual is at a greater risk of heart disease. While triglyceride levels are indeed controversial as an independent risk factor for heart disease, epidemiological studies do suggest that in combination with hyperinsulinemia, hypertriglyceridemia indeed becomes a serious risk factor.

Other Specific Types of Diabetes Mellitus

There are several physiological situations wherein an individual presents the signs of diabetes mellitus, such as hyperglycemia, but the etiology does not allow it to be classified as either type 1 or type 2. These include (1) genetic defects in pancreatic β cell, thereby reducing the secretion of insulin; (2) genetic defects in the insulin receptor, thereby reducing the action of insulin; (3) diseases of the exocrine pancreas; and (4) drug- and chemical-induced diabetes mellitus.

Genetic Defects of the β Cell, Insulin, and Insulin Receptors

There are several forms of diabetes mellitus associated with a specific genetic anomaly (monogenetic aberrations) that directly result in alterations in β cell function. Because β cell destruction or insulin resistance are not the primary etiological factors, these genetic defects do not easily fall into either type 1 or 2. While most have been nuclear DNA-related, mitochondrial DNA defects have also been identified. The nuclear DNA-related forms are autosomal dominant aberrations and typically manifest in a mild hyperglycemia, usually before the age of 25. They are often called maturity-onset diabetes of the young (MODY). Typically there is a reduction in insulin secretion, but there is no change in the action of the insulin hormone itself. The defects that have been isolated at this point have three genetic loci: (1) hepatic nuclear factor (HNF)-1α gene located on chromosome 12; (2) glucokinase gene located on chromosome 7p; and (3) HNF-4α gene located on chromosome 20q. The mutation to HNF-1α is the most common form and may actually be present in as many as 2 to 5% of type 2 diabetes cases. HNF-1α is a transcription factor that is known to be involved in the tissue-specific regulation of the expression of several liver recognized genes. It also serves as a weak transactivator of the insulin-I gene. HNF-4α is a member of the steroid/thyroid hormone receptor superfamily and an upstream regulator of HNF-1α expression. Glucokinase is involved in the phosphorylation of glucose to form glucose 6-phosphate, whose metabolism is believed to be involved in the secretion of insulin.

Other genetic anomalies associated with the development of diabetes have been identified that, again, do not fit the criteria for inclusion into the type 1 or 2 categories. For instance, aberrations in the insulin hormone itself can result in mild to pronounced hyperglycemia. Leprechaunism and Rabson-Mendenhall syndrome are two pediatric disorders characterized by diabetes as a result of a defect in the insulin receptor.

Gestational Diabetes Mellitus

Beyond genetic disposition, drug, toxin, or chemical injury may result in diabetes, as can trauma and pancreatitis. Pregnancy may also result in the development of diabetes. The incidence in the U.S. is estimated at 4% of all pregnancies or 135,000 cases annually. The percentage of incidence is indeed broad, ranging from 1 to 14%, depending on the population studied. The term *gestational diabetes mellitus (GDM)* is applied to any degree of hyperglycemia experienced during pregnancy. Maternal complications more common for these individuals include hypertension and increased rate of ceasarian delivery. Hyperglycemia as a result of deterioration of glucose tolerance does appear to occur normally during pregnancy and in particular during the 3rd trimester.

Diagnostic Criteria for Diabetes Mellitus

The diagnostic criteria for diabetes mellitus continue to evolve. The most recent criteria were published by the Expert Committee mentioned above. There are three ways to diagnose diabetes mellitus, as presented in Table 18.1. A positive finding relative to the criteria must be confirmed on a subsequent day, again, by any of the three criteria. A typical oral glucose tolerance test is presented in Figure 18.1.

TABLE 18.1
Criteria for the Diagnosis of Diabetes Mellitus

1. Symptoms of diabetes plus casual plasma glucose concentration ≥ 200 mg/100 ml (1.1 μmol/l). "Casual" is defined as any time of day without regard to time since last meal. The classic symptoms of diabetes include polyuria, polydipsia, unexplained weight loss, or
2. Fasting plasma glucose ≥ 126 mg/100 ml (7.0 μmol/l). "Fasting" is defined as no caloric intake for at least 8 h, or
3. 2-hour plasma glucose ≥ 200 mg/100 ml during an oral glucose tolerance test. The test should be performed as described by WHO, using a glucose load of 75 g of anhydrous glucose dissolved in water

In addition to those individuals meeting the criteria, as listed in Table 18.1, there are many individuals who have fasting glucose levels below 126 mg/100 ml but above what would be considered normal (≥110 mg/100 ml). These individuals are considered to have intermediate fasting glucose (IFG) levels. Thus, normal glucose tolerance is considered a fasting plasma glucose <110 mg/100 ml, IFG is ≥110 yet <126 mg/100 ml, and the provision of the diagnosis of diabetes mellitus when fasting glucose is ≥ 126 mg/100 ml.

When considering the oral glucose tolerance test as a diagnostic tool, a 2-h post-glucose load <140 mg/100 ml is considered normal glucose tolerance and ≥140 yet <200 mg/100 ml is considered IGT, and last, >200 mg/100 ml is considered a diagnostic indicator of diabetes mellitus. The utilization of a 2-h postglucose test is common practice because it has been

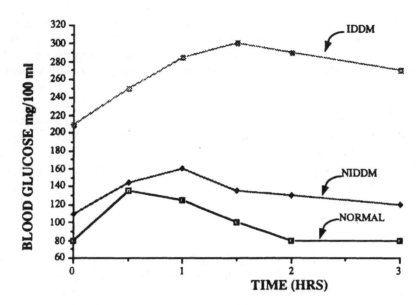

FIGURE 18.1
Normal and diabetic glucose—time curves of an oral glucose tolerance test (OGTT).

defined as a cutoff point whereby the association to microvascular diseases increases dramatically.

Glycosylated hemoglobin A_{1c} (Hb A_{1c}) is another blood test utilized for diabetes screening and monitoring. During the typical life-span of a RBC, which is about 120 days, glucose can nonenzymatically attach to hemoglobin molecules. The resulting glycohemoglobin is a relatively stable complex, allowing for a direct relationship between blood glucose levels and the level of Hb A_{1c}. Thus, Hb A_{1c} provides an effective tool for monitoring blood glucose levels over time and can be particularly useful in evaluating efficacy of treatment as well as an individual's adherence to treatment. In nondiabetic adults, the level of Hb A_1 is 2.2 to 4.8, and in children it is about 1.8 to 4.0. A good control treatment protocol will result in a level of 2.5 to 6.0, while a Hb A_{1c} greater than 8.0 reflects poor control.

Medical Complications Associated with Diabetes Mellitus

Few clinical disorders compare to diabetes mellitus for causing such widespread aberrations. Common sites of lesions include the pancreas, blood vessels, kidneys, nervous tissue and the eyes. Before the advent of insulin therapy, the complications resulting from long-term poorly controlled diabetes mellitus were not as significant as they are today. This is largely because of the dim prognosis for a short survival time for individuals with type 1 diabetes mellitus. The reader is referred to other resources in the Suggested Readings for a more thorough review of the mechanisms of pathophysiology associated with diabetes mellitus.

Diabetic Neuropathy

Diabetic neuropathy is believed to be the most common of neuropathy in the Western world. It is also perhaps the most common complication associated with diabetes mellitus occurring in both type 1 and type 2. The underlying cause is vague in nature. It may be due to vascular or metabolic mechanisms, or a combination of both. There are two stages: (1) the *subclinical stage*, which presents slowed motor and sensory impulse conduction, and (2) the *clinical stage*, in which significant symptomology is present, possibly concomitant to marked neurological deficits.

It appears that early changes, such as axonal degeneration, are most noticeable in unmyelinated peripheral nerves. With time, metabolic and structural abnormalities develop as well, causing segmental loss of myelin. The spinal cord is often a site of demyelination. Signs and symptoms of diabetic neuropathy include reduction in motor nerve conduction and sensory perception. There may be recovery of more normalized neural activity if good glucose control occurs.

Retinopathy

As the retina of the eye is on a per weight basis the most metabolically active tissue in the human body, it is particularly vulnerable to microvascular disease. Uncontrolled diabetes mellitus results in changes in the blood vessel resulting in ischemia which damages the tissue. There is a strong association between the severity of the injury and the individual's age and duration of diabetes mellitus. Retinopathy is very common in diabetes mellitus and individuals with type 2 appear to develop the pathology more rapidly. There are three stages of retinopathy. Increased retinal capillary permeability characterizes *Stage I* or *nonproliferative retinopathy*, along with the formation of microaneurysms, dilation of veins, and superficial flame shaped and deep blotting hemorrhages. *Stage II* or *preproliferative retinopathy* presents progressive damage due to ischemia that leads to retinal infarcts. *Stage III* or *proliferative diabetic retinopathy* is the product of new blood vessel formation and the formation of fibrous tissue within the retina and optic disc.

Diabetic Nephropathy

Diabetes mellitus is the most common cause of end-stage renal disease in the western world. Approximately 30% and 5 to 10% of individuals with type 1 and type 2 diabetes mellitus, respectively, have increased levels of nitrogenous waste in their blood (uremia). Early signs include the detection of small to progressively increasing amounts of albumin in the urine or albuminuria, decreased creatinine clearance, and hypertension.

Diabetic nephropathy develops over time. Several pathological changes occur in nephrons, including a thickening of the basement membrane (basal laminae) associated with the glomerulus along with the development of atherosclerotic-like lesions in the glomerular region (glomerulosclerosis). Lesions and hyalination of the afferent and efferent arterioles also occur. Diabetic nephropathy is preventable with appropriate insulin treatment in type 1 diabetes mellitus.

Pancreatic Degeneration

Progressive accumulation of *hyalin* in the islets is common. Hyalin is a glassy, translucent material assumedly derived from eosinophils. While hyalinization of pancreatic parenchyma is recognized in both type 1 and 2 diabetes mellitus, it is more prevalent in type 2.

Medical Nutritional Therapy for Diabetes Mellitus

The most recent recommendations made by the American Diabetes Association for nutritional management of diabetes were published in 1997. The overall goal of nutritional therapy for diabetes is to assist individuals in achieving and maintaining metabolic control, to reduce the risk of both acute and long-term complications of diabetes, and to improve general health through proper nutrition. A more complete summary of the goal is listed in Table 18.2.

TABLE 18.2
Goals of Nutrition Therapy for Patients with Diabetes Mellitus

1. Maintenance of blood glucose levels as close to normal as possible. This is to be accomplished by proper diet in combination with insulin, oral glucose-lowering drugs, and physical activity
2. Achievement of optimal serum lipids levels
3. Dietary energy should be appropriate for achieving or maintaining reasonable weights for adults, normal rates of growth and development for children and adolescents, and optimal nutrition during pregnancy and lactation or recovery from catabolic illness
4. Prevention and treatment of the acute complications of diabetes such as severe hypo- or hyperglycemia, renal disease, autonomic neuropathy, hypertension, hyperlipidemia, and cardiovascular disease
5. Improvement in overall health through optimal nutrition

For the treatment of type 1 diabetes mellitus, the emphasis of nutritional therapy should consider the following factors: (1) provision of adequate energy to achieve a normal body weight or as close as possible for adults or to allow normal growth and development in children and adolescence, (2) coordination of food intake, especially carbohydrate, with insulin injections and physical activity to maintain blood glucose within a respectable range and to also prevent hypoglycemia.

For treatment of type 2 diabetes mellitus, the emphasis of nutritional therapy should be focused on achieving normal, or as close as possible, blood glucose and serum lipid levels, as well as blood pressure and body weight. As obesity, especially intraabdominal obesity, is closely associated with the development of insulin resistance and type 2 diabetes, weight reduction is an extremely important component of nutritional therapy. Also, as mentioned previously, obesity is strongly associated with the signs of syndrome X (i.e., hypertension, hyperlipidemia) which places the individual at greater risk of heart disease and stroke. Weight reduction resulting in a reduction in total and intraabdominal body fat is associated with improved glycemic control and more favorable blood lipids and blood pressure measurements. Weight loss should be obtained by combination of a mild hypocaloric diet in combination with physical activity.

Historical Recommendations

Historically the recommendations for the energy nutrient composition of the diet for diabetes has changed considerably. Before the 1920s, and the advent of insulin therapy, individuals, mostly children, were placed on starvation diets and the prognosis was death within a few months to a year or so. However, after insulin therapy became available, starvation was replaced by a carbohydrate restriction to 20% of total calories, while individuals strived to achieve normal growth or maintain a normal body weight. In the 1950s, the recommendations for energy nutrient contributions to total energy intake were modified again to 40% from carbohydrate, 40% from fat, and 20% from protein. In the early 1970s, the recommendations were modified yet again to increase the carbohydrate contribution to 45% and decrease fat contribution to 35% of total energy, while the protein recommendation did not change. Then in 1986, the recommendations were further modified by the American Diabetes Association to reduce the fat contribution to 30%, with saturated fat contributing 10% or less of total calories. This modification was made with respect to the relationship between diets high in fat and saturated fat and dyslipidemia and cardiovascular disease.

At this time there is still debate as to the best percentages of total energy contribution of carbohydrate, protein, and fat. Considerations include the effect of energy nutrients upon glycemic index and control of serum lipids. Therefore, the most current guidelines set by the American Diabetes Association do not make specific recommendations but require that patients be evaluated individually.

While little controversy exists as to appropriate amount of protein for individuals with diabetes, more discussion is focused upon how the remaining 80 to 90% of the energy should be divided between carbohydrate and fat. As mentioned above, one of the most significant considerations for dietary recommendations is reducing an individual's risk of heart disease. It is also recommended that dietary cholesterol not exceed 300 mg daily. If dietary fat is limited to less than 30% of total energy, then the remaining nonprotein energy must be carbohydrate.

Carbohydrates

At one time, it was common practice to restrict dietary carbohydrates. Even up until the 1950s, it was recommended that carbohydrates contribute less than 20% of the energy to the diet of an individual diagnosed with diabetes mellitus. As mentioned above, these recommendations were eventually increased to 40% of energy and then 45% in 1971. Prior to the 1970s, the recommendations for carbohydrate intake mostly considered the impact of this energy nutrient dietary carbohydrate upon glucose control. However, as more became known about chronic degenerative diseases and the relationship between diet, diabetes, and their etiology, the recommendations for carbohydrate intake also had to consider the other energy nutrients (i.e., fat) as well. The recommendations for carbohydrate were increased to 50 to 60% of total energy to accommodate the updated recommendations for fat (<30% of total calories).

Complex vs. Simple Carbohydrates

For decades, it was assumed that because of the relatively complex nature of starch molecules to simpler sugars, they would be digested more slowly and therefore absorbed more slowly and evenly after a meal. As the control of postprandial hyperglycemia is an important consideration in the management of diabetes mellitus, and in conjunction with the purported desirable digestion/absorption attributes of starch, early recommendations were to limit simple carbohydrates, especially sucrose. Therefore, foods, such as candies and cakes, with sucrose in their recipe, or the use of table sugar were discouraged in the management of diabetes mellitus. However, in the mid 1970s it was reported that glycemic effect associated with ingested glucose, which requires no digestion, and more complex carbohydrates similar to those found in bread, rice, and potatoes were not substantially different as expected. Nevertheless, these were isolated carbohydrate sources, and when considering intact food, several factors (i.e., fat and fiber content, rate of gastric emptying) will influence the glycemic effect of endowed carbohydrate-containing food. This led to the development of the *glycemic index*. The glycemic index was developed as a way of classifying different carbohydrate-containing foods, based upon their glycemic response. The glycemic response of the different carbohydrate-containing foods was originally compared to glucose but later changed to a white bread of known composition.

The glycemic index of a food is the incremental blood glucose area after consumption divided by the corresponding area after consumption of the reference white bread in an amount providing an equivalent amount of carbohydrate as the test food. The glycemic index has some limitations. First, there can be large variations in glycemic response between individuals. Second, differences in cooking and other methods of preparation can also effect the glycemic index of a food. Last, humans tend to eat food in combination with other food items, thereby nullifying the glycemic index predictability associated with a given carbohydrate-containing food.

In the years that followed, researchers began to isocalorically substitute sucrose and other simple carbohydrates for complex carbohydrates in the diet. This allowed researchers to investigate simple sugars, as a percentage of carbohydrate and energy within a single meal or a diet, for several days to weeks to determine if they negatively impacted glycemic control. In studies substituting sucrose for complex carbohydrates up to 25% of energy in a single meal, researchers reported that there was no adverse effects on glycemic index. Meanwhile, researchers also reported that long-term (several weeks) substitution of complex carbohydrates with sucrose, to reach as high as 38% of total energy also had no adverse effect upon glycemia. Based upon the results of clinical investigations of this nature, the American Diabetes Association concluded that the restriction of dietary sucrose and other simple carbohydrates for glycemic control is not justified. However, whether or not the restriction of sucrose with regard to lipemia in individuals with diabetes mellitus is justified is still unclear.

Fructose

The substitution of fructose for sucrose or glucose in foods has long been considered, as fructose ingestion is associated with a lower effect on blood glucose. Furthermore, insulin is not necessary for its metabolism. Some researchers have actually reported that postprandial glucose responses were lowered when fructose is isocalorically substituted for other carbohydrates in a meal. However, one negative effect of higher fructose intakes is the potentially adverse influence on serum lipids. While total serum cholesterol and triglycerides may remain unchanged, LDL-cholesterol may be increased. Therefore, substitution of sucrose with fructose may not be beneficial. However, individuals with diabetes mellitus need not avoid natural foods containing fructose, such as fruits, vegetables, and honey.

Protein

For those individuals diagnosed with diabetes at an earlier age, protein intake must be adequate to ensure proper growth and development. The recommended protein intake for most individuals with diabetes is 10 to 20% of total energy. This is adequate for growth and development provided adequate energy intake. Protein intake should be restricted to 0.8 g/kg body weight in individuals with diabetes and who are in the onset of renal failure. Protein intake may be further reduced to 0.6 g/kg body weight as glomerular filtration rate

(GFR) declines. Oppositely, in situations where additional protein is necessary such as the treatment of obesity with very-low-calories-diets, pregnancy and catabolic diseases may increase protein needs.

Total Fat

As mentioned above, general recommendations for protein for adults is 10 to 20% of total energy. Thus the remaining 80 to 90% of energy is to be divided between carbohydrate and fat, provided alcohol consumption is minimal to absent. Furthermore, if saturated fats and polyunsaturated fats are to contribute less than 10% and as much as 10% of total energy, respectively, the remaining 60 to 70% of energy is to be split between monounsaturated fats and carbohydrate. However, the practical distribution between carbohydrate and fat may need to be individualized based upon nutrition assessment and treatment goals.

The recommendation for an individual may consider that person's desired blood lipid and body weight and composition. For individuals diagnosed with diabetes mellitus, as well as nondiabetic individuals with more normalized blood lipids, body weight, and composition, general recommendations are for less than 30% of total energy to be derived from fat. However, if weight loss and reduction of body fat content are desired outcomes, then a reduction of total fat intake, in conjunction with exercise, is recommended.

The *Step I* diet guidelines as established by the National Cholesterol Education Program (NCEP) in America may be prescribed for individuals with diabetes mellitus with elevated total cholesterol and LDL-cholesterol levels. Similar to general recommendations above, the Step I diet guidelines limit total fat intake to 30% of total calories and cholesterol to 300 mg daily. The contribution of saturated fat is limited to 10%, while recommendations for monounsaturated and polyunsaturated fats are 10 to 15% and 10%, respectively. The NCEP's *Step II* diet guidelines are even more restrictive, and are prescribed when the Step I guidelines are unsuccessful or the dyslipidemia is treated more aggressively. The Step II diet guidelines limit saturated fat to 7% of total calories and reduce cholesterol intake to less than 200 mg daily.

Alcohol

Alcohol is metabolized primarily in hepatocytes. It does not require the presence of insulin to be metabolized. However, this lack of dependence upon insulin does not necessarily offer an advantage. In fact, alcohol consumption and the production of its breakdown product acetyl CoA can promote gluconeogenesis and ketogenesis. Further, alcohol is calorically dense and nutrient void. Therefore, excessive alcohol consumption can promote obesity as well as exacerbate clinical manifestations of uncontrolled diabetes. In addition, a small number of individuals utilizing sulfonurea drugs in treatment of diabetes experience higher levels of these substances in their circulation; alcohol consumption can bring about distressing symptoms.

Sweeteners

In addition to sucrose and fructose, other sweeteners include nutritive sweeteners such as corn syrup, fruit juice and concentrate, honey, molasses, dextrose, sorbitol, mannitol, and xylitol; and nonnutritive sweeteners such as saccharin, aspartame, and acesulfame K.

While substituting fruit juices and fruit juice concentrates for sucrose can improve the nutritional content of the diet, at this time there does not seem to be an advantage to improve glycemic response. The use of sugar alcohols, such as mannitol and sorbitol, may reduce the glycemic response associated with a food when substituted for sucrose as a sweetener. However, the excessive use of sugar alcohols may result in a laxative effect.

Fiber

Soluble fibers, such as from legumes, oats, and some fruits and vegetables, have demonstrated the ability to hinder glucose absorption from the lumen of the small intestine. In theory this could reduce postprandial hyperglycemia. However, in 1995 the American Diabetes Association stated that the clinical significance of this effect was probably nominal and should not be considered a focal part of diabetes management. Therefore, the recommendations for fiber intake are not different than the population at large. However, this is not meant to belittle the clinical significance of an adequate fiber intake for individuals with diabetes mellitus. This is especially true for soluble fibers that have been shown to reduce total cholesterol and LDL-cholesterol levels which can be elevated in diabetes.

Vitamins and Minerals

At this time, there are no recommendations for vitamin or mineral supplements for individuals with diabetes mellitus. However, researchers have reported that individuals with diabetes mellitus have lower serum vitamin C levels and that 1 gram of supplemental ascorbic acid can reduce the level of glycosylated hemoglobin by 18%. It may be that ascorbic acid inhibits glycosylation of hemoglobin in a competitive manner. Furthermore, supplemental doses of vitamin C (2 g/d) for 3 weeks also lower erythrocyte sorbitol levels by 44.5% and is believed to reduce capillary fragility as well. Thus, vitamin C supplementation may be a viable adjunctive therapy.

Chromium deficiency in experimental animals has resulted in hyperglycemia, which appears to be correctable by reintroduction of chromium. Elevations in serum cholesterol and triglyceride levels are also correctable by a reintroduction of chromium. However, it is assumed that most individuals with diabetes mellitus are not chromium deficient. This belief is confirmed by several research investigations in which chromium supplementation to individuals with type 2 diabetes failed to reduce hyperglycemia or improve insulin intolerance.

The Exchange System of Meal Planning

The Exchange System of Meal Planning was developed by the American Diabetes Association and the American Dietetic Association. This system allows individuals to plan their diet based upon an appropriate caloric intake to allow for weight management, as well as to promote healthy eating. The Exchange System also promotes regular physical activity, goal setting, and lifestyle changes conducive to healthy eating and achieving goals for eating, body weight, and body composition.

Under the Exchange System, foods are comprised of three groups (carbohydrate, meat and meat substitutes, and fat groups), with associated subgroups. All foods in these groups are listed with serving sizes. The subgroups have associated grams of carbohydrate, protein, and fat, as well as caloric content. These are presented in Table 18.3. The carbohydrate group has five subgroups, which include starch, fruit, milk, vegetables, and other carbohydrates, including high-sugar foods or "sweets." The starch group includes cereals, grains, pastas, breads, crackers, starchy vegetables (i.e., baked beans, corn, green peas, potatoes, squash, and yams) and starchy foods (i.e., pancakes, waffles, stuffing, and corn bread). Fruits include fruits and fruit juices. Milk is subdivided into skim, low-fat, and whole milk, as these variations will vary the fat and energy content. The "other" carbohydrate list includes a variety of cakes, cookies, doughnuts, ice creams, syrup, and yogurt. The carbohydrate, fat, and energy content will vary between items in this subgroup.

TABLE 18.3
The Exchange List for Meal Planning

Food Group/List	Carbohydrates	Protein	Fat	Kilocalories
Carbohydrates				
Starch	15	3	1 or less	80
Fruit	15	—	—	60
Milk				
Skim milk	12	8	0–3	90
Low-fat milk	12	8	5	120
Whole milk	12	8	8	150
Other carbohydrates	15	Varies	Varies	Varies
Vegetables	5	2	—	25
Meat and meat substitutes				
Very lean	—	7	0–1	35
Lean	—	7	3	55
Medium-fat	—	7	5	75
High-fat	—	7	8	100
Fat	—	—	5	45

The meat and meat substitutes include those foods that contain both protein and fat. One meat exchange is equivalent to 1 ounce of meat, fish, poultry, or cheese or 1/2 cup of dried beans. Based upon their fat content, meats are subdivided into very lean, lean, medium-fat and high-fat meats. While one exchange of each will contain approximately 7 g of protein and no appreciable carbohydrate, the variation in fat content drastically influences the energy content. For instance, the energy content of one exchange of very lean meat, lean meat, medium-fat meat, and high-fat meat are approximately 35, 55, 75, and 100 kcal, respectively.

The fats group includes saturated, monounsaturated, and polyunsaturated fat sources. The monounsaturated fat list includes avocados and olives; nuts such as almonds, peanuts, and pecans; peanut butter and sesame seeds; and oils such as canola, olive, and peanut oils. The polyunsaturated fat list includes margarine (30 to 50% fat), nuts such as walnuts, oils such as corn, soybean, and safflower oils, and pumpkin and sunflower seeds. The saturated fat list includes bacon, butter, lard, shortening, coconut, cream cheese, and sour cream.

The Exchange System instructional booklets also provide lists of so-called "free foods." Free foods are those food or drink items that contain less than 20 kcal or less than 5 g of carbohydrate per serving. Free foods are to be limited to three servings daily if they contain energy (i.e., fat-free cream cheese, salsa, fat-free margarine, catsup, pickles, and sugar-free syrup) or may be unrestricted if the calorie content is nominal (i.e., sugar-free gum, lemon juices, tea, coffee, diet soft drinks, seasoning, mustard, and sweeteners such as aspartame, saccharin, and acesulfame K. In addition, the foods that are relatively high sources of sodium (>400 mg per serving) are indicated.

Carbohydrate Counting

Carbohydrate counting is a method of meal planning for individuals with diabetes mellitus that has become extremely popular in western Europe and is gaining in popularity in the U.S. Because the primary energy nutrient influencing blood glucose, and therefore insulin requirements, is carbohydrate, carbohydrate counting focuses only on the amount of carbohydrate ingested daily. Carbohydrate counting allows for greater precision in estimating carbohydrate consumption than does the Exchange System. Currently the American Dietetic Association offers three booklets to assist in carbohydrate counting. These booklets provide guidance at three progressive levels and include (1) "Getting Started"; (2) "Moving On"; and (3) "Using Carbohydrate/Insulin Ratios".

Non-Nutritional Medical Therapy

Insulin Therapy

Insulin is required therapy for individuals with type 1 diabetes mellitus. Some individuals with type 2 diabetes may also require either long-term or periodic exogenous insulin therapy. These individuals include those that have failed to adequately control hyperglycemia by diet and oral hypoglycemic agents alone, or individuals experiencing acute injury, pregnancy, stress, or infection.

Insulin is available from either animal or human resources. Cow (bovine) or pig (porcine) insulin, derived from pancreatic tissue extracts, was the insulin resource for decades. However, these resources were immunogenic to humans, bovine insulin more so than porcine insulin, and antiinsulin antibodies that delayed and/or limit the immunogenic effect of animal insulin had to be developed. Recently, human insulin made available via recombinant DNA techniques in bacterial cultures has become a primary resource in countries such as the U.S. Here the human insulin gene is inserted into a bacterial vector and expressed in large quantities. Human insulin produced by recombinant DNA technique does not have an associated immunogenic effect.

There are three general types of pharmacological insulin that are separated based upon onset time and peak activity and duration of activity.

1. **Rapid-acting insulin** can have an effect as quickly as 15 min (*lispro*) after injection. Lispro (Humalog) has a peak and duration of activity of about 30 to 60 min and 1 to 2 h, respectively. Lispro is actually a human insulin analog in which the basic amino acid sequencing is slightly altered by reversing two amino acids (lysine and proline) in sequence at positions 28 and 29 on the β chain of insulin. Because of its immediate impact, lispro should be taken immediately prior to a meal. Other rapid-acting insulin include Humulin R, Regulin, Semilenti, and Velosulin R. They are virtually the same; however the names differ due to different manufacturers. These insulins are derived from bovine, porcine, or human resources. Their onset to activity is approximately ½ to 1 h, with a peak between 2 to 4 h and a duration of 3 to 7 h.

2. **Intermediate-acting insulin** includes Humulin L, Lente, NPH, Insulatard N, and Insulatard. These insulins are detected in the blood within 2 h with a peak around 11 h and a duration of activity of about 18 to 24 h.

3. **Long-acting insulin** includes Humulin U and Ultralente. The onset of activity is between 2 to 6 h, with a peak activity that is minimal and a duration of 24 to 36 h. Long-acting insulin is rarely used except in special needs, because of the difficulty associated with predicting onset, peaks, and duration.

While a detailed description of insulin's structure and function can be found in Chapter 11, some of the most outstanding functions include stimulation of glucose transport in muscle and adipocytes, increased amino acid uptake in muscle cells and enhanced protein synthesis, inhibition of hormone-sensitive lipase in adipocytes, and promotion of glycogen synthesis, glycolysis, and fatty acid synthesis. Exogenous insulin is delivered by regular injection with disposable syringes or by continuous subcutaneous insulin infusion (CSII), via an insulin pump. The insulin pump is a relatively small device, easily worn on a belt with a subcutaneous abdominal needle attachment. An individual can initiate a timely, programmed flow of insulin, with regard to food intake, by pushing buttons on the pump device.

The long-acting insulins became available in the 1930s as *protamine* was added to the insulin molecule along with zinc. The former substance prolonged the action of insulin, while the latter substance enhanced its stability. Then, in the early 1940s, intermediate-acting insulins were introduced as Hagedorn modified the long-acting protamine-zinc insulin (PZI) form to produce a neutral protamine insulin complex. It was called NPH for neutral protamine Hagedorn. The different insulin types are presented in Table 18.4.

TABLE 18.4
Pharmacological Aspects of Select Insulin

Insulin	Onset of Action	Peak Action	Duration of Activity	Source
Rapid-acting				
Humalog (lispro)	15 min	$1/2$–1 h	1–2 h	H
Regular	$1/2$–1 h	2–3 h	3–6 h	H
Regular	$1/2$–2 h	3–4 h	4–6 h	A
Intermediate-acting				
Lente	3–4 h	4–12 h	12–18 h	H
Lente	4–6 h	8–14 h	16–20 h	A
NPH	2–4 h	4–10 h	10–16 h	H
NPH	4–6 h	8–14 h	16–20 h	A
Long-acting				
Ultralente	6–10 h	None	18–20 h	H
Ultralente	8–14 h	Minimal	24–36 h	A

Sources are denoted as human (H) and animal (A).

Oral Antidiabetic Agents

Oral antidiabetic agents include sulfonurea drugs that stimulate the release of preformed insulin from the pancreas as well as having an effect upon glucose transport. These drugs include Tolbutamide (Orinase), Chloropropamide (Diabinese), Tolazamide (Tolinase), Glyburide (Diabeta, Micronase), and Glipizide (Glucotrol and Glucotrol XL). The initial dosage prescribed is the least amount determined to be effective in individuals maintaining the ability to secrete insulin. If this level is ineffective, the prescription dose is increased thereafter every 1 to 2 weeks until glycemic control is achieved. About 65 to 75% of individuals with type 2 diabetes demonstrate satisfactory control on the initial prescription dosage. Side effects are not common, however, the potential for hypoglycemia should monitored. Weight gain may be experienced in some individuals and should also be monitored.

Another oral agent prescribed for individuals with type 2 diabetes mellitus is Metformin. Metformin, prescribed either alone or in combination with sulfonylurea agents, decreases blood glucose levels by increasing cellular glucose utilization. This drug is not associated with weight gain or hypoglycemia.

Thiazolidinediones, such as troglitazone, are another group of drugs prescribed in the treatment of type 2 diabetes. These drugs have been shown to decrease insulin resistance. They have also been shown to reduce both fasting and postprandial hyperglycemia and hyperinsulinemia. Other drugs, namely, α-glucosidase inhibitors appear to decrease postprandial hyperglycemia by competitively inhibiting intestinal brush border carbohydrate digestive enzyme activity. The use of specific oral antidiabetic agents is individualized and often these agents are used in combination.

Suggested Reading

The Expert Committee on the Diagnosis and Classification of Diabetes Mellitus, Report of the Expert Committee on the Diagnosis and Classification of Diabetes Mellitus, Diabetes Care, 20 (7): 1183–1197, 1997.

19

Osteoporosis and Nutrition

Osteoporosis is a skeletal disorder in which a chronic imbalance in bone turnover results in an excessive loss of bone mineral and matrix. This renders bone more susceptible to fracture. Osteoporosis is a major health issue in countries such as the U.S. where it affects as many as 25 million individuals, including about 1 out of 4 women over the age of 60. The complications associated with osteoporosis, such as hip fracture, make this disorder the 12th leading cause of death in the U.S. Each year, about 260,000 American women will suffer hip fractures as a result of osteoporosis.

The major risk factors for osteoporosis are (1) age, as bones become less dense; (2) sex, since women have less bone tissue and also potentially experience more bone loss later in life due to menopause; and (3) race as caucasian and Asian women are more susceptible than African-American and Hispanic women.

Bone Tissue

Bone Structure

All 206 bones in the human body are classified based upon shape, either long, short, flat, or irregular. Bones of different shapes contain varying proportions of the two basic types of osseous tissue: *compact* bone and *cancellous* or spongy bone. Compact bone is dense and presents a smooth and homogenous appearance. On the other hand, cancellous bone is composed of trabeculae, which are tiny needle-like or flat pieces of bone. The trabeculae form a network that houses bone marrow (Figures 19.1 and 19.2).

While cancellous bone is honeycomb by design, compact bone contains a very organized structure. Compact bone contains a multitude of small structural units called osteons or Haversian systems. Electron microscopy reveals that each osteon is a system of concentric tubes (lamella) separated by thin regions called lacunae. Within lacunae, osteocytes are present, and lacunae are connected to each other, as well as the central canal, by very thin canals called canaliculi. The innermost lamella in an osteon surrounds a thin canal that houses nerve fibers and blood vessels. Small canals running through adjacent lamellae and connecting with the central canal at a right angle are called Volkmann's canals. Lamellae are constructed largely of collagen fibers in a manner such that adjacent lamellae contain collagen fibers running in an antiparallel fashion.

Bone material contains both an organic matrix (30%) and calcium salt mineral deposits (70%). The matrix is largely collagen fibers; in fact, about 90 to 95% of the matrix may be attributable to collagen. Collagen provides incredible tensile strength to bone. The remaining portion of the matrix is a homogeneous medium called *ground substance*. Ground substance is made up of extracellular fluid plus proteoglycans. Proteoglycans are composed of proteins plus glycosaminoglycan (GAG), polysaccharide-based molecules such as *chondroitin sulfate*. *Hyaluronic acid* is another GAG found in bone matrix; however, it is not bound to proteins.

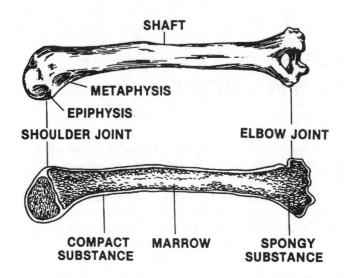

FIGURE 19.1

The humerus: the long bone of the upper arm. The top diagram presents the three parts of a long bone: (1) the shaft (the long part of the bone); (2) the metaphysis (the end of the shaft, or diaphysis, where it joins the epiphysis), and (3) the epiphysis (the rounded end).

Bone mineral deposits are largely crystalline salts with each crystal being about 400 Å long, 10 to 30 Å thick, and about 100 Å wide. Thus, bone mineral crystals have the shape of a long flat plate. Calcium and phosphate are the principal minerals in bone crystals, which are called *hydroxyapatite*. These minerals form a basic salt unit with the chemical formula of $Ca_{10}(PO_4)_6(OH)_2$. Calcium phosphate deposits (i.e., $CaHPO_4 \cdot 2H_2O$ and $Ca_3(PO_4)_2 \cdot 3H_2O$) are also found to a lesser degree. Magnesium, potassium, and sodium ions are also present in bone matrix associated with hydroxyapatite crystals.

The concentration of calcium and phosphate in the extracellular fluid is more than adequate to allow for the formation of hydroxyapatite in bone. In fact, this would occur in all

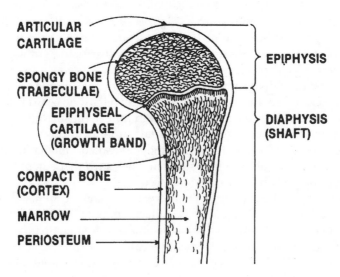

FIGURE 19.2

Diagram of the longitudinal section of a bone.

tissue if it were not for inhibiting substances such as pyrophosphate that prevent precipitation. These inhibitors are either not present in bone, or bone-forming cells (osteoblasts) secrete inhibitors of these substances.

The initial stage of bone formation is the secretion of collagen monomer molecules and ground substances by osteoblastic bone cells. Collagen monomers rapidly polymerize by cross-linking to form mature collagen fibers. The resulting tissue is similar to cartilage. In the formation of this tissue some *osteoblasts* become entrapped in tissue spaces, such as lacunae, and become osteocytes. Once mature collagen fibers are formed, calcium phosphate salts can begin to be deposited on the surfaces of these large molecular structures. With time and as the calcium phosphate salt concentration associated with collagen fibers increases, hydroxyapatite crystals begin to form. These complexes are actually developed over a period of days to weeks to months. Not all of the calcium salts are destined to become part of hydroxyapatite crystals. As much as 20 to 30% remains uncrystalized and can serve as an easily dissolved and readily available source of calcium when serum calcium levels are low.

Bone Turnover

Bone is continuously turned over. This is to say, bone is continuously being made, while at the same time it is being broken down. If there is a balance between the actions of the bone-forming osteoblasts and cells that dissolve bone, called *osteoclasts*, then bone is maintained over time. However, an imbalance in these activities can result in either an increase or decrease in bone. This is particularly important during growth as osteoblast activity must be greater than osteoclast activity.

Osteoblasts are generally found on the surfaces of bone and within bone cavities. It has been estimated that osteoblasts are active on 3 to 5% of bone surface area at any given moment. Conversely, osteoclasts, which are larger than osteoblasts and are probably derived from monocytes or monocyte-like cells produced in bone marrow, continuously reabsorb bone. It is estimated that osteoclasts are constantly active on about 1% of bone surfaces. Parathyroid hormone is principally involved in controlling osteoclast activity. The manner in which osteoclasts are able to reabsorb bone seems to be by stretching out villus-like projections of their plasma membrane along the surface of bone which then secrete proteolytic enzymes and acids (i.e., citric acid and lactic acid). The proteolytic enzymes digest bone matrix protein, such as collagen, while the acids dissolve mineral salts. Increased levels of parathyroid hormone are associated with increased osteoclast activity of this nature.

One of the greatest factors influencing the rate of bone deposition is physical stress. Bone is deposited relative to the compressional load the bone must endure. Perhaps this point is most obvious during bone fracture immobilization or protracted exposure to zero gravity in space. If an individual experiences a fractured leg and must walk with a cast on that leg and without putting weight on the leg, that leg can experience as much as a 25 to 30% loss of bone calcium over a period of several weeks. However, the opposite leg, which still must bear weight and thus endure compression stress, will not experience significant change in mineralization. Astronauts, such as the Russian Cosmonauts, existing for long periods of time at zero gravity in a space station, experienced significant reduction in bone density as well.

Total bone mass turnover in adults is about 15% annually. While single and dual photon absorptiometry easily indicates changes in bone density over time, certain biochemical markers can also be measured. Fasting urine calcium/creatine (Ca/Cr) levels are based on the concept that the concentration of calcium in the urine in a fasting state reflects bone resorption operations. This measure assumes the absence of influential clinical situations such as idiopathic hypercalcemia. Typically this indicator becomes elevated after menopause and remains elevated for several years thereafter. Fasting hydroxyproline/creatinine (OHpr/Cr) excretion is also a good independent measurement of bone resorption. The peak increase in fasting OHpr/Cr typically occurs within the first 2 to 3 years after menopause. Both Ca/Cr and OHPr/Cr levels return to premenopausal levels after estrogen therapy.

Other newer measures of bone turnover rate belong to a class of compounds called *cross-links* (pyridinium cross-links), which are also measured in the urine. The level of urinary pyridinoline is elevated by roughly 60 to 80% after menopause and the level of deoxypryidinoline increases by about 50 to 60%. Serum indices of bone turnover include osteocalcin, bone alkaline phosphatase, and carboxyterminal propeptide of type I collagen.

Bone Density and Peak Bone Mass

During periods of growth and into the 3rd decade of human life, bone deposition exceeds bone resorption. However, after a very brief plateau period, bone resorption begins to exceed bone deposition. During the very brief plateau period, an individual is said to be at peak bone mass (PBM). PBM is typically experienced within the range of 25 to 35 years of age, with an average of 28.3 to 29.5 years.

Generally males have a greater PBM than females because of a larger frame size. For instance, it would not be unusual for a man to have as much as 15% greater bone density and 30% greater bone mass than an age-matched female. Along with gender, heredity also appears to influence bone density. In age-matched individuals, Hispanics and those of African descent tend to have a greater bone density as well as bone mass than individuals of western European descent. This might be related to the relatively greater skeletal muscle mass. Also, within families, daughters of premenopausal osteoporotic women tend themselves to have a lower bone density in comparison to age-match daughters of non-osteoporotic women.

Bone loss after PBM is estimated at about 1.2% annually. Bone losses are experienced in both men and women and occur in both cortical bone and trabecular bone; however, their rate of loss is not identical. The loss of trabecular bone may be greater than cortical bone, especially in women. After menopause, the loss of both bone types continues and is accelerated in women. As much as 2 to 3% losses of bone per year can be experienced for the first 5 to 10 years after menopause. The rate of bone loss will then slow to less than or up to 1% in the years that follow. Here, again, in the postmenopausal period, there are greater losses experienced within trabecular bone. Throughout a woman's life, she may lose up to 45 to 50% of her bone mass while men may only experience half of that, losing 20 to 30% of their bone mass. The actual loss of bone is a combination of deterioration of both the organic matrix and mineral deposits. Osteoclastic proteolytic enzymes and acid secretions dismantle collagen fibers and dissolve mineral complexes. This results in losses in bone density and mass and tensile strength, rendering bone more susceptible to fracture.

Pregnancy and Lactation

During a typical full-term pregnancy, about 30 g of calcium will be transferred to the fetus. To compensate for this stress upon maternal calcium status, the efficiency of intestinal absorption can double and renal excretion of calcium will decrease. While it is believed that a woman with good calcium status and dietary intake throughout pregnancy will not have her own skeleton compromised, a woman in poor status may lose as much as 3% of her bone mineral during a pregnancy. Also, a woman with good calcium status may, at least theoretically, experience an increase in bone density during the last trimester of pregnancy due to increased estrogen levels and increased mechanical stress upon bone provided by the pregnancy-associated weight gain. Research in this area is not entirely clear. However, it does seem that a well-nourished woman in good calcium status during pregnancy will either not experience bone loss or have only slight losses at skeletal regions that have both corticol and trabecular bone.

During lactation there is a significant demand on maternal calcium for breast milk. If the skeleton was the exclusive source of calcium, there would be approximately a 4 to 6% reduction in skeletal calcium. However, calcium is transferred from maternal serum to breast milk. It is not clear whether lactation will result in bone mineral reduction in women with good calcium intake and status. However, if there is a reduction, preliminary research indicates that the mineral may be recovered with weaning and the reestablishment of menses.

Osteoporosis

Osteoporosis, as defined by a recent consensus of involved scientists, is a disease characterized by low bone mass and microarchitectural deterioration of bone tissue, leading to enhanced bone fragility and a consequent increase in fracture risk. Osteoporosis results from deficits in the normal composition of bone. This is to say that the minerialization and matrix is not abnormal, but is simply deficient in amount and distribution. Thus, osteoporosis will differ somewhat from osteomalacia in that the latter is due largely to gross undermineralization. Most individuals with osteoporosis do not experience excessive loss of minerals relative to matrix. However, it should be mentioned that some individuals do demonstrate a decrease in the calcium to phosphate ratio, as well as carbonate, and these same people typically have increased bone content of sodium and magnesium. This emphasizes the fact the osteoporosis can be highly individualized.

The diagnosis for high-risk individuals includes history, physical examination, laboratory tests, and the most telling, bone mass quantification. Again, the most significant risk factors include age, female gender, postmenopausal state, Caucasian or Asian ancestry, lower lean body mass, and poor calcium status. Laboratory measurements should include serum calcium and phosphate, alkaline phosphatase, thyroxine, parathyroid hormone, and a 24-h urine and creatinine. Bone mass can be quantified by single and dual photon absorpiometry, computer tomography, and X-ray densitometry. Bone mass quantification will allow for a baseline assessment, especially at menopause, as well as provide information as to the rate of bone mass reduction.

Osteoporosis Classification

Like many disorders, the etiology and manifestations of osteoporosis are not ubiquitous, and therefore researchers have applied a classification system in which the major factors are sex, age at which fractures occur, and the kinds of bones involved. There are two types (I and II) of osteoporosis according to this classification scheme. There are also a couple of other osteoporotic disorders that do not necessarily fall into these two classes. These disorders affect younger individuals and may or may not be associated·with a rare genetic disorder or be secondary to drug therapy or another disease process.

Type I or postmenopausal osteoporosis occurs in elderly women and primarily involves trabecular bone. Typically these individuals are 15 to 20 years postmenopausal. Fractures are experienced in the distal radius and/or as painful debilitating "crush" fractures of the lumbar vertebrae. The bone mass of lumbar vertebrae of type I osteoporotic women may be a third lower than age-match women not experiencing osteoporosis.

Type II osteoporosis is sometimes called age-associated osteoporosis, and it is not limited to the female gender. These individuals are usually greater than 70 years of age and both types of bone are affected. Fractures are experienced in the hip and vertebrae and "wedge" fractures of the thoracic vertebrae result in pain and slumping of the head. Spinal deformities can result in losses of height between 10 to 25 cm (4 to 10 in.). While occurring in both sexes, those individuals diagnosed with type II osteoporosis are mostly women. Women not only experience the typical bone losses associated with aging but also the accelerated losses associated with the years following menopause. Furthermore, women also experience lower PBM than men: therefore manifestations of excessive bone loss would begin earlier in women, whereas many men may die prior to complications. Hip fractures are very common in type II osteoporosis, as nearly 1 out of 5 women before the age of 80 and half of women beyond the age of 80 may endure a pelvic fracture.

As mentioned above, there appears to be a heredity linked to bone density. There are strong associations for gender and race and also within families. Recent investigations suggest that a genetic variation in the vitamin D receptor may account for a significant portion of the variation in bone density among women. Researchers are now investigating this area.

Menopause and Estrogen

Natural menopause is a period of time that marks the irreversible cessation of a woman's menstrual activity. Typically this occurs between 35 to 58 years of age with 25% of women experiencing menopause before the age of 47, 50% by the age 50, 75% by age 52, and 95% by age 55. Menses may stop suddenly, or it may taper off monthly until a final cessation, or the periods between menses may become longer until final cessation. Menopause may also be induced surgically by removal of the ovaries. Symptoms associated with menopause develop shortly after the final menses and may last for several months to years and vary in severity. These symptoms include hot flashes, nervousness, vasomotor instability, chills, fatigue, apathy, depression, palpitation, vertigo, headache, crying, numbness, tingling, myalgia, and urinary disturbances such as incontinence.

Bone loss follows an exponential pattern in the years that follow menopause. The rate of bone loss is greater after artificial menopause than natural menopause. This is most likely attributable to the sudden and complete cessation of estrogen production in the artificial menopause, while the natural menopause may allow for a tapering of estrogen secretion. For instance, after surgical removal of the ovaries, a woman may experience about a 20% loss of trabecular bone during the first 12 to 18 months. The rate of cortical bone loss is about 2 to 3%. The difference in extent of bone loss is probably related to the increased surface area of trabecular bone, thereby allowing for greater resorption. After natural menopause, women experience greater losses in trabecular bone, with vertebral trabecular bone enduring as much as a 50% loss in density at the close of 5 years after menopause. However, after several years past menopause the rate of bone loss slows to about 1% annually.

Estrogen

Estrogen is a class of steroid hormones associated with female reproductive activities, but they have an impact on many other organ systems as well. Estrogen is mainly involved in the promotion of proliferation and growth of certain cells and is principally responsible for the development of most secondary sexual characteristics of the female body. The three estrogens found in significant quantity in the human plasma are *β-estradiol*, *estrone*, and *estriol*. Dehydroepiandrosterone (DHEA) produced by the adrenal glands and converted to estrogen in peripheral tissue is also a source of estrogen. Furthermore, the placenta of pregnant women can also secrete estrogen. β-Estradiol is the primary estrogen secreted by the female ovaries along with smaller amounts of estrone. Most of the estrone formed is actually derived from precursor molecules such as DHEA in peripheral tissue. Estriol is created from β-estradiol and estrone in the liver. β-Estradiol is about 10 times as potent as estrone and 80 times as potent as estriol. Thus, β-estradiol is considered the major estrogen form in humans.

Another class of female sex hormones is the *progestins*. This class of sex hormones includes progesterone and 17α-hydroxyprogesterone, with the former being considered the most physiologically significant. Progesterone is secreted primarily by ovaries and the adrenal glands in relatively small amounts in the first half of the ovarian cycle, and in relatively higher amounts by the corpus luteum of the ovaries in the latter half of each ovarian cycle. The liver is largely responsible for degrading progesterone to other inactive steroid forms such as pregnanediol, which is filtered by nephrons and voided in urine.

Medical, Nutritional, and Behavioral Prevention and Treatment of Osteoporosis

Hormone Replacement Therapy

Hormone replacement therapy (HRT) includes exogenous estrogen provision, with or without progesterone. Estrogen is a powerful antiresorption factor. Researchers have demonstrated its effectiveness in relieving menopausal conditions, such as rapid bone loss and potentially reducing the risk of cardiovascular disease morbidity and mortality. While its short-term use has been deemed safe and is certainly effective, some scientists question its safety with prolonged use (>10 years). At this time, it is not clear whether estrogen therapy is directly related to breast cancer; also, long-term estrogen use is probably associated with an increased incidence of endometrial cancer. However, the risk of the latter is markedly lowered by the addition of progesterone. Age and/or elapsed time from menopause may be important in the efficacy of estrogen therapy. For instance, there is experimental evidence that women who are 15 to 20 years past menopause may not benefit from estrogen therapy due to the slowed rate of bone turnover at that point. Side effects of estrogen therapy may include bloating, tenderness to breasts, and vaginal bleeding.

With regard to osteoporosis, estrogen therapy can prevent the loss of both cortical and trabecular bone as well as decrease the occurrence of hip fractures. It is appropriate to begin therapy in the perimenopausal period, during menopause, or shortly after menopause. Routine Pap smears and mammography are strongly recommended. In postmenopausal women utilizing estrogen therapy, the rate of bone resorption and formation return to premenopausal values. Most of the effect of estrogen is attributable to its antiresorptive effects on bone. However, estrogen may also improve calcium balance by increasing intestinal absorption and renal tubule reabsorption.

Research has demonstrated that estrogen therapy initiated within 3 years of menopause can definitely stop bone resorption and perhaps increase bone density to some degree. Not many studies have been conducted in this area, but those that have demonstrate the efficacy of estrogen therapy as well as the importance of the timing of initiation of therapy. It seems that women who initiate estrogen therapy within 3 to 4 years postmenopause are able to regain bone loses prior to the onset of therapy, whereas those women who initiate therapy after 6 years were unable to regain lost bone.

The goal of estrogen therapy is use the smallest dosage possible which is able to prevent bone loss and result in the least number of side effects. The major side effects are vaginal bleeding, stimulation of endometrial tissue, fluid retention, and mastalgia (pain in the breasts). Estrogen is available in transdermal patches as well as oral estrogens. For the transdermal estrogen, the minimal dose needed to retard a mean decrease in spinal density was 50 µg. However, since that was a statistical mean, some of the women on this dose may actually experience small losses in bone. Therefore, a slightly higher dosage may be appropriate for some women or as a general prescription level.

The efficacy of oral estrogen therapy, either in combination dosages or provided with calcium supplements, has been tested. At doses of 4.0/2.0 mg, 2.0/1.0 mg, and 1.0/0.5 mg of 17β-estradiol/estriol (Trisequens) compared to a placebo, there was a 1.5% increase in bone density on the highest doses vs. an 0.8% increase on the medium dose and 0% change on the lowest dose. In comparison, there was a –2.0% change in bone density in the placebo group. Bone density was measured in the distal radius. Another investigation demonstrated that 17β-estradiol at 2.0, 1.0, and 0.5 mg in conjunction with a calcium supplement allowing for an intake greater than 1500 mg of calcium daily, resulted in changes in spine density at +2.0%, +3.0%, and +1.0%, respectively, in comparison to –2.0% measured in control women. While 0.5 mg may be regarded as the minimal dose required, as per data collected in this study, it should be recognized again that these percentages are statistical means and some of the women experienced bone loss at these levels. For instance, about one third of the women receiving 0.5 mg actually experienced bone loss, as did about one fifth of the women receiving 1.0 mg.

While conjugated estrogen is recommended alone for women without a uterus, conjugated estrogen and progesterone therapy are recommended for women with an intact uterus. Caution should be applied when utilizing progesterone or progestational agents as long-term therapy. Progesterone is known as a mitogen or a substance that promotes cell mitosis. Also, progesterone therapy may adversely alter serum lipid profiles by decreasing HDL. Furthermore, it is not clear how progesterone influences the development of breast and endometrial cancer. There is preliminary evidence to suggest that the combination of estrogen and progesterone increases the risk of breast cancer.

Exercise

Without a doubt, weight-bearing activity is essential for bone health. In the absence of weight-bearing physical activity, there is a marked reduction in bone mass as well as poor bone development in youth. With regard to osteoporosis, the effects of weight-bearing exercise can be discussed in three stages: (1) in young adults prior to reaching PBM; (2) adulthood, prior to menopause for women; and (3) perimenopausal and postmenopause periods for women.

There is evidence that during periods of growth during youth the human skeleton is the most responsive to the mechanical stress of physical activity, therefore contributing to a greater PBM. However, during puberty, vigorous training programs can actually reduce bone accruement by disrupting hormonal cyclicity and delay the progression of puberty for girls. The result can actually be the attainment of a lower PBM than expected. During prepubertal periods of growth, the skeleton appears to be particularly receptive to weight-bearing activity.

In the young adult, cross-sectional studies have continuously demonstrated that athletes or active women have a greater bone mineral density than age-matched controls. Common sites of measurement include the humerus, radius, calcaneous, and femoral neck. One exception is swimmers. College swimmers have reduced bone mineral density, as determined by assessment of the lower vertebrae, than other age-matched athletes and controls. However, as alluded to above, for women, the hypertrophic effect on bone by weight-bearing activity can only occur in a normal hormonal milieu. Bone hypertrophic processes are blunted in amenorrheic females and women with a history of menstrual irregularities

A woman's bone density upon reaching menopause is extremely important in determining her risk of osteoporotic fractures in the ensuing years. Therefore, the rate of bone loss during her mature adult years becomes very important. In general, active women have a higher bone density than inactive women; however, body weight is an important factor. For instance, women runners can have greater density of the radial midshaft and middle phalanx of their fingers, but a lower calcaneal density in comparison to age-matched controls of a greater body weight. Therefore, while activity is a very influential factor in increasing or maintaining bone density, the effect of a greater body weight is important as well, even in a high-impact area such as the heel bone.

At this point in understanding the effects of exercise in preventing or slowing the rate of bone loss in mature adults there are not a lot of definitive answers. For instance, only a couple of studies have actually evaluated the effect of training in a longitudinal (over time) manner. Most of the reports are cross-sectional. In fact, one of the first longitudinal investigative efforts found that there was not the predicted benefit of a 9-month structured weight-training program for beginners by premenopausal women despite a significant increase in muscular strength. However, since the women were novice weight-trainers, some scientists believe that the weights utilized may not have been enough to produce an effect or that the training period was too short. This argument is supported by numerous cross-sectional studies whereby premenopausal weight-training women have greater bone densities than age-matched sedentary women.

In postmenopausal women, there are a few important considerations with regard to the benefit of activity. Among those of the greatest consideration are: (1) the determination of the initial risk of osteporotic fractures at menopause; (2) how effective weight-training is in preventing osteoporotic fractures in this population; and (3) whether or not estrogen-replacement therapy will be utilized. Women whose bone mineral density is 2 SD below the mean for a young adult female are at double the risk for fracture as those women whose bone mineral density is 1 SD below the mean. The risk is doubled for a woman who is 1 SD below the mean, when a standard deviation represents about a 10% lower bone mineral density.

Cross-sectional studies have indeed indicated that Masters runners have greater bone mineral densities than age-matched runners, while the level of difference reported has been variable. It does not seem at this time that exercise can offset the detrimental effect of the lack of estrogen production upon bone mass, regardless of age. This is supported by studies involving Masters athletes and amenorrheic younger athletes.

Calcitonin–Salmon Therapy

While a relatively new therapy, preliminary investigations have demonstrated that calcitonin–salmon (Calcimar, Miacalcin) might be an effective treatment of osteoporosis. Calcitonin–salmon may decrease osteoclast receptors resulting in decreased osteoclast activity and bone resorption. Some research also suggests that calcitonin may also increase bone formation. Not only is this therapy purported to stabilize bone density, it is also reported to reduce pain and increase mobility. Currently this treatment is available in an injectable form, but the production of nasal sprays may expand its marketability.

Disintegrins

Osteoclasts produce a class of transmembrane heterodimeric glycoproteins called integrins. The purpose of these proteins appears to be to facilitate the binding of osteoclasts to various molecular substrates. In order to construct these quartenary protein structures, osteoclasts must express α_v, α_2, β_1, and β_3 subunits. The $\alpha_v\beta_3$ integrin is of particular interest with regard to osteoporosis as this integrin mediates osteoclast binding to bone matrix proteins containing RGD (Arg-Gly-Asp) consensus sequences. These sequences are found in matrix proteins such as vitronectin (VTN) and fibronectin, osteoponin, and von Willebrand factor. Because this integrin binds to a specific protein sequence, as in VTN, it is also called VTN receptor or VTR. The binding of osteoclasts to matrix proteins is a key event in osteoclastic activity.

Disintegrins typically are monomeric proteins with molecular masses ranging from 5 to 8 kDa. An outstanding characteristic is also the presence of an Arg-Gly-Asp (RGD) sequence near their carboxyl terminus. Disintegrins found in snake venom, such as echistatin (ECS) and kistrin, have been known to inhibit osteoclast attachment. Another disintegrin found in snake venom, contortrostatin (CTS), a dimeric protein having a mass of approximately 13.5 kDa, has also been shown to decrease osteoclast attachment and activity. Therefore, disintegrin therapy to prevent resorptive activity in osteoporosis at this time appears to holds promise.

Calcium

It is currently believed that an optimal calcium intake during preadolescence and adolescence can support the formation of a greater PBM and possibly a greater bone mineral density at menopause. While the cross-sectional reports of the influence of age, weight, height, and pubertal status upon bone density are consistent and well understood, the influence of calcium intake is less clear. There have been positive reports as well reports of researchers failing to determine an association between dietary calcium intake and bone density. Longitudinal studies, performed for 10 and 15 years, also failed to find a true relationship between varied calcium intake and bone density. However, significant associations were identified for smoking and exercise. Interestingly, investigations with monozygotic twin pairs determined that a twin supplemented with calcium during prepubertal years demonstrated significant increases in bone measurements in comparison to their placebo-supplemented twin. However, this result was not carried through to the pubertal years. It is possible that the type of calcium supplement used in some investigations is a factor. For example, calcium salts such as calcium citrate malate (CCM) have a better fractional absorption relative to calcium carbonate (36% vs. 26%). In fact, there has been a report that 12-year-old females presented significant increases in bone density after supplementing their diet with CCM in comparison to a placebo. The level of calcium intake that could result in a higher PBM is 1200 to 1500 mg/d, as suggested by the National Institutes of Health Consensus Conference Panel.

It is still uncertain whether calcium supplementation is effective in slowing the rate of calcium resorption from bone in postmenopausal women, but preliminary data appear promising. There are at least three considerations for the potential effectiveness of calcium supplementation in this population. First, their current calcium intake; second, their age and years postmenopause; and last, the form of calcium salt used as a supplement. Preliminary research suggests that women receiving <400 mg of calcium in their diet can significantly slow the rate of bone mineral loss from the spine, femoral neck, and radius with calcium citrate malate supplementation. However, postmenopausal women currently receiving between 400 to 650 mg of calcium in their diet were unable to slow the rate of bone density loss with a calcium carbonate or calcium citrate malate supplement. Another investigation produced results suggesting that postmenopausal women (>3 years) currently consuming >750 milligrams calcium daily could slow the rate of bone loss with 1000-mg supplements of either calcium lactate or calcium gluconate. Researchers have also investigated the influence of calcium supplementation in conjunction with vitamin D in postmenopausal women with some promising results. It appears that calcium and vitamin D supplementation at levels of 1200 mg and 20 µg (800 IU) may reduce the number of fractures in this population and may actually increase bone mineral density.

Vitamin D

Active vitamin D, as well as intermediates and metabolites, tends to decrease as humans age. Interestingly, within the elderly population, those individuals who lead a more active lifestyle had higher vitamin D levels than more sedentary individuals. Whether or not vitamin D supplementation by postmenopausal women is beneficial has not received as much attention as calcium. Currently available information from research investigations suggest that vitamin D supplementation or therapy may have merit. Researchers have reported that elderly subjects given a dose of 3750 to 7500 µg annually experienced a significant reduction in fractures. Furthermore, other researchers have reported that supplementing vitamin D at a dose of 10 µg daily demonstrated improvements in bone mineral density. This investigation also included the combination of calcium and vitamin D supplements as mentioned above. Again, the combination of vitamin D and calcium resulted in a slight, yet significant, increase in bone density.

Sodium Fluoride

Sodium fluoride (NaF) is believed to stimulate osteoblastic activity in bone and therefore increase bone density. However, preliminary research regarding the efficacy of NaF therapy in osteoporotic women suggested that the incidence of hip fractures actually increases with NaF use. It seems that NaF may increase the density of the axial skeleton, but at the expense of the appendicular skeleton. Thus, NaF is not a common mode of treatment of osteoporosis.

Zinc

Zinc is an important mineral involved in bone growth and bone formation. It is now known that there is an inverse relationship between urinary zinc content and changes in bone mineral density. Furthermore, as mentioned above, exercise is believed to be beneficial to skeletal health, while extreme training may be detrimental to health. Stress fractures are common and in women who become amenorheric, bone density can actually decrease. Excessive sweating can result in increased zinc loss and zinc deficiency is also related to hypogonadism and bone loss. Therefore, it is feasible to speculate that some of the detrimental effects associated with chronic strenuous training may be related to a compromised zinc status. At this time there are preliminary data to suggest that zinc supplementation can reduce some of the detrimental effects and a zinc supplement may be warranted in these individuals if dietary intake is inadequate.

Suggested Readings

Drinkwater, B.L., Physical activity, fitness, and osteoporosis, in *Physical Activity, Fitness and Health*, Bouchard, C., Shepard, R.J., and Stephens, T., Eds., Human Kinetics Publishers, Champaign, IL, 1994.

Farley, J.J., Wergedal, J.E., and Hall, S.L., Calcitonin has direct effects on the proliferation and differentiation of human osteoblast-line cells in vitro, *J. Bone Miner. Res.*, 4 (Suppl. 1), s278, 1989.

Gennari, C., Comparative effects on bone mineral content of calcium and calcium plus salmon calcitonin given in two different regimens in postmenopausal osteoporosis, *Curr. Ther. Res.*, 38, 455, 1985.

Hough, J.C., Osteoporosis, in *Primary Care Geriatrics: A Case-based Approach*, Ham, R.J. and Sloane, P.D., Eds., Mosby-Year Book, St. Louis, MO, 1997.

Puu, K.K. and Chan, M.B., Analgesis effect of intranasal salmon calcitonin in the treatment of postmenopausal osteoporosis, *Clin. Ther.*, 11, 205, 1989.

Sowers, M., Nutritional advances in osteoporosis and osteomalacia, in *Present Knowledge in Nutrition*, 7th ed., Ziegler, E.E. and Filer, L.J., Eds., ILSI Press, Washington, D.C., 1996.

Tilyard, M.W., Treatment of postmenopausal osteoporosis with calcitriol or calcium, *N. Engl. J. Med.*, 321, 293, 1989.

Rencken, M.L., Chestnut, C.H., and Drinkwater, B.L., Bone density at multiple skeletal sites in amenorrheic athletes, *J. Am. Med. Assoc.*, 276, 238, 1996.

Keen, A.D., Drinkwater, B.L., No gain in vertebral bone density over 10 years in previously amenorrheic athletes, abstracted, *J. Bone Miner. Dens.*, 10 (Suppl.), S243, 1995.

Cumming, D.C., Exercise-associated amenorrhea, low bone density, and estrogen replacement therapy, *Arch. Int. Med.*, 156, 2193–2195, 1996.

Hergenroeder, A.C., Klish, W.J., Smith, E.O., et al., A randomized clinical trial of bone mineral density changes in young women with hypothalmic amenorrhea treated with oral contraceptive pills, *Med. Sci. Sports Exer.*, 27, S94, 1995.

Eastell, R., Treatment of osteoporosis: drug therapy, *N. Eng. J. Med.*, 338(11), 736–746, 1998.

Kanis, J.A., Melton, L.J., III, Christinsen, C., et al., The diagnosis of osteoporosis, *J. Bone Miner. Res.*, 9, 1137–1141, 1994.

Shimegi, S., Yanagaita, M., Okano, H., et al., Physical exercise increases bone mineral density in postmenopausal women, *Endocr. J.*, 41, 49–56, 1994.

Murkies, A.L., Wilcox, G., and Davis, S.R., Phytoestrogens (*Clinical Review '92*), *J. Clin. Endocrinol. Metab.*, 83, 297–303, 1998.

Scientists spotlight phytoestrogens for better health, *Tufts Diet Nutr. Lett.*, 12(12), 3–6, 1995.

Dwyer, J.T., Goldin, B.R., Saul, N., Gualteri, L., Barakat, S., and Adlercreutz, H., Tofu and soy drinks contain phytoestrogens, *J. Am. Diet. Assoc.*, 94(7), 739–743, 1994.

Helferich, B., Dietary estrogens: a balance of risk and benefit, *Food Technol.*, 1996, 168.

Boonen, S., Vanderschueren, D., Cheng, X.G., Verbeke, G., Dequeker, J., Geusens, P., Broos, P., and Boullion, R., Age-related (type II) femoral neck osteoporosis in men: biochemical evidence for both hypervitaminosis D-androgen deficiency-induced bone resorption, *J. Bone Miner. Res.*, 12(12), 2119–26, 1997.

Groff, L.J., Gropper, S.S., and Hunt, S.M., *Advanced Nutrition and Human Metabolism*, 2nd ed., West Publishing, St. Paul, MN, 1995.

Hosking, D., Chilvers, C.E., Christiansen, C., Raven, P., Wasnich, R., Ross, P., McClung, M., Blaske, A., Thompson, D., Daley, M., and Yates, A.J., Prevention of bone loss with aldronate in postmenopausal women under 60 years of age. Early postmenopausal Intervention Cohort Study Group, *N. Engl. J. Med.*, 338(8), 485–492, 1998.

Looker, A.C., Orwell, E.S., Johnston, C.C., Lindsay, R.L., Wahner, H.W., Dunn, W.L., Calvo, M.S., Harris, T.B., and Heyse, S.P., Prevalence of femoral bone density in older U.S. women from NHANES III, *J. Bone Miner. Res.*, 12(11), 1761–1768, 1997.

Mackerras, D. and Lumley, T., First and second year effects in trials of calcium supplementation on the loss of bone denisty in postmenopausal women, *Bone*, 16, 527–533, 1997.

Melton, L.J., Epidemiology of spine osteoporosis, *Spine*, 22 (24 Suppl.), S2–S11, 1997.

Mortensen, L., Charles, P., Bekker, P.J., Digennaro, J., and Johnston, C., Risedronate increases bone mass in an early postmenopausal population: two years of treatment plus one year of follow-up, *J. Clin. Endocrinol. Metab.*, 83, 396–402, 1997.

Murkies, A., Phytoestrogens—what is the current knowledge?. (review), *Aust. Fam. Physician*, 27 (Suppl. 1), S47–51, 1998.

Tamatani, M., Morimoto, S., Nakajima, M., Fukuo, K., Onishi, T., Kitano, S., Niinobu, T., and Ogihara, T., Decreased circulating levels of vitamin K and 25-hydroxyvitamin D in osteopenic elderly men, *Metabolism*, 47(2), 195–199, 1998.

Tsai, Ks., Cheng, W.C., Chen, C.K., Sanchez, T.V., Su, C.T., Chieng, P.U., and Yang, R.S., Effect of bone area on spine density in Chinese men and women in Taiwan, *Bone*, 16, 547–551, 1997.

20

Nutrition Research: Past, Present, and Future

Nutrition Research in the 20th Century

The 20th century has certainly been an epoch for science in general. Along with great strides in so many disciplines, the expansion of nutrition knowledge has been astounding. At the beginning of the century, work conducted on food and food components was carried out by only a handful of scientists. As the century progressed into the first few decades of the 20th century, many of the vitamins were discovered, their structures defined, and synthesis techniques developed. The metabolic mechanisms of macronutrients, namely, proteins, lipids and carbohydrates, as well as energy metabolism in general became the subject of intense research. Furthermore, efforts for defining the requirements for the essential amino acids were taking place. The scientists who carried out such research came from a wide variety of disciplines including organic and inorganic chemistry, agricultural chemistry, physiological chemistry, medicine, and animal sciences. Some of the initial assessments of the energy content of foods were performed by Atwater at the Agriculture Experiment Station in Connecticut. Today, a bomb calorimeter is utilized to combust foods and food components to determine their energy content (Figure 20.1)

Much of the stimulus for nutrition research at the beginning of the century was simple curiosity and the love of science by men and women. The involvement of the federal government became more evident during World War II, and was partially motivated by the high rate of rejection of military conscripts due to nutrition-related conditions. This observation led to the establishment of the first Recommended Dietary Allowances (RDA) for the U.S. in 1941. After that the RDAs continued to be modified and formed the impetus to continue Federal involvement with nutrition research. However, long before the first RDAs were established, federally sponsored research in nutrition was occurring through the system of land grant institutions created by the Morrill Act. Modern nutrition evolved from the agriculture, medical, and basic sciences into a discipline of its own. Therefore, nutrition as a science may be viewed as a relative newcomer, but one that has certainly left its mark on the scientific community. The "father of nutrition," E.G. McCollum, introduced the laboratory rat as a useful model in scientific research. Poultry scientists used chicks as a research model and as such made contributions to medical sciences. Much of the research on fiber began with animal scientists studying forage and feeds of livestock.

Research pertaining to minerals and their composition in the human diet and physiological roles, took form in the 20th century. Some of the earlier mineral research efforts were more focused upon the major minerals, namely, calcium, phosphorus, sodium, potassium, chloride, and magnesium. However, some work relating to the role of iron and the development of deficiency is certainly apparent in the earlier decades of the century. Later on, as the 1960s and 1970s arrived, the conquest of space allowed for a rapid advance in technology. In tandem with the explosion of Space Age technology, came the ability to detect small quantities of trace elements such as zinc, selenium, iron, copper, and iodide. While the role of iodine in goiter was already known as well as the potential for selenium toxicity, there

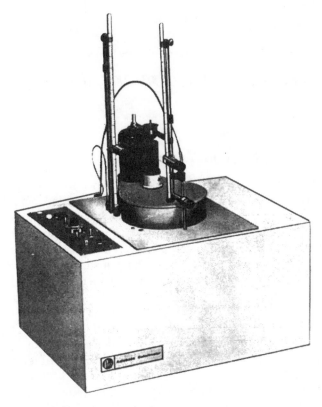

FIGURE 20.1

A bomb calorimeter. This laboratory tool is used to determine the gross energy endowed to a food or food component.

was very limited information on the requirements of many trace elements in optimizing human health. In any event, newer technologies such as neutron activation and atomic absorption spectrophotometry (AAS) allowed for detecting trace elements in the parts per billion range. An explosion of research in the area of trace elements occurred in the latter portions of the 20th century, due to the availability of these newer technologies. In addition, modern biology evolved as a science, where the molecular aspects of life were not only explored, but could be altered in the lab. In tandem, scientists began to discover that many nutrients function not only as cofactors or coenzymes, but also at the gene level.

Perhaps a defining moment in nutrition research came during the 1970s when the U.S. Senate Select Committee on Health and Human Needs first met and devised Dietary Guidelines for the U.S. This committee was chaired by South Dakota Senator George McGovern, and its findings became known as the McGovern Report. The findings of the committee revealed that the etiology of many of the most prevalent chronic diseases in the U.S. and Western societies, including heart disease and cancer, had a large nutrition component. The report was an initial attempt to offer dietary advice (in addition to the RDAs and food groups) to the public to help reduce the incidence of chronic illnesses and optimize health.

Another significant event in the 1970s was the publication of Charles Butterworth's "Skeleton in the Hospital Closet," which documented poor nutritional practices at American hospitals. He described a general failure in monitoring patient weight and food intake, as well as the documentation of dietary deficiencies in patients leaving the hospital where none existed at the time of admission. This article clearly caused major concern among the health care community. The failure to adequately educate physicians on nutrition was singled out as a very important omission in medical education, one that unfortunately is still common today. Butterworth's article has often been referred to as the Magna Carta of nutrition research in the latter part of the 20th century.

Regardless of how nutrition evolved during the 20th century, certain tools, technologies and approaches were used to discover the nutrients and define their functions. The approaches, ranging from epidemiology to molecular biology, are seemingly as varied as the nutrients themselves. Nutrition counseling and education remain a major portion of the nutrition field. Nutrition is not only a science, but a clinical area of practice, where both clinical and research instruments and methodologies are used to discover new information. The purpose of the remainder of this chapter is to consider the tools and methodologies used in the nutritional sciences. The new emerging areas are considered and examples given in several instances.

Determination of Nutrient Requirements

There are several acceptable approaches in determining nutrient requirements as summarized in Table 20.1. For humans, precise requirements depend on age, gender, activity level, and health status, just to name a few. Epidemiological surveys can be used in which the intake of nutrients and the incidence of particular clinical signs of deficiency or tissue level of the nutrient under investigation are evaluated. For example, one can estimate the dietary intake of niacin from food records, diet histories, and a 24-h recall. Insight could also be obtained by determining if the clinical signs of pellagra are revealed. However, this approach is limited in that the stores of niacin must be depleted before the clinical signs are often apparent. Evaluation of serum levels in conjunction with dietary intake may be more useful in such a situation.

Balance studies are another approach in which subjects in a metabolic ward may be fed graded levels of a particular nutrient and balance determined as intake – output. A zero, or slightly positive balance may be considered the requirement. However, such studies are expensive to conduct and may not evaluate interorgan distribution of the nutrient at zero

TABLE 20.1
Summary of Methods used to Determine Nutrient Requirements

Human Studies

Epidemiology surveys: diet records, diet histories, 24-hr recalls, blood and urine chemistries
Metabolic balance studies: metabolic ward or free-living

Animal Studies

Feeding of defined diets, varying levels or particular nutrient and examining:
Body weights
Blood levels of nutrients
Tissue/blood enzyme activities
Physiological function of organ systems
Tolerance to physiological stress
Gene expression

balance. Furthermore, extrapolation to other ages is often the case and certainly may not consider age-related differences in requirements. For instance, a balance study conducted with adults may have the results extrapolated to adolescents or children. Animal studies have also been utilized in the determination of nutrient requirements. The classic "feed them and weigh them" method was used to identify the essentiality of nutrients. Animal studies proved useful in determining how nutrients function as well as the determining specific deficiency symptoms that may prove useful when evaluating humans.

The evaluation of the intake of specific nutrients is not always clear. Population studies may use diet histories based on food frequencies, 3- or 7-day diet records, or 24-h recalls. In all cases, an estimation of portion sizes, how food was prepared and stored are evaluated. The 24-h recall is not considered accurate on an individual basis, but is useful in estimating the nutrient intakes of large samples of 70 to 100 subjects, or more. The diet history is considered the most accurate tool for estimating nutrient intake, especially on an individual basis and often used both in scientific research and clinical settings. Weighed food intakes are also a possibility, but take more time and subject compliance. In all cases, food items are coded and entered into a nutrient database program where many nutrient values are usually based upon USDA Handbook Number 8.

As alluded to above, requirements for humans may be determined using a metabolic ward where facilities are available to measure intake as well as urinary and fecal output. More sophisticated studies include excretion of nutrients in sweat and body hair. However, studies using free-living subjects are valuable in that subjects are able to participate in their usual activities and may provide proof to be more insightful in a practical sense.

Blood levels of nutrients are often used to assess nutrient status. While this approach is indeed informative, there are several drawbacks that must be recognized. One major drawback is that blood levels of a particular nutrient may not reflect diet intake. A good example of this is blood calcium levels, which are tightly regulated by calcitonin, vitamin D, and parathyroid hormone. In addition to simple blood levels, the activities of nutrient-dependent enzymes often serve as good indicators of status.

One critical area of research is the determination of methodology necessary to accurately assess nutrient status in humans. For obvious reasons, sampling of tissue in humans is problematic when compared with experimental animals. For instance, while liver samples are often used in animals to assess nutrient status of vitamins, minerals, and other food components (via the concentration of the nutrient or some enzyme activity), in humans, blood and urine are often the only tissues available. The use of hair and saliva has proved to be of limited value in assessing nutrient status. Functional indices of organ systems, immune function, and response to a physiological challenge are subjects of ongoing research and may prove valuable in allowing the proper assessment of nutrient status.

Clinical indicators of nutrient status and the use of anthropometric measures, such as triceps skinfold, midarm circumference, and abdominal fat using magnetic imaging resonance, CAT scans, and bioelectrical impedance assessment, are all useful in assessing nutritional states. It is important that studies designed to answer questions using humans as subjects use methods that are as accurate and precise as well as feasibly possible. Each nutrient must be evaluated in terms of what is the best measure of status. It is clear that each nutrient has different parameters appropriate for measuring status. For instance, serum zinc levels may be a good measure for zinc status, but serum calcium levels would be worthless for calcium status. However, the use of serum ionized calcium levels is a good measure of the physiologically active pools of calcium. Again, each nutrient has its own unique set of variables.

Nutrition Laboratory Research

Nutrition research has clearly been advanced by discoveries made in the modern scientific laboratory. This is to say that there are standard tools and pieces of equipment, as well as principles, utilized by nutrition researchers to advance the understanding of nutrient properties and functions. Also, today nutrition researchers are in the era of molecular biology, thereby allowing for discovery of how nutrients function at the gene level. The classic interpretation on how nutrients function was that most of the vitamins and minerals were cofactors or coenzymes for certain organic compounds, such as an enzyme. For example, riboflavin is part of FAD, which is associated with key enzymes involved in the oxidation of energy nutrients. Also, copper is a cofactor for the electron transport enzyme cytochrome c oxidase. However, we now know that nutrients such as vitamins A and D have nuclear receptors that are activated by these nutrients and the receptor–nutrient complex can then bind to specific elements in the promoter region of a gene. Zinc, through zinc fingers, and leucine via leucine zippers, also demonstrate functionality at the gene level.

While the rat has been used as a model for a lot of nutrition research, other animals such as mice, gerbils, guinea pigs, rabbits, and swine may be used. Nonhuman primates are used, but the cost is rather high and availability of animals is variable. It is important that the "correct" animal model be used for studying specific nutrients. Here correctness implies applicability to humans. A classic example is the guinea pig for vitamin C research or a rabbit for lipoprotein investigation. However, research on nutrients does not have to be conducted only with humans and animals. The use of tissue and cell culture techniques has provided researchers with more powerful tools in which to evaluate and discover new roles of nutrients. The ability to transfect certain tissues and cell lines with specific genes and examine nutrient effects upon gene expression is equally powerful. The use of Northern and Western blotting techniques to evaluate mRNA and specific proteins in tissues in response to nutrients is a common tool in today's nutrition laboratory.

Laboratory Tools

The modern laboratory used to study human nutrition will vary from one investigator to the next, depending upon the field of expertise of the investigator. However, much of what is used is not unlike that used by other life scientists. The tools are summarized in Table 20.2. The centrifuge, for instance, is a work horse of modern laboratories. The modern centrifuge can "spin" at incredible speeds and generate a force in excess of 100,000 times that of gravity. Centrifugation is used to separate organelles and macromolecules, the scratch material for cells. Cells that comprise tissues or organs are first disrupted via grinding (homogenization), osmotic shock, ultrasonic vibration, or forcing the cells through microorifices. Broken cells are then rotated or spun at high speeds within centrifugation tubes. Cell components are separated on the basis of size/density. Large particles will migrate under centrifugal force faster than smaller ones. At *low speed*, nuclei and unbroken cell debris go to the bottom of the tube and form the pellet, with the upper liquid layer referred to as the supernatant. At even higher speeds, mitochondria may be pelleted. Centrifugal speed may be defined as:

Low speed	1,000 times gravity for 10 min
Medium speed	20,000 times gravity for 20 min
High speed	80,000 times gravity for 1 h
Very high speed	150,000 times gravity for 3 h

When the supernatant is sequentially removed and recentrifuged at higher speeds, this is commonly referred to as sequential centrifugation, or (another term) cell fractionation. At ultracentrifugation speeds, friction is reduced for the rotor by use of a vacuum. Also, the vacuum helps maintain refrigerated temperatures in most modern centrifuges.

The laboratory spectrophotometer is another work horse. Compounds absorb light at a particular wavelength — that is an inherent physical property of every compound known. By placing the compound in the path of light at a particular wavelength, absorbency can be determined (Figure 20.2). Atomic absorption spectrophotometry is a particular instrument where minerals at a very small level may be determined. This instrument has been responsible for the trace element research explosion of the last part of the 20th century.

TABLE 20.2
Laboratory Tools Commonly used in Nutrition Research

1. Spectrophotometry
   a. Can measure absorbency of particular compounds
   b. Atomic absorption spectrophotometry (AAS) can measure absorbency of minerals
2. Centrifugation
   a. Separates organelles and macromolecules based on mass when rotated at high speeds
   b. Higher speeds will "pellet" smaller mass particles
3. Chromatography
   a. Partition — compounds in a mixture are separated on the basis of their solubility in solvents
   b. Column — mixture of compounds are separated by passing them in a solution through a column containing a porous matrix. Matrix may be charged (ion-exchange) or separation may be based on size (gel permeation chromatography)
4. Electrophoresis
   a. Normally used to separate proteins or peptides and the basis of charge and mass.
   b. Sodium-dodecyl-sulfate (SDS) is a detergent that gives proteins a strong negative charge. Proteins when mixed with SDS migrate to the + end when placed in an electrical field.
   c. Polyacrylamide gel — a matrix which a protein mixture passes through during electrically induced migration.
   d. β-Mercaptoethanol — strong reducing agent; breaks SH groups and proteins into constitutive peptide subunits
5. Isoelectric focusing
   a. Proteins separated based on a pH gradient.
   b. Proteins when placed in both a pH gradient and electric field will migrate to the pH at which they are neutral (isoelectric point)

Separation of Compounds

Compounds may be separated by a variety of techniques. One of the oldest and more common techniques utilizes chromatography. In partition chromatography, compounds are in a mixture of solvents such as water and alcohol. Paper or silica plates are placed in a tank with the solvent touching at the bottom of the plate or paper. As the solvent migrates upward, the molecules separate in the sample according to their relative solubility in the

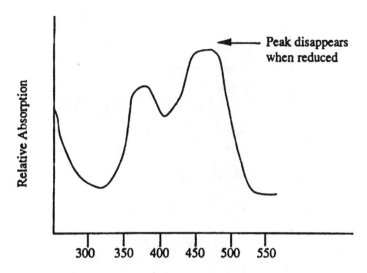

FIGURE 20.2
Absorption spectra for riboflavin. The peak wavelength absorption for riboflavin can be greatly diminished if the substance is reduced.

two solvents. Amino acids are examples of compounds that can be separated by partition chromatography.

Column chromatography utilizes a column, packed with a porous solid matrix, to separate out components of a mixture, typically a class of substances. A solution containing the desired substance will be added at the top of the column. The matrix will vary, depending on the substance to be separated. For instance, some matrices will separate proteins based upon charge. Fatty acids will be separated, based on relative solubility or polarities. Gel permeation chromatography is a common technique used to separate substances or particles on the basis of size. Here, a good example is the lipoproteins. Agarose beads endowed with microscopic pores can be used to separate HDL, LDL, and VLDL from one another. HDL are smaller in size, whereas chylomicrons and VLDL are larger. The HDL particles will pass through the pores of the agarose beads, whereas the larger chylomicrons and VLDLs will go around the beads because they are too large to go into the pores. This means that the HDL particles will be retarded and take a longer time to exit the separation column.

A powerful tool in the laboratory, particularly when working with proteins, is the use of electrophoresis. Here, compounds are separated on the basis of charge and size properties. Proteins are endowed with both positive and negative charges depending on the mixture of amino acids in their composition. If proteins are placed within an electric field they will migrate, depending on their size, shape, and charge.

A common technique often used in laboratories is sodium-dodecyl sulfate polyacrylamide gel electrophoresis or SDS-PAGE. SDS is a detergent that, when mixed with proteins, gives them a strong negative charge. The proteins when applied to the acrylamide gel matrix will migrate to the positive (+) end of the gel. β-Mercaptoethanol is a strong reducing agent and is also added in order to break sulfhydryl bonds. This will allow proteins to be broken into their individual subunits. With SDS, shape is not important since proteins are unfolded at low pH. Proteins of the same molecular weight have similar migration properties. Larger proteins are retarded by the acrylamide gel. Distinct bands representing the peptides are formed. A dye known as Coomassie blue is added to the gel to visualize the protein (Figure 20.3).

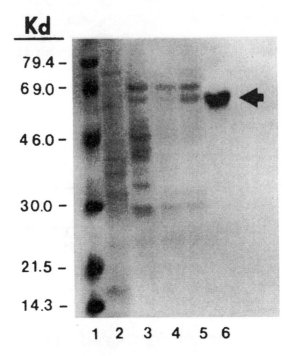

FIGURE 20.3
Separation or purification of proteins using SDS-PAGE. Lane 1 contains a standard solution endowed with proteins of specific molecular weights. These are called markers. This allows a size reference for samples added to the other lanes.

A related technique, called isoelectric focusing, is commonly applied in many laboratories as well. Separation of proteins is performed at low pH, where the carboxylic acid groups of proteins tend to be uncharged and their nitrogen-containing basic groups are fully charged, giving most proteins a net positive charge. At high pH, the carboxylic groups are negatively charged and the basic amino groups tend to be uncharged, giving most proteins a net negative charge. At its isoelectric charge, a protein has no net charge since the positive and negative charges balance. Therefore, when a tube with a fixed pH gradient is subjected to an electrical field, each protein will migrate until it forms a sharp band at its isoelectric pH.

Western Blotting

Western blotting allows for an estimation of protein quantity. Here, the use of antibodies can identify and quantify the protein or peptide of particular interest. First, the proteins are separated by SDS-PAGE. Next, the proteins are electrically transferred to a nitrocellulose or another type of membrane. The membrane is then immersed in a buffer solution that contains an antibody against the protein of interest. This antibody is often referred to as the *primary antibody*. The primary antibody will then bind to the protein. Next, the membrane is rinsed with a buffer and is then immersed in a solution containing a secondary antibody. This antibody is in essence directed against the species in which the primary antibody was produced. For instance, if a protein (antigen) from a rat is injected into a rabbit, the rabbit will produce an antibody to the rat protein. The secondary antibody will react against the primary antibody produced in the rabbit (antirabbit antibody). The secondary antibody may be associated with a dye, a radioactive isotope, or an enzyme that will react in some fashion with a dye allowing for the production of an image. The presence of color and intensity determines the presence and amount of protein, respectively, that was originally present on the gel.

Tools Used to Examine Gene Expression

One of the most rapidly developing areas of science technology is molecular biology. Certainly nutrition science has benefited as much as any other scientific field, as it has allowed for numerous discoveries of how certain nutrients function at the gene level. While scientists have long appreciated that the genetic code is *transcribed* to mRNA which is *translated* to build proteins, many of the factors influencing the "turning on" and "turning off" of genes are still being elucidated and will be for years to come. Also, once a primary protein has been translated, posttranslational activities can greatly manipulate the final protein. Nutrition scientists are now becoming more suitably trained to investigating these and other molecular biological effects as well as the influence of nutrients and nutrition states. Some of the tools used are summarized in Table 20.3.

TABLE 20.3
Summary of Commonly used Molecular Biology Tools

1. Western blot—detects proteins or peptides using antibodies
2. Northern blot—detects mRNA using labeled cDNA probes (gene expression)
3. Southern blot—detects DNA or presence of a gene, using labeled cDNA
4. Polymerase chain reaction (PCR)—amplification of DNA using a "thermocycler"
5. Cell culture—growing of individual cells in a medium capable of supporting growth
6. Transfection studies—insertion of DNA into cells to examine function and response
7. Transgenic animals—animals, usually murine, genetically altered, that either overexpress a particular gene, or are unable to express a particular gene (knock-out)
8. Transmission electron microscopy—capable of magnifying up to 100,000×

As discussed in Chapter 1, DNA is composed of two strands of polynucleotides that are complementary base-paired. Cytosine bonds with guanine while adenosine bonds with thymidine (Figure 1.9). This simple property has been greatly exploited by molecular biological laboratory techniques to quantify mRNA levels as well as the presence of DNA genes. The two complementary DNA strands can be artificially separated by high heat. Heat will dissociate the hydrogen bonds that hold the strands together and thus the single polynucleotide strands become independent. This is commonly referred to as *denaturation*. Furthermore, when mRNA, coding for a specific protein of interest is isolated, a corresponding strand of DNA, or the complementary strand (cDNA), can be synthesized from the RNA using the enzyme found in viruses. This enzyme is called *reverse transcriptase*. After formation of the cDNA, a strand of DNA, complementary to cDNA, can be produced by adding the nucleotides ATP, CTP, GTP, TTP. The enzyme *DNA polymerase* must also be added. Thus, the cDNA strand serves as the *template* for the formation of the second strand. One must keep in mind that one strand of DNA runs from the 5' (pronounced "5 prime") to the 3' direction. This refers to the position of the phosphate groups on the ribose sugar. The phosphate groups connect the strand by bonding to these two carbons on adjacent ribose groups (Figure 1.8). The second DNA strand must run in the opposite direction, or 3' to 5'. When the nucleotide sequence of DNA or RNA is written out, it is usually conventional to write it from the 5' to the 3' direction.

Northern and Southern Hybridizations

How does molecular biology information help us to understand how nutrients influence gene expression? When a gene is turned on or expressed by an upstream promoter region of DNA, mRNA will be synthesized in the nucleus and migrate to the cell cytoplasm. The ability to measure the mRNA transcribed from a particular gene of interest provides insight to its expression. After a particular nutrition situation is created, the appropriate tissue is ground up or homogenized to begin the extraction procedure for RNA. The RNA is then isolated from the homogenized tissue by chemical methods. Furthermore, the various mRNAs and other RNAs become separated from each other on the basis of size, which in this case is the number of base pairs. Homogenate samples are loaded into wells of an agarose gel that is positioned in an electrical field. The RNA in their respective lanes will migrate toward the positive end of the field as RNA is negatively charged. After this occurs, the RNA on the gel is transferred to a membrane, composed of nitrocellulose, vinyl, or nylon. This transfer is performed by a purely passive mechanism. Here the wet blot is placed under the gel and a membrane is placed on top of the gel. The ends of the wet blot are placed in a buffer and the membrane is situated under a stack of paper towels or similar material (Figure 20.4). The buffer will migrate through the gel, up to the membrane and continue to the paper towels. While this occurs, the RNA is gently transferred to the positively charged membrane. The membrane now contains the RNA of interest. This technique is referred to as a *Northern blot*.

Once a Northern blot is created, one can proceed to determine which one of the literally thousands of mRNAs that have been transferred to the membrane is the one of interest. This is where the cDNA that corresponds to the particular mRNA becomes an important tool. When cDNA for a particular gene is created to be subsequently introduced into a Northern blot, it is called a cDNA *probe*. The cDNA can be labeled by various methods to contain ^{32}P in its nucleotides, which makes it radioactive. The labeled DNA probe is separated from its template DNA by heating to a high temperature (~95°C), which allows for denaturation. The cDNA probe is then placed in a salt solution along with the membrane, again at an elevated temperature (~65°C). Depending on conditions (time, temperature, and salt concentration), the cDNA will align with the complementary base pairs of the mRNA of interest. This is referred to as hybridization or *Northern hybridization*. The more mRNA of interest that is present, the more cDNA that will hybridize. After the reaction has occurred, the membrane is washed several times in various salt solutions to remove nonspecific binding of the cDNA probe. Next, the membrane is placed against photographic film that is exposed to the radioactive ^{32}P. The more radioactivity present, the greater the size of the band that will be present when the film is developed. For example, if one wishes to determine whether dietary zinc influences intestinal metallothionein of, say, a rat, they could conduct an experiment by first feeding various zinc levels in the diet and removing the small intestine. Next they would obtain the RNA and conduct Northern blots and hybridization experiments.

If instead of RNA a scientist chooses to extract DNA from a tissue, it can also be electrophoresed, then blotted to a membrane, and the membrane then probed with a radioactive cDNA; this would detect the actual gene present. This procedure is referred to as *Southern blotting and hybridization*. Looking at the various methods described above, one may view these tools as simply examining protein synthesis at various cell levels: DNA, mRNA, and peptides, respectively. These tools are extremely powerful in that very small levels of material can be detected in many cases.

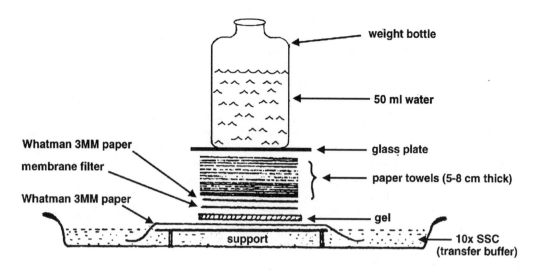

FIGURE 20.4
Standard assembly for capillary transfer of nucleic acids (DNA and RNA) from an agarose gel onto nitrocellulose or nylon membrane filters.

Polymerase Chain Reaction

The polymerase chain reaction (PCR) is another tool that is becoming more commonly used in laboratories today. In this technique, small quantities of DNA are introduced into a tube containing small oligonucleotide bases (10 to 12 bases in length) that correspond to the 5′ end of one strand and the 3′ end of the second DNA strand. These primers are designed to anneal to the respective ends of the DNA molecules when they are separated. Also added to the tube are the nucleotides ATP, CTP, GTP, and TTP and DNA polymerase. The entire mixture is placed in an instrument termed a "thermocycler" which will change the temperature of the contents such that the DNA will become denatured to become single stranded. Next, the temperature changes again to allow the primers to anneal to the ends of each single strand. At the correct temperature, the DNA polymerase will add nucleotides to a growing chain, using the single DNA strand as a template. After the second strand is synthesized and annealed to form the new DNA molecules, this completes the first cycle. The process is repeated over and over allowing for the generation of much more DNA. Normally 30 or more cycles are executed. The end result is a large amplification of small samples of DNA.

A slight variation of this technique is reverse transcriptase PCR or RT-PCR. Here, mRNA is the starting material and DNA is synthesized with reverse transcriptase. After the DNA is produced, the reverse transcriptase is inactivated and then PCR amplification occurs. The DNA can be added to a gel and transferred to a membrane; or the DNA may be made radioactive first and added to the gel. A Southern blot and hybridization can be performed to quantify the initial levels of message initially present. This can allow for the detection of very small levels of mRNA, whereas Northern techniques generally are unable to detect such small amounts.

Transgenic Animal Models

Animal species that have been altered genetically are becoming more common in nutrition research. Whether it is the presence of a powerful promoter linked to a gene of interest, or the deletion of a gene by blocking an exon sequence, *transgenic* models offer nutrition new insights into how nutrients function. A transgenic model in which the gene of interest is no longer expressed is called a *knock-out* model. For example, the peroxisomal proliferating activating receptor-alpha (PPARα) is not expressed in one knock-out mouse model. This nuclear receptor is critical in the oxidation of fatty acids, since it is believed to bind to the promoters of such genes as medium-chain acyl dehydrogenase and carnitine palmityl CoA translocase I. Without PPARα, the expression of these genes is markedly decreased and fatty acid oxidation is significantly impaired. Fat accumulates within tissue as a result. How specific fatty acids are handled when these enzymes are not functioning may be studied in such a model. Another example of a transgenic mouse presents an overexpression of Cu/Zn-superoxide dismutase. Does this strain have increased copper and zinc requirements? Is this strain more protected against free radical injury as a result of this overexpression? Such models offer us insights to answer these fundamental questions on the entire organism. Also, in addition to a model being a whole-body knock-out or overexpression of a gene, it is possible to create such models wherein the altered genetic events are isolated to one or more organs.

Cell Cultures

Cell lines may also be manipulated genetically. The addition of specific DNA sequences into cells is termed *transfection*. Specific cell lines that lack the expression of a particular gene can be transfected with DNA containing the gene promoter as well as the gene to study how various nutrients may interact with the expression of a gene. Rapidly dividing cells can easily take up such DNA. In other cases, where the cells are nonprolific, viruses may be used to insert DNA sequences. In either case, nutrient function at the cell level and at the cell–gene level, as well as how a specific nutrient functions, may be studied and provide definitive results.

Histology

Visual examination of tissue subjected to various nutrient conditions can lead to novel discoveries on structure–function relationships. Organs and tissues often reveal pathology, as well as the nature of a pathology, which lends insight into the underlying influence of nutrients or nutritional state. The light microscope is a powerful tool even in today's laboratory. The use of antibodies to label or tag particular compounds, similar to the principles used for Western blotting, may also be applied. Cell localization of particular proteins as affected by nutrient manipulation is often used as well. In addition to the use of immunohistochemistry with the use of antibodies, *in situ* hybridization techniques are available in which a labeled cDNA can be hybridized to a tissue. Of course this can provide quantitative information such as the Northern blot, as well as localization within tissues as to where the change in potential transcript expression may be occurring. For instance, the small intestine is a complex organ composed of many tissues. Performing a Northern hybridization on the total RNA may allow one to gain insight as to a change in a transcript, but combining this technique with the tools of microscopy can provide insight as to where within the small intestine the change is occurring.

A major advance has been the use of transmission electron microscopy (TEM). Several electron micrographs were presented in this text. However, the number of nutritionists using this powerful tool is limited. The electron microscope can allow the viewing of cell details not visible by the light microscope since magnification of over 100,000× are not uncommon. For instance, the electron microscope allows one to view in detail cell organelles, such as mitochondria, that are not normally seen by a light microscope.

Furthermore, the organizational structure of the extracellular matrix can be viewed in great detail as well as macrophages and their interaction with cells and other matter. For instance, the electron microscope has allowed nutritionists to determine that copper deficiency resulted in a proliferation of mitochondria in the heart and was the contributing factor to the enlargement. A related tool, the scanning electron microscope, allows cells to be viewed in a 3-dimensional perspective.

Evolving Information on Nutrient Function

The tireless efforts of nutrition scientists, coupled with ever-improving scientific tools and techniques, has allowed for a seemingly continuous evolution of information on the functional roles of nutrients and the ramifications of various nutritional states. Nutrition textbooks almost seem to be outdated as soon as they are published. For example, it was not too long ago that calcium was recognized merely for its involvement in bone health, blood clotting, and muscle contraction. However, in the mid-1960s, there were a series of published investigations that indicated human populations living in *hard water* areas had a lower incidence of heart disease compared to populations living in *soft water* areas. The hard water contains appreciable amounts of calcium and magnesium and this suggested even more roles for calcium. Some studies suggested that if water hardness changed over time, the incidence of heart disease changed according to the water hardness. While much of this was observational, a definite role for this was not certain. Although it was recognized that calcium in itself is important for muscle contraction and the heart, a direct nutritional role in the prevention of cardiomyopathy was to remain unclear. Later, in the 1980s it was discovered that there was a lower association between pregnancy and/or its symptomology was less severe in women whose diets were sufficient in calcium. Further investigation suggested that calcium supplements could lower the blood pressure and decrease the incidence of toxemia of pregnancy in high risk women. Following this series of investigations, researchers discovered that administration of calcium supplements or foods high in calcium to individuals with chronic hypertension could lower blood pressure. Some animal studies have suggested that calcium may exert its blood pressure lowering effect through blocking the reabsorption of sodium in the kidney tubules and therefore enhancing urinary sodium excretion. While the exact mechanism is still uncertain, however, this is a good example of new discoveries of nutrients having specific functions outside of classically known functions.

How Do Nutritionists Make New Discoveries with Such an Array of Diverse Tools?

The methods used to study nutrition can vary tremendously. One may ask, how does one get to learn and know all of these techniques? Is a single person or a laboratory able to *do it all* in studying how a particular nutrient functions? The current and future state of research, not only in nutrition, but in all science, suggests that it is unlikely and not possible to become an expert in all of these techniques. Today's laboratory researcher needs to be aware of the potential powers provided by and limitations associated with each of the methods described above. However, more important is the issue that nutritionists work with other scientists who do possess the skills in the technique of interest that may be used to answer the question of interest. Team-building, networking, collaborating — call it what you wish. However, one thing is indeed true, the future of nutrition research calls for multidisciplinary approaches to answer scientific questions posed. One can discern rather quickly that the team approach to scientific inquiry is indeed popular today by simply looking at the multiauthored publications appearing in premier scientific journals.

Finally, the goal of nutrition is like that of other scientific disciplines, to ask the right questions and seek out the truth in an objective fashion. Nevertheless, use of tools and technology cannot take the place of generating the right questions, nor interpret the data or results. Only the person trained and experienced in the particular area can do this. Therefore collaborative efforts are a necessity.

Suggested Readings

Wildman, R.E.C., Basic tissue preparation for electron microscopy assessment of rodents, in *Trace Elements in Laboratory Rodents*, Watson, R.R., Ed., CRC Press, Boca Raton, FL, 1996.

Kaufman, P.B., Wu, W., Kim, D., and Cseke, L.J., *Handbook of Molecular and Cellular Methods in Biology and Medicine*, CRC Press, Boca Raton, FL, 1995.

Alberts, B., Bray, D., Lewi, J., Raff, M., Roberts, K., and Watson, J.D., *Molecular Biology of the Cell*, Garland, New York, N.Y., 1995.

Robyt, J.F. and White, B.J., *Biochemical Techniques: Theory and Practice*, Waveland Press, Prospect Heights, IL, 1987.

Manchenko, G.P., *Handbook of Detection of Enzymes on Electrophoretic Gels*, CRC Press, Boca Raton, FL, 1994.

Dykstra, M.J., *A Manual of Applied Techniques for Biological Electron Microscopy* Plenum Press, New York, N.Y., 1993.

Gelehrter, T.D. and Collins, F.S., *Principles of Medical Genetics*, Williams & Wilkins, Baltimore, MD, 1990.

21

Nutrition in the 21st Century

Throughout his existence, man has pondered the relationship between food and his body. Ancient medicine men and charlatans used plants in attempts to treat or prevent illnesses long before we could even begin to understand atoms, molecules, enzymes, hormones, and cells. Perhaps the field of nutrition dates back this far. However, despite its long existence, without doubt the most remarkable strides in understanding nutrition have occurred within the 20th century. This is largely due to advances in scientific investigative techniques concomitant with an extraordinarily enhanced ability to share information among scientists. In the last couple of decades alone, the importance of more novel areas of nutrition has really began to reveal itself. Topics such as fibers, eicosanoids, *trans* fatty acids, lipoprotein metabolism, nutrition supplements, and phytochemicals are now common conversations among nutritionists. What will the hot topics of the early 21st century be? What, in the year 2020, will be what phytochemicals and omega-3 polyunsaturated fatty acids are today?

Just as it would have been difficult to foresee 25 years ago the interest in eicosanoids, it is somewhat difficult for us to envision nutrition research 25 years in the future. One thing is clear however, the ability to objectively investigate nutrition-based factors will not be a limiting factor in the quest for this understanding. For instance, molecular biological assessment, such as Southern, Northern, and Western blotting allows scientists to assess human operations at the level of genes, mRNA, and proteins. Light and electron microscopy allow scientists the power of high magnification visualization of cell ultrastructure and tissue structure. Furthermore, clinical and laboratory equipment and machines such as MRI, CAT scans, dual photon absorptiometry, metabolic carts, electro- and echocardiographs, gamma counters, scintillation counters, spectrophotometers, centrifuges, and electrophoresis will leave very few aspects of the human body beyond scrutiny.

Nutrition Past

Paleolithic Diet

Now that humans have modernized investigation to a point whereby the potential exists to thoroughly investigate nutrition, it may be a good idea to look back in time at the origins of diet. It only makes sense in the "survival of the fittest" scenario of evolution that to a given point humans survived based upon the foods we were able to acquire. Thus, the development of the human genome is harmonious with diet throughout evolution.

Paleolithic nutrition studies of man's diet as he evolved. The story actually begins before man was man. More than 55 million years ago, a small insect-eating mammal climbed into the trees of the forests that developed during the late Cretaceous period (some 94 to 64 million years ago). Its descendants began to eat edible plants, and evolution allowed for the development of characteristics that allowed plant-based substances to be the major component of its diet. As examples, natural selection yielded hands more suitable for grasping branches and handing its components (i.e., leaves, fruits). Also, visual acuity increased, allowing for greater depth perception and color recognition. Motor skills also increased as well. Thus, our distant ancestors were able to maneuver throughout the forest canopy and identify and acquire fruits and leaves. The development of these characteristics is associated with the development of the enlarged brain characteristic of primates who are descendants of the earlier mammalian form.

Paleonutritionists believe that human DNA has made very little evolutionary progress over the last 10,000 to 100,000 years relative to the incredible changes in foods during this time. During this earlier period, human ancestors were eating a diet that largely consisted of wild game and vegetation (fruits, vegetables, roots, leaves), and perhaps still some insects. However, the years that followed the development of agriculture and the domestication of animals vastly changed the human diet. It is believed that agriculture began to develop about 10,000 years ago. It is also now believed that prior to agriculturization the human form was taller and much more lean than present-day man. To maintain a larger and leaner frame during strenuously active times, it has been estimated that about 3000 kcal/d was the average consumption for an adult male. The industrialization of work greatly reduced caloric expenditure. For instance, the utilization of mechanized farming in Japan has reduced the estimated daily work expenditure by more than half.

The estimated energy contribution of carbohydrates, protein, and fat was 41, 37, and 22%, respectively. Cholesterol intake is estimated to have been about 480 mg daily. The contribution of wild game to the paleolithic diet was about 30 to 35% of total mass, while the remainder of the sustenance was provided by fruits, vegetables, roots, legumes, nuts, and other noncereals. Wild game was a considerable component of the paleolithic diet. However, the composition of this meat differs significantly from domesticated animal products today. For example, wild game is much more lean with a lower proportion of the hypercholesterolemic fatty acids lauric (12:0), myristic (14:0), and palmitic (16:0) acids and a higher proportion of essential fatty acids.

The total protein intake of the paleolithic diet far exceeds current human recommendations. For example, the RDA for protein is 0.8 g/kg body weight and it is generally recommended that protein provides 12 to 15% of total energy. This contrasts with the greater than 30% of energy as protein consumed by human ancestors. In comparison to other primates, such as chimpanzees, gorillas, baboons, and howler monkeys in the wild, protein intake ranges from 1.6 to 5.9 g/kg body weight. Veterinary recommendations for primates in captivity also exceed human recommendations. It is difficult to argue that during human evolution from his primate ancestors, when he was further developing the skills necessary to increase his carnivorous consumption, man evolved to be harmed by a protein-rich diet. While it is indeed true that higher protein diets are linked to diseases such as heart disease and certain cancers, the epidemiological data require some scrutiny. Findings that a higher protein intake is linked to colon and breast cancer are not always consistent. Furthermore, the high protein diets positively correlated to heart disease in some countries are typically part of high fat–high saturated fat diet and lower in nutrient- and phytochemical-rich fruits and vegetables. On the other hand, some research suggests that a high protein diet in conjunction with a low fat and vegetable-rich diet may actually raise HDL-cholesterol levels while lowering total cholesterol and triglyceride levels.

The carbohydrate contribution to the paleolithic diet was mostly fruits, vegetables, and roots, while very little contribution was derived from cereal grains and refined sugars. In the U.S. today, less than one fourth of carbohydrates is derived from fruits and vegetables.

Human preagricultural ancestors are believed to have consumed three times the vegetables and fruits as Westerners today. This substantially increased the fiber intake as well as the phytochemical consumption. Fiber is believed to possibly exceed 100 g/d. One interesting potential result of a diet higher in protein and lower in carbohydrate sources such as potatoes, bread, rice, pasta, and refined sugars, is a lowering of the glycemic index. Some researchers have speculated that the relatively higher glycemic indexes of foods today have contributed to the development of type 2 diabetes mellitus.

It is estimated that fruits, roots, legumes, nuts, and other noncereals provided 65 to 70% of the average forager's substistence base, with the remaining largely from animals. Furthermore, these foods were consumed within the same day of their gathering and with minimal to no processing. This means that these foods experienced minimal losses in vitamins, phytochemicals, and minerals relative to their energy content. Thus, the high consumption of nutrient-rich foods, in conjunction with a greater total food intake, resulted in the consumption of vitamins, minerals, and other beneficial substances in levels that for most individuals today can only be achieved by supplementation. For instance, the consumption of vitamin E may have been three times greater, while the consumption of calcium was more than double the current American intake. Carotene consumption was also probably double the current intake by Americans. Fiber consumption is estimated to potentially be in excess of 100 g daily, while in the U.S., where fiber consumption averages less than one fifth of that amount, this level may appear extremely high. However, other cultures do indeed have fiber intakes exceeding 50 g daily. Individuals in rural China may consume as much as 77 g daily, while an intake of 60 to 120 g of fiber have been estimated for rural Africans. Furthermore, an adult chimpanzee, which is one of the species most closely related to man, may ingest 200 g of fiber a day. Since one of the speculative concerns of consuming a high fiber diet is an increased presence of phytate in the digestive tract, it is important to realize that most of the phytate consumed in diets common to countries such as America, come via cereal grains.

Therefore, the Paleolithic diet certainly provides nutritionists with something to think about. Furthermore, the paleolithic diet probably provides a template for modern dietary design.

Aging

Certainly one aspect of nutrition that will have to be expanded is the understanding of how to optimally nourish the human body as it ages, as well as the influence of nutrition upon the aging process itself. Globally the percentage of the population attributed to individuals over the age of 65 is increasing. Humans are simply living longer. For example, the life expectancy for a female born today is 79 years and for a male about 72 years of age. Much of this increased life expectancy is the result of a decrease in infectious diseases as well as improvements in the medical management of diseases.

The aging process is complex. There are indeed several factors that have been purported to be involved in the aging process. These include reductions in DNA telemeres via telemerase enzymes; excessive free radical damage to DNA, proteins, and cellular structures; failure of cells to properly turnover leading to the accumulation of "deadened tissue," and the glycation of cellular structure and functional components. Some intriguing insight to the aging process is provided in a rare genetic disorder called Werner's syndrome. In this disease, individuals are characterized by premature graying of the hair and early onset of heart disease. The individual is the genetic recipient of two defective copies of the *helicase* enzyme. Helicase functions in the nucleus of cells by splitting the two complementary strands of DNA to allow for replication of DNA for cell reproduction. Apparently helicase is also necessary for DNA repair operations as well. As DNA sustains point mutations from mutagens (i.e., free radicals, toxins, or radiation), DNA repair proteins recognize the mutations and attempts to repair them. However, helicase is needed to separate the DNA leading and lagging strands to allow the repair to take place. Thus, mutations and damage can be "un-fixed" and cells become dysfunctional and age. One interesting feature of Werner's syndrome is that brain cells and some other tissue appear resistant to the damage and dysfunction associated with other tissue.

Physical and Physiological Changes

There are several physical and physiological changes that occur with aging. For instance, the number of active cells in the human body is decreased. Organ size and function also decline. In America, on average, there are decreases in bone mass and lean body mass which occur as body weight and percentage body fat increases. For muscle mass, humans seem to follow a linear pattern of decline, losing about 2 to 3% a decade during aging. The rate of skeletal muscle mass can be slowed by resistance training. Body fat accumulates, more so in the central and truncal regions than subcutaneously. Thus, more fat appears in the abdomen, buttocks, and thighs as humans age. Body weight follows a different pattern of change with aging. Weight gain continues until around 60 to 70 years of age, and then declines as energy intake wanes. Basal metabolic rate decreases during aging as well, with most of the change related to an increase in the ratio of adipose tissue to skeletal muscle. Also, along with aging, there is a decreased sense of smell, taste, sight, and hearing. One interesting feature of advancing age is the nature of skin cells to express more collagenase, which breaks down collagen and allows for wrinkling. Other tissue, such as endothelium and digestive mucosal cells, produce a lot of the inflammation-triggering interleukin 1 (IL-1), which can damage tissue.

Functional Foods

Without question more and more dollars are being spent to better understand chemical components of foods that may provide benefit to humans by either helping to prevent disease or to help treat and/or recover from disease. These factors are called *nutraceuticals*, and have been discussed in Chapter 14. The father of medicine himself, Hippocrates, included food as part of treatment of disease. The terms *functional foods*, "nutraceuticals," and *designer foods* are often used interchangeably. The term "nutraceutical" was probably first officially defined by the Foundation for Innovation in Medicine. It is applied to "any substance considered a food or part of a food that provides medical or health benefits, including the prevention and treatment of disease." Nutraceuticals can range from a food in general to isolated compounds and supplements. Also, genetically altered foods (designer foods) can also be included — for example, the genetic alteration of a tomato to have a greater lycopene content.

Without question, nutraceuticals will surely be a hot area of nutrition in the early part of the 21st century. Concomitant to an increased funding for nutrition research by federal and private groups, food companies are investing millions of dollars in the research and development of functional foods. It is estimated that as more and more of these products are marketed over the next couple years, consumers will spend in excess of $10 billion.

Suggested Readings

Bidlack, W.R. and Wang, W., Designing functional foods, in *Modern Nutrition in Health and Disease*, Shils, M.E., Olson, J.A., Shike, M., and Ross, A.C., Eds., Williams & Wilkins, Baltimore, MD, 9th ed., 1999.

Eaton, S.B., Eaton, S.B., and Konner, M.J., Paleolithic nutrition revisted: a twelve-year retrospective on its nature and implications, *Eur. J. Clin. Nutr.*, 51, 207–216, 1997.

Wolf, B.M., Potential role of raising dietary protein intake for reducing risk of atherosclerosis, *Can. J. Cardiol.*, 1 (Suppl. G), 127G–131G, 1995.

Concar, D., Death of old age, *New Scientist*, June 22, 1996, p. 24–29.

Simopoulos, A.P., Omega-3 fatty acids, Part I: Metabolic effects of omega-3 fatty acids and essentiality, in *Lipids in Human Nutrition*, Spiller, G., Ed., CRC Press, Boca Raton, FL, 1996.

Appendix A
Common Food Additives

TABLE A-1
Terms Used to Describe the Functions of Food Additives

Term	Function
Anticaking agents and free-flow agents	Substances added to finely powdered or crystalline food products to prevent caking.
Antimicrobial agents	Substances used to preserve food by preventing growth of microorganisms and subsequent spoilage, including fungicides, mold and yeast inhibitors, and bacteriocides.
Antioxidants	Substances used to preserve food by retarding deterioration, rancidity, or discoloration due to oxidation.
Colors and coloring adjuncts	Substances used to impart, preserve, or enhance the color or shading of a food, including color stabilizers, color fixatives, and color-retention agents.
Curing and pickling agents	Substances imparting a unique flavor and/or color to a food, usually producing an increase in shelf-life stability.
Dough strengtheners	Substances used to modify starch and gluten, thereby producing a more stable dough.
Drying agents	Substances with moisture-absorbing ability, used to maintain an environment of low moisture.
Emulsifiers and emulsifier salts	Substances which modify surface tension of two (or more) immiscible solutions to establish a uniform dispersion of components. This is called an emulsion.
Enzymes	Substances used to improve food processing and the quality of the finished food.
Firming agents	Substances added to precipitate residual pectin, thus strengthening the supporting tissue and preventing its collapse during processing.
Flavor enhancers	Substances added to supplement, enhance, or modify the original taste and/or aroma of a food, without imparting a characteristic taste or aroma of its own.
Flavoring agents and adjuvants	Substances added to impart or help impart a taste or aroma in food.
Flour treating agents	Substances added to milled flour, at the mill, to improve its color and/or baking qualities, including bleaching and maturing agents.
Formulation aids	Substances used to promote or produce a desired physical state or texture in food, including carriers, binders, fillers, plasticizers, film-formers, and tableting aids.
Fumigants	Volatile substances used for controlling insects or pests.
Humectants	Hygroscopic substances incorporated in food to promote retention of moisture, including moisture-retention agents and antidusting agents.
Leavening agents	Substances used to produce or stimulate production of carbon dioxide in baked goods to impart a light texture, including yeast, yeast foods, and calcium salts.
Lubricants and release agents	Substances added to food contact surfaces to prevent ingredients and finished products from sticking to them.
Nonnutritive sweeteners	Substances having less than 2% of the energy value of sucrose per equivalent unit of sweetening capacity.

(continues)

TABLE A-1 (continued)
Terms Used to Describe the Functions of Food Additives

Term	Function
Nutrient supplements	Substances which are necessary for the body's nutritional and metabolic processes.
Nutritive sweeteners	Substances having greater than 2% equivalent unit of sweetening capacity.
Oxidizing and reducing agents	Substances which chemically oxidize or reduce another food ingredient, thereby producing a more stable product.
pH control agents	Substances added to change or maintain active acidity or alkalinity, including buffers, acids, alkalis, and neutralizing agents.
Processing aids	Substances used as manufacturing aids to enhance the appeal or utility of a food or food component, including clarifying agents, clouding agents, catalysts, flocculents, filter aids, and crystallization inhibitors.
Propellants, aerating agents, and gases	Gases used to supply force to expel a product or used to reduce the amount of oxygen in contact with the food in packaging.
Sequestrants	Substances which combine with polyvalent metal ions to form a soluble metal complex to improve the quality and stability of products.
Solvents and vehicles	Substances used to extract or dissolve another substance.
Stabilizers and thickeners	Substances used to produce viscous solutions or dispersions, to impart body, improve consistency, or stabilize emulsions, including suspending and bodying agents, setting agents, gelling agents, and bulking agents.
Surface-active agents	Substances used to modify surface properties of liquid food components for a variety of effects, other than emulsifiers but including solubilizing agents, dispersants, detergents, wetting agents, rehydration enhancers, whipping agents, foaming agents, and defoaming agents.
Surface-finishing agents	Substances used to increase palatability, preserve gloss, and inhibit discoloration of foods, including glazes, polishes, waxes, and protective coatings.
Synergists	Substances used to act or react with another food ingredient to produce a total effect different or greater than the sum of the effects produced by the individual ingredients.
Texturizers	Substances which affect the appearance or feel of the food.

Source: From Ensminger et al., *Foods and Nutrition Encyclopedia*, 2nd ed., CRC Press, Boca Raton, FL, 1994, 11.

TABLE A-2
Common Food Additives

Name	Function[a]	Food Use and Comments
Acetic acid	pH control; preservative	Acid of vinegar is acetic acid. Miscellaneous and/or general purposes; many food uses; GRAS additive.
Adipic acid	pH control	Buffer and neutralizing agent; use in confectionery; GRAS additive.
Ammonium alginate	Stabilizer and thickener; texturizer	Extracted from seaweed. Widespread food use; GRAS additive.
Annatto	Color	Extracted from seeds of *Bixa crellana*. Butter, cheese, margarine, shortening, and sausage casings; coloring foods in general.
Arabinogalactan	Stabilizer and thickener; texturizer	Extracted from Western larch. Widespread food use; bodying agent in essential oils, nonnutritive sweeteners, flavor bases, nonstandardized dressings and pudding mixes.
Ascorbic acid (Vitamin C)	Nutrient; antioxidant; preservative	Widespread use in foods to prevent rancidity, browning; used in meat curing; GRAS additive.
Aspartame	Sweetener; sugar substitute	Soft drinks, chewing gum, powdered beverages, whipped toppings, puddings, gelatin, and tabletop sweetener.
Azodicarbonamide	Flour treating agent	Aging and bleaching ingredient in cereal flour.
Benzoic acid	Preservative	Occurs in nature in free and combined forms. Widespread food use; GRAS additive.
Benzoyl peroxide	Flour treating agent	Bleaching agent in flour; may be used in some cheeses.
Beta-apo-8' carotenal	Color	Natural food color. General use not to exceed 30 mg/lb or pt of food.
BHA (butylated hydroxyanisole)	Antioxidant; preservative	Fats, oils, dry yeast, beverages, breakfast cereals, dry mixes, shortening, potato flakes, chewing gum, and sausage; often used in combination with BHT; GRAS additive.
BHT (butylated hydroxytoluene)	Antioxidant; preservative	Rice, fats, oils, potato granules, breakfast cereals, potato flakes, shortening, chewing gum, and sausage; often used in combination with BHA; GRAS additive.
Biotin	Nutrient	Rich natural sources are liver, kidney, pancreas, yeast, and milk; vitamin supplement; GRAS additive.
Calcium alginate	Stabilizer and thickener; texturizer	Extracted from seaweed. Widespread food use; GRAS additive.
Calcium carbonate	Nutrient	Mineral supplement; general purpose additive; GRAS additive.
Calcium lactate	Preservative	General purpose and/or miscellaneous use; GRAS additive.
Calcium phosphate	Leavening agent; sequestrant; nutrient	General purpose and/or miscellaneous use; mineral supplement; GRAS additive.
Calcium propionate	Preservative	Bakery products, alone or with sodium propionate; inhibits mold and other microorganisms; GRAS additive.
Calcium silicate	Anticaking agent	Used in baking powder and salt. GRAS additive.

(continues)

TABLE A-2 (continued)
Common Food Additives

Name	Function[a]	Food Use and Comments
Canthaxanthin	Color	Widely distributed in nature. Color for foods; more red than carotene.
Caramel	Color	Miscellaneous and/or general purpose use in foods for color; GRAS additive.
Carob bean gum	Stabilizer and thickener	Extracted from bean of carob tree (locust bean). Numerous foods like confections, syrups, cheese spreads, frozen desserts, and salad dressings; GRAS additive.
Carrageenan	Emulsifier; stabilizer and thickener	Extracted from seaweed. A variety of foods, primarily those with a water or milk base.
Cellulose	Emulsifier; stabilizer and thickener	Component of all plants. Inert bulking agent in foods; may be used to reduce energy content of food; used in foods which are liquid and foam systems.
Citric acid	Preservative; antioxidant; pH control agent; sequestrant	Widely distributed in nature in both plants and animals. Miscellaneous and/or general purpose food use; used in lard, shortening, sausage, margarine, chili con carne, cured meats, and freeze-dried meats; GRAS additive.
Citrus Red No. 2	Color	Coloring skins of oranges.
Cochineal	Color	Derived from the dried female insect, *Coccus cacti*; raised in West Indies, Canary Islands, southern Spain, and Algiers; 70,000 insects to 1 lb. Provides red color for such foods as meat products and beverages.
Corn endosperm oil	Color	Source of xanthophyll for yellow color. Used in chicken feed to color yolks of eggs and chicken skin.
Cornstarch	Anticaking agent; drying agent; formulation aid; processing aid; surface-finishing agent	Digestible polysaccharide used in many foods often in a modified form; these include baking powder, baby foods, soups, sauces, pie fillings, imitation jellies, custards, and candies.
Corn syrup	Flavoring agent; humectant; nutritive sweetener; preservative	Derived from hydrolysis of cornstarch. Employed in numerous foods, e.g., baby foods, bakery products, toppings, meat products, beverages, condiments, and confections; GRAS additive.
Dextrose (glucose)	Flavoring agent; humectant; nutritive sweetener; synergist	Derived from cornstarch. Major uses of dextrose are confections, wine, and canned products; used to flavor meat products; used in production of caramel; variety of other uses.
Diglycerides	Emulsifiers	Uses include frozen desserts, lard, shortening, and margarine; GRAS additive.
Dioctyl sodium sulfosuccinate	Emulsifier; processing aid; surface active agent	Employed in gelatin dessert, dry beverages, fruit juice drinks, and noncarbonated beverages with cocoa fat; used in production of cane sugar and in canning.
Disodium guanylate	Flavor enhancer	Derived from dried fish or seaweed.
Disodium inosinate	Flavor adjuvant	Derived from seaweed or dried fish; sodium guanylate is a by-product.

TABLE A-2 (continued)
Common Food Additives

Name	Function[a]	Food Use and Comments
EDTA (ethylenediamine-tetraacetic acid)	Antioxidant; sequestrant	Calcium disodium and disodium salt of EDTA employed in a variety of foods including soft drinks, alcoholic beverages, dressings, canned vegetables, margarine, pickles, sandwich spreads, and sausage.
FD&C colors: Blue No. 1 Red No. 40 Yellow No. 5	Color	Coloring foods in general including dietary supplements.
Gelatin	Stabilizer and thickener; texturizer	Derived from collagen by boiling skin, tendons, ligaments, bones, etc. with water. Employed in many foods including: confectionery, jellies, and ice cream; GRAS additive.
Glycerine (glycerol)	Humectant	Miscellaneous and general purpose additive; GRAS additive.
Grape skin extract	Color	Colorings for carbonated drinks, beverage bases, and alcoholic beverages.
Guar gum	Stabilizer and thickener; texturizer	Extracted from seeds of the guar plant of India and Pakistan. Employed in such foods as cheese, salad dressings, ice cream, and soups.
Gum arabic	Stabilizer and thickener; texturizer	Gummy exudate of acacia plants. Used in variety of foods; GRAS additive.
Gum ghatti	Stabilizer and thickener; texturizer	Gummy exudate of plant growing in India and Ceylon. A variety of food uses; GRAS additive.
Hydrogen peroxide	Bleaching agent	Modification of starch and bleaching tripe; GRAS bleaching agent.
Hydrolyzed vegetable (plant) protein	Flavor enhancer	To flavor various meat products.
Invert sugar	Humectant; nutritive sweetener	Main use in confectionery and brewing industry.
Iron	Nutrient	Dietary supplements and food; GRAS additive.
Iron-ammonium citrate	Anticaking agent	Used in salt.
Karraya gum	Stabilizer and thickener	Derived from dried extract of *Sterculia urens*, found primarily in India. Variety of food uses; a substitute for tragacanth gum; GRAS additive.
Lactic acid	Preservative; pH control	Normal product of human metabolism. Numerous uses in foods and beverages; a miscellaneous general purpose additive; GRAS additive.
Lecithin (phosphatidylcholine)	Emulsifier; surface active agent	Normal tissue component of the body; edible and digestible additive naturally occurring in eggs; commercially derived from soybeans. Margarine, chocolate, and wide variety of other food uses; GRAS additive.
Mannitol	Anticaking; nutritive sweetener; stabilizer and thickener; texturizer	Special dietary foods; GRAS additive; supplies 1/2 the energy of glucose; classified as a sugar alcohol or polyol.

(continues)

TABLE A-2 (continued)
Common Food Additives

Name	Function[a]	Food Use and Comments
Methylparaben	Preservative	Food and beverages; GRAS additive.
Modified food starch	Drying agent; formulation aid; processing aid; surface finishing agent	Digestible polysaccharide used in many foods and stages of food processing; examples include baking powder, puddings, pie fillings, baby foods, soups, sauces, candies, etc.
Monoglycerides	Emulsifiers	Widely used in foods such as frozen desserts, lard, shortening, and margarine; GRAS additive.
MSG (monosodium glutamate)	Flavor enhancer	Enhances the flavor of a variety of foods including various meat products; possible association with the Chinese restaurant syndrome.
Papain	Texturizer	Miscellaneous and/or general purpose additive; GRAS additive; achieves results through enzymatic action; used as meat tenderizer. Heat inactivated.
Paprika	Color; flavoring agent	To provide coloring and/or flavor to foods; GRAS additive.
Pectin	Stabilizer and thickener; texturizer	Richest source of pectin is lemon and orange rind; present in cell walls of all plant tissues. Used to prepare jellies and jams. GRAS additive.
Phosphoric acid	pH control	Miscellaneous and/or general purpose additive; used to increase effectiveness of antioxidants in lard and shortening. GRAS additive.
Polyphosphates	Nutrient; flavor improver; sequestrant; pH control	Numerous food uses; most polyphosphates and their sodium, calcium, potassium, and ammonium salts. GRAS additive.
Polysorbates	Emulsifiers; surface-active agent	Polysorbates designated by numbers such as 60, 65, and 80; variety of food uses including baking mixes, frozen custards, pickles, sherbets, ice creams, and shortenings.
Potassium alginate	Stabilizer and thickener; texturizer	Extracted from seaweed. Wide usage; GRAS additive.
Potassium bromate	Flour treating agent	Employed in flour, whole wheat flour, fermented malt beverages, and to treat malt.
Potassium iodide	Nutrient	Added to table salt or used in mineral preparations as a source of dietary iodine.
Potassium nitrite	Curing and pickling agent	To fix color in cured products such as meats.
Potassium sorbate	Preservative	Inhibits mold and yeast growth in foods such as wines, sausage casings, and margarine; GRAS additive.
Propionic acid	Preservative	Mold inhibitor in breads and general fungicide; GRAS additive; used in manufacture of fruit flavors.
Propyl gallate	Antioxidant; preservative	Used in products containing oil or fat; employed in chewing gum; used to retard rancidity in frozen fresh pork sausage.

TABLE A-2 (continued)

Common Food Additives

Name	Function[a]	Food Use and Comments
Propylene glycol	Emulsifier, humectant; stabilizer and thickener; texturizer	Miscellaneous and/or general purpose additive; uses include salad dressings, ice cream, ice milk, custards, and a variety of other foods; GRAS additive.
Propylparaben	Preservative	Fungicide; controls mold in sausage casings; GRAS additive.
Saccharin	Nonnutritive sweetener	Special dietary foods and a variety of beverages; baked products; tabletop sweeteners.
Saffron	Color; flavoring agent	Derived from plant of western Asia and southern Europe. All foods except those where standards forbid; to color sausage casings, margarine, or product branding inks.
Silicon dioxide	Anticaking agent	Used in feed or feed components, beer production, production of special dietary foods, and ink diluent for marking fruits and vegetables.
Sodium acetate	pH control; preservative	Miscellaneous and/or general purpose use; meat preservation; GRAS additive.
Sodium alginate	Stabilizer and thickener; texturizer	Extracted from seaweed. Widespread food use; GRAS additive.
Sodium aluminum sulfate	Leavening agent	Baking powders, confectionery, and sugar refining.
Sodium benzoate	Preservative	Variety of food products; margarine to retard flavor reversion; GRAS additive.
Sodium bicarbonate	Leavening agent; pH control	Miscellaneous and/or general purpose uses; separation of fatty acids and glycerol in rendered fats; neutralize excess and clean vegetables in rendered fats, soups and curing pickles; GRAS additive.
Sodium chloride (salt)	Flavor enhancer; formulation acid; preservation	Used widely in many foods; GRAS additive.
Sodium citrate	pH control; curing and pickling agent; sequestrant	Evaporated milk; miscellaneous and/or general purpose food use; accelerate color fixing in cured meats; GRAS additive.
Sodium diacetate	Preservative; sequestrant	An inhibitor of molds and rope forming bacteria in baked products; GRAS additive.
Sodium nitrate (Chile saltpeter)	Curing and pickling agent; preservative	Used with or without sodium nitrite in smoked or cured fish, and cured meat products.
Sodium nitrite	Curing and pickling agent; preservative	May be used with sodium nitrate in smoked or cured fish, cured meat products, and pet foods.
Sodium propionate	Preservative	A fungicide and mold preventative in bakery products; GRAS additive.
Sorbic acid	Preservative	Fungistatic agent for foods, especially cheeses; other uses include baked goods, beverages, dried fruits, fish, jams, jellies, meats, pickled products, and wines; GRAS additive.

(continues)

TABLE A-2 (continued)
Common Food Additives

Name	Function[a]	Food Use and Comments
Sorbitan monostearate	Emulsifier; stabilizer and thickener	Widespread food usage such as whipped toppings, cakes, cake mixes, confectionery, icings, and shortenings.
Sorbitol	Humectant; nutritive sweetener; stabilizer and thickener; sequestrant	A sugar alcohol or polyol. Used in chewing gum, meat products, icings, dairy products, beverages, and pet foods. Provides less energy than sucrose.
Sucrose	Nutritive sweetener; preservative	The most widely used additive; used in beverages, baked goods, candies, jams and jellies, and other processed foods.
Tagetes (Aztec marigold)	Color	Source is flower petals of Aztec marigold. To enhance yellow color of chicken skin and eggs, incorporated in chicken feed.
Tartaric acid	pH control	Occurs free in many fruits; free or combined with calcium, magnesium, or potassium. Used in soft drinks industry, confectionery products, bakery products, and gelatin desserts.
Titanium dioxide	Color	For coloring foods generally, except standardized foods; used for coloring ingested and applied drugs.
Tocopherols (Vitamin E)	Antioxidant; nutrient	To retard rancidity in foods containing fat; used in dietary supplements; GRAS additive.
Tragacanth gum	Stabilizer and thickener; texturizer	Derived from the plant *Astragalus gummifer* or other Asiatic species of *Astragalus*. General purpose additive.
Turmeric	Color	Derived from rhizome of *Curcuma longa*. Used to color sausage casings, margarine, or shortening and ink for branding or marking products.
Vanilla	Flavoring agent	Used in various bakery products, confectionery and beverages; natural flavoring extracted from cured, full grown unripe fruit of *Vanilla panifolia*; GRAS additive.
Vanillin	Flavoring agent and adjuvant	Widespread confectionery, beverage, and food use; synthetic form of vanilla; GRAS additive.
Yellow prussiate of soda	Anticaking agent	Employed in salt.

[a] Function refers to those defined in Table .
Source: Adapted from Ensminger et al., *Foods and Nutrition Encyclopedia*, 2nd ed., CRC Press, Boca Raton, FL, 1994, 13–18.

Appendix B
Growth Charts

To use the growth curves shown in Figures B-1 through B-4, it is necessary to determine the percentile which corresponds most closely to the data from the infant that was measured. A simple procedure follows:

1. Locate and mark the height or weight of the infant on the vertical scale in the left margin of the appropriate chart. If the value of the measurement falls between the values marked on the scale, its placement should be estimated as accurately as possible.

2. With the aid of a ruler, draw a light, horizontal line across the chart, starting from the marked value for height or weight.

3. Using a procedure similar to step 1 (above), locate and mark the age of the child on the horizontal scale at the bottom of the chart.

4. Draw a vertical line on the chart, starting from the marked value for age.

5. Circle the point at which the horizontal and vertical lines intersect on the chart and note the percentile curve which is closest to the intersection.

Values which fall between the 5th and 95th percentiles are considered to be within the normal range. However, there should not be a wide discrepancy between the percentiles for height and weight. Sometimes, a pediatrician will not diagnose and treat an otherwise healthy infant until a clear-cut trend of growth abnormality is indicated by measurements taken at 2 or more consecutive monthly or bimonthly visits. Some typical interpretations of deviant growth measurements follow:

- **Short height for age, or low weight for age or height** — A low value of height for age suggests the possibility of an acute or chronic illness or a nutritional deficiency. This may also be the case when height for age is above the 10th percentile but weight for height is less than the 5th percentile. It is likely that any illness of sufficient severity to cause notable weight loss will result in a decrease in the ratio of weight to height.

  When measurements of height (or length) and weight have been made before the time of the current evaluation, they should be analyzed to determine the past rate of growth. When feasible, the child should be followed with sequential measurements so that rate of growth (more sensitive than single measurements in detecting abnormalities) may be recorded.

- **Excess weight for age, or height** — In the case of infants with weight for age or length greater than the 95th percentile, the emphasis should be placed on avoiding further excessive weight gain. With a caloric intake of approximately 40 to 43 kcal/lb/day (90 to 95 kcal/kg/day), one may anticipate that gain in fat-free tissue will continue at a normal rate, whereas increase in body content of fat will not occur or will occur only at a slow rate. The major aim should be directed to the correction of any patterns of overeating that may have been associated with the previous abnormal gain in weight.

It is noteworthy that the measurement of weight gain has the weakness of not indicating the composition of the gain. For example, the building up of body protein in muscle is accompanied by 3 to 4 parts of water to 1 of protein, whereas fat deposition is not accompanied by water and is much higher in caloric value than muscle tissue.

Other Means of Assessing Infant Development and Nutritional Status

The measurement of growth is only part of the assessment of infant development. Pediatricians also look for signs of inherited or congenital disorders and nutritional deficiencies. For example, special attention is paid to general features such as pallor, apathy, and irritability Similarly, the skin is examined carefully for signs of rickets.

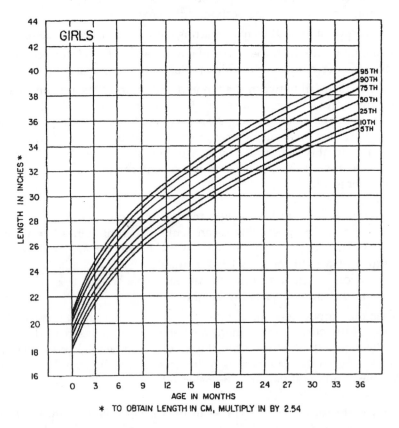

FIGURE B-1
Lengths (heights) of girls by age percentiles from birth, to 36 months. (Source: *NCHS Growth Curves for Children, Birth–18 Years, United States*, U.S. Department of HEW).

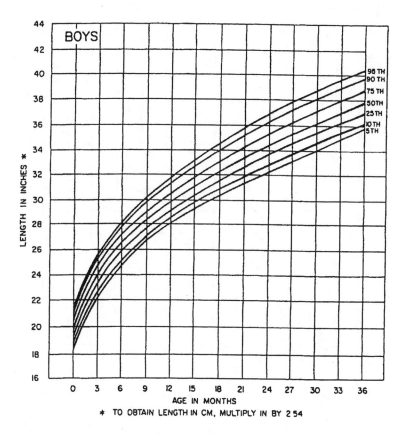

FIGURE B-2

Lengths (heights) of boys by age percentiles from birth to 36 months. (Source: *NCHS Growth Curves for Children, Birth–18 Years, United States*, U.S. Department of HEW).

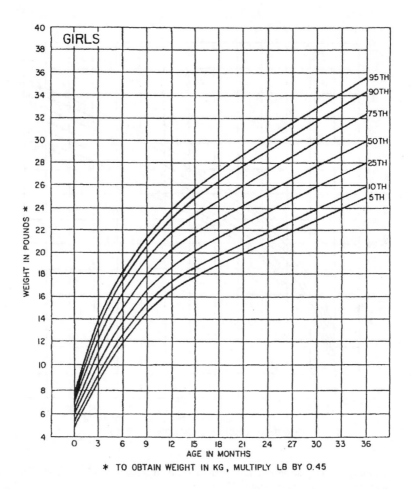

FIGURE B-3
Weights of girls by age percentiles from birth to 36 months. (Source: *NCHS Growth Curves for Children, Birth–18 Years, United States*, U.S. Department of HEW).

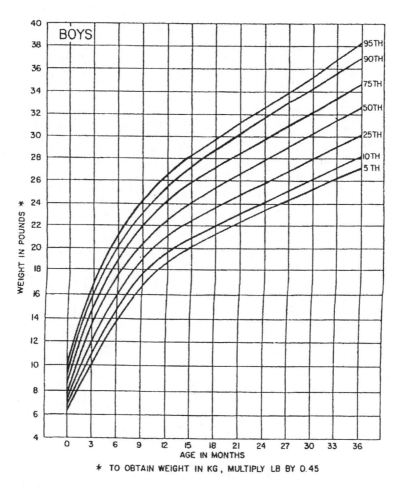

FIGURE B-4

Weights of boys by age percentiles from birth to 36 months. (Source: *NCHS Growth Curves for Children, Birth–18 Years, United States*, U.S. Department of HEW).

Appendix C
Vitamins

TABLE C-1
Vitamins

Functions	Deficiency and Toxicity Symptoms	Sources	Comments
Fat-Soluble Vitamins			
Vitamin A Helps maintain normal vision in dim light — prevents night blindness and xerophthamia. Essential for body growth. Necessary for normal bone growth and normal tooth development. Is an essential component of nuclear transcription factors and, as such, has an important role in cell replication gene expression and embryogenesis.	Deficiency symptoms — Night blindness (nyctalopia), xerosis, and xerophthalmia. Stunted bone growth, abnormal bone shape, and paralysis. Unsound teeth, characterized by abnormal enamel, pits, and decay. Rough, dry, scaly skin — a condition known as follicular hyperkeratosis (it looks like "gooseflesh"); increased sinus, sore throat, and abscesses in ears, mouth, or salivary glands; increased diarrhea and kidney and bladder stones. Reproductive disorders, including poor conception, abnormal embryonic growth, placental injury, and death of the fetus. Toxicity — Toxicity of Vitamin A is characterized by loss of appetite, headache, blurred vision, excessive irritability, loss of hair, dryness and flaking of skin (with itching), swelling over the long bones, drowsiness, diarrhea, nausea, and enlargement of the liver and spleen.	Liver, carrots, dark-green leafy vegetables. Yellow vegetables — pumpkins, sweet potatoes, squash (winter). Yellow fruits — apricots, peaches. Some seafoods (crab, halibut, oysters, salmon, swordfish), milk and milk products, eggs. Supplemental sources — Synthetic Vitamin A, cod and other fish liver oils.	The forms of Vitamin A are: alcohol (retinol), ester (retinyl palmitate), aldehyde (retinal or retinene), and acid (retinoic acid). Retinol, retinyl palmitate, and retinal are readily converted from one form to other forms. Retinoic acid fulfills some of the functions of Vitamin A, but it does not function in the visual cycle. β carotene found in vegetables serves as a Vitamin A precursor.

(continues)

517

TABLE C-1 (continued)
Vitamins

Vitamins	Functions	Deficiency and Toxicity Symptoms	Sources	Comments
Vitamin D	Increases calcium absorption from the small intestine. Promotes growth and mineralization of bones. Promotes sound teeth. Increases absorption of phosphorus through the intestinal wall, and increases resorption of phosphates from the kidney tubules. Maintains normal level of citrate in the blood. Protects against the loss of amino acids through the kidneys.	Deficiency symptoms — Rickets in infants and children, characterized by enlarged joints, bowed legs, knocked knees, outward projection of the sternum (pigeon breast), a row of beadlike projections on each side of the chest at the juncture of the rib bones and joining (costal) cartilage (called rachitic rosary), bulging forehead, pot belly, and delayed eruption of temporary teeth and unsound permanent teeth. Osteomalacia in adults, in which the bones soften, become distorted, and fracture easily. Tetany, characterized by muscle twitching, convulsions, and low serum calcium. Toxicity — Excessive Vitamin D may cause hypercalcemia (increased intestinal absorption, leading to elevated blood calcium levels), characterized by loss of appetite, excessive thirst, nausea, vomiting, irritability, weakness, constipation alternating with bouts of diarrhea, retarded growth in infants and children, and weight loss in adults.	D-fortified foods — Milk (400 IU/qt) and infant formulas. Other foods to which Vitamin D is often added include: breakfast and infant cereals, breads, margarines, milk flavorings, fruit and chocolate beverages, and cocoa. Supplemental sources — Fish liver oils (from cod, halibut, or swordfish); irradiated ergosterol or 7-dehydro-cholesterol such as viosterol. Exposure to sunlight or sunlamp — Converts the Vitamin D precursor to active Vitamin D.	Vitamin D includes both D_2 (ergocalciferol, calciferol, or viosterol) and D_3 (cholecalciferol). Vitamin D is unique among vitamins because it can be formed in the body and in certain foods by exposure to ultraviolet rays, and the active compound of Vitamin D $(1, 25\text{-}(OH)_2\text{-}D_3)$ functions as a hormone.
Vitamin E (Tocopherols)	As an antioxidant which protects body cells from free radicals formed from the unsaturated fatty acids. Maintains the integrity of red blood cells by its action as a suppressor of free radicals.	Deficiency symptoms — Newborn infants (especially the premature). Anemia caused by shortened life span of red blood cells, edema, skin lesions, and blood abnormalities. Patients unable to absorb fat have low blood and tissue tocopherol levels, decreased red blood cell life span, and increased urinary excretion of creatine.	Vegetable oils (except coconut oil), alfalfa seeds, margarine, nuts (almonds, Brazil nuts, filberts, peanuts, pecans), sunflower seed kernels. Good sources — Asparagus, avocados, beef and organ meats, blackberries, butter, eggs, green leafy vegetables, oatmeal, potato chips, rye, seafoods (lobster, salmon, shrimp, tuna), tomatoes.	There are 8 tocopherols and tocotrienols, of which α-tocopherol has the greatest Vitamin E activity.

As an agent essential to cellular respiration, primarily in heart and skeletal muscle tissues.	Toxicity — Vitamin E is relatively nontoxic. Some persons consuming daily doses of more than 300 IU of Vitamin E have complained of nausea and intestinal distress. Excess intake of Vitamin E appears to be excreted in the feces.	Supplemental sources — Synthetic alpha-tocopherol acetate, wheat germ, wheat germ oil.	
Vitamin K Vitamin K is essential for the synthesis in the liver of four bloodclotting proteins: 1. Factor II, prothrombin 2. Factor VII, proconvertin 3. Factor IX, Christmas factor 4. Factor X, Stuart-Power. Its action is on the posttranslational carboxylation of glutamic acid residues.	Deficiency symptoms —1. Delayed blood clotting, 2. Hemorrhagic disease of newborn. Vitamin K deficiency symptoms are likely in 1. Newborn infants. 2. Infants born to mothers receiving anticoagulants. 3. Obstructive jaundice (lack of bile). 4. Fat absorption defects (celiac disease, sprue). 5. Anticoagulant therapy or toxicity. Toxicity — The natural forms of Vitamin K_1 and K_2 have not produced toxicity even when given in large amounts. However, synthetic menadione and its various derivatives have produced toxic symptoms in rats and jaundice in human infants when given in amounts of more than 5 mg daily.	Vitamin K is fairly widely distributed in foods and is available synthetically.	Two forms: K_1 (phylloquinone, or phytylmenaquinone), and K_2 (manequinones), multiprenyl-manequinones. Vitamin K is synthesized by bacteria in the intestinal tracts of human beings and other species. There are several synthetic compounds, the best known of which is menadione, formerly known as K_3.
Water-Soluble Vitamins **Biotin** Biotin functions as a coenzyme mainly in decarboxylation-carboxylation and in deamination reactions.	Deficiency symptoms — The deficiency symptoms in man include a dry scaly dermatitis, loss of appetite, nausea, vomiting, muscle pains, glossitis (inflammation of the tongue), pallor of skin, mental depression, a decrease in hemoglobin and red blood cells, a high cholesterol level, and a low excretion of biotin; all of which respond to biotin administration. Toxicity — There are no known toxic effects.	Rich sources — Cheese (processed), kidney, liver, soybean flour. Good sources — Cauliflower, chocolate, eggs, mushrooms, nuts, peanut butter, sardine and salmon, wheat bran. Supplemental sources — Synthetic biotin, yeast (brewer's torula), alfalfa leaf meal (dehydrated). Considerable biotin is synthesized by the microorganisms in the intestinal tract.	Avidin, found in raw egg white, binds biotin making it unavailable. Avidin is destroyed by cooking.

(continues)

TABLE C-1 (continued)
Vitamins

Functions	Deficiency and Toxicity Symptoms	Sources	Comments
Choline 1. As part of the neurotransmitter acetyl choline, transmits nerve impulses. 2. Is essential for one of the membrane phospholipids (phosphatidylcholine). 3. Serves as a methyl donor.	Deficiency symptoms — Poor growth and fatty livers are the deficiency symptoms in most species except chickens and turkeys. Chickens and turkeys develop slipped tendons (perosis). In young rats, choline deficiency produces hemorrhagic lesions in the kidneys and other organs. Toxicity — No toxic effects have been observed.	Rich sources — Egg yolk, eggs, liver (beef, pork, lamb). Good sources — Soybeans, potatoes (dehydrated), cabbage, wheat bran, navy beans, alfalfa leaf meal, dried buttermilk, dried skimmed milk, rice polish, rice bran, whole grains (barley, corn, oats, rice, sorghum, wheat), hominy, turnips, wheat flour, blackstrap molasses. Supplemental sources — Yeast (brewers', torula), wheat germ, soybean lecithin, egg yolk lecithin, and synthetic choline and choline derivatives.	The classification of choline as a vitamin is debated because it does not meet all the criteria for vitamins, especially those of the B vitamins. The body manufactures choline from methionine, with the aid of folacin and Vitamin B-12.
Folacin/Folate (Folic acid) Folacin coenzymes are responsible for the following important functions: 1. The formation of purines and pyrimidines which, in turn, are needed for the synthesis of the nucleic acids DNA and RNA. 2. The formation of heme, the iron-containing protein in hemoglobin. 3. The interconversion of the three-carbon amino acid serine from the two-carbon amino acid glycine. 4. The formation of the amino acids tyrosine from phenylalanine and glutamic acid from histidine.	Deficiency symptoms — Megaloblastic anemia (of infancy), also called macrocyticanemia (of pregnancy), in which the red blood cells are larger and fewer than normal, and also immature. The anemia is due to inadequate formation of nucleoproteins, causing failure of the megaloblasts (young red blood cells) in the bone marrow to mature. The hemoglobin level is low because of the reduced number of red blood cells, and the white blood cell, blood platelet, and serum folate levels are low. Other symptoms include a sore, red, smooth red tongue (glossitis), disturbances of the digestive tract (diarrhea), and poor growth. Toxicity — Normally, no toxicity.	Rich sources — Liver and kidney. Good sources — Avocados, beans, beets, celery, chickpeas, eggs, fish, green leafy vegetables (such as asparagus, broccoli, Brussels sprouts, cabbage, cauliflower, endive, lettuce, parsley, spinach, turnip greens), nuts, oranges, orange juice, soybeans, and whole wheat products. Supplemental sources — Yeast, wheat germ, and commercially synthesized folic acid (pteroyl-glutamic acid, or PGA).	There is no single vitamin compound with the name folacin; rather, the term "folacin" is used to designate folic acid and a group of closely related substances which are essential for all vertebrates, including man. Ascorbic acid, vitamin B_{12}, and Vitamin B_6 are essential for the activity of the folacin coenzymes. Folacin deficiencies are thought to be a health problem in the U.S. and throughout the world. Infants, adolescents, and pregnant women are particularly vulnerable. The folacin requirement is increased by tropical sprue, certain genetic disturbances, cancer, parasitic infection, alcoholism, and oral contraceptives.

5. The formation of the amino acid methionine from homocysteine.
6. The synthesis of choline from ethanolamine.
7. The conversion of nicotinamide to N-methylnicotinamide, one of the metabolites of niacin that is excreted in the urine.

Raw vegetables stored at room temperature for 2–3 days lose as much as 50–70% of their folate content. Between 50 and 95% of food folate is destroyed in cooking. Intestinal synthesis provides some folacin.

Niacin (Nicotinic acid; nicotinamide) is a constituent of two important coenzymes in the body, nicotinamide adenine and dinucleotide (NAD) and nicotinamide adenine dinucleotide phosphate (NADP). These coenzymes function as reducing equivalent (H^+) acceptors or donors.

Generally speaking, niacin is found in animal tissues as nicotinamide and in plant tissues as nicotinic acid. Both forms are of equal niacin activity.
Rich sources — Liver, kidney, lean meats, poultry, fish, rabbit, corn flakes (enriched), nuts, peanut butter, milk, cheese, and eggs, although low in niacin content, are good antipellagra foods, because their niacin is in available form. Enriched cereal flours and products are good sources of niacin.
Supplemental sources — Both synthetic nicotinamide and nicotinic acid are commercially available. For pharmaceutical use, nicotinamide is usually used; for food nutrification, nicotinic acid is usually used. Also, yeast is a rich natural source of niacin.

Deficiency symptoms — A deficiency of niacin results in pellagra, the symptoms of which are: dermatitis, particularly of areas of skin which are exposed to light or injury; inflammation of mucous membranes, including the entire gastrointestinal tract, which results in a red, swollen, sore tongue and mouth, diarrhea, and rectal irritation; and psychic changes, such as irritability, anxiety, depression, and in advanced cases, delirium, hallucinations, confusion, disorientation, and stupor.
Toxicity — Only large doses of niacin, sometimes given to an individual with mental illness, are known to be toxic. However, ingestion of large amounts may result in vascular dilation, or "flushing" of the skin, itching, liver damage, elevated blood glucose, elevated blood enzymes, and/or peptic ulcer.

An average mixed diet in the U.S. provides about 1% protein as tryptophan. Thus, a diet supplying 60 g of protein contains about 600 mg of tryptophan, which will yield about 10 mg of niacin (on the average, 1 mg of niacin is derived from each 60 mg of dietary tryptophan).
Niacin is the most stable of the B-complex vitamins. Cooking losses of a mixed diet usually do not amount to more than 15–25%.

Pantothenic acid (Vitamin B_3)
Pantothenic acid functions as part of two enzymes — coenzyme A (CoA) and acyl carrier protein (ACP). CoA functions in the following important reactions:

Deficiency symptoms — The symptoms: irritableness and restlessness; loss of appetite, indigestion, abdominal pains, nausea; headache; sullenness, mental depression; fatigue, weakness; numbness and tingling of hands and feet, muscle

Organ meat (liver, kidney, and heart), cottonseed flour, wheat bran, rice bran, rice polish, nuts, mushrooms, soybean flour, salmon, blue cheese, eggs, buckwheat flour, brown rice, lobster, sunflower seeds.

Coenzyme A, of which pantothenic acid is a part, is one of the most important substances in body metabolism. It functions in acetyl group transfer and thus is important to fatty acid synthesis and degradation.

(continues)

TABLE C-1 (continued)
Vitamins

Functions	Deficiency and Toxicity Symptoms	Sources	Comments
Pantothenic acid (Vitamin B₃) (*continued*) 1. The formation of acetylcholine, a substance of importance in transmitting nerve impulses. 2. The synthesis of porphyrin, a precursor of heme, of importance in hemoglobin synthesis. 3. The synthesis of cholesterol and other sterols. 4. The steroid hormones formed by the adrenal and sex glands. 5. The maintenance of normal blood sugar, and the formation of antibodies. 6. The excretion of sulfonamide drugs. ACP, along with CoA, required by the cells in the synthesis of fatty acids.	cramps in the arms and legs; burning sensation in the feet; insomnia; respiratory infections; rapid pulse; and a staggering gait. Also, in these subjects there was increased reaction to stress; increased sensitivity to insulin, resulting in low blood sugar levels; increased sedimentation rate for erythrocytes; decreased gastric secretions; and marked decrease in antibody production. Toxicity — Pantothenic acid is relatively nontoxic. However, doses of 10–20 g per day may result in occasional diarrhea and water retention.	Supplemental sources — Synthetic calcium pantothenate is widely used as a vitamin supplementation. Yeast is a rich natural supplement. Intestinal bacteria synthesize pantothenic acid, but the amount and availability is unknown.	
Riboflavin (Vitamin B₂) Riboflavin is an integral part of the coenzymes FAD and FMN. These coenzymes accept or donate reducing equivalents.	Deficiency symptoms — Unlike all the other vitamins, riboflavin deficiency is not the cause of any severe or major disease of man. Rather, riboflavin often contributes to other disorders and disabilities such as beriberi, pellagra, scurvy, keratomalacia, and nutritional megaloblastic anemia. Riboflavin deficiency symptoms are: sores at the angles of the mouth (angular stomatitis); sore, swollen, and chapped	Rich sources — Organ meats (liver, kidney, heart). Good sources — Corn flakes (enriched), almonds, cheese, eggs, lean meat (beef, pork, lamb), mushrooms (raw), wheat flour (enriched), turnip greens, wheat bran, soybean flour, bacon, cornmeal (enriched). Supplemental sources — Yeast (brewers', torula). Riboflavin is the only vitamin present in significant amounts in beer.	Riboflavin is destroyed by light; and by heat in an alkaline solution.

lips (cheilosis); swollen, fissured, and painful tongue (glossitis); redness and congestion at the edges of the cornea of the eye; and oily, crusty, scaly skin (seborrheic dermatitis).

Toxicity — There is no known toxicity of riboflavin.

Thiamin
(Vitamin B_1)
As a coenzyme in transketolation (keto-carrying).
In direct functions in the body, including (1) maintenance of normal appetite, (2) the tone of the muscles, and (3) a healthy mental attitude.

Moderate thiamin deficiency symptoms include fatigue; apathy (lack of interest); loss of appetite; nausea; moodiness; irritability; depression; retarded growth; a sensation of numbness in the legs; and abnormalities of the electrocardiogram. Severe thiamin deficiency of long duration culminates in beriberi, the symptoms of which are polyneuritis (inflammation of the nerves), emaciation and/or edema, and disturbances of heart function.

Toxicity — None.

Thiamin is found in a large variety of animal and vegetable products but is abundant in few.

Rich sources — Lean pork, sunflower seed, corn flakes (enriched), peanuts, safflower flour, soybean flour.

Good sources — Wheat bran, kidney, wheat flour (enriched), rye flour, nuts (except peanuts, which are a rich source), whole wheat flour, cornmeal (enriched), rice (enriched), white bread (enriched), soybean sprouts.

Supplemental sources — Thiamin hydrochloride, thiamin mononitrate, yeast (brewers', torula), rice bran, wheat germ, and rice polish.

Enriched flour (bread) and cereal which were initiated in 1941 have been of special significance in improving the dietary level of thiamin in the U.S.

Vitamin B_6
(Pyridoxine; pyridoxal; pyridoxamine)
Vitamin B_6 functions as a coenzyme (pyridoxal phosphate)
a. Transamination
b. Decarboxylation
c. Transsulfuration
d. Tryptophan conversion to nicotinic acid.

Deficiency symptoms — In adults, greasy scaliness (seborrheic dermatitis) in the skin around the eyes, nose, and mouth, which subsequently spread to other parts of the body; a smooth, red tongue; loss of weight; muscular weakness; irritability; mental depression. In infants, the deficiency symptoms are irritability, muscular twitchings, and convulsions.

Rice bran, wheat bran, sunflower seeds, avocados, bananas, corn, fish, kidney, lean meat, liver, nuts, poultry, rice (brown), soybeans, whole grain.

Supplemental sources — Pyridoxine hydrochloride is the most commonly available synthetic form, and yeast (torula, brewers'), rice polish, and wheat germ are used as natural source supplements.

In rats, the three forms of Vitamin B_6 have equal activity, and it is assumed that the same applies to man. Processing or cooking foods may destroy up to 50% of the B_6. Because Vitamin B_6 is limited in many foods, supplemental B_6 with synthetic pyridoxine hydrochloride may be indicated, especially for infants and during pregnancy and lactation.

(continues)

TABLE C-1 (continued)
Vitamins

Functions	Deficiency and Toxicity Symptoms	Sources	Comments
e. Absorption of amino acids. f. The conversion of glycogen to glucose 1-phosphate. g. The conversion of linoleic acid to arachidonic acid.	Toxicity — B_6 is relatively nontoxic, but, large doses may result in sleepiness and be habit-forming when taken over an extended period.		
Vitamin B_{12} (Cobalamins) 1. Synthesis or transfer of single carbon units. 2. Biosynthesis of methyl groups ($-CH_3$), and in reduction reactions such as the conversion of disulfide (S–S) to the sulfhydryl group (-SH).	Deficiency symptoms — Vitamin B_{12} deficiency in man may occur as a result of (1) dietary lack, which sometimes occurs among vegetarians who consume no animal food, or (2) deficiency of intrinsic factor due to pernicious anemia, total or partial removal of the stomach by surgery, or infestation with parasites such as the fish tapeworm. The common symptoms of a dietary deficiency of Vitamin B_{12} are sore tongue, weakness, loss of weight, back pains, tingling of the extremities, apathy, and mental and other nervous abnormalities. Anemia is rarely seen in dietary deficiency of B_{12}. In pernicious anemia, the characteristic symptoms are abnormally large red blood cells, lemon-yellow pallor, anorexia, prolonged bleeding time, abdominal discomfort, loss of weight, glossitis, an unsteady gait, and neurological disturbances, including stiffness of the limbs, irritability, and mental depression. Without treatment death follows. Toxicity — No toxic effects of Vitamin B_{12} are known.	Liver and other organ meats — kidney, heart, muscle meats, fish, shellfish, eggs, and cheese. Supplemental sources — Cobalamin, of which there are at least three active forms, produced by microbial growth; available at the corner drugstore. Some B_{12} is synthesized in the intestinal tract of human beings. However, little of it may be absorbed.	Plants cannot manufacture Vitamin B_{12}. Vitamin B_{12} is the largest and the most complex of all vitamin molecules. Vitamin B_{12} is the only vitamin that requires a specific gastrointestinal factor for its absorption (intrinsic factor), and the absorption of Vitamin B_{12} in the small intestine requires about 3 hours.

Vitamin C
(Ascorbic acid)
Formation and maintenance of
collagen, the substance that binds
body cells together.
Metabolism of the amino acids
tyrosine and tryptophan.
Absorption and movement of iron.
Metabolism of fats and lipids and
cholesterol control. Sound teeth and
bones.
Strong capillary walls and healthy
blood vessels.
Metabolism of folic acid.

Deficiency symptoms — Early symptoms,
called latent scurvy: loss in weight,
listlessness, fatigue, fleeting pains in the
joints and muscles, irritability, shortness
of breath, sore and bleeding gums, small
hemorrhages under the skin, bones that
fracture easily, and poor wound healing.
Scurvy—Swollen, bleeding and ulcerated
gums; loose teeth; malformed and weak
bones, fragility of the capillaries with
resulting hemorrhages throughout the
body; large bruises; big joints, such as the
knees and hips, due to bleeding into the
joint cavity; anemia; degeneration of
muscle fibers, including those of the
heart; and tendency of old wounds to
become red and break open. Sudden
death from severe internal hemorrhage
and heart failure.
Toxicity — Adverse effects reported of
intakes in excess of 8 g per day (more
than 100 times the recommended
allowance) include nausea, abdominal
cramps, and diarrhea; absorption of
excessive amounts of iron; destruction of
red blood cells; increased mobilization of
bone minerals; interference with
anticoagulant therapy; formation of
kidney and bladder stones; inactivation
of Vitamin B_{12}; rise in plasma cholesterol;
and possible dependence upon large
doses of Vitamin C.

Natural sources of Vitamin C occur
primarily in fruits (especially citrus
fruits) and leafy vegetables — acerola
cherry, *camu-camu*, and rose hips, raw,
frozen, or canned citrus fruit or juice,
oranges, grapefruit, lemons, and limes;
guavas, peppers (green, hot), black
currants, parsley, turnip greens, poke
greens, and mustard greens.
Good sources — Green leafy vegetables:
broccoli, Brussels sprouts, cabbage
(red), cauliflower, collards, kale, lamb's-
quarter, spinach, Swiss chard, and
watercress. Also, cantaloupe, papaya,
strawberries, and tomatoes and tomato
juice (fresh or canned).
Supplemental sources — Vitamin C
(ascorbic acid) is available wherever
vitamins are sold.

All animal species appear to require
Vitamin C, but dietary need is limited
to humans, guinea pigs, monkeys, fruit
bats, birds, certain fish, and certain
reptiles.
Of all the vitamins, ascorbic acid is the
most unstable. It is easily destroyed
during storage, processing, and
cooking; it is water-soluble, easily
oxidized, and attacked by enzymes.

Note: Some nutritionists include inositol, coenzyme Q (ubiquinone), the bioflavinoids, and carnitine as essential nutrients or as vitamins. While these compounds are essential to normal metabolism, the needs for them as essential nutrients can depend on the physiologic state of the consumer. Premature infants require carnitine in the diet because they do not synthesize adequate amounts. Similarly, inositol is synthesized in the body; however, there may be instances where that synthesis is inadequate. Ubiquinone and the bioflavinoids have yet to be shown as essential dietary ingredients for humans. Some drugs interfere with vitamin use.

Appendix D
Minerals

TABLE D-1

Minerals as Essential Dietary Components: Macrominerals

Function	Deficiencies and Toxicity Symptoms	Sources	Comments
Calcium (Ca) The primary function of calcium is to build the bones and teeth and to maintain the bones. Other functions are: 1. Blood clotting. 2. Muscle contraction and relaxation, especially the heartbeat. 3. Nerve transmission. 4. Cell wall permeability. 5. Enzyme activation. 6. Secretion of a number of hormones and hormone-releasing factors.	Deficiency symptoms: 1. Stunting of growth. 2. Poor quality bones and teeth. 3. Malformation of bones — rickets. The clinical manifestations of calcium-related diseases are: 1. Rickets in children. 2. Osteomalacia, the adult counterpart of rickets. 3. Osteoporosis, a condition of too little bone, resulting when bone resorption exceeds bone formation. 4. Hypercalcemia, characterized by high serum calcium. 5. Tetany, characterized by muscle spasms and muscle pain. 6. Kidney stones. Toxicity — Normally, the small intestine prevents excess calcium from being absorbed. However, a breakdown of this control may raise the level of calcium in the blood and lead to calcification of the kidneys and other internal organs. High calcium intake may cause excess secretion of calcitonin and very dense bones. High calcium intakes have also been reported to cause kidney stones.	Cheeses, wheat-soy flour, blackstrap molasses, milk, and milk products.	Calcium is the most abundant mineral in the body. It comprises about 40% of the total mineral present; 99% of it is in the bones and teeth. Generally, nutritionists recommend a calcium–phosphorus ratio of 1.5:1 in infancy, decreasing to 1:1 at 1 year of age and remaining at 1:1 throughout the rest of life; although they consider ratios between 2:1 and 1:2 as satisfactory.

(continues)

527

TABLE D-1 (continued)

Minerals as Essential Dietary Components: Macrominerals

Function	Deficiencies and Toxicity Symptoms	Sources	Comments
Phosphorus (P) Essential for bone formation and maintenance. Important in the development of teeth. Essential for normal milk secretion. Important in building muscle tissue. As a component of nucleic acids (RNA and DNA), which are important in genetic transmission and control of cellular metabolism. Maintenance in many metabolic functions especially: 1. Energy utilization; 2. Phospholipid formation; 3. Amino acid metabolism; protein formation; 4. Enzyme systems.	Deficiency symptoms — General weakness, loss of appetite, muscle weakness, bone pain, and loss of calcium. Severe and prolonged deficiencies of phosphorus may be manifested by rickets, osteomalacia, and other phosphorus related diseases. Toxicity — There is no known phosphorus toxicity per se. However, excess phosphate consumption may cause hypocalcemia (a deficiency of calcium in the blood).	Cocoa powder, cottonseed flour, fish flour, peanut flour, pumpkin and squash seeds, rice bran, rice polish, soybean flour, sunflower seeds, wheat, and bran.	Phosphorus comprises about 1/4 the total mineral matter in the body. Eighty percent of the phosphorus is in the bones and teeth in inorganic combination with calcium. Normally, 70% of the ingested phosphorus is absorbed. Generally, nutritionists recommend a calcium–phosphorus ratio of 1.5:1 in infancy, decreasing to 1:1 at 1 year of age, and remaining at 1:1 throughout the rest of life, although they consider ratios between 2:1 and 1:2 as satisfactory.
Sodium (Na) Helps to maintain the balance of water, acids, and bases in the fluid outside the cells. As a constituent of pancreatic juice, bile, sweat, and tears. Associated with muscle contraction and nerve functions. Plays a specific role in the absorption of carbohydrates.	Deficiency symptoms — Reduced growth, loss of appetite, loss of body weight due to loss of water, reduced milk production of lactating mothers, muscle cramps, nausea, diarrhea, and headache. Excess perspiration and salt depletion may be accompanied by heat exhaustion. Toxicity — Salt may be toxic when (1) a high intake is accompanied by a restriction of water, (2) when the body is adapted to a chronic low salt diet, or (3) when it is fed to infants or others whose kidneys cannot excrete the excess in the urine.	Table salt, processed meat products, and pickled/cured products.	Deficiencies of sodium may occur when there has been heavy, prolonged sweating, diarrhea, vomiting, or adrenal cortical insufficiency. In such cases, extra salt should be taken.

Chlorine (Cl)

Plays a major role in the regulation of osmotic pressure, water balance, and acid-base balance.

Required for the production of hydrochloric acid in the stomach; this acid is necessary for the proper absorption of Vitamin B_{12} and iron, for the activation of the enzyme that breaks down starch, and for suppressing the growth of microorganisms that enter the stomach with food and drink.

Deficiency symptoms — Severe deficiencies may result in alkalosis (an excess of alkali in the blood), characterized by slow and shallow breathing, listlessness, muscle cramps, loss of appetite, and, occasionally, by convulsions.

Deficiencies of chloride may develop from prolonged and severe vomiting, diarrhea, pumping of the stomach, injudicious use of diuretic drugs.

Toxicity — An excess of chlorine ions is unlikely when the kidneys are functioning properly.

Table salt (sodium chloride) and foods that contain salt.

Persons whose sodium intake is severely restricted (owing to diseases of the heart, kidney, or liver) may need an alternative source of chloride; a number of chloride-containing salt substitutes are available for this purpose.

Magnesium (Mg)

Constituent of bones and teeth.

Essential element of cellular metabolism, often as an activator of enzymes involved in phosphorylated compounds and of high energy phosphate transfer of ADP and ATP.

Involved in activating certain peptidases in protein digestion.

Relaxes nerve impulse, functioning antagon-istically to calcium which is stimulatory.

Deficiency symptoms — A deficiency of magnesium is characterized by (1) muscle spasms (tremor, twitching) and rapid heartbeat; (2) confusion, hallucinations, and disorientation; and (3) lack of appetite, listlessness, nausea, and vomiting.

Toxicity — Magnesium toxicity is characterized by slowed breathing, coma, and sometimes death.

Rich sources — Coffee (instant), cocoa powder, cottonseed flour, peanut flour, sesame seeds, soybean flour, spices, wheat bran, and wheat germ.

Overuse of such substances as "milk of magnesia" (magnesium hydroxide) or "Epsom salts" (magnesium sulfate) may lead to deficiencies of other minerals or even to toxicity.

Potassium (K)

Involved in the maintenance of proper acid-base balance and the transfer of nutrients in and out of individual cells.

Relaxes the heart muscle — action opposite to that of calcium which is stimulatory.

Required for the secretion of insulin by the pancreas in enzyme reactions involving the phosphorylation.

Deficiency symptoms — Potassium deficiency may cause rapid and irregular heartbeats and abnormal electrocardiograms; muscle weakness, irritability, and occasionally paralysis; and nausea, vomiting, diarrhea, and swollen abdomen. Extreme and prolonged deficiency of potassium may cause hypokalemia, culminating in the heart muscles stopping.

Dehydrated fruits, molasses, potato flour, rice bran, seaweed, soybean flour, spices, sunflower seeds, and wheat bran.

Potassium is the third most abundant element in the body, after calcium and phosphorus, and it is present in twice the concentration of sodium

(continues)

TABLE D-1 (continued)

Minerals as Essential Dietary Components: Macrominerals

Function	Deficiencies and Toxicity Symptoms	Sources	Comments
Potassium (K) (continued)	Toxicity — Acute toxicity from potassium (known as hyperpotassemia or hyperkalemia) can result when kidneys are not functioning properly. The condition may prove fatal due to cardiac arrest.		
Cobalt (Co) The only known function of cobalt is that of an integral part of Vitamin B_{12}, an essential factor in the formation of red blood cells.	A cobalt deficiency as such has never been produced in humans. The signs and symptoms that are sometimes attributed to cobalt deficiency are actually due to lack of Vitamin B_{12}, characterized by pernicious anemia, poor growth, and occasionally neurological disorders.	Cobalt is present in many foods.	Cobalt is an essential constituent of Vitamin B_{12} and must be ingested in the form of vitamin molecules inasmuch as humans synthesize little of the vitamin. (A small amount of Vitamin B_{12} is synthesized in the human colon by *E. coli*, but absorption is very limited.)
Copper (Cu) Facilitating the absorption of iron from the intestinal tract and releasing it from storage in the liver and the reticuloendothelial system. Essential for the formation of hemoglobin, although it is not a part of hemoglobin as such. Constituent of several enzyme systems. Development and maintenance of the vascular and skeletal structures (blood vessels, tendons, and bones). Structure and function of the central nervous system. Required for normal pigmentation of hair. Component of important copper-containing proteins. Reproduction (fertility).	Deficiency symptoms — Deficiency is most apt to occur in malnourished children and in premature infants fed exclusively on modified cow's milk and in infants breast-fed for an extended period of time. Deficiency leads to a variety of abnormalities, including anemia, skeletal defects, demyelination and degeneration of the nervous system, defects in pigmentation and structure of the hair, reproductive failure, and pronounced cardiovascular lesions. Toxicity — Copper is relatively nontoxic to monogastric species, including man. The recommended copper intake for adults is in the range of 2–3 mg/day. Daily intakes of more than 20–30 mg over extended periods would be expected to be unsafe.	Black pepper, blackstrap molasses, Brazil nuts, cocoa, liver, and oysters (raw).	Most cases of copper poisoning result from drinking water or beverages that have been stored in copper tanks and/or pass through copper pipes. Dietary excesses of calcium, iron, cadmium, zinc, lead, silver, and molybdenum plus sulfur reduce the utilization of copper.

Fluorine (F)
Constitutes 0.02–0.05% of the bones and teeth. Necessary for sound bones and teeth. Assists in the prevention of dental caries.

Deficiency symptoms — Excess dental caries. Also, there is indication that a deficiency of fluorine results in osteoporosis in the aged.
Toxicity — Deformed teeth and bones, and softening, mottling, and irregular wear of the teeth.

Fluorine is found in many foods, but seafoods and dry tea are the richest food sources.
Fluoridation of water supplies to bring the concentration of fluoride to 1 ppm.

Large amounts of dietary calcium, aluminum, and fat will lower the absorption of fluorine.
Fluoridation of water supplies (1 ppm) is the simplest and most effective method of providing added protection against dental caries.

Iodine (I)
The sole function of iodine is making the iodine-containing thyroid hormones.

Deficiency symptoms — Iodine deficiency is characterized by goiter (an enlargement of the thyroid gland at the base of the neck), coarse hair, obesity, and high blood cholesterol.
Iodine-deficient mothers may give birth to infants with a type of dwarfism known as cretinism, a disorder characterized by malfunctioning of the thyroid gland, goiter, mental retardation, and stunted growth. A similar disorder of the thyroid gland, known as myxedema, may develop in adults.
Toxicity — Long-term intake of large excesses of iodine may disturb the utilization of iodine by the thyroid gland and result in goiter.

Among natural foods the best sources of iodine are kelp, seafoods, and vegetables grown in iodine-rich soils and iodized salt. Stabilized iodized salt contains 0.01% potassium iodide (0.0076% I), or 76 mcg of iodine per gram.

Certain foods (especially plants of the cabbage family) contain goitrogens, which interfere with the use of thyroxine and may produce goiter. Fortunately, goitrogenic action is prevented by cooking.

Iron (Fe)
Iron (heme) combines with protein (globin) to make hemoglobin, the iron-containing compound in red blood cells which transports oxygen. Iron is also a component of enzymes which are involved in energy metabolism.

Deficiency symptoms — Iron-deficiency (nutritional) anemia, the symptoms of which are: paleness of skin and mucous membranes, fatigue, dizziness, sensitivity to cold, shortness of breath, rapid heartbeats, and tingling of the fingers and toes.
An excess of iron in the diet can tie up phosphorus in an insoluble iron–phosphate complex, thereby creating a deficiency of phosphorus.

Red meat, egg yolk, and dark green, leafy vegetables.

About 70% of the iron is present in the hemoglobin, the pigment of the red blood cells. The other 30% is present as a reserve store in the liver, spleen, and bone marrow.

Manganese (Mn)
Formation of bone and the growth of other connective tissues.

Deficiency symptoms — No clear deficiency disease in man has been reported.

Rice (brown), rice bran and polish, walnuts, wheat bran, and wheat germ.

In average diets, only about 45% of the ingested magnesium is absorbed. The manganese content of plants is dependent on soil content.

(continues)

TABLE D-1 (continued)

Minerals as Essential Dietary Components: Macrominerals

Function	Deficiencies and Toxicity Symptoms	Sources	Comments
Manganese (Mn) (continued) Blood clotting. Insulin action. Cholesterol synthesis. Activator of various enzymes in the metabolism of carbohydrates, fats, proteins, and nucleic acids.	Toxicity — Toxicity in man as a consequence of dietary intake has not been observed. However, it has occurred in workers (miners and others) exposed to high concentrations of manganese dust in the air. The symptoms resemble those found in Parkinson's and Wilson's disease.		
Molybdenum (Mo) As a component of three different enzyme systems which are involved in the metabolism of carbohydrates, fats, proteins, sulfur-containing amino acids, nucleic acids (DNA and RNA), and iron. As a component of the enamel of teeth.	Deficiency symptoms — Naturally occurring deficiency in man is not known. Molybdenum-deficient animals are especially susceptible to the toxic effects of bisulfite, characterized by breathing difficulties and neurological disorders. Severe molybdenum toxicity in animals (molybdenosis), particularly cattle, occurs throughout the world wherever pastures are grown on high-molybdenum soils. The symptoms include diarrhea, loss of weight, decreased production, fading of hair color, and other symptoms of copper deficiency.	The concentration of molybdenum in food varies considerably, depending on the soil in which it is grown. Most of the dietary molybdenum intake is derived from organ meats, whole grains, leafy vegetables, legumes, and yeast.	The utilization of molybdenum is reduced by excess copper, sulfate, and tungsten. In cattle, a relationship exists between molybdenum, copper, and sulfur. Excess molybdenum will cause copper deficiency. However, when the sulfate content of the diet is increased, the symptoms of toxicity are avoided inasmuch as the excretion of molybdenum is increased.
Selenium (Se) Component of the enzyme glutathione peroxidase, the metabolic role of which is to protect against oxidation of polyunsaturated fatty acids and resultant tissue damage.	Deficiency symptoms — There are no clear-cut deficiencies of selenium, because this mineral is so closely related to vitamin E that it is difficult to distinguish deficiency due to selenium alone. Toxicity — Poisonous effects of selenium are manifested by (1) abnormalities of the hair, nails, and skin; (2) garlic odor on the breath; (3) intensification of selenium toxicity by arsenic or mercury; and (4) higher than normal rates of dental caries.	The selenium content of plant and animal products is affected by the selenium content of the soil and animal feed, respectively. Brazil nuts, butter, flour, fish, lobster, and smelt.	The high selenium areas are in Great Plains and the Rocky Mountain states — especially in parts of the Dakotas and Wyoming.

Zinc (Zn) Needed for normal skin, bones, and hair. As a component of several different enzyme systems which are involved in digestion and respiration. Required for the transfer of carbon dioxide in red blood cells; for proper calcification of bones; for the synthesis and metabolism of proteins and nucleic acids; for the development and functioning of reproductive organs; for wound and burn healing; for the functioning of insulin; and for normal taste acuity.	Deficiency symptoms — Loss of appetite, stunted growth in children, skin changes, small sex glands in boys, loss of taste sensitivity, lightened pigment in hair, white spots on the fingernails, and delayed healing of wounds. In the Middle East, pronounced zinc deficiency in man has resulted in hypogonadism and dwarfism. In pregnant animals, experimental zinc deficiency has resulted in malformation and behavioral disturbances in offspring. Toxicity — Ingestion of excess soluble salts may cause nausea, vomiting, and purging.	Beef, liver, oysters, spices, and wheat bran.	The biological availability of zinc in different foods varies widely; meats and seafoods are much better sources of available zinc than vegetables. Zinc availability is adversely affected by phytates (found in whole grains and beans), high calcium, oxalates (in rhubarb and spinach), high fiber, copper (from drinking water conveyed in copper piping), and EDTA (an additive used in certain canned foods).

Adapted from Ensminger et al., *Foods and Nutrition Encyclopedia*, 2nd ed., CRC Press, Boca Raton, FL, 1994, pp. 1511–1521.

Appendix E
Sweetening Agents, Sugar Substitutes

Name	Sweetness[a]	Classification	Uses	Comments
Acesulfame-K (sold under brand Sunette)	130	Nonnutritive; artificial.	As a tabletop sweetener, chewing gum, dry beverage mixes, and puddings.	This is actually the potassium salt of the 6-methyl derivative of a group of chemicals called oxathiazinone dioxides. Approved by the FDA in 1988.
Aspartame	180	Nutritive; artificial.	It is in most diet sodas. Also used in cold cereals, drink mixes, gelatin, puddings, toppings, dairy products, and at the table by the consumer; not used in cooking due to lack of stability when heated.	Composed of the two naturally occurring amino acids, aspartic acid and phenylalanine; sweeter than sugar, therefore less required, hence fewer calories.
Cyclamate	30	Nonnutritive; artificial.	Used as a tabletop sweetener and in drugs in Canada and 40 other countries.	Discovered in 1937. FDA banned all cyclamate-containing beverages in 1969 and all cyclamate-containing foods in 1970. Cyclamate safety is now being re-evaluated by the FDA.
Dulcin (4-ethoxy-phenyl-urea)	250	Nonnutritive; artificial.	None.	Not approved for food use in the U.S.; used in some European countries. Also called Sucrol and Valzin.
Fructose (levulose)	1.7	Nutritive; natural.	Beverages, baking, canned goods; anywhere invert sugar or honey may be used.	A carbohydrate; a monosaccharide; naturally occurs in fruits; makes up about 50% of the sugar in honey; commercially found in high-fructose syrups and invert sugars; contributes sweetness and prevents crystallization.
Glucose (dextrose)	0.7	Nutritive; natural.	Primarily in the confection, wine, and canning industries; and in intravenous solutions.	Glucose acts synergistically with other sweeteners.

(continues)

Name	Sweetness[a]	Classification	Uses	Comments
Glycine	0.8	Nutritive; natural.	Permissible to use to modify taste of some foods.	A sweet-tasting amino acid. Tryptophan is also a sweet-tasting amino acid.
Mannitol	0.7	Nutritive; natural.	Candies, chewing gums, confections, and baked goods; dietetic foods.	A sugar alcohol or polyhydric alcohol (polyol); occurs naturally in pineapples, olives, asparagus, and carrots; commercially prepared by the hydrogenation of mannose or glucose; slowly and incompletely absorbed from the intestines; only slightly metabolized, most excreted unchanged in the urine; may cause diarrhea.
Miraculin	—	Nutritive; natural.	None.	Actually a taste-modifying protein rather than a sweetener; after exposing tongue to miraculin, sour lemon tastes like sweetened lemon; responsible for the taste changing properties of mircale fruit, red berries of *Synsepalum dulcificum*, a native plant of West Africa; first described in 1852; one attempt made to commercialize by a U.S. firm but FDA denied approval and marketing was stopped.
Monellin	3,000	Nutritive; natural.	None; only a potential low-calorie sweetener.	Extract of the pulp of the light red berries of the tropical plant *Dioscoreophyllum cumminsii*; also called Serendipity Berry; first protein found to elicit a sweet taste in man; first extracted in 1969; potential use limited by lack of stability; taste sensation is slow and lingering; everything tastes sweet after monellin.

Name	Sweetness[a]	Classification	Uses	Comments
Neohesperidin dihydrochalone (Neo DHC, NDHC)	1,250	Nonnutritive; artificial.	None approved; potential for chewing gum, mouthwash, and toothpaste.	Formed from naringen isolated from citrus fruit; slow to elicit the taste sensation; lingering licoricelike aftertaste; animal studies indicate not toxic.
P-4,000 (5-nitro-2-propoxy-aniline)	4,100	Nonnutritive; artificial.	None approved.	Derivative of nitroaniline; used as a sweetener in some European countries but banned in the U.S. due to toxic effects on rats; no bitter aftertaste; major drawback of P-4000 is powerful local anesthetic effect on the tongue and mouth. Used in the Netherlands during German occupation and during Berlin blockade.
Phyllodulcin	250	Natural.	None approved.	Isolated from *Hydrangea macrophylla* Seringe in 1916; displays a lagging onset of sweetness with licorice aftertaste; not well studied; possible market for hard candies, chewing gums, and oral hygiene products.
Saccharin (*O*-benzo-sulfimide)	500	Nonnutritive; artificial.	Used in beverages, as a tabletop sweetener, and in cosmetics, toothpaste, and cough syrup. Used as a sweetener by diabetics.	Both sodium and calcium salts of saccharin used; passes through body unchanged; excreted in urine; originally a generally recognized as safe (GRAS) additive. Subsequently, saccharin was classed as a carcinogen based on experiments with rats. However, recent experiments indicate that saccharin causes cancer in rats, but not in mice and people.

(continues)

Name	Sweetness[a]	Classification	Uses	Comments
Sorbitol	0.6	Nutritive; natural.	Chewing gum, dairy products, meat products, icing, toppings, and beverages.	A sugar alcohol or polyhydric alcohol (polyol); occurs naturally in many fruits commercially prepared by the hydrogenation of glucose; many unique properties besides sweetness; on the FDA list of generally recognized as safe (GRAS) food additives; the most widely used sugar alcohol; slow intestinal absorption; consumption of large amounts may cause diarrhea.
SRI Oxime V (Perilla sugar)	450	Nonnutritive; artificial.	None approved.	Derived from extract of *Perilla namkinensis*; clean taste; needs research; used as sweetening agent in Japan.
Stevioside	300	Nutritive; natural.	None approved.	Isolated from the leaves of the wild shrub, *Stevia rebaudiana* Bertoni; used by the people of Paraguay to sweeten drinks; limited evidence suggests nontoxic to humans. Rebaudioside A is isolated from the same plant, and it is said to taste superior to stevioside. Its chemical structure is very similar to stevioside, and it is 190 times sweeter than sugar.
Sucrose (brown sugar, liquid sugar, sugar, table sugar, white sugar) (Also see SUGAR.)	1.0	Nutritive; natural.	Many beverages and processed foods; home use in a wide variety of foods.	The chemical combination of the sugars fructose and glucose; one of the oldest sweetening agents; most popular and most available sweetening agent; occurs naturally in many fruits; commercially extracted from sugarcane and sugar beets.
Thaumatins	1,600	Nutritive; natural	None.	Source of sweetness of the tropical fruit from the plant *Thaumatococcus daniellii*; enjoyed by inhabitants of western Africa; doubtful commercial applications.

Name	Sweetness[a]	Classification	Uses	Comments
Xylitol (Also see XYLITOL.)	0.8	Nutritive; natural	Chewing gums and dietetic foods.	A sugar alcohol or polyhydric alcohol (polyol); occurs naturally in some fruits and vegetables; produced in the body; commercial production from plant parts (oat hulls, corncobs, and birch wood chips) containing xylans — long chains of the sugar xylose; possible diarrhea; one British study suggests xylitol causes cancer in animals.

[a] Sweetness relative to sucrose.
Adapted from Ensminger et al., *Foods and Nutrition Encyclopedia*, 2nd ed., CRC Press, Boca Raton, FL, 1994, pp. 2082–2087.

Appendix F
Normal Clinical Values for Blood

TABLE 32

Normal Clinical Values for Blood

	Common Units or SI Units
Ammonia	22–39 μmol/l
Calcium	8.5–10.5 mg/dl or 2.25–2.65 mmol/l
Carbon dioxide	24–30 meq/l or 24–29 mmol/l
Chloride	100–106 meq/l or mmol/l
Copper	100–200 μg/dl or 16–31 μmol/l
Iron	50–150 μg/dl or 11.6–31.3 μmol/l
Lead	50 μg/dl or less
Magnesium	1.5–2.0 meq/l or 0.75–1.25 mmol/l
P CO_2	35–40 mmHg
pH	7.35–7.45
Phosphorus	3.0–4.5 mg/dl or 1–1.5 mmol/l
PO_2	75–100 mmHg
Potassium	3.5–5.0 meq/l or 2.5–5.0 mmol/l
Sodium	135–145 meq/l or 135–145 mmol/l
Acetoacetate	<2 mmol
Ascorbic acid	0.4–15 mg/dl or 23–85 μmol/l
Bilirubin	0.4–0.6 mg/dl or 1.71–6.84 μmol/l
Carotinoids	0.8–4.0 mg/ml
Creatinine	0.6–1.5 mg/dl or 60–130 μmol/l
Lactic acid	0.6–1.8 meq/l or 0.44–1.28 mmol/l
Cholesterol	120–220 mg/dl or 3.9–7.3 mmol/l
Triglycerides	40–150 mg/dl or 6–18 mmol/l
Pyruvic acid	0–0.11 meq/l or 79.8–228.0 μmol/l
Urea nitrogen	8–25 mg/dl or 2.86–7.14 mmol/l
Uric acid	3.0–7.0 mg/dl or 0.18–0.29 mmol/l
Vitamin A	0.15–0.6 μg/dl
Albumin	3.5–5.0 g/dl
Insulin	6–20 μU/dl
Glucose	70–100 mg/dl or 4–6 mmol/l

Appendix G
Some Common Medicinal Plants

Common and Scientific Name	Description	Production	Part(s) of Plant Used	Reported Uses
Agrimony *Agrimonia gryposepala*	Small yellow flowers on a long spike; leaves hairy and at least 5 in. (13 cm) long, narrow and pointed; leaf edges toothed; a perennial.	Needs good soil and sunshine; grows in New England and Middle Atlantic states.	Whole plant including roots.	A tonic, alterative, diuretic, and astringent; infusions from the leaves for sore throats; treatment of kidney and bladder stones; root for jaundice.
Aletris root (whitetube stargrass) *Aletris farinosa*	Grasslike leaves in a flat rosette around a spike-like stem; white to yellow tubular flowers along stem.	Moist locations in woods, meadows, or bogs; New England to Michigan and Wisconsin; south to Florida and west to Texas.	Leaves; roots.	Poultice of leaves for sore breast; liquid from boiled roots for stomach pains, tonic, sedative, and diuretic.
Alfalfa *Medicago sativa*	Very leafy plant growing 1–2 ft (30–61 cm) high; small green leaves; bluish-purple flowers; deep roots.	A legume cultivated widely in the U.S.	Leaves.	Powdered and mixed with cider vinegar as a tonic; infusions for a tasty drink; leaves may also be used green.
Aloe vera *Aloe barbadensis*	A succulent plant with leathery sword-shaped leaves, 6–24 in. (15–61 cm) long.	A semidesert plant which grows in Mexico and Hawaii; temperature must remain above 50°F (10°C); can be a house plant.	Mucilaginous juice of the leaves.	Effective on small cuts and sunburn; speeds healing; manufactured product for variety of cosmetic purposes.
Angelica *Angelica atropurpurea*	Shrub growing to 8 ft (2.4 m) high; stem purplish with 3 toothed leaflets at tip of each leaf stem; white or greenish flowers in clusters at end of each stalk.	Grows in rich low soil near streams and swamps and in gardens; from New England west to Ohio, Indiana, Illinois, and Wisconsin; south to Delaware, Maryland, West Virginia, and Kentucky.	Roots; seeds.	Small amount of dried root or seeds for relief of flatulence; roots for the induction of vomiting and perspiration; roots for treatment of toothache, bronchitis, rheumatism, gout, fever, and to increase menstrual flow.

(continues)

543

Common and Scientific Name	Description	Production	Part(s) of Plant Used	Reported Uses
Anise (Anise seed) *Pimpinella anisum*	Annual plant, 1–2 ft (30–61 cm) high; belongs to carrot family; small white flowers on long hairy stalk; lower leaves egg-shaped; upper leaves feathery.	Grown all over the world; grows wild in countries around the Mediterranean; much is imported to U.S.	Seed.	As a hot tea to relieve flatulence or for colic.
Asafetida *Ferula* sp.	A coarse plant growing to 7 ft (2.1 m) high with numerous stem leaves; pale green-yellow flowers; flowers and seeds borne in clusters on stalks; large fleshly root; tenacious odor.	Indigenous to Afghanistan, but some species grow in other Asiatic countries.	Gummy resin from the root.	As an antispasmodic; to ward off colds and flu by wearing in a bag around the neck.
Bayberry (Southern wax myrtle) *Myrica cerifera*	Perennial shrub growing to 30 ft (9.2 m) high; waxy branchlets; narrow evergreen leaves tapering at both ends; yellowish flowers; fruits are grayish berries.	Grows in coastal regions from New Jersey, Delaware and Maryland to Florida, Alabama, Mississippi, and Arkansas.	Root bark; leaves and stems.	Decoction of root bark to treat uterine hemorrhage, jaundice, dysentery, and cankers; leaves and stems boiled and used to treat fevers; decoction of boiled leaves for intestinal worms.
Bearberry *Arctostaphylos uva-ursi*	Creeping evergreen shrub with stems up to 6 in. (15 cm) high; reddish bark; bright green leaves, 1 in. (3 cm) long; white flowers with red markings, in clusters; smooth red fruits.	Grows in well-drained soils at higher altitudes; from Oregon, Washington, and California, to Colorado and New Mexico.	Leaves.	As a diuretic; also boiled infusions used as a drink to treat sprains, stomach pains, and urinary problems; poison oak inflammations treated with leaf decoction by pioneers.

Common and Scientific Name	Description	Production	Part(s) of Plant Used	Reported Uses
Black cohosh *Cimicifuga racemosa*	Perennial shrub growing to 9 ft (2.7 m) or more in height; leaf has 2 to 5 leaflets; plant topped with spike of slender candlelike, white or yellowish flowers; rhizome gnarled and twisted.	Grows throughout eastern U.S.; commercial supply from Blue Ridge Mountains.	Rhizomes and roots.	Infusion and decoctions used to treat sore throat, rheumatism, kidney trouble, and general malaise; also used for "women's ailments" and malaria.
Black walnut *Juglans nigra*	A tree growing up to 120 ft (36.6 m) high; leaflets alternate 12 to 23 per stem, finely toothed and about 3–3.5 in. (8–9 cm) long; nut occurs singly or in clusters with fleshy, aromatic husk.	Native to a large section of the rich woods of eastern and midwestern U.S.	Bark; nut husk; leaves.	Inner bark used as mild laxative; husk of nut used for treating intestinal worms, ulcers, syphilis, and fungus infections; leaf infusion for bedbugs.
Blackberry (brambleberry, dewberry, raspberry) *Rubus*	Shrubby or viny thorny perennial; numerous species; large white flowers; red or black fruit.	Grows wild or in gardens throughout the U.S.; wild in old fields, waste areas, forest borders, and pastures.	Roots; root bark, leaves; fruit.	Infusion made from roots used to dry up runny noses; infusion from root bark to treat dysentery; fruit used to treat dysentery in children; leaves also used in similar manner.
Blessed thistle *Cnicus benedictus*	Annual plant growing to 2 ft (61 cm) high; spiny tooth, lobed leaves; many-flowered yellow heads.	Grows along roadsides and in waste places in eastern and parts of southwestern U.S.	Leaves and flowering tops in full bloom; seeds.	Infusions from leaves and tops for cancer treatment, to induce sweating, as a diuretic, to reduce fever, and for inflammations of the respiratory system; infusion of tops as Indian contraceptive; seeds induce vomiting.

(continues)

Common and Scientific Name	Description	Production	Part(s) of Plant Used	Reported Uses
Boneset; *Eupatorium perfoliatum*	Perennial bush growing to 5 ft (1.5 m) in height; heavy stems with leaves opposite; purplish to white flowers borne in flat heads.	Commonly found in wet areas such as swamps, rich woods, marshes, and pastures; grows from Canada to Florida and west to Texas and Nebraska.	Leaves; flowering tops.	Infusions made from leaves used for laxative and treatment of coughs and chest illnesses — a cold remedy; Negro slaves and Indians used it to treat malaria.
Borage *Borago officinalis*	Entire plant not over 1 ft (30 cm) high; nodding heads of starlike flowers grow from clusters of hairy obovate leaves.	Introduced in U.S. from Europe; occasionally grows in waste areas in northern states; cultivated widely in gardens.	Leaves.	Most often used as an infusion to increase sweating, as a diuretic, or to soothe intestinal tract; can be applied to swellings and inflamed areas for relief.
Buchu *Rutaceae*	Low shrubs with angular branches and small leaves growing in opposition; flowers from white to pink.	Grown in rich soil in warm climate of South Africa.	Dried leaves.	Prepared as tincture or infusion; used for genitourinary diseases, indigestion, edema, and early stages of diabetes.
Buckthorn *Rhamnus purshiana*	Deciduous tree growing to 25 ft (7.6 m) high; leaves 2–6 in. (5–15 cm) long; flowers small greenish yellow; fruit globular and black, about 1/4 in. (6 mm) across.	Grows usually with conifers along canyon walls, rich bottom lands, and mountain ridges in western U.S.	Bark; fruit.	Bark used as a laxative and tonic; fruit (berries) used as a laxative.
Burdock *Arctium minus*	Biennial or perennial growing 5–8 ft (1.5–2.4 m) high; large leaves resembling rhubarb; tube-shaped white and pink to purple flowers in heads; brown bristled burrs contain seeds.	Grows in wastelands, fields, and pastures throughout the U.S.	Root.	Infusion of roots for coughs, asthma, and to stimulate menstruation; tincture of root for rheumatism and stomachache.

Common and Scientific Name	Description	Production	Part(s) of Plant Used	Reported Uses
Calamus (Sweet flag) *Acorus calamus*	Perennial growing 3–5 ft (1.0–1.5 m) high; long narrow leaves with sharp edges; aromatic leaves; flower stalk 2–3 in. (3–8 cm) long and clublike; greenish-yellow flowers.	Grows in swamps, edges of streams and ponds from New England west to Oregon and Montana, and from Texas east to Florida and north.	Rhizomes.	Root chewed to clear phlegm (mucous) and ease stomach gas; infusions to treat stomach distress; considered useful as tonic and stimulant.
Catnip *Nepeta cataria*	Perennial growing to 3 ft (1 m) in height; stem downy and whitish; leaves heart-shaped, opposite, coarsely toothed and 2–3 in. (3–8 cm) long; tubular, whitish with purplish marked flowers in compact spikes.	Grows wild along fences, roadsides, waste places, and streams in Virginia, Tennessee, West Virginia, Georgia, New England, Illinois, Indiana, Ohio, New Mexico, Colorado, Arizona, Utah, and California; readily cultivated in gardens.	Entire plant.	Infusions for treating colds, nervous disorders, stomach ailments, infant colic, and hives; smoke relieves respiratory ailments; poultice to reduce swellings.
Celery *Apium graveolens*	A biennial producing flower stalk second year; terminal leaflet at end of stem; fruit brown and round.	Cultivated in California, Florida, Michigan, New York, and Washington.	Seeds.	As an infusion to relieve rheumatism and flatulence (gas); to act as a diuretic; to act as a tonic and stimulant; oil from seeds used similarly.
Chamomile *Anthemis nobilis*	Low-growing, pleasantly strong-scented, downy, and matlike perennial; daisylike flowers with white petals and yellow center.	Cultivated in gardens; some wild growing which escaped from gardens.	Leaves and flowers.	Powdered and mixed with boiling water to stimulate stomach, to remedy nervousness in women, and stimulate menstrual flow, also a tonic; flowers for poultice to relieve pain; Chamomile tea known as soothing, sedative, completely harmless.

(continues)

Common and Scientific Name	Description	Production	Part(s) of Plant Used	Reported Uses
Chaparral *Croton corynbulosus*	Shrubby perennial plant of the Spurge family.	Grows in dry rock areas from Texas west.	Flowering tips.	Infusions act as laxative; some claims as cancer treatment.
Chickweed *Stellaria media*	Annual growing 12–15 in. (30–38 cm) high; stems matted to somewhat upright; upper leaves vary but lower leaves ovate; white, small individual flowers.	Grows in shaded areas, meadows, wasteland, cultivated land, thickets, gardens, and damp woods in Virginia to South Carolina and Southeast.	Entire plant in full bloom.	Poultice made to treat sores, ulcers, infections, and hemorrhoids.
Chicory *Cichorium intybus*	Easily confused with its close relative the dandelion; in bloom bears blue or soft pink blooms not resembling dandelion.	Introduced from Europe, now common wild plant in U.S.; some grown in gardens.	Roots; leaves.	No great medicinal value; some mention of diuretic, laxative, and tonic use; mainly added to give coffee distinctive flavor.
Cinnamon *Cinnamomum zeylanicum*	An evergreen bush or tree growing to 30 ft (9 m) high.	A native plant of Sri Lanka, India, and Malaysia; tree kept pruned to a shrub; bark of lower branches peeled and dried.	Bark.	Treatment for flatulence, diarrhea, vomiting, and nausea.
Cleaver's herb (Catchweed bedstraw) *Galium aparine*	Annual plant; weak reclining bristled stem with hairy joints; leaves in whorls of 8; white flowers in broad, flat cluster; bristled fruit.	Grows in rich woods, thickets, seashores, waste areas, and shady areas from Canada to Florida and west to Texas.	Entire plant during flowering.	To increase urine formation; to stimulate appetite; to reduce fever; to remedy Vitamin C deficiency; also used to remove freckles.

Common and Scientific Name	Description	Production	Part(s) of Plant Used	Reported Uses
Cloves *Syzygium aromaticum*	Dried flower bud of a tropical tree which is a 30-ft (9 m) high red flowered evergreen.	Tree native to Molucca, but widely cultivated in tropics; flower bud picked before flower opens and dried.	Flower bud.	To promote salivation and gastric secretion; to relieve pain in stomach and intestines; applied externally to relieve rheumatism, lumbago, toothache, muscle cramps, and neuralgia; clove oil used, too; infusions with clove powder relieves nausea and vomiting.
Colt's foot (Canada wild ginger) *Asarum canadense*	Low-growing stemless perennial; heart-shaped leaves; flowers near root, brown and bell-shaped.	Found in moist woods from Maine to Georgia and west to Ohio.	Roots; leaves.	Infusion of root to relieve flatulence; powdered root to relieve flatulence, induce sweating, and to relieve aching head and eyes; leaves substitute for ginger.
Comfrey *Symphytum officinale*	A perennial which reaches about 2 ft (61 cm) in height; leaves are large and broad at base but lancelike at terminal; fine hair on leaves; tail-shaped head of white to purple flowers at terminal.	Prefers a moist environment; a European plant now naturalized in the U.S.	Roots; leaves.	Numerous uses including treatments for pneumonia, coughs, diarrhea, calcium deficiency, colds, sores, ulcers, arthritis, gallstones, tonsils, cuts and wounds, headaches, hemorrhoids, gout, burns, kidney stones, anemia, and tuberculosis; used as a poultice, infusion, powder, or in capsule form.

(continues)

Common and Scientific Name	Description	Production	Part(s) of Plant Used	Reported Uses
Dandelion *Taraxacum officinale*	Biennial growing 2–12 in. (5–30 cm) high; leaves deeply serrated forming a basal rosette in spring; yellow flower but turns to gray upon maturing.	Weed throughout the U.S.; the bane of lawns.	Flowers; roots; green leaves.	Root uses include diuretic, laxative, tonic, and to stimulate appetite; infusion from flower for heart troubles; paste of green leaves and bread dough for bruises.
Echinacea (Purple echinacea) *Echinacea purpurea*	Perennial from 2–5 ft (0.6–1.5 m) high; alternate lance-shaped leaves; leaf margins toothed; top leaves lack stems; purple to white flower.	Grows wild on road banks, prairies, and dry, open woods in Ohio to Iowa, south to Oklahoma, Georgia, and Alabama.	Roots.	Treatment of ulcers and boils, syphilis, snakebites, skin diseases, and blood poisoning; used as powder and in capsules.
Eucalyptus *Eucalyptus globulus*	Tall, fragrant tree growing up to 300 ft (92 m) high; reddish-brown stringy bark.	Native to Australia but grown in other semitropical and warm temperate regions.	Leaves and oil distilled from leaves.	Antiseptic value; inhaled freely for sore throat; asthma relief; local application to ulcers; used on open wounds.
Eyebright (Indian tobacco) *Lobelia inflata*	Branching annual growing to 3 ft (1 m) high with leaves 1–3 in. (3–8 cm) long; small violet to pinkish-white flowers in axils of leaves; seed capsules at base of flower containing many tiny brown seeds.	Roadside weed of eastern U.S, west to Kansas.	Entire plant in full bloom or when seeds are formed.	Treatment of whooping cough, asthma, epilepsy, pneumonia, hysteria, and convulsion; alkaloid extracted for use in antismoking preparations.
Fenugreek *Trigonella foenum-graceum*	Annual plant similar to clover in size.	Native to the Mediterranean regions and northern India; widely cultivated; easily grown in home gardens.	Seed.	Poultice for wounds; gargle for sore throat.
Flax (Linseed) *Linum usitatissimum*	Herbaceous annual; slender upright plant with narrow leaves and blue flowers; grows to about 2 ft (61 cm) high.	Originated in Mediterranean region; cultivated widely for fiber and oil.	Seed.	Ground flaxseed mixed with boiling water for poultice on burns, boils, carbuncles, and sores; internally as a laxative.

Common and Scientific Name	Description	Production	Part(s) of Plant Used	Reported Uses
Garlic *Allium sativum*	Annual plant growing to 12 in. (30 cm) high; long, linear, narrow leaves; bulb composed of several bulblets.	Throughout the U.S. under cultivation; some wild.	Entire plant when in bloom; bulbs.	Fresh poultice of the mashed plant for treating snake bite, hornet stings, and scorpion stings; eaten to expel worms, treat colds, coughs, hoarseness, and asthma; bulb expressed against the gum for toothache.
Gentian (Sampson snakeroot) *Gentiana villosa*	Perennial with stems growing 8–10 in. (20–25 cm) high; opposite ovate, lance-shaped leaves; pale blue flowers.	Grows wild in swampy areas Florida west to Louisiana, north to New Jersey, Pennsylvania, Ohio, and Indiana.	Rhizomes and roots.	Treatment of indigestion, gout, and rheumatism; induction of vomiting; aid to digestion; a tonic.
Ginger *Zingiber officinale*	Perennial plant; forms irregular-shaped rhizomes at shallow depth.	Native to southeastern Asia; now grown all over tropics.	Rhizome.	An expectorant; treatment of flatulence, colds, and sore throats.
Ginseng *Panax quinquefolia*	Hollow stems solid at nodes; leaves alternate; root often resembles shape of a man; small, inconspicuous flowers; vivid, shiny, scarlet berries.	Grows in eastern Asia, Korea, China, and Japan; some grown in United States.	Root.	As a tonic and stimulant; treatment of convulsions, dizziness, vomiting, colds, fevers, headaches, and rheumatism; commonly believed to be an aphrodisiac.
Goldenrod *Solidago odora*	Grows 18–36 in. (46–91 cm) high with narrow leaves scented like anise; inconspicuous head with 6 to 8 flowers.	Grows throughout the U.S..	Leaves.	Infusions from dried leaves as aromatic stimulant, a carminative, and a diuretic.

(continues)

Common and Scientific Name	Description	Production	Part(s) of Plant Used	Reported Uses
Goldenseal *Hydrastis canadensis*	Perennial growing to about 1 ft (30 cm) high; one stem with 5 to 7 lobed leaves near top; several single leafstalks topped with petalless flowers; raspberry-like fruit but inedible.	Grows in rich, shady woods of southeastern and midwestern U.S.; grown under cultivation in Washington.	Roots; leaves, and stalks.	Root infusion as an appetite stimulant and tonic; root powder for open cuts and wounds; chewing root for mouth sores; leaf infusion for liver and stomach ailments.
Guarana *Paullinia cupana*	Climbing shrub of the soapberry family; yellow flowers; pear-shaped fruit; seed in 3-sided, 3-celled capsules.	Grows in South America, particularly Brazil and Uruguay.	Seeds.	Stimulant; seeds high in caffeine.
Hawthorn *Crataegus oxycantha*	Hardy shrub or tree depending upon growth conditions; small, berry fruit; cup-shaped flowers with 5 parts; thorny stems.	Originally grown throughout England as hedges; also grows wild; some introduced in the U.S.	Berry.	Tonic for heart ailments such as angina pectoris, valve defects, rapid and feeble heart beat, and hypertrophied heart; reverses arteriosclerosis.
Hop *Humulus lupulus*	Twining, perennial growing 20 ft (6 m) or more; 3 smooth-lobed leaves 4–5 in. (10–13 cm) long; membranous, conelike fruit.	Grows throughout the U.S.; often a cultivated crop.	Fruit (hops).	Straight hops or powder used; hot poultice of hops for boils and inflammations; treatment of fever, worms, and rheumatism; as a diuretic; as a sedative.
Horehound (White horehound) *Marrubium vulgare*	Shrub growing to 3 ft (1 m) in height; fuzzy ovate-round leaves which are whitish above and gray below; foliage aromatic when crushed.	Grows wild throughout most of U.S. in pastures, old fields, and waste places, except in arid Southwest.	Leaves and small stems; bark.	Decoctions to treat coughs, colds, asthma, and hoarseness; other uses include treatment for diarrhea, menstrual irregularity, and kidney ailments.

Common and Scientific Name	Description	Production	Part(s) of Plant Used	Reported Uses
Huckleberry (Sparkleberry) *Vaccinium arboreum*	Shrub or tree growing to 25 ft (7.6 m) high; leathery; shiny, thick leaves; white flowers; black berries; other species.	Grows wild in woods, clearings, sandy and dry woods in Virginia, Georgia, Florida, Mississippi, Indiana, Illinois, Missouri, Texas, and Oklahoma.	Leaves, root bark, and berries.	Decoctions of leaves and root bark to treat sore throat and diarrhea; drink from berry for treating chronic dysentery.
Hyssop *Hyssopus officinalis*	Hardy, fragrant, bushy plants belonging to the mint family; stem woody; leaves hairy, pointed, and about 1/2 in. (20 mm) long; blue flowers in tufts.	Grows in various parts of Europe including the Middle East; some grown in U.S.	Leaves.	Infusions for colds, coughs, tuberculosis, and asthma; an aromatic stimulant; healing agent for cuts and bruises.
Juniper (Common juniper) *Juniperus communis*	Small evergreen shrub growing 12–30 ft (3.7–9.2 m) high; bark of trunk reddish-brown and tends to shred; needles straight and at right angles to branchlets; dark, purple, fleshy berrylike fruit.	Widely distributed from New Mexico to Dakotas and east; dry areas.	Fruit (berries).	Used as a diuretic, to induce menstruation, to relieve gas, and to treat snake bites and intestinal worms.
Lemon balm *Melissa officinalis*	Persistent perennial growing to 1 ft (30 cm) high; light green, serrated leaves; lemon smell and taste to crushed leaves.	Wild in much of the U.S.; grown in gardens.	Leaves.	Infusion used as a carminative, diaphoretic, or febrifuge.
Licorice (Wild licorice) *Glycyrrhiza lepidota*	Erect perennial growing to 3 ft (1 m) high; pale yellow to white flowers at end of flower stalks; brown seed pods resemble cockleburs.	Grows wild on prairies, lake shores, and railroad right-of-ways throughout much of the U.S.	Root. **Caution:** Licorice raises the blood pressure of some people dangerously high, due to the retention of sodium.	Root extract to help bring out phlegm (mucus); treatment of stomach ulcers, rheumatism, and arthritis; root decoctions for inducing menstrual flow, treating fevers, and expulsion of afterbirth.

(continues)

Common and Scientific Name	Description	Production	Part(s) of Plant Used	Reported Uses
Marshmallow *Althaea officinalis*	Stems erect and 3–4 ft (0.9–1.2 m) high with only a few lateral branches; roundish, ovate-cordate leaves 2–3 in. (5–8 cm) long and irregularly toothed at margin; cup-shaped, pale-colored flowers.	Introduced into U.S. from Europe; now found on banks of tidal rivers and brackish streams; grew wild in salt marshes, damp meadows, by ditches, by the sea, and banks of tidal rivers from Denmark south.	Root.	Primarily a demulcent and emollient; used in cough remedies; good poultice made from crushed roots.
Motherwort *Leonurus cardiaca*	Perennial growing 5–6 ft (1.5–1.8 m) high; lobed, dented leaves, 5 in. (13 cm) long; very fuzzy white to pink flowers.	Grows wild in pastures, waste places, and road-sides from northeastern states west to Montana and Texas, south to North Carolina and Tennessee.	Entire plant above ground.	Used as a stimulant, tonic, and diuretic; Europeans used for asthma and heart palpitation; usually taken as an infusion.
Mullein (Aaron's rod) *Verbascum thapsus*	At base, a rosette of woody, lance-shaped, oblong leaves with a diameter of up to 2 ft (61 cm); yellow flowers along a clublike spike arising from the rosette to a height of up to 7 ft (2.1 m).	Grows wild throughout the U.S. in dry fields, meadows, pastures, rocky or gravelly banks, burned areas, etc.	Leaves; roots; flowers.	Infusions of leaves to treat colds and dysentery; dried leaves and flowers serve as a demulcent and emollient; leaves smoked for asthma relief; boiled roots for croup; oil from flowers for earache; local applications of leaves for hemorrhoids, inflammations, and sunburn.
Nutmeg *Muristica fragrans*	Evergreen tree growing to about 25 ft (7.6 m) high; grayish-brown, smooth bark; fruit resembles yellow plum, the seed of which is known as nutmeg.	Native to Spice Islands of Indonesia; now cultivated in other tropical areas.	Seed.	For the treatment of nausea and vomiting; grated and mixed with lard for hemorrhoid ointment.

Common and Scientific Name	Description	Production	Part(s) of Plant Used	Reported Uses
Papaya *Carica papaya*	Small tree seldom above 20 ft (6.1 m) high; soft, spongy wood; leaves as large as 2 ft (61 cm) in diameter and deeply cut into 7 lobes; fruit oblong and dingy green-yellow.	Originated in South American tropics; now cultivated in tropical climates.	Leaves.	Dressing for wounds, and aid for digestion; contains proteolytic enzyme, papain, used as a meat tenderizer.
Parsley *Petroselinum crispum*	Biennial which is usually grown as an annual; finely divided, often curled, fragrant leaves.	Originated in the Mediterranean area; now grown worldwide.	Leaves; seeds; roots.	As diuretic with aromatic and stimulating properties.
Passion flower (Maypop passion-flower) *Passiflora incarnata*	Perennial vine growing to 30 ft (9.2 m) in length; alternate leaves composed of 3 to 5 finely toothed lobes; showy, vivid, purple, flesh-colored flowers; smooth, yellow ovate fruit 2–3 in. (5–8 cm) long.	Grows wild in West Indies and southern U.S.; cultivated in many areas.	Flowering and fruiting tops.	Crushed parts for poultice to treat bruises and injuries; other uses include treatment of nervousness, insomnia, fevers, and asthma.
Peppermint *Mentha piperita*	Perennial growing to about 3.5 ft (1 m) high; dark, green, toothed leaves; purplish flowers in spike-like groups.	Originated in temperate regions of the Old World where most is still grown; grows in shady damp areas in many areas of the U.S.; grown in gardens.	Flowering tops; leaves.	Infusions for relief of flatulence, nausea, headache, and heartburn; fresh leaves rubbed into skin to relieve local pain; extracted oil contains medicinal properties.
Plantain *Plantago* sp.	Low perennial with broad leaves; flowers on erect spikes.	Grows wild throughout the U.S. in poor soils, fields, lawns, and edges of woods.	Leaves; seeds; root.	Infusion of leaves for a tonic; seeds for laxative; soaking seeds provides sticky gum for lotions; fresh, crushed leaves to reduce swelling of bruised body parts; fresh, boiled roots applied to sore nipples.

(continues)

Common and Scientific Name	Description	Production	Part(s) of Plant Used	Reported Uses
Pleurisy root (Butterfly milkweed) *Asclepias tuberosa*	Leafy perennial growing to 3 ft (1 m) high; alternate leaves which are 2 to 6 in. (5–15 cm) long and narrow; bright orange flowers in a cluster; root spindle-shaped with knotty crown.	Grows in sandy, dry soils; pastures, roadsides, and gardens; south to Florida and west to Texas and Arizona.	Root.	Small doses of dried root as a diaphoretic, diuretic, expectorant, and alterative; ground roots fresh or dried for poultice to treat sores.
Queensdelight *Stillingia sylvatica*	Perennial growing to 3 ft (1 m) high; contains milky juice; leathery, fleshy, stemless leaves; yellow flowers.	Grows wild in dry woods, sandy soils, and old fields; Virginia to Florida, Kansas, and Texas, north to Oklahoma.	Root.	Treatment of infectious diseases; as an alterative.
Red clover *Trifolium pratense*	Biennial or perennial legume less than 2 ft (61 cm) high; 3 oval-shaped leaflets form leaf; flowers globe-shaped and rose to purple colored.	Throughout U.S.; some wild, some cultivated.	Entire plant in full bloom.	Infusions to treat whooping cough; component of salves for sores and ulcers; flowers as sedative; to relieve gastric distress and improve the appetite.
Rosemary *Rosmarinus officinalis*	Low-growing perennial evergreen shrub; leaves about 1 in. (3 cm) in height; orange-yellow flowers; white, shiny seeds.	Native to Mediterranean region; now cultivated in most of Europe and the Americas.	Leaves.	Used as a tonic, astringent, diaphoretic, stimulant, carminative, and nervine.
Saffron (Safflower) *Carthamus tinctorius*	Annual with alternate spring leaves; grows to 3 ft (1 m) in height; orange-yellow flowers; white, shiny seeds.	Wild in Afghanistan; cultivated in the U.S., primarily in California.	Flowers; seeds; entire plant in bloom.	Paste of flowers and water applied to boils; flowers soaked in water to make a drink to reduce fever, as a laxative, to induce perspiration, to stimulate menstrual flow, and to dry up skin symptoms of measles.

Common and Scientific Name	Description	Production	Part(s) of Plant Used	Reported Uses
Sage (Garden sage) *Salvia officinalis*	Fuzzy perennial belonging to the mint family; leaves with toothed edges; terminal spikes bearing blue or white flowers in whorls.	Originated in the Mediterranean area where it grows wild and is cultivated; grown throughout the United States, some wild.	Leaves.	Treatment for wounds and cuts, sores, coughs, colds, and sore throat; infusions used as a laxative and to relieve flatulence; major use for treatment of dyspepsia.
Sarsaparilla *Smilax* sp.	Climbing evergreen shrub with prickly stems; leaves round to oblong; small, globular berry for fruit.	Grown in tropical areas of Central and South America and in Japan and China.	Root.	Primarily an alterative regarded as an aphrodisiac; for colds and fevers; to relieve flatulence; best used as an infusion.
Sassafras *Sassafras album*	Tree growing to 40 ft (12.2 m) high; leaves may be 3-lobed, 2-lobed, mitten-shaped, or unlobed; yellowish-green flowers in clusters; pea-sized, 1-seeded berries in fall.	Originated in New World; grows in New England, New York, Ohio, Illinois, and Michigan, south to Florida and Texas; grows along roadsides, in woods, along fences, and in fields.	Root bark.	Sassafras was formerly used for medical purposes, but the use of the roots was banned by the FDA because of their carcinogenic qualities.
Saw palmetto *Serenoa serrulata*	Low-growing fan palm; whitish bloom covers sawtoothed, green leaves; flowers in branching clusters; fruit varies in size and shape.	Grows in warm, swampy, low areas near the coast.	Fruit (berries).	To improve digestion; to treat respiratory infections; as a tonic and as a sedative.
Senna (Wild senna) *Cassia marilandica*	Perennial growing to 6 ft (1.8 m) in height; alternate leaves with leaflets in pairs of 5 to 10; bright yellow flowers.	Grows along roadsides and in thickets from Pennsylvania to Kansas and Iowa, south to Texas and Florida.	Leaves.	Infusions primarily employed as a laxative.
Skullcap *Scutellaria lateriflora*	Perennial growing 1–2 ft (30–61 cm) high; toothed, lance-shaped leaves; blue or whitish flowers.	Native to most sections of the U.S.; prefers moist woods, damp areas, meadows, and swampy areas.	Entire plant in bloom.	Powdered plant primarily a nervine.

(continues)

Common and Scientific Name	Description	Production	Part(s) of Plant Used	Reported Uses
Spearmint *Mentha spicata*	Perennial resembling other mints; grows to 3 ft (1 m) in height; pink or white flowers borne in long spikes.	Throughout the U.S. in damp places; cultivated in Michigan, Indiana, and California.	Above-ground parts.	Primarily a carminative; administered as an infusion through extracted oils.
Tansy *Tanacetum vulgare*	Perennial growing to 3 ft (1 mg) in height; pungent fernlike foliage with tops of composite heads of buttonlike flowers.	Grown or escaped into the wild in much of the U.S.	Leaves and flowering tops.	Infusions used as stomachic, emmenagogue, or to expel intestinal worms; extracted oil induced abortion often with fat results; poultice for sprains and bruises.
Valerian *Valeriana officinalis*	Coarse perennial growing to 5 ft (1.5 m) high; fragrant, pinkish-white flowers opposite pinnate leaves.	Native to Europe and Northern Asia; cultivated in the U.S.	Root.	As a calmative and as a carminative.
Witch hazel *Hamamelis virginiana*	Crooked tree or shrub 8–15 ft (2.4–4.6 m) in height; roundish to oval leaves; yellow, threadlike flowers; fruits in clusters along the stem eject shiny, black seeds.	Found in damp woods of North America from Nova Scotia to Florida and west to Minnesota and Texas.	Leaves, bark, and twigs.	Twigs, leaves, and bark basis for witch hazel extract which is included in many lotions for bruises, sprains, and shaving; bark sometimes applied to tumors and skin inflammations; some preparations for treating hemorrhoids.
Yerba santa *Eriodictyon californicum*	Evergreen shrub with lance-shaped leaves.	Part of flora of the west coast of the U.S.	Leaves.	As an expectorant; recommended for asthma and hay fever.

From Ensminger et al., *Foods and Nutrition Encyclopedia*, 2nd ed., CRC Press, Boca Raton, FL, 1994, pp. 1432–1441.

Index

A

Abetalipoproteinemia, 120, 177
Absorption, *See* Digestion and absorption; specific nutrients
Accutane, 167
ACE inhibitors, 419
Acesulfame-K, 85, 462, 535
Acetaldehyde, 315, 316
Acetate, alcohol metabolite, 315, 316
Acetic acid, 95, 100, 220, 505
Acetoacetate, 142, 312, 541
Acetyl CoA, 16, 17, 223, 301, 304–305, 316, 318
  alcohol metabolism and, 462
  cholesterol synthesis and, 114
  fatty acid metabolism and, 101—102, 309, 312, 353
  myocardial metabolism, 412, 413
  pantothenic acid and, 220
  terpenoid metabolism and, 448
Acetyl CoA carboxylase, 102
Acetylcholine, 23, 344
  choline precursor, 377
  enteric nervous system, 65
  gastrointestinal secretions and, 73, 75
Acid-base balance, protein function, 137
Acid detergent method, 90
Acid hydroxylases, lysosomal, 8
Acrodermatitis enteropathica, 257
Actin, 26, 45, 127, 136, 140, 344
Action potential, 23, 64, 230
Acyl carnitine, 309
Acyl carrier protein (ACP), 223
Acyl CoA, 309, 353, 414
Acyl CoA dehydrogenase, 309
Acylcarnitine, 370, 414
Adaptive thermogenesis, 288–289
Additives, *See* Food additives
Adenine, 10
Adenosine, 10
  caffeine and, 361, 362
Adenosine diphosphate, *See* ADP
Adenosine monophosphate, *See* AMP
Adenosine triphosphate, *See* ATP
Adequate intake (AI), 44
Adipic acid, 505
Adipocytes, 327–328, *See* Adipose tissue; Body fat
Adipose tissue, 321, 327–328, *See also* Body fat
  distribution of, 331–332
  glycogen content, 87
  hypertrophy and hyperplasia, 327–328, 333
  liposuction, 342
Adipsin, 327

ADP (adenosine diphosphate), 16, 81
Adrenocorticrotropic hormone (ACTH), 136
Aerating agents, 504
Age, and obesity, 337–338
Agglutination inhibitors, 380, *See* Anticoagulants
Aging, 499–500
  bone and, 500
  calcium absorption and, 228
Agriculture, 498
Agrimony, 543
Alanine, 126, 127, 140
  biosynthesis, 139
  fasting energy metabolism, 318
  gluconeogenic precursor, 307
  muscle metabolism, 355
Alanine amino transferase (ALT), 202
Alanine cycle, 350
Alanine transaminase, 385
Albumin, 45, 46, 135
  copper transport and, 266
  normal blood values, 541
Alcohol (ethanol)
  cancer and, 449
  cardiovascular health and, 430
  cellular detoxification sites, 7, 9
  diabetes and, 462
  folate absorption and, 207
  hypertension and, 430
  ketone body production, 310
  oxidation, 315–316
  pregnancy and, 402
  substrate for ATP formation, 16
Alcohol dehydrogenase, 315
Aldehyde oxidase, 280
Aldosterone, 33, 99, 155, 241
Aletris root, 543
Alfalfa, 543
Algal polysaccharides, 47
Alkalating agents, 438
Alkaloids, 439
Allergic reactions, 408–409
Allicin, 429
Allinase, 380
Allium compounds, 380, 440
Allylic sulfides, 447–448
Aloe vera, 543
Alpha (α)-helix, 127
Aluminum hydroxide, 232
Alzheimer's disease, 377
Amine oxidases, 266
Amino acids, 10, 123–127
  classification, 123

copper absorption and, 266
degradation, 140–142
energy metabolic pathways, 137
essential, 124, *See* Essential amino acids
exercise and, 354–355
fasting energy metabolism, 318, 319
fed state energy metabolism, 317
glucogenic, 137, 140, 307
intake requirements, 146–147
  infants, 407
  protein RDA and, 43
ketogenic, 137, 140, 310
Krebs cycle intermediates and, 141
limiting, 124, 133, 148
metabolism and function, 135–143
nickel and, 281
nitrogen disposal, 142, 147
precursors, 137
protein synthesis, 12
sequence and protein structure, 127–128
substrate for ATP formation, 16
supplements, possible harmful effects, 149
synthesis of, 139–140
transport and absorption, 131
vitamin B$_6$ and transamination, 202
vitamin C and, 185
Amino acid score, 134
Aminolevulinic acid, 202, 204
Aminopeptidases, 130
Aminopterin, 210
Aminotransferases, 138
Ammonia
  amino acid metabolism, 138
  normal blood values, 541
  urea cycle, 143
Ammonium alginate, 505
AMP (adenosine monophosphate), 16, 81, *See also*
    Cyclic AMP
Amygdalin, 383, 450
Amylase, 70, 73, 89, 91–92
Amylopectin, 47, 86
Amylose, 47, 86
Android obesity, 331–332
Androstenedione, 379
Anemia
  iron and, 250, 252
  vitamin B$_{12}$ and, 212, 216
  zinc toxicity, 259
Angelica, 543
Angina pectoris, 369
Angiotensin, 158, 418, 419
Angiotensin converting enzyme (ACE), 418, 419
Angiotensinogen, 327
Animal carbohydrates, 46–47, 86–87
Animal fat, 106
Animal models, 487
  flavonoids and mammary tumors, 446
  nutrient requirements determination, 486
  transgenic models, 493–494
Animal protein, 129, 45–46
Anise, 544

Annatoo, 505
Anthocyanins, 53, 55
Anthoxanthins, 55, 379
Anthropometry, 322, 324
Antibiotics, vitamin K and, 181
Antibodies, 137
  Western blotting, 490
Anticaking agents, 503
Anticoagulants, 88
Antidepressants, 388
Antidiuretic hormone (ADH), 33, 155–156, 158, 241,
    418
Antiemetic, 380–381
Antigens, 409
Antimetabolites, 438
Antimicrobial agents, 503
Antioxidants, 503
  carotenoids, 166, 429
  coenzyme Q10 (ubiquinone), 376
  copper and superoxide dismutase, 267–268
  gingko preparations, 382
  glutathione peroxidase, 270–272
  vitamin C, 182, 185, 444
  vitamin E, 176, 428
Aphrodisiac, 390
Apipex-P, 341
Apoferritin, 248
Apoprotein B-100, 120
Apoproteins, 117, 119, 120
Apoptosis, 447
Appetite, 55–57
Apricots, 54
Arabinogalactan, 505
Arabinose, 80, 90
Arachidic acid, 100
Arachidonic acid (AA), 104, 113–114
Arginase, 277
Arginine, 125, 139, 141
  supplementation, 369, 390
Arginosuccinate, 143
Arsenic, 282, 430
Ascorbate, 182–183, *See* Vitamin C
Ascorbic acid, 505, *See* Vitamin C
  normal blood values, 541
Asparagine, 126, 139, 141
Aspartame, 85, 462, 505, 535
Aspartate, 139, 141
Aspartate amino transferase (AST), 202
Aspartic acid, 126, 369–370, 391
Aspirin, 114
Astaxanthin, 54
Atherosclerosis, 411, 418, *See also* Heart disease
  dietary guideline, 425–429
Athletic performance-enhancing supplements, 360,
    See also Supplements and nutraceuticals
  arginine, 369
  aspartic acid, 369
  bicarbonate loading, 362
  caffeine, 361–362
  carbohydrate supercompensation, 360–361

carnitine, 370–371
chromium, 372–373
coenzyme Q10 (ubiquinone), 375–376
creatine, 374–375
DHEA, 379
glycerol, 382
glycogen loading, 360–361
ornithine, 384–385
pyruvate, 386
sports drinks, 363–364
vanadium, 388–389
Atomic absorption spectrophotometry, 484, 488
ATP (adenosine triphosphate), 15–16, 81, 233, 234, 283
  creatine phosphate and regeneration of, 374
  enteric nervous system, 65
  fed-state energy metabolism, 317
  Krebs cycle and, 16–19, 305
  magnesium interaction, 236
  mitochondria and, 9
  muscle and, 27, 343, 345, 355
  myocardial metabolism, 413
  protein synthesis and, 13, 15
Autoimmune disorders, 452
Autonomic nervous system, enteric nervous system, 65
Avidin, 217
Azodicarbonamide, 505

B

Bacterial fermentation products, 95
Bananas, as potassium source, 240
Basal metabolic rate (BMR), 286–287
  aging and, 500
Bayberry, 544
Bearberry, 544
Benedectin, 206
Benign prostate hyperplasia, 387
Benign tumors, 433
Benzoic acid, 505
Benzoyl peroxide, 505
Beriberi, 190, 429
Beta-apo-8' carotenal, 505
β-cells, 452
  genetic defect, 455
Betaine, 138, 377
β-pleated sheet, 127
BHA, 505, 505
Bicarbonate, 74, 241, 242
  saliva, 71
Bilabolide, 381
Bile acids (or bile), 74–76, 112
  blood cholesterol and, 122
  calcium absorption and, 228, 446
  cholesterol in, 76
  fiber and, 95–95, 97, 426
  lipid digestion and, 110, 111, 112
  precursor amino acids, 137
  saponin complexes, 386
  vitamin E component, 175
Bile-sequestering agents, 122

Bilirubin, 76
  normal blood values, 541
Bioelectrical impedance analysis (BIA), 322, 324–325
Biological value, 133–134
Biotin, 42, 46, 48, 216–218, 243, 359, 505, 519
  absorption, 217
  deficiency, 218, 519
  intestinal microflora and, 37
  metabolism and function, 217–218
  recommended intake, 218
Birth weight, 405
Bitot's spots, 167
Bixin, 54, 371
Blackberry, 545
Black cohosh, 545
Black walnut, 545
Bladder cancer, 448
Blessed thistle, 545
Blood, 29–30, *See* Erythrocytes
Blood circulation, 27–30
Blood pressure, 30–31, *See also* Hypertension
Blood sugar, 80
Body composition, 321–342, *See also* Body fat; Lean body mass; Obesity
  adipose tissue, 327–328, *See also* Adipose tissue
  assessment methods, 322–325
  elemental level, 321
  essential fat, 321
  futile cycle systems, 334
  mediators of energy homeostasis, 334–337
  pregnancy and, 399
  variations, 325–327
Body density, 323
Body fat, 99, *See also* Adipose tissue; Body composition; Obesity
  adipocytes, 327–328, *See also* Adipose tissue
  densitometry, 323
  distribution of, 331–332
  energy homeostasis, 333–334
  essential fat, 321
Body mass index (BMI), 331
Body weight, *See* Body composition; Obesity; Weight gain; Weight loss
  growth charts, 511–516
Bomb calorimeter, 483, 484
Bombesin, 56
Bone, 21–22, 469–480, *See also* Osteoporosis
  aging effects, 500
  calcitonin-salmon therapy, 478
  calcium and, 226, 229, 231, 478–479
  classification, 469
  density, 472
  disintegrins and, 478
  estrogen and, 474, 475
  exercise and, 476–477, 480
  fluoride and, 274, 479
  lactation and, 473
  magnesium content, 235, 236
  menopause and, 474
  peak bone mass, 472, 477
  pregnancy and, 472–473

silicon and, 282
  sodium content, 241
  structure and composition, 469–471
  turnover, 22, 471–472
  vitamin D and, 172, 479
  zinc and, 256, 479–480
Bone Gla protein (BGP), 181, 229
Bone loss, *See* Bone; Osteoporosis
Bone marrow, essential fat, 321
Bone marrow transplantation, 439
Bone morphogenetic proteins (BMPs), 328
Boneset, 546
Borage, 546
Boric acid, 279
Boron, 278–279, 370, 391
Bowman-Birk inhibitor (BBI)
Bowman's capsule
Brain, 23
  ketone bodies and, 310
  protein malnourishment and, 149
  riboflavin status, 193
Bran, 90, 97
Bread making, 46
Breast cancer
  alcohol and, 449
  bone marrow transplantation, 439
  caffeine and, 448–448
  dietary fat and, 442, 443
  dietary fiber and, 443
  estrogen and, 475, 476
    flavonoids and phytoestrogens, 447
  obesity and, 441
  protein intake and, 498
  risk factors, 439
  vitamin E and, 445
Breast milk, 45, 107, 403, 404, *See also* Lactation; Milk
  fatty acids composition, 404
  nutrient content variations, 404
  vitamin C content, 186
  vitamins and minerals, 407
  water composition, 157
Brown adipose tissue (BAT), 334
Brunner's glands, 74
Buchu, 546
Buckthorn, 546
Burdock, 546
Burning feet syndrome, 223
Butterworth, Charles, 484
Butylated hydroxyanisole (BHA), 505
Butylated hydroxytoluene (BHT), 505
Butyric acid, 95, 107
B vitamins, 182, *See* specific vitamins

C

Cabbage, 367
Cadmium, 249
Caffeic acid, 187
Caffeine, 361–362
  cancer and, 448–449
  pregnancy and, 403

Calamus, 547
Calbinden, 172, 228
Calcimar, 478
Calcitonin-salmon therapy, 478
Calcium, 49, 225, 226–231, 495, 527, 541
  absorption, 227–228
  bile acids and, 446
  blood levels, 228–229, 486
  blood pressure regulation, 419
  bone and, 226, 229, 231, 470, 478–479
    bone loss prevention and treatment, 478–479
    osteoporosis risk, 473
  cancer and, 446
  deficiency, 231, 527
  dietary sodium and excretion, 243
  heart disease and, 495
  hypertension and, 495
  intracellular and extracellular concentration, 22
  iron absorption and, 248
  lactation demand, 473
  muscle fiber activity and
  phosphorus absorption and, 232
  physiological role, 229
  pregnancy and, 402, 472, 495
  recommended intake, 42, 230–231
  sources, 226–227, 527
  supplements, 226–227
  toxicity, 231, 527
  vitamin D and, 172
Calcium acetate, 226–227
Calcium alginate, 505
Calcium-binding protein (CBP), 228, 230
Calcium carbonate, 226–227, 479, 505
Calcium citrate, 226–227
Calcium citrate malate, 227, 478, 479
Calcium/creatine urine level, 471
Calcium gluconate, 226–227, 479
Calcium ion channels, 26, 230
Calcium lactate, 226–227, 479, 505
Calcium oxalate, 186
Calcium phosphate, 229, 505
Calcium propionate, 505
Calcium silicate, 505
Calmodulin, 230
Caloric restriction, 339–340, 441
Calorimetry, 283–285
Calsequestrin, 230
Campesterol, 426
Cancer, 433–450, *See also* specific types
  chemoprevention, 440
  genetic alterations, 435–436
  inheritance, 436, 439
  mortality rate, 433
  nutrient/nutraceutical associations (preventive,
    ameliorative, or carcinogenic), 447
    alcohol, 449
    allylic sulfides (garlic and onions), 447–448
    caffeine (coffee), 448–449
    calcium, 446
    β-carotene, 445
    carotenoids, 371

coffee and caffeine, 448–449
DHEA, 377
dietary fat, 441–443
dietary fiber, 97, 443
dithiolthiones, 446
energy intake, 441
estrogen, 475, 476
flavonoids, 446–447
folate, 212
fruits and vegetables, 444
iron overload, 253
laetrile, 383
phytoestrogens, 385, 446–447
protein intake, 498
selenium, 445–446
soy products, 387
terpenoids, 448
vitamin C, 444–445
vitamin E, 445
nutritional concerns of conventional therapies, 450
risk factors, nonnutritive, 439–440
physical activity, 443
smoking, 440–441
stages, 436–437
treatment, 437–439
tumors, 433
unproven oral treatments, 449–450
Canola oil, 107
Canthaxanthin, 55, 162, 506
Capillaries, 29
Capsanthin, 54
Caramels, 53, 506
Carbamoyl phosphate, 143
Carbohydrate counting, 465
Carbohydrate supercompensation (glycogen loading), 360–361
Carbohydrates (and carbohydrate metabolism), 79–97
animal flesh, 47, 86–87
ATP formation substrate, 16
caffeine and, 362
complex and simple, 460–461
diabetes and, 460–461
dietary fiber, 88–91, 96
dietary guidelines for disease risk reduction, 426
dietary restriction, 460
digestion, 76, 91–94
disaccharides, 84–85
energy substrate utilization, 16
epimers, 81
exercise and, 349–352
food sources, 46–48, 80
Golgi apparatus and, 7
high-carbohydrate meals, 352
infant requirements, 407
intolerance, 92
monosaccharides, 80–84
myocardial tissue, 412
oligosaccharides, 84
paleolithic diet, 498
phosphorylation, 82
polysaccharides, 85–88

proportion of human mass, 2
RDA, 79
stores, 349
structural function, 87
Carbon, 1
Carbon dioxide (CO_2), 17, 217, 242, 30, 305, 415, 541
Carboxyeptidases, 130
Carboxylases, biotin and, 217–218
Cardiac hypertrophy, 415–417, 429
Cardiac muscle, 230, *See* Cardiovascular system; Heart
Cardiac output, 30
Cardiolipin, 9
Cardiovascular system, 27–30, 411–431; *See also* Heart disease; Hypertension
energy metabolism, 412–414
hypertrophic state, 415
ischemic state, 414
phytoestrogens and, 385
selenium toxicity, 292
Carnitine, 185, 370–371, 391–392
cardiac hypertrophy and, 415
Carnitine acyltransferase, 414
Carnitine-palmitoyl transferase I, 309
Carob bean gum, 506
α-Carotene, 54, 160, 371
structure, 162
β-Carotene, 54, 55, 160, 371, *See also* Carotenoids
absorption, 163
anticancer effects, 445
cardiovascular health and, 429
structure, 162
γ-Carotene, 54, 160, 371
structure, 162
Carotenes, 53, 160, *See* Carotenoids; specific carotenes
Carotenoids, 160, *See also* Vitamin A; specific carotenes, carotenoids
anticancer effects, 445
antioxidant activity, 166, 429
cardiovascular health and, 429
color, 53–53
dietary sources, 160–161
digestion and absorption, 161–163
excretion, 166
food sources
function, 165–166
normal blood values, 541
nutrient interactions, 166
paleolithic diet, 499
plasma transport, 164
retinal conversion, 164
ripening and, 55
structures, 162
suggested reading, 392
supplements, 371–372
synthetic, 55
Carrageenan, 506
Carrots, 53, 54
Cartilage, 277
Casein, 45, 133, 134
CAT scan, 322

Catalase, 249, 250, 316
Catecholamines, 293–294, *See also* Epinephrine;
        Norepinephrine; Serotonin
    exercise effects, 348–349
Catechol-*O*-methyl transferase (COMT), 294
Catnip, 547
Celery, 547
Cell culture, 487, 494
Cell fractionation, 488
Cell proliferation, vitamin A analogs and, 166
Cell structure, 2–10
    nucleus and genetic aspects, 10–12
    organelles, 4–10, *See also* Mitochondria
    plasma membrane, 3–4
Cellular retinoid binding proteins (CRBPs), 163–165
Cellulose, 47, 87, 88, 89, 91, 96, 506
Central nervous system (CNS, 22
Centrifugation, 487–488
Ceruloplasmin, 135, 249, 266
Chamomile, 547
Chaparral, 548
Chelates, 49
Chemical score, 134
Chemoprevention, 440
Chemotherapy, 437, 438, 450
Chenodeoxycholic acid, 112
Chewing, 59, 69
Chickweed, 548
Chicory, 548
Children and infants, 405–409, *See* Infant nutrition
    growth charts, 511–516
    obesity in, 337–338
Chitin, 87
Chlorambucil, 438
Chloride (or chlorine), 49, 229, 529
    absorption, 240–241
    intracellular and extracellular concentration, 22
    normal blood values, 541
    physiological function, 241
    recommended intake, 242
    saliva, 71
    sources, 238, 529
    sports drinks, 363
    sweat composition, 155
    tissue and fluids content, 241
    toxicity, 529
Chloride shift, 242
Chlorophyll, 53, 55
Chloropropamide, 466
Cholecalciferol, 167
Cholecystokinin, 56, 65, 67, 68, 75, 110, 335
Cholesterol, 99
    bile acids and, 76, 96
    DHEA synthesis and, 377
    digestion and absorption, 112–113
    HDL-cholesterol, 120–121
        DHEA and, 379
        dietary fat and, 420
        low-fat diet and, 338
    LDL-cholesterol, 120–121, *See also* Cholesterol,
        blood

atherosclerosis and, 421–423
    clinical intervention considerations, 423–425
    dietary fat and, 420
    low-fat diet and, 338
    soy products and, 426
    plasma membrane, 3–4
    saponin complexes, 386
    steroidal derivatives, 114, 116
    synthesis, 6, 114, 116
Cholesterol, blood
    atherosclerosis and, 421–423
    clinical intervention considerations, 423–425
    dietary cholesterol and, 420
    dietary fat and, 420
    dietary fiber and, 90, 426
    dietary guidelines for disease risk reduction,
        425–429
    garlic and, 380, 429
    HDL and LDL and health implications, 120–122,
        See also under Cholesterol
    heart disease risk and, 417, 420–423
    hypercholesterolemia treatment, 121–122
        nicotinic acid, 199–200
    low-fat diet and, 338
    normal blood values, 541
    saponins and, 386
    soy products and, 387, 426–427
Cholesterol, dietary, 48, 420
    blood cholesterol and, 420
    content of selected foods, 108–109
    nutritional requirement, 109
    paleolithic diet, 498
    recommended intake for diabetes, 463
Cholesterol esterase, 111
Cholestyramine, 122
Cholic acid, 112
Choline, 376–377, 520
Chondroitin sulfate, 7, 22, 87–88, 277, 372, 392, 469
Chromaffin cells, 293
Chromatography, 488–489
Chromium, 42, 249, 275–276, 372–373, 392
    deficiency, 463
    supplementation, 276
    toxicity, 373
Chromium picolinate, 372, 373
Chylomicrons, 113, 117, 119, 120, 163, 169, 174, 179, 353
    separation techniques, 489
Chyme, 72
Chymotrypsin, 130
Chymotrypsinogen, 130
Cigarette smoking, *See* Smoking
Cimetidine, 69
Cinnamon, 548
Cis-fatty acids, 102–103
Citrate
    fatty acid synthesis and, 312
    Krebs cycle metabolite, 306
Citric acid, 246, 506
Citric acid cycle, 16, *See* Krebs cycle
Citrulline, 143
Citrus fruits, 368

Citrus Red No.2, 506
Cleaver's herb, 548
Clotting factor V, 268
Clotting factors, 136, 179–181, 268
Cloves, 549
Coagulation, *See also* Anticoagulants; Clotting factors
   calcium and, 230
   copper and, 268
   vitamin K function, 179–181
Cobalamin, 212
Cobalt, 212, 278, 430, 530
Cochineal, 506
Codons, 12
Coenzyme A (CoA), pantothenic acid and, 220
Coenzyme athletic performance system (CAPS), 376
Coenzyme Q (CoQ), 19, 393
Coenzyme Q10 (ubiquinone), 375–376
Coffee, 448–449
Colestipol, 122
Colipase, 76, 111
Collagen, 46, 127, 136, 266
   bone, 22, 469, 471
   precursor amino acids, 137
   silicon and, 282
   vitamin C and, 184
Colloidal suspension, 151
Colon, 63
   digestive processes, 77
   excess dietary fiber effects, 97
Colon cancer (or colorectal cancer), 439, 441, 442, 448, 498
   calcium and, 446
   dietary fiber and, 97, 443
   dietary fruits and vegetables and, 444
   vitamin E and, 445
Colonic microflora, *See* Gut microflora
   calcium absorption and, 228
   fiber metabolism, 89
Color, 52–55
Coloring agents, 503
Colostrum, 45, 131, 403
Colt's foot, 549
Column chromatography, 489
Comfrey, 549
Compensatory hyperinsulinemia, 455
Complete proteins, 133
Complex carbohydrates, 460–461
Computerized axial tomography (CAT), 322
Conformal radiotherapy, 438
Conjugases, 207
Conjugated dienoic derivatives of linoleic acid (CLA), 442
Connective tissue, 21
Contortrostatin, 478
Copper, 42, 249, 264–269, 530
   absorption, 265–266, 279
   ascorbate deactivation, 183
   deficiency, 249, 256, 268, 271, 429, 530
   enzymes, 264, 266–268, 487
   genetic anomalies, 268–269
   iron metabolism and, 265
   metabolism and function, 266–268
   mineral interactions, 265
   molybdenum interaction, 279
   normal blood values, 541
   recommended intake, 268
   sources, 265, 530
   toxicity, 266, 269, 530
   transport and distribution, 266
Cori cycle, 350
Corn endosperm oil, 506
Corn oil, 107
Corn starch, 47, 506
Corn syrup, 47, 363, 462, 506
Corticotropin-releasing hormone, 136
Cortisol, 33, 99, 294–295, 318
   exercise effects, 348
Coumestans, 385
Cow's milk, *See* Milk
C-peptide, 290
CPT-11, 438
Creatine, 137, 393
   bone turnover measures, 471–472
   supplementation, 374–375
Creatine monohydrate, 450
Creatine phosphate, 233, 344, 355, 374
Creatinine, normal blood values, 541
Crocin, 371
Crude fiber method, 90
Cryptoxanthin, 54, 160, 162, 371
Crypts of Lieberkuhn, 63
Cuproenzymes, 264, 266–268, 487
Curing agents, 503
Cyanide, 383–384
Cyanocobalamin, 212
Cyanogenic compounds, 450
Cyclamate, 535
Cyclic AMP (cAMP), 293
   glucagon and, 33
Cyclooxygenase, 113–114
Cyclophosphamide, 438
Cysteine, 126, 140, 142
   coenzyme A metabolism, 220
Cysteine-rich protein (CRIP), 255
Cystic acne therapy, 167, 401
Cystinuria, 132
Cytochrome, 249
Cytochrome c, 19, 376
Cytochrome c oxidase, 268, 487
Cytochrome oxidase, 267
Cytochrome P$_{450}$ system, 249, 315
Cytochrome reductase, 193
Cytoplasm, 3, 4
Cytosine, 10
Cytosol, 4

D

Daidzein, 380, 387, 447
Dairy products, as calcium source, 226
Dandelion, 550
Deamination, 138–139

Dehydration, 151, 158, 360
Dehydroascorbic acid, 182
Dehydroepiandrosterone (DHEA), 99, 377–379, 394, 475
Delta- (Δ-) desaturases, 104
Delta (Δ) system of fatty acid nomenclature, 101
Denaturation, 491
Densitometry, 322–324
Deoxycorticosterone, 241
Deoxyribonucleic acid, *See* DNA
Deoxyribose, 10
Desaturation, 102
Designer foods, 500
DEXA, 322
Dexfenfluramine, 341
Dextrose, 462, 506, *See* Glucose
DHA, 104, 368, 427
Diabetes mellitus, 339, 418, 451–467
   associated medical conditions, 457–458
   β-cell defect, 455
   definition and classification, 451
      type I (insulin dependent), 451, 452–453
      type II (noninsulin dependent), 451, 453
   diagnostic criteria, 456–456
   genetic insulin anomalies, 456
   gestational diabetes, 456
   glycemic index, 499
   inheritance, 452
   insulin resistance, 453, , 454–455
   insulin therapy, 465–466
   nutritional management, 459–465
      alcohol, 462
      carbohydrates, 460–461
      exchange system of meal planning, 463–464
      fat, 462
      fiber, 463
      fructose, 461
      historical recommendations, 459–460
      minerals, 463
      protein, 461–462
      sweeteners, 462–463
      vitamins, 463
   obesity and, 339, 453, 459
   oral antidiabetic agents, 466–467
Diabetic nephropathy, 458
Diabetic neuropathy, 457–458
Diabetic retinopathy, 458
Diallyl sulfide (DAS), 447
Dialysis patients, 371
Dietary fat, *See* Fat, dietary
Dietary fiber, *See* Fiber
Dietary reference intakes, 43–44
Diet history, 486
Diet-induced thermogenesis, 288
Difluormethylornithine (DFMO)
Digestibility of proteins, 134
Digestion and absorption, *See also* specific nutrients
   bacterial fermentation products, 95
   bile secretion, 75, *See also* Bile acids
   carbohydrate, 76, 91–94
   carotenoids and vitamin A, 161–163

dietary fiber and, 90
enterocytes and, 76–77
esophageal transit, 71–72
large intestine and, 77
lipids, 76, 110–113
mastication and saliva, 69–71
pancreatic secretions, 74–75, 110–113, 130
proteins, amino acids, and peptides, 129–132
small intestine and, 73, 74–76
water and, 76
Diglycerides, 99, 506
Dihydrobiopterin, 185
Dihydroxyacetone, 80, 386
Dioctyl sodium sulfosuccinate, 506
Dipeptide, 128
Diphosphatidylglycerol, 9
Direct calorimetry, 283–284
Disaccharides, 46, 84–85
Disintegrins, 478
Disodium guanylate, 506
Disodium inosinate, 506
Distal tubule, 155
Dithiolthiones, 446
Diuretics, 419
DNA, 2, 10–12, 80, 491
   aging and free radical effects, 499–500
   complementary DNA (cDNA), 491, 492
   evolution, 498
   mitochondrial, 11
   polymerase chain reaction, 493
   repair dysfunction, 436
DNA polymerase, 491
Docetaxel, 439
Docosahexaenoic acid (DHA), 104, 368, 427
Dopamine, 23, 65, 293
   precursor amino acids, 137
   vitamin C and, 185
Dopamine β-hydroxylase (DBH), 294
Dopamine hydroxylase, 267
Dough strengtheners, 503
Doxorubicin, 438
Drug therapy
   cholesterol reduction, 425
   diabetes, *See* Insulin
   obesity, 340–341
   hypertension, 419
Drying agents, 503
Dulcin, 535

E

Echinacea, 379, 395, 550
Echistatin, 478
EDTA, 248, 507
Egg allergies, 409
Egg proteins, 46, 133, 134
Egg white consumption, and biotin deficiency, 216, 218
Eicosanoids, 113
   synthetic pathways, 105
Eicosapentaenoic acid (EPA), 104, 368, 427

Elaidic acid, 103
Elastin, 127, 136
Electrolytes, 238–244, *See* Chloride; Potassium;
        Sodium
    ethanol abuse and, 430
    intracellular and extracellular concentration, 22
    ion channels, 23
    pancreatic secretions, 74
    saliva components, 71
    sports drinks, 363
    sweat composition, 155, 241
Electron microscopy, 494–495
Electron transport chain, 16–19, 249–250, *See also*
        Krebs cycle
Electrophoresis, 119, 489
Elements, 1–2
Emulsifiers, 503
Emulsifying lipoproteins, 46
Emulsions, 151
Endocrine system, 32–34
Endometrial cancer, 440, 441, 475
Endoplasmic reticulum, 4, 6–7, 13
End-stage renal disease, 371, 458
Endurance training
    endocrine adaptation, 348–349
    muscle adaptations, 346–347
Energy allowances, 39
Energy metabolism, 283–319, *See also* ATP;
        Carbohydrate; Lipids
    adaptive thermogenesis, 288–289
    adipocytes and, 327
    alcohol oxidation, 315–316
    amino acids, 137, 140, 141, 307, 310, 317–319, *See*
        Amino acids
    basal metabolic rate, 286–287
    calorimetry, 283–285
    cardiac hypertrophy and, 415
    cardiac ischemia and, 414
    catecholamines and, 293–294
    chemical mediators of energy homeostasis, 334–335
    coenzyme A and pantothenic acid involvement, 220
    components of, 285–286,
    coordinated metabolism during exercise, 355–356
    cortisol and, 294–295
    electron transport chain and oxidative
        phosphorylation, 15–19
    energy balance feedback loops, 332
    energy intake and expenditure regulation, 33–334
    exercise effects, 349–357
    glucagon and, 292–293
    glucose production, 307–309, *See* Gluconeogenesis
    glycogen synthesis and degradation, 303–304, *See*
        Glycogen
    glycolysis, 298–302, *See* Glycolysis
    infant requirements, 406
    insulin and, 290–292, 334–335, *See* Insulin
    ketone body production, 309, 310–312
    Krebs cycle, 16–19, 304–307, *See* Krebs cycle
    leptin and, 336
    lipids and, 99, *See* Fatty acids
        fatty acid synthesis, 312–314

    molecular control of fat metabolism, 314–315
    major metabolic pathways, 295–316
    mitochondria function, 9–10
    myocardial tissue, 412–414
    neuroendocrine mediators of energy homeostasis,
        335–337
    pentose phosphate pathway, 102, 190, 292, 304
    pregnancy and, 400
    protein and, *See* Amino acids; Protein
    substrate utilization, 316–319, *See also* specific
        substrates
        fasting state, 316, 318–319
        fed state, 316, 317–318
        glucose transport, 295–298
    thermal effect of activity, 287
    thermal effect of food, 288
    tissue and organ contributions, 286
    total energy expenditure, 283–285
Enkephalins, 65
Enteric nervous system, 64–66
Enterochromaffin cells, 63
Enterocytes, 63, 76–77
Enterokinase, 74, 130
Enterooxyntin, 73
Enzymatic method of fiber analysis, 91
Enzymes, 503, *See also* specific enzymes, types
    classifications and functions, 135
    digestive, 74–75, 110–113, 130
    metal cofactors, 49, *See also* specific metals
        copper, 264, 266–268, 487
        magnesium, 236
        molybdenum, 280
        zinc, 254–257
EPA (Eicosapentaenoic acid), 104, 368, 427
Ephedrine, 341
Epidermal growth factor (EGF), 328
Epimers, 81
Epinephrine, 33
    energy metabolism and, 293–294
    enteric nervous system, 65
    exercise effects, 348–349
    glycogenolysis and, 303
    precursor amino acids, 137
Epithelial tissue, 19
erb$_i$, 435
Erectile dysfunction, 390
Ergocalciferol, 167
Ergogenic practices, *See* Athletic performance-
        enhancing supplements
Erythrocytes, 29–30, *See also* Hemoglobin
    selenium (in glutathione peroxidase) and, 271
Erythropoietin, 32
Erythrose, 80
Erythrulose, 80
Esophageal cancer, 440, 449
Esophagus, 71–72
Essential amino acids, 43, 124
    determining protein requirements, 148
    infant requirements, 407
    intake requirements, 146, 407
    protein quality, 132–133

Essential fat, 321
Essential fatty acids, 99, 103–104, 110, *See also* Linoleic
    acid; Linolenic acid
  food sources, 107
  paleolithic diet, 498
Essential nutrients, 38
Estimated average requirement (EAR), 44
Estradiol, 475, 476
Estriol, 475
Estrogen, 33, 99
  bone loss and, 474, 475
    replacement therapy, 475–476
  calcium absorption and, 228
  cancer and, 475, 476
  fiber binding, 443
  phytoestrogen properties, 385, 447
Estrone, 475
Ethacrynic acid, 207
Ethanol, *See* Alcohol
Eucalyptus, 550
Eukaryotic initiation factor (eIF), 146
Evolution, 1
  paleolithic diet, 497–499
Exercise and physical activity, 343–364
  bone health and, 476–477, 480
  cancer risk and, 443
  carbohydrate metabolism, 349–352
  cardiac hypertrophy and, 416
  cardiac output and, 30
  catecholamine levels and, 348–349
  coordinated energy metabolism, 355–356
  high-carbohydrate meals, 352
  hormonal adaptation, 347–349
  immune system and, 443
  insulin and, 348, 454
  lipid metabolism, 352–354
  minerals and, 359
  muscle adaptations, 346–347
  nitrogen balance, 355
  obesity and sedentary lifestyle, 332
  obesity in children and, 338
  performance-enhancing ergogenic practices, *See*
    Athletic performance-enhancing supplements
  protein and amino acid metabolism, 354
  thermal effect of activity, 287
  total energy expenditure (, 407), 343
  vitamins and, 357–359
  water and, 359–360
  weight loss program, 338
Exchange system of meal planning, 463–464
Exons, 12
Extrinsic pathway, 179
Eyebright, 550

F

FABP, 113, 309, 413
Factor X, 179
Factorial method, 143
FAD, 191, 192, 487
FADH$_2$, 16–19, 305, 309

Fastin, 341
Fasting state energy metabolism, 318–319
Fast-twitch (FT) fibers, 345, 353
Fat, *See* Adipose tissue; Body fat; Fatty acids; Lipids;
    Triglycerides
Fat, dietary, 48, 106–110
  anticarcinogenic fatty acid (CLA), 442
  blood cholesterol and, 420
  breast milk and, 107
  cancer risk and, 441–443
  diabetes and, 462
  essential fatty acids, 99, 103–104, 110, *See also*
    Linoleic acid; Linolenic acid
  Exchange System of Meal Planning, 464
  fatty acids synthesis and, 102
  food content, 108–109
  guidelines for cholesterol and heart disease risk
    reduction, 425–429
  immune response and, 442
  infant requirements, 407
  low-fat diets, 338
  Mediterranean diet, 427–428
  nutritional requirements, 109–110
  obesity and, 328, 340
  paleolithic diet, 498
  saturated and unsaturated fatty acids, 106–107
Fat-free mass (FFM), 321
Fatty acid binding protein (FABP), 113, 309, 413
Fatty acid oxidation, 309–310, 412
  cardiac hypertrophy and, 415
  exercise effects, 352–354
  fed state energy metabolism, 317
  glucose transport inhibition, 297
  insulin resistance and, 454
  ketone body production, 309, 310
  peroxisomes and, 9
  starvation and, 319
Fatty acid peroxidation, 113
Fatty acids, 48, 99–101, *See also* Lipids; specific types
  activation, 413
  bacterial fermentation products, 95
  blood cholesterol and, 420
  breast milk composition, 404
  chain length, 100
  cis vs. *trans*, 102–103
  dietary, *See* Fat, dietary
  digestion, 110–113
  elongation and desaturation, 102
  exercise and metabolism, 352–354
  magnesium absorption and, 236
  muscle metabolism, 356
  myocardial metabolism, ischemia, 414
  myocardial uptake and utilization, 413
  nickel and, 281
  omega (Ω) and delta (Δ) nomenclature, 101
  oxidation, *See* Fatty acid oxidation
  saturation and unsaturation, 100–101
  separation techniques, 489
  types, 48
Fatty acid synthase (FAS), 102, 223, 312
Fatty acid synthesis, 101–102, 312–314

biotin and carboxylase-catalyzed reactions, 218
fed state energy metabolism, 317
insulin and, 292
FD&C colors, 507
Fecal nitrogen, 133
Fecal vitamin E, 175
Fecal water loss, 156
Fed state energy metabolism, 317–318
Feeding regulation, 334
Fenfluramine, 341
Fen-phen, 341
Fenton reaction, 252–253
Fenugreek, 550
Ferritin, 246, 247, 248, 254
Ferroxidase, 266
Fetal alcohol syndrome, 402
Fetal hemoglobin, 135
Fetal nutrition, 399–400
Fiber, 47
    analysis of, 90–91
    bile acids and, 95–96, 97, 426
    bran content, 97
    cancer and, 439, 443
    diabetes and, 463
    dietary guidelines for disease risk reduction, 426
    digestion and, 90
    fecal bulk and composition, 96
    food sources, 88–89
    gut microflora and, 94–95
    hydration, 95
    monosaccharides in, 81
    negative consequences of excess, 97
    paleolithic diet, 499
    physical and physiological properties, 94–97
    soluble and insoluble, 88–89
Fibrin, 127, 136
Fibrinogen, 136
Fibroblast growth factors (FGFs), 328
Fibronectin, 478
Fibrous proteins, 127
Firming agents, 503
Fish allergy, 409
Fish oils, 48, 107, 368, 427
    anti-cancer properties, 442
Fish proteins, 46
Flatulence producers, 85
Flavin adenine dinucleotide (FAD), 191, 192, 487
Flavin mononucleotide (FMN), 191, 192
Flavonoids, 53, 55, 379–380, 385, 395, 440
    cancer and, 446–447
Flavoring additives, 503
Flax, 550
Flour treating agents, 503
Fluoridated water, 273–274
Fluoride (or fluorine), 42, 273–276, 479, 531
    absorption, 274
    metabolism and function, 274
    recommended intake, 274
    sources, 273–274
    toxicity, 274
Fluorosis, 274

Fluorouracil, 438
Foam cells, 422
Folate (folic acid), 48, 206–212, 520
    absorption, 207
    cancer and, 212
    deficiency, 210–212, 401, 423, 520
    exercise and, 359
    function, 209–210
    infant requirements, 407
    methyl-folate trap, 210, 215
    pregnancy and, 401
    recommended intake, 41, 210
    sources, 206–207, 520
    supplementation, 212
    toxicity, 212, 520
    transport and metabolism, 208–209
Follicle-stimulating hormone (FSH), 136
Food, 37
    allergies and intolerances, 408–409
    nutrient sources, 44–49
Food additives, 54, 57, 505–510
    terminology, 503–504
Foot drop syndrome, 191
Formulation aids, 503
fos, 166
Free-flow agents, 503
Free radicals
    aging effects, 499
    carotenoid interactions, 166
    dietary fiber and, 96
    eicosanoid synthesis and, 113
    iron overload and, 252–253
    vitamin C and, 444
    vitamin E and, 176
Fructose, 80, 363, 535
    absorption of, 93
    diabetes and, 461
    relative sweetness, 85
Fruit juice, as sweetener, 462–463
Fruit ripening, 55
Fruits and vegetables, and cancer prevention, 444
Fumarate, 142, 143
Fumigants, 503
Functional foods, 500
Funk, Casimir, 159, 187
Furosemide, 207
Futile cycle systems, 334, 386

G

GABA, 65, 202
Gag reflex, 408
Galactans, 90
Galactose, 80, 89, 93
Galactouronic acid, 90
Galanin, 336
Gall bladder, 75–76
γ-aminobutyric acid (GABA), 65, 202
Gamma globulins, 131
Garlic, 380, 429, 447, 551

Gases, 504
Gas exchange method of indirect calorimetry, 284
Gastric-releasing peptide (GRP), 65
Gastric acid, *See* Hydrochloric acid
Gastric emptying, 73
Gastric inhibitory polypeptide (GIP), 67–69
Gastrin, 67–68, 73
Gastrointestinal system, 59–64
    blood supply, 66–67
    dietary fiber and, 97
    digestive processes, 72–77, *See also* Digestion and
        absorption
    endocrine and paracrine substances, 65, 67–69
    enteric nervous system, 64–66
    movements, 66
    smooth muscle and motility, 64
Gastroplasty, 342
Gatorade, 363
GBE, 382
Gel permeation chromatography, 119, 489
Gelatin, 507
Gemcitabine, 438
Gender, and obesity, 337
Genes, 10, 14
    cancer and, 435–436
    expression, 491–494
    risk factors for heart disease, 411
Genistein, 380, 387, 427, 447, 447
Gentian, 551
Gestational diabetes, 456
Ginger, 380–381, 395, 551
Gingko biloba, 381–382, 395
Ginseng, 551
Glipizide, 466
Globular proteins, 127
Gloss, 52
Glucagon, 33, 136, 292–293
    appetite effects, 56
    exercise effects, 348
    fasting energy metabolism, 318
    glycogenolysis and, 303
    insulin:glucagon ratio, 293, 317
Glucocorticoids, 257, 294
Glucogenic amino acids, 137, 140
Glucokinase, 291, 298, 455
Gluconeogenesis, 307–309
    cortisol and, 295
    fasting energy metabolism, 318
    fed state energy metabolism, 317–318
    insulin and, 292
    weight loss and, 339
Glucose (and glucose metabolism), 80, 506, 535, *See
        also* Gluconeogenesis; Glycolysis
    absorption, 76–77, 93
    adaptive cardiac hypertrophy, 415
    ascorbate derivative, 182
    biosynthesis, *See* Gluconeogensis
    blood sugar, 80
    dietary, diabetes and, 460
    exercise and, 349–351
    fasting energy metabolism, 318

fed state energy metabolism, 317
    intolerance, 455
    myocardial metabolism, ischemia, 414
    myocardial uptake and utilization, 413
    relative sweetness, 85
    sports drinks, 363
    transport into cells, 295–298
Glucose, blood, *See also* Hyperglycemia
    diabetes diagnostic criteria, 456
    exercise effects, 348
    glycemic index, 461
    insulin effects, 291–292, *See also* Insulin
    normal values, 541
Glucose-alanine cycle, 350
Glucose 1-phosphate, 303
Glucose 6-phosphate, 82, 295, 298, 317, 318, 413,
        455
Glucose tolerance factor (GTF), 199, 275, 276, 372
Glucose tolerance test, 456
Glucose transport proteins, 291–292, 295–297
    GLUT1, 296
    GLUT2, 296, 297, 304
    GLUT3, 296, 297
    GLUT4, 291, 296, 297, 317, 349, 351, 454
    GLUT5, 296, 297
    GLUT7, 296, 297, 303
Glucostasis theory, 333
Glutamate, 141, *See also* Glutamic acid
    biosynthesis, 139
    folate and, 210
Glutamate-arginine, 369
Glutamate dehydrogenase, 138, 142
Glutamic acid, 125, *See also* Glutamate
    folate and, 206
Glutamine, 125, 141
    muscle metabolism, 355
γ-Glutamylcarboxypeptidases, 207
Glutathione, 176
Glutathione peroxidase, 250, 269–272
Glutathione-*S*-transferase, 380, 446, 448
Gluten, 46
Glyburide, 466
Glycemic index, 461, 499
Glyceraldehyde, 80
Glycerine, 507
Glycerol, 396, 507
    hyperhydration, 382
    lipid digestion and absorption, 112–113
    supplementation, 382–383
Glycine, 126, 127, 137, 536
    enteric nervous system, 65
    metabolism, 140
Glycocalyx, 4
Glycocholic acid, 112
Glycogen (and glycogen metabolism), 2, 86–87, 303
    animal flesh, 46
    caffeine and, 362
    cortisol and, 295
    degradation, 303–304
    exercise effects, 349–352
    fasting energy metabolism, 318, 319

fed state energy metabolism, 317
glycogenolysis, 293, 303, 454
insulin and, 292, 454
loading, 360–361
synthesis, 303
tissue content, 87
Glycolipids, 99
Glycolysis, 16, 292, 298–300
fate of pyruvate, 300–302
myocardial metabolism, 413
reactions (table), 302
Glycoproteins, 13
allergens, 409
vitamin A and, 166
Glycosaminoglycans, 87–88, 372, 469
Glycosylated hemoglobin, 457, 463
Glycyrrhizin, 384
Goblet cells, 63
Goiter, 259, 264
Goldenrod, 551
Goldenseal, 552
Golgi apparatus, 4, 7–8
Gonadotropin-releasing hormone, 136
Grain-derived nutrients, 368
polishing/refining and nutrient loss
magnesium, 235
riboflavin, 191–192
thiamin, 186, 190
vitamin B$_6$, 200
starches, 86
Grape skin extract, 507
Green tea, 367
Ground substance, 22, 469
Growth charts, 511–516
Growth hormone, 33, 253, 136
arginine and, 369
exercise and, 348
ornithine supplementation and, 385
Growth hormone releasing hormone (GHRH), 136
GTP, 17, 233
Guanine, 10
Guanosine, 10
Guanosine triphosphate (GTP), 17, 165
Guarana, 552
Guar gum, 507
Gum arabic, 507
Gum ghatti, 507
Gums, 47, 88, 89, 90, 95, 507
Gustation, 50–52
Gut microflora, 37, 77
calcium absorption and, 228
fiber and, 89, 94–95
Gynoid obesity, 331–332

H

Hair follicle differentiation, 172
Hard water, 419, 495
Harris and Benedict equation, 287
Hartnup disease, 132
Hawthorn, 552

HDL, *See* High-density lipoprotein
Heart, 27, 29, *See also* Heart disease
selenium toxicity, 273
Heart disease, 411
alcohol and, 430
calcium and, 495
carotenoids and, 371
clinical intervention, 423–425
cobalt toxicity, 278
coenzyme Q10 (ubiquinone) and, 376
DHEA and, 377
dietary fiber and, 90
dietary guidelines, 425–429
flavonoids and, 380
hypertrophy, 415–417, 429
iron and, 254
ischemia, 414
protein intake and, 498
risk factors, 417–423
atherosclerosis, 421–423
cholesterol, 121–122, 420–423, *See also* Cholesterol, blood
hypertension, 417–419, *See also* Hypertension
vitamin and mineral deficiency, 429
Heat exhaustion, 360
Height and weight charts, 511–516
Helicase, 499
Hemagglutination inhibitors, 46
Hematocrit, 29
Heme, 49, 53, 245
Hemicellulose, 47, 81, 88, 89, 91, 96
Hemochromatosis, 250–251
Hemoglobin, 30, 135, 248
fetal, 135
glycosylated, diabetes and, 457, 463
iron deficiency and, 250
vitamin B$_6$ and, 204
Hemolytic anemia, 259
Hemosiderin, 246, 249
Heparin, 88
Hepatic lipase, 121
Hepatic tocopherol transfer protein (HTTP), 174
Hepatocellular carcinoma, 253
Herbal fen-phen, 341
Herbs, 368–369, 543–558
Hesperidin, 55, 380
Hexokinases, 291, 298
Hexose monophosphate shunt, 102, 190
High biological value proteins, 133
High blood pressure, *See* Hypertension
High-density lipoprotein (HDL), 117–118
HDL-cholesterol, 120–121
DHEA and, 379
dietary fat and, 420
low-fat diet and, 338
separation techniques, 489
vitamin E absorption and transport, 174
High-fructose corn-syrup, 47, 80
Hip fracture, 469, 474
Hippocrates, 329, 500
Histamine, 23, 69, 73, 124, 125, 140, 141, 210

Histology, 494–495
Historical recommendations, 459–460
HLA, 452
HLA-linked hemochromatosis, 250–251, 253
HMB, 383, 396
HMG-CoA, 114, 116, 121, 312, 448
HMG-CoA reductase inhibitors, 122, 425, 429, 448
Homocysteine, 138, 140, 141, 215, 423
Honey, 462
Hop, 552
Horehound, 552
Hormone replacement therapy, 475–476
Hormones, 32–34, 136, *See* specific hormones
    gastrointestinal secretions, 65, 67–69
    receptors, 33
Hospital nutrition practices, 484
Huckleberry, 553
Humalog, 465, 466
Human calorimetry, 283–284
Human insulin, 465
Human milk fats, 107
Humectants, 503
Humulin R, 465
Hunger and appetite, 55–57
Hyalin, 458
Hyaluronic acid, 7, 87, 469
Hydration of fiber, 95
Hydrochloric acid (HCl), 72, 130, 242
    iron absorption and, 246
Hydrogen, 1
Hydrogenated oils, 48
Hydrogen breath test, 95
Hydrogen peroxidase, 249
Hydrogen peroxide, 176, 268, 316, 507
Hydrolyzed vegetable protein, 507
Hydroxyapatite, 22, 229, 274, 470
Hydroxyl radical, 176, 252
Hydroxylysine, 125, 137, 140
β-Hydroxy-β-methylbutyrate (HMB), 383, 396
3-Hydroxy-3-methylglutaryl CoA, *See* HMG CoA
17α-Hydroxyprogesterone, 475
Hydroxyproline, 125, 127, 137, 140, 282, 472
Hypercholesterolemia, *See* Cholesterol, blood
Hyperglycemia, *See also* Diabetes mellitus; Glucose, blood
    chromium deficiency and, 463
    gestational diabetes, 456
    postprandial, complex and simple carbohydrates and, 460
    type II diabetes, 453
Hyperplasia, 433
Hypertension, 411, 417–419
    calcium and, 495
    cardiac hypertrophy and, 416
    ethanol and, 430
    fish oil and, 427
    obesity and, 339–340
    pregnancy and, 419
    treatment approaches, 419
Hyperzincaemia, 257
Hypochlorous acid, 250

Hypochromic microcytic anemia, 250
Hypothalamus, 23
    appetite control, 56
    energy intake regulation, 334, 335
    hormones, 136
    osmoreceptors, 156
    thirst sensation and, 157
Hyssop, 553

I

Immune system
    dietary fat and, 442
    food allergies, 409
    physical activity and, 443
    protein function, 137
    vitamin B_6 and, 204, 205
    vitamin C and, 444
Immunoglobulins, 45
Immunostimulants, 379
Indirect calorimetry, 284–285
Infant nutrition, 404–409
    adverse food reactions, 408–409
    carbohydrate, 407
    growth and development, 405
    growth charts, 511–516
    iron overload, 252
    lipid, 407
    phosphorus, 234
    protein, 130–131, 149, 406–407
    transition to solid food, 408
    vitamins and minerals, 407–408
Infrared interactance, 322
In situ hybridization, 494
Inosine, 376
Inositol hexaphosphate (IP_6), 388, *See* Phytate
Insensible water losses, 156
Insoluble fibers, 88–89
Insulatard, 465
Insulin, 33, 136, 290–292, 466
    appetite and, 56
    chromium and, 275, 276, 372
    cortisol interactions, 295
    energy homeostasis, 334–335
    exercise effects, 348, 349, 351
    fasting energy metabolism, 318
    fatty acid synthesis and, 312
    fed state energy metabolism, 317
    genetic defects, 456
    glucagon ratio, 293, 317
    glycolysis and, 298
    normal blood values, 541
    therapy, 465–466
    vanadium and, 281
Insulin-dependent diabetes mellitus (IDDM, type I diabetes), 451, *See* Diabetes mellitus; Type I diabetes
Insulin-like growth factor 1 (IGF-I), 369, 379
Insulin-like growth factors (IGFs), 328
Insulin pump, 466
Insulin receptor, 292, 454

defects, 456
Insulin resistance, 327, 454–455
    obesity and, 453
    weight loss and, 339
Integrins, 478
Internal radiation therapy (IRT), 438
International Olympic Commit, 407 (IOC), banned
        substances, 379
Intestinal microflora, *See* Gut microflora
Intracrinology, 378
Intrinsic factor, 73, 212
Intrinsic pathway, 179
Introns, 12
Invert sugar, 507
Iodine (or iodide), 259–264, 483, 531
    absorption, 261
    deficiency, 264
    metabolism and function, 261–263
    recommended intake, 42, 263
    sources, 259–261
Iodized salt, 261
Iodothyronine deiodinase, 271
Iron, 38, 49, 245–254, 507, 531
    absorption, 246–248
    ascorbate deactivation, 183
    binding protein, 249
    calcium and, 228, 248
    copper and, 265
    deficiency, 166, 250, 402, 408, 531
    distribution in body, 248
    exercise and, 359
    infant requirements, 408
    metabolism and function, 248–250
    normal blood values, 541
    pregnancy needs, 402
    protein binders, 46
    recommended intake, 42, 250
    sources, 245–248, 531
    storage proteins, 246
    supplementation, 367
    toxicity ("overload"), 245, 250–254, 430, 531
        carcinogenic effect, 254–254
    vitamin C and, 183, 185, 248
    zinc absorption and, 255
Iron-ammonium citrate, 507
Ischemia, 411
Isoelectric focusing, 490
Isoflavones, 385, 387, 427, 440, 447
Isolated soy protein (ISP), 46
Isoleucine, 124, 141
    intake requirements, 146
    nickel and, 281
Isoniazid, 199
Isoprenoids, 53
Isoprostane, 113
Isoretinoin, 167, 401
Isothiocyanates, 440

J

jun, 166

Juniper, 553

K

Kallikrein, 70
Karraya gum, 507
Keratin, 127, 136
Keshan disease, 269
Ketogenic amino acids, 137, 140
α-Ketoglutarate, 142, 202
Ketone bodies, 140, 295, 309, 310–312, 319
Kidney, 31–32, 155, 418
    electrolyte balance and, 241
    selenium toxicity, 273
Kidney disease, 371, 418, 458
    carnitine supplementation and, 371
    diabetic nephropathy, 458
Kidney stones, 186, 231, 269, 280
Kistrin, 478
Knock-out models, 494
Krebiozen, 449
Krebs cycle, 16–19, 199, 304–307
    amino acids and, 139, 141
    thiamin and, 189–190
Kwashiorkor, 149

L

Laboratory methods, 483, 487–496
    body composition assessment, 322–325
    calorimetric methods, 283–285
    cell cultures, 487, 494
    centrifugation, 487–488
    energy content, 483
    gene expression, 491
    histology, 494–495
    lipoprotein separation, 119
    molecular biology tools for studying gene
        expression, 491–494
    polymerase chain reaction, 493
    separation techniques, 488–490
    trace element measurement, 484
    transgenic animal models, 493–494
    Western blotting, 490–491
Lactase, 92
Lactate, 300–301, *See also* Lactic acid
    cardiac hypertrophy and, 415
    fed state energy metabolism, 317
    gluconeogenic precursor, 307
    muscle production in response to exercise, 349–350
    myocardial uptake and utilization, 413
Lactate dehydrogenase (LDH), 300, 415
Lactation, 403–405
    bone and, 473
    calcium demand, 473
    energy demands, 403
    maternal dietary fat composition and, 107
    nutrient content variations, 404
    RDAs for vitamins and minerals, 40–42
    recommended intakes, *See* recommended intakes
        for specific nutrients

Lactic acid, 507, *See also* Lactate
  bicarbonate loading and, 362
  iron absorption and, 246
  normal blood values, 541
Lactic acid cycle, 350
Lactobacillus acidophilus, 92
Lactobacillus bifidus, 403
β-Lactoglobulin, 45
Lactose, 80, 84–85
  intolerance, 92
  relative sweetness, 85
Laetrile, 383–384, 396, 450
Lard, 106, 107
Large intestine, *See* Colon
Laryngeal cancer, 449
Lauric acid, 420
Laxatives, 243
LDL, *See* Low-density lipoprotein
L-Dopa, 268
Lead, 430, 541
Lean body mass (LBM), 321, 325–326
  aging and, 500
  creatine supplementation and, 374–375
  HMB and, 383
  ornithine supplementation and, 385
  vanadium and, 388
Leavening agents, 503
Lecithin (phosphatidyl choline), 105, 106, 110, 111, 377, 507
Lecithin-cholesterol acyltransferase (LCAT), 121
Legumes, 85, 86, 93
Lemon balm, 553
Lente, 465, 466
Leprechaunism, 456
Leptin, 327, 333, 335–337, 454
Leucine, 124, 126
  intake requirements, 146
  metabolism, 142
  nickel and, 281
  vitamin B$_{12}$ and isomerization, 215
Leucine zippers, 487
Leukemias, bone marrow transplantation and, 439
Leukocytes, 29
Leukopenia, 212
Leukotrienes, 113–114
Licorice, 384, 396, 553
Lignans, 385, 440, 447
Lignin, 47, 88, 90, 91, 95, 95, 96
Liminoids, 440
Limiting amino acids, 124, 133, 148
Limolin, 448
Limonene, 448
Limonoids, 448
Lingual lipase, 70, 110
Linoleic acid, 48, 99, 104, 107
  conugated dienoic derivatives, 442
  infant requirements, 407
Linolenic acid, 99, 104, 110
Linseed, 107, 550
Lipase inhibitor, 341

Lipids, 99–122, *See also* Cholesterol; Fat, dietary; Fatty acids; Lipoproteins; Phosopholipids; Triglycerides
  digestion, 76, 110–113
  eicosanoid precursors, 113–114
  energy metabolism, 99
  exercise and, 352–354
  food sources, 48, 106–110, *See* Fat, dietary
  general properties and nomenclature, 99–106
  insulin and, 292
  malabsorption, 177
  myocardial metabolism, ischemia, 414
  myocardial uptake and utilization, 413
  oxidation, *See* Fatty acid oxidation
  peroxidation, 113
    iron and, 253
  plasma membrane, 3
  proportion of body mass, 1
  site of synthesis, 6
  steroidal derivatives, 114–116
Lipoprotein lipase, 117, 119, 309, 318, 353, 454
Lipoproteins, 116–121
  cholesterol component and health implications, 120–122
  emulsifying, 46
  metabolism of, 119–120
  muscle metabolism, 353, 354
  separation methods, 119, 489
Lipostasis theory, 333
Lipoxygenase, 113–114
Lispro, 465, 466
Liver
  carbohydrate store, 349, *See* Glycogen
  glycogen content, 87
  insulin absorption, 292
  iron overload, 252–253
  lipoproteins, 117
  vitamin B$_{12}$ content, 214–215
  vitamin E storage, 175
Loop of Henle, 155
Lovastatin, 122, 425
Low-calorie diet, 339–340
Low-density lipoprotein (LDL), 117–118, 120
  LDL-cholesterol, 120–121, *See also* Cholesterol, blood
    atherosclerosis and, 421–423
    clinical intervention considerations, 423–425
    dietary fat and, 420
    low-fat diet and, 338
    soy products and, 426
    tocopherol transport, 174
Low-fat diets, 338
Low-protein diet, 146–147
Lubricants, 503
Lung, 30
Lung cancer, 440, 445, 448
Lutein, 54, 371
Luteinizing hormone (LH), 136
Lycopene, 54, 55, 162, 371, 440
Lysine, 124, 125
  intake requirements, 146

limiting, 148
metabolism, 142
Lysolecithin, 111–112
Lysosomes, 4, 8
Lysyl oxidase, 266

M

Macrophages
  activators, 379
  atherosclerosis and, 421
Magnesium, 49, 225, 235–238, 529
  absorption, 236
  bone, 470
  calcium absorption and, 227
  deficiency and toxicity, 237–238, 529
  enzymes, 236
  excretion, 236
  normal blood values, 541
  phosphorus absorption and, 232
  physiological roles, 236–237
  recommended intake, 42, 237
  sources, 235, 529
  tissue content, 236
Magnetic resonance imaging (MRI), 322
Ma huang, 341
Malabsorption, 177
Malignant tumors, 433
Malondialdehyde, 253
Maltase, 92
Maltose, 84, 85
Manganese, 42, 249, 277–278, 531–532
  enzyme cofactor, 277
  recommended intake, 278
Mannans, 90
Mannitol, 85, 462–463, 507, 536
Mannose, 89
MAO inhibitors, 294, 388, 390
Marasmus, 149
Margarines, 107
Marine oils, 48, 107, *See* Fish oils
Marshmallow, 554
Mast cells, 88
Mastication, 59, 69
Matrix Gla protein, 229
Maturity-onset diabetes of the young, 455
McCollum, E. G., 483
McGovern Report, 484
Meat, Exchange System of Meal Planning, 464
Meats, 44
Medicinal botanicals, 37, 543–558, *See* specific plants
Mediterranean diet, 427–428
Megaloblastic macrocytic anemia, 210
Melanin, 268
Melanocytes, 268
Melanocyte-stimulating hormone (MSH), 136
Melanoidins, 53
Membrane polarization, 23
Membrane potential, 242
Menadinone, 178
Menaquinones, 178

Menke's disease, 268–269, 429
Menopausal and postmenopausal women, 228, 370
  bone and, 472, 474
  estrogen replacement therapy, 475–476
  obesity and, 337
3–Mercaptopicolinic acid {MPA}
Messenger RNA (mRNA), 11, 12, 491, 492
Metabolic rate, 283, 286–287
  adaptive thermogenesis, 288–289
  thermal effect of food, 288
Metalloenzymes, 49, *See* Enzymes
Metallothionein, 255, 266
Metals, 245–282, *See* Minerals; Trace elements; specific metals
Metastasis, 433
Metformin, 467
Methionine, 124, 126, 127, 138, 141, 215, 243
  intake requirements, 146
  limiting, 148
Methionine synthase, 210
Methotrexate, 210, 438
Methylcobalamin, 214, 215
Methyl-folate trap, 210, 215
4-O-Methyl glucuronic acids, 90
2-Methyl histidine, 140
Methylmalonyl CoA, 215
Methylparaben, 508
Miacalcin, 478
Micelle, 112
Michaelis-Menton constant, 146
Microcytic anemia, 259
Microsomal ethanol-oxidizing system, 315
Microvilli, 63
Milk
  allergens, 409
  emulsion, 151
  fats, 48, 107
  human, *See* Breast milk
  lactose intolerance, 92
  mineral content, 49
  proteins, 45, 133
  sugar, 84, *See* Lactose
  sunlight exposure and riboflavin content, 191
  vitamin D, 169
Minerals, 225–282, 527–523, *See also* specific minerals, trace elements
  body composition, 321, 326
  bone, 470
  classic interpretation of nutrient function, 487
  diabetes and, 463
  dietary fiber and, 96, 97
  exercise and, 359
  food sources, 49, *See* specific minerals
  heart disease and, 495
  major, 225–244
  minor (trace elements), 245–282
  pregnancy needs, 402
  RDAs 42
  research, 483
Miraculin, 536
Mirosterol, 447

Mitochondria, 4, 9–10
  fatty acid oxidation, 309
  iron overload, 253
  muscle content, 347
  myocardial activity, 412
Modified food starch, 508
Molasses, 462
Molecular biology tools, 491–494
Molecules, 1–2
Molybdenum, 42, 279–280, 532
Molybdopterin, 280
Monellin, 536
Monoamine oxidase, 266, 294, 388, 390
Monoglycerides, 508
Monosaccharides, 46, 80–84
  absorption of, 93
Monosodium glutamate (MSG), 508
Monounsaturated fatty acids, 100–101
  dietary guidelines for disease risk reduction,
    425–426
  recommended intake for diabetes, 463
Motherwort, 554
Motilin, 65, 67, 69
Motor neurons, 343
Mouth, 69
MRI, 322
MSG, 508
Mucilages, 47, 88, 89, 90, 95
Mucin, 70
Mucopolysaccharides, 87
Mucus, 7, 87
Mullein, 554
Muscle, 19–21, 25–27
  adaptation to strength training, 346
  calcium ion function, 230
  carbohydrates stores, 349
  contractile proteins, 136
  exercise and carbohydrate metabolism, 349–352
  exercise and lipid metabolism, 352–354
  fiber hypertrophy, 346
  fibers, 343–345
  gastrointestinal smooth muscle, 64
  glycogen content, 87
  innervation, 343
  iron function, 249
  mitochondrial content, 347
  protein metabolism, 354–355
  proteins, 45, 129
  wasting, 149
  water composition, 153
  zinc content, 256
myc_1, 435
Myeloperoxidase, 249, 250
Myocardial infarction, 254, 411
Myocardial tissue, 230
Myoelectric migrating complexes, 69
Myofibrils, 26
Myoglobin, 53, 248, 249
Myosin, 26–27, 45, 127, 136, 344
Myosin ATPase, 345
Myristic acid, 420

N

N-acetyl galactosamine, 277
NAD (nicotinamide adenine dinucleotide), 81,
    198–199, 296, 301, 305, 306, 309
NADH, 16–19, 199, 301, 305, 306, 309
NADH dehydrogenase, 193
NADP (nicotinamide adenine dinucleotide
    phosphate), 81, 196, 198, 199
NADPH, 102, 304, 314
National Cholesterol Education Program, 425, 462
Neohesperidin dihydrochalon e, 537
Nephrons, 31–32
Nephropathy of diabetes, 458
Nervous tissue, 21, 22–25
Neuropathy of diabetes, 457–458
Neuropeptide Y (NPY), 335, 336
Neurotensin, 65, 67, 69
Neurotransmitters, 23, 65
  calcium and synaptic release, 230
Neutral fiber method, 90
Neutron activation, 484
Niacin, 48, 195–200, 485, 521
Niacin, 521
  biosynthesis, 197, 198
  deficiency, 195–196, 199, 521
  digestion and absorption, 197–198
  pharmacological use, 199–200
  recommended intake, 41, 199
  sources, 197, 521
  toxicity, 200, 521
Nickel, 249, 281–282
Nicotinamide, 196–199, *See* Niacin
Nicotinamide adenine dinucleotide, *See* NAD
Nicotinamide adenine dinucleotide phosphate, *See*
    NADP
Nicotinic acid, 199–200
Niemann-Pick disease, 106
Nitric acid, 369
Nitrogen, 1
  biological value, 133–134
  dietary protein quality, 132–134
  excretion, 133, 142
  intake requirements, 143
  urea acid cycle enzymes and, 147
Nitrogen balance, 143, 145
  exercise and, 355
Nitrosamines, 445, 449
Nomilin, 448
Noninsulin-dependent diabetes mellitus (NIDDM,
    type II diabetes), 451, *See* Diabetes mellitus;
    Type II diabetes
Nonsteroidal antiinflammatory drugs, 114
Norepinephrine, 23, 293
  exercise effects, 348
  precursor amino acids, 137
  reuptake inhibitor and obesity treatment, 341
  vitamin C and, 185
Northern blot, 492, 494
Northern hybridization, 492
NPH, 465, 466

Nucleic acids, 80, *See* DNA; RNA
  proportion of body mass, 2
Nucleosides, 10
Nucleotides, 10
Nucleus, 3
Nutmeg, 554
Nutraceuticals, 37, 367–398, 500, *See* Supplements and
      nutraceuticals; specific plants, substances
  food sources, 368
  medicinal botanicals, 37, 543–558, *See* specific
      plants
Nutritional supplements, *See* Supplements and
      nutraceuticals
Nutrients, 38, *See* Minerals; Vitamins
  food sources of, 44–49
  recommended intakes, 38–44
  status assessment, 485–486
Nutrition, defined, 1
Nutrition Labeling Regulation, 147
Nutrition research, 483–496
  laboratory methodology, 483, 487–496, *See*
      Laboratory methods
  multidisciplinary approaches, 495
  nutrient function, 495
  nutrient requirements determination, 485–486

O

Obesity, 321, 328–333
  adipocytes and, 327
  adipose tissue distribution, 331–332
  body mass index (BMI), 331
  cancer risk and, 441
  children and, 337–338
  definition and prevalence, 330–331
  diabetes and, 339, 453, 459
  diet therapy, 339–340
  dyslipidemia, 338
  fatty acid synthesis and, 102
  financial implications, 329
  gender and, 337
  genetic influences, 332–333
  heart disease risk and, 417
  history of, 329
  hypertension and, 339–340
  lifestyle and, 332
  liposuction, 342
  mortality correlation, 328
  neuroendocrine influences, 335–337
  pharmacological treatment, 340–341
  related diseases, 338–339
  surgical treatment, 342
1,25-(OH)$_2$D$_3$, *See* Vitamin D
25-(OH)D$_3$, *See* Vitamin D
Oils, 48, 106
  fish, 48, 107, 368, 427, 442
  vitamin E content, 173–174
OKG, 384
Oleic acid, 48, 103, 107, 427
Olfaction, 50, 52
Oligosaccharides, 84

Olive oil, 107, 428
Oltipraz, 440
Omega-3 (Ω-3) fatty acids, 104, 312, 427, 440
  immune response and anticarcinogenic effects, 442
Omega-6 (Ω-6) fatty acids, 104, 312
  immune response and, 442
Omega (Ω) system of fatty acids nomenclature, 101
4-O-methyl glucuronic acids, 90
Oncogenes, 435
Onions, 367, 447
Opsin, 137, 165
Oral cancer, 440, 448, 449
Oral cavity, 69–71
Organelles, 4–10, *See also* Mitochondria
Organic matrix, 22
Organosulfur compounds, 447
Organ systems, 21
Orlistat, 341
Ornithine, 138, 384–385
Ornithine-α-ketoglutarate (OKG), 384
Orphan receptors, 314
Osmoreceptors, 156
Osmotic pressure, protein and, 137
Osteoarthritis, 372
Osteoblasts, 22, 471
Osteocalcin, 181, 229
Osteoclasts, 22, 471, 478
Osteomalacia, 172, 229, 231
Osteoponin, 478
Osteoporosis, 229, 231, 469–480, *See also* Bone
  classification, 473–474
  diagnosis, 473
  prevention and treatment, 475–480
    calcitonin-salmon therapy, 478
    calcium, 478–479
    disintegrins, 478
    exercise, 476–477
    fluoride, 479
    vitamin D, 479
    zinc, 479–480
  risk factors, 469, 473
Oxalates, 186, 226, 227
Oxalic acid, 254
Oxaloacetate, 143, 189, 312
Oxidative phosphorylation, 9–10, 18
Oxidizing agents, 504
Oxygen, 1
Oxyntic cells, 72
Oxyntic glands, 62
Oxytocin, 241

P

P-4,000, 537
Paclitaxel, 439
Paleolithic diet, 243, 497–499
Palm oil, 54
Palmitate, 312, 353, 415
Palmitic acid, 48, 102, 107, 420
Pancreatic cancer, 448
Pancreatic degeneration, 458

Pancreatic enzymes, 74–75, 110–113, 130
Pancreatic polypeptide, 69
Pancreatitis, 130
Pantothenate salts, 220
Pantothenic acid, 42, 48, 218–223, 312, 521–522
    absorption, 220
    deficiency, 223
    metabolism and function, 220–223
    recommended intake, 223
    sources, 219–220
Pantothenol, 220
Papain, 508
Papaya, 555
Paprika, 508
Paraaminobenzoic acid (PABA), 206
Parasympathetic nervous system, 65
Parathyroid hormone (PTH), 229, 237, 471
Parsley, 555
Partition chromatography, 488
Passion flower, 555
Peach carotenoids, 54
Peak bone mass, 472, 477
Pectins, 47, 88, 89, 90, 95, 96, 426, 508
Pellagra, 195–196, 199
Pentose phosphate pathway, 102, 190, 292, 304
Pentoses, 80
Peppermint, 555
Pepsin, 73, 129–130
Pepsinogen, 72, 73, 130
Peptidases, 131–132
Peptide YY, 69
Peptides, 128
    absorption, 131–132
Performance-enhancing practices, *See* Athletic
        performance-enhancing supplements
Peripheral artery disease, 371
Peristalsis, 66, 72
Pernicious anemia, 212, 216
Peroxidases, 249–250
Peroxide, 176, *See* Hydrogen peroxide
Peroxisome proliferator-activated receptors (PPARs),
    314, 328, 494
Peroxisomes, 4, 8–9, 414
Peroxy radical, 176
Persicaxanthin, 371
Peyer's patches, 63
pH
    control agents, 504
    normal blood values, 541
Phenolics, 427–428, 440
Phenteramine, 341
Phenylalanine, 124, 125, 185
    intake requirements, 146
    metabolism, 142
Phenylalanine hydroxylase, 185
Phenylbutazone, 207
Phenylethanolamine-*N*-methyltransferase (PNMT)
Phosphate, *See* Phosphorus
Phosphatidyl choline (lecithin), 105, 106, 110, 111, 377,
    507

Phosphenolpyruvate-carboxykinase (PEPCK), 277,
    314, 350
Phosphofructokinase 1 (PFK1), 298, 413
Phospholipase, 111
Phospholipids, 48, 99, 105–106
    plasma membrane, 3
    site of synthesis, 6
    vitamin B$_6$ and, 204
Phosphoric acid, 508
Phosphorus (or phosphate), 225, 232–234, 528
    absorption, 232
    bone, 470
    calcium absorption and, 227
    deficiency, 234, 528
    normal blood values, 541
    physiological roles, 233–234
    recommended intake, 42, 234
    serum levels, 233
    sources, 232, 528
    toxicity, 234, 528
    vitamin D and, 172
Phosphorylase, 303, 318
Phosphorylation, 82
Photosynthesis, 79
Phyllodulcin, 537
Phylloquinone, 178
Physical activity, *See* Exercise and physical activity
Phytalin, 70
Phytates, 49, 226, 227, 232, 254, 266, 387
Phytic acid, 388
Phytobezoars, 97
Phytochemicals, 37, *See* Nutraceuticals
Phytoestrogens, 385, 443
    cancer and, 446–447
Pickling agents, 503
Pigments, 53–55
Pituitary hormones, 136
Plantain, 555
Plants, 37
    derived foods, 44
    mineral content, 49
Plasma, 29, 153
Plasma membrane, 3–4
Plasma proteins, 135
Plasma volume, and exercise, 359–360
Plasmogens, 105
Platelet-activating factor (PAF) antagonists, 382
Platelet-derived growth factor (PDGF), 421, 423, 435
Platelets, 29
Pleurisy root, 556
PO$_2$, 541
Polished rice, thiamin deficiency and, 186, 190
Polyacetylene, 440
Polymerase chain reaction, 493
Polypeptide, 128
Polyphosphates, 508
Polysaccharides, 85–88
Polysorbates, 508
Polyunsaturated fatty acids (PUFAs), 100–101
    blood cholesterol and, 420

dietary guidelines for disease risk reduction, 425–426
essential fatty acids, 103–104
fatty acid synthase enzymes, 312
fish oils, 48, 107, 368, 427, 442
omega-3, 104, 312, 427, 440, 442
omega-6, 104, 312, 442
recommended intake for diabetes, 463
saturated fatty acid ratio (P/S) ratio, 106–107
Pondimin, 341
Postmenopausal women, *See* Menopausal and postmenopausal women
Potassium, 49, 225, 529
absorption, 240–241
blood pressure and, 419
bone, 470
deficiency, 243, 529
intracellular and extracellular concentration, 22
membrane polarization, 23
normal blood values, 541
physiological function, 241
recommended intake, 242
saliva, 71
sodium ratio, 49
sources, 240, 529
tissue and fluid content, 241
toxicity, 530
Potassium alginate, 508
Potassium bromate, 508
Potassium iodide, 508
Potassium nitrite, 508
Potassium sorbate, 508
Potassium-sparing diuretics, 419
Pravastatin, 425
Preadipocyte factor-1 (Pref-1), 328
Pregnancy, 399–403
alcohol consumption and, 402
body composition changes, 399
bone and, 472–473
caffeine and, 403
calcium and, 472, 495
fetal metabolism and nutrition, 399
gestational diabetes, 456
ginger contraindication, 381
hypertension, 419
insulin secretion, 291
mineral needs, 402
obesity and, 337
protein needs, 400
RDAs for vitamins and minerals, 40–42
recommended intakes, *See* recommended intakes for specific nutrients
vitamin B_6 and, 206
vitamin needs, 400–401
water requirements, 157
Pregnenolone, 377
Premenstrual syndrome (PMS), vitamin B_6 and, 205–26
Primary protein structure, 127
Processing aids, 504
Progesterone, 33, 475, 476

Progestins, 475
Proinsulin, 290
Prolactin, 33, 136
Prolactin-inhibiting hormone, 136
Prolactin-releasing hormone, 136
Proline, 125, 127, 139, 141, 282
Propellants, 504
Propionate, 312
Propionic acid, 508
Propionyl-L-carnitine, 371
Propionyl CoA, 220
Proprionic acid, 95
Propyl gallate, 508
Propylene glycol, 509
Propylparaben, 509
Prosky method, 91
Prostacyclin, 428
Prostaglandins, 113–114
Prostate, 387
Prostate cancer, 440, 441, 442, 445, 447, 448
Protamine, 466
Protease inhibitors, 387, 440
Protein, 123–150, *See also* Amino acids; Lipoproteins
body composition, 321
cancer and, 498
definition, 128
denaturing, 129
dietary fiber and, 96
digestibility, 134, 147–148
digestion and absorption, 129–132
energy needs, 400
excess, 148–149
food content, 129
heart disease and, 498
infants, 406–407
pregnancy, 400
intake requirement, 143–148
low protein diet, 146–147
malnutrition, 166
mass of, 127
metabolism and function, 135–138
muscle wasting, 149
paleolithic diet, 498
plasma membrane, 4
proportion of body mass, 1
quality, 132–134, 147
RDA, 43
recommended intake for diabetes, 460, 461–462
sources, 45–46
structures, 127–128
synthesis, 10
genetic level processes, 11, 12–15
turnover, 354–355
undernutrition, 149–150
vitamin B_{12} binding, 214
Western blotting, 490
Protein efficiency ratio (PER), 134
Protein-energy malnutrition (PEM), 149
Protein-sparing modified fasts (PSMF), 340
Proteoglycans, 7, 22, 372, 469
Prothrombin, 179, 277

Protooncogenes, 435
Proximal convoluted tubule, 155
Pulmonary artery, 30
Purines, 10
Pyridoxal phosphate, 200–206, *See* Niacin
Pyridoxine, 200
Pyridoxol, 200
Pyrimidines, 10
Pyrophosphate, 16, 471
Pyruvate, 17
   amino acids and, 140, 142
   fasting energy metabolism, 318
   gluconeogenesis and, 307
   glycolysis product, 298–302
   muscle metabolism, 355
   normal blood values, 541
   suggested reading, 396
   supplementation, 385–386
Pyruvate dehydrogenase, 301, 317, 413
Pyruvate kinase, 298

Q

Queensdelight, 556
Quercetin, 55, 380, 446
Quinones, 440

R

Rabson-Mendenhall syndrome, 456
Race
   diabetes and, 453
   hypertension and, 418
Radiation therapy, 438, 450
Raffinose, 85, 93
RBCs, *See* Erythrocytes
RDAs, *See* Recommended Dietary Allowances
Rebound scurvy, 186
Recommended Dietary Allowances (RDAs), 38–44,
      483, *See also* recommended intakes for specific
      nutrients
Red blood cells, *See* Erythrocytes
Red clover, 556
Reducing agents, 504
Redux, 341
Reference protein, 133
Refined grains, nutrient loss
   magnesium, 235
   riboflavin, 191–192
   thiamin, 186, 190
   vitamin B$_6$, 200
Regulin, 465
Renal cancer, 441
Renal disease, *See* Kidney disease
Renin-angiotensin system, 158, 418
Research, *See* Laboratory methods; Nutrition research
Resistance training, 287, *See also* Weight training
Respiratory quotient (RQ), 284–285
   exercise response, 351
Resting energy expenditure (REE), 286
Resting potential, 23

Retinal, 160, 164, 165
Retinoic acid, 160, 166
   cell binding proteins, 164
   receptor, 314
   toxicity, 167
Retinoid X receptor (RXR), 171
Retinol, 160, 161, 163, *See also* Vitamin A
   cell binding proteins, 164
   toxicity, 167
Retinopathy, 458
Reverse transcriptase PCR, 493
Rhodopsin, 165
Ribitol, 80
Riboflavin (vitamin B$_2$), 48, 191–195, 279, 487, 522
   absorption and transport, 192
   deficiency, 194
   metabolism and functions, 192–193
   recommended intake, 41, 194
   sources, 191–192
   toxicity, 194
Ribonucleic acid, *See* RNA
Ribose, 80–81
Ribosomal RNA (rRNA), 11
Ribosomes, 6, 12–13
Ribulose, 80
Ribulose 5–phosphate, 304
Rickets, 172, 231
Ripening, 55
RNA, 2, 11–12, 80
   extraction and analytical methods, 492
RNA polymerases, 11, 12
Rosemary, 556

S

Saccharin, 85, 462, 509, 537
S-adenosyl methionine (SAM), 138
Safflower oil, 107
Saffron, 509, 556
Sage, 557
Saliva, 59, 70–71
Salivary glands, iodide absorption, 261
Salt, 238, 418–419, 509, *See also* Chloride; Sodium
   iodized, 261, 264
Saponins, 386
Sarcomeres, 26344
Sarcoplasmic reticulum, 26, 344
Sarsaparilla, 557
Sassafras, 557
Saturated fatty acids, 100–101, 106
Saw palmetto, 387, 397, 557
Scanning electron microscopy, 495
Scurvy, 182, 185
SDS-PAGE, 489, 490
Secondary protein structure, 127
Secretin, 65, 67, 68, 75
Secretory vesicles, 8
Sedatives, 389
Selenium, 250, 269–273, 532
   absorption, 269–270
   deficiency, 269, 272, 532

metabolism and function, 270–271
nutrient interactions, 271
recommended intake, 42, 272
sources, 269, 532
toxicity, 272–273, 483, 532
Selenoprotein P, 270
Semilenti, 465
Senna, 557
Senses, 50–55
Sensory neurons, 22
Sequential centrifugation, 119, 488
Sequestrants, 504
Serine, 126, 139, 140
Serotonin, 23
    gastrointestinal secretion, 65, 67, 65, 67
    precursor amino acids, 137
    reuptake inhibitor and obesity treatment, 341
Serum proteins, 45
Sesquiterpenes, 389
Shivering thermogenesis, 289
Sibutramine, 341
Silicon, 282
Silicon dioxide, 509
Simvastatin, 425
Sitosterol, 388, 426
Skeletal muscle, 25–27, *See also* Muscle
    caffeine and, 362
    calcium function, 230
    coordinated energy metabolism, 355–356
    energy metabolism, 286
        fed state, 317
    exercise and carbohydrate metabolism, 349–352
    exercise and lipid metabolism, 352–354
    glucose transport, 297
    glycogen content, 87
    glycogenolysis, 293
    lactate production, 349–350, *See also* Lactate
    muscle fibers, 343–345
    protein content, 129
    protein metabolism, 354–355
    water composition, 153
    zinc content, 256
Skeletal system, 21–22, *See* Bone
Skin cancer, 437
Skinfold thickness, 322, 324
Skullcap, 557
Slow-twitch (ST) fibers, 345, 353
Slow waves, 64
Small intestine, 59, 62–63, 73, 74–76, 92
Smell, 50, 52
Smoking, 417, 420
    cancer risk and, 440
    vitamin C metabolism and, 444
Smooth muscle, 64
    calcium ion and contraction, 230
Snake venom, 478
Sodium, 49, 225, 528
    absorption, 240–241
    bone, 470
    calcium excretion and, 243
    deficiency, 243, 528

dietary, heart disease risk and, 418–419
digestion process and, 77
excess consumption, 243
intracellular and extracellular concentration, 22
normal blood values, 541
physiological function, 241
potassium ratio, 243
recommended intake, 242
saliva, 71
sources, 238–239, 528
sports drinks, 363
sweat composition, 155
tissue and body fluids content, 241
toxicity, 528
Sodium acetate, 509
Sodium alginate, 509
Sodium aluminum sulfate, 509
Sodium benzoate, 509
Sodium bicarbonate, 509
Sodium borate, 279
Sodium chloride, 238, 509, *See also* Chloride; Salt;
        Sodium
Sodium citrate, 509
Sodium diacetate, 509
Sodium fluoride, 479
Sodium nitrate, 509
Sodium nitrite, 509
Sodium propionate, 509
Soft water, 495
Soil mineral content, 49
Solubility, 151
Soluble fibers, 88–89
Solvents, 504
Somatostatin, 56, 68, 136
Sorbic acid, 509
Sorbitan monostearate, 510
Sorbitol, 85, 462–463, 510, 538
Southern blotting and hybridization, 492
Southgate fractionation system, 90
Soybean oil, 104, 107
Soy products, 46, 380, 387–388, 397
    guidelines for disease risk reduction, 426–427
Spearmint, 568
Specific dynamic action (SDA), 288
Spectrophotometry, 488
Sphingolipids, 106, 204
Sphingomyelin, 106
Sphingomylinase, 106
Spike potential, 64
Sports, *See* Athletic performance-enhancing
        supplements; Exercise and physical activity
Sports drinks, 363–364
SRI Oxime V, 538
Stabilizers, 504
Stachyose, 85, 93
Starch, 47, 85–86
    digestion, 92, 93–94
    Exchange System of Meal Planning, 464
Starvation
    energy metabolism, 316, 319
    ketone body formation, 310, 319

Stearic acid, 48, 102, 107
Stellate cells, 165
Stem cells, 327–328
Step I diet, 462
Step II diet, 462
Steroids, 33, 99, 114–116
Stevioside, 538
St. John's Wort, 341, 388, 397
Stomach, 59–62
    digestive process, 72–73
    protein digestion, 129
    stapling, 342
Stomach cancer, 440
Strength training, *See also* Weight training
    chromium supplementation and, 373
    muscle adaptations, 346
    vanadium and, 389
Stress response, 293
Stroke, 411
Structural polysaccharides, 87
Substance P, 65
Succinate dehydrogenase, 193
Succinyl CoA, 141, 220
Sucrase, 92
Sucrose, 79, 80, 84, 510, 538
    diabetes and, 460, 462–463
    relative sweetness, 85
Sugars, 79, *See also* Carbohydrates; Glucose; specific
        sugars
    disaccharides and oligosaccharides, 84–85
    epimers, 81
    food sources, 46
    intolerance, 92
    monosaccharides, 80–84
    sweetness of, 85, 535–539
Sulfates, 49
Sulfinpyazone, 207
Sulfonurea drugs, 462, 466, 467
Sulfur, 225, 243
Sunflower oil, 107
Sunlight
    riboflavin and, 191
    vitamin D and, 168–169
Superoxide dismutase, 266, 277, 494
Superoxide radical, 176, 267–268
Supplements and nutraceuticals, 367–398, 500, *See also*
        Athletic performance-enhancing
        supplements; specific substances
    food sources, 368
    medicinal botanicals, 37, 543–558, *See* specific
        plants
    minerals, *See* specific minerals
    vitamins, *See* specific vitamins
Surface-active agents, 504
Surface-finishing agents, 504
Surgery, cancer, 450
Surgical intervention, 437
Swallowing, 71
Sweat, 153–154
    electrolyte content, 241
    exercise and, 359

water loss, 156–157
Sweet flag, 547
Sweeteners, 47, 85, 462, 503, 509, 535–539
    diabetes and, 462–463
Sweetness, 85, 535–539
Sympathetic innervation, enteric nervous system, 65
Synapse, 23
Syndrome X, 417, 455
Synergists, 504
Szyent-Gyorgyi, Albert, 182, 200

T

Tagetes, 510
Tallow, 106
Tamoxifen, 440
Tannic acid, 187
Tannins, 254
Tansy, 568
Tartaric acid, 246, 510
Taste, 50–52
Taste buds, 50–52
Taurine, 137, 138
Taurocholic acid, 112
Terpenes, 440
Tertiary structure, 127
Testosterone, 33, 99
    boron stimulation, 370
    DHEA-stimulated increase, 379
Tetrahydrofolate, 438
Tetrahydropterin, 185
Texturizers, 504
Thaumatins, 538
Thermal effect of activity, 287
Thermal effect of food, 288
Thermogenesis, 288–289
Thermogenin, 334
Thiamin (vitamin B_1), 48, 186–191, 243, 523
    absorption and transport, 188–189
    deficiency, 187, 190, 429, 523
    exercise and, 358
    metabolism and functions, 189–190
    recommended intake, 41, 190
    sources, 187, 523
    toxicity, 191
Thiazolidinediones, 314, 467
Thionein, 255, 256, 265–266
Thirst, 157
Threonine, 124, 126, 140, 141, 146, 148
Threose, 80
Thromboplastin, 179
Thromboxane A_2, 380
Thromboxanes, 113–114, 380
Thymidine, 10
Thymine, 10
Thyroid gland, iodine deficiency and, 259
Thyroid hormone, 33, 137, 261–264, 271
    adaptive thermogenesis and, 289
    iodide absorption, 261
    T_3 receptor, 166
Thyroid-stimulating hormone (TSH), 136, 262

Thyrotropin, 262
Thyrotropin-releasing hormone (TRH), 136, 262
Thyroxine (T₄), 261–262, 271, *See* Thyroid hormone
Tissue, 19–21
Titanium dioxide, 510
Tobacco, *See* Smoking
Tocopherol, 173, 510, 518, *See also* Vitamin E
β-Tocopherol, 177
α-Tocopherol, 174, *see also* Vitamin E
  equivalents, 177
Tocotrienols, 173, 177, *See also* Vitamin E
Tolazamide, 466
Tolbutamide, 466
Tolerable upper intake level (UL), 44
Topoisomerase inhibitors, 438
Total body potassium (TBK), 322
Total energy expenditure (TEE), 283–285, 343, 406
Toxicity, *See* toxicity for specific substances
Tolerable upper intake level (UL), 44
Trace elements, 49, 245–282, *See* Minerals; specific
    elements
  research methods, 483–484
Tragacanth gum, 510
Training, *See* Exercise and physical activity
Transamination, 138–139, 202
Transcobalamin II, 214
Transcription, 11
Transcription factors, 166, 257, 314
  cancer and, 435
Transcuprin, 266, 268
Transducin, 165
Trans-fatty acids, 48, 102–103, 107, 109, 420
Transfection, 494
Transfer RNA (tRNA), 11, 12
Transferrin, 135, 247–248, 249, 251–252
Transferrinemia, 251–252
Transforming growth factors (TGFs), 328, 435
Transgenic animal models, 493–494
Translation, 12
Transmission electron microscopy, 494
Tricarboxylic acid cycle (TCA), *See* Krebs cycle
Triglycerides, 16, 99, *See also* Fatty acids
  exercise and, 352–354
  food, 106
  muscle metabolism, 356
  myocardial tissue, 412
  normal blood values, 541
  simple and mixed, 106
Triiodothyronine (T₃), 261–262, 271, *See* Thyroid
    hormone
Triiodothyronine receptor, 166
Troglitazone, 467
Tropocollagen, 184
Tropomyosin, 26, 45, 136, 344
Troponins, 26, 136
Trypsin, 74, 130
Trypsin inhibitor, 130
Trypsinogen, 74, 130
Tryptophan, 124, 125, 127, 137, 140
  intake requirements, 146
  limiting, 148

  metabolism, 142
  niacin and, 197, 198, 199
Tuberculosis treatment, 205
Tubulin, 439
Tumor necrosis factor α (TNFα), 327, 454
Tumor suppressor genes, 436
Turmeric, 510
Type I diabetes, 451, 452–453, *See* Diabetes mellitus
  insulin therapy, 465–466
Type II diabetes, 339, 499, 451, 453, *See* Diabetes
    mellitus
Tyrosine, 125, 137, 185
  biosynthesis, 139
  copper and metabolism, 268
  intake requirements, 146
  metabolism, 142
Tyrosine hydroxylase, 268
Tyrosine kinase inhibitor, 427

U

Ubiquinol, 19
Ubiquinone, 176, 375–376
Ubiquitin, 223
UDP-glucose, 303
UDP-glucuronic acid, 277
Ultracentrifugation, 119
Ultrafiltrate, 32
Uncoupling protein, 334
Underwater weighing, 322–323
Unsaturated fatty acids, 48
Uracil, 11
Urea, 142, 541
Urea cycle, 143, 147
Uric acid, 280, 541
Urinary nitrogen, 133
Urine, 155–156

V

Vagovagal reflex, 73, 75
Vagus nerve, 65, 72
Valepotriates, 389
Valerian, 389, 398, 568
Valine, 124, 126, 141
  intake requirements, 146
  nickel and, 281
Vanadium, 280–281, 388–389, 397
Vanilla, 510
Vanillin, 510
Van Soest method, 90
Vasoactive inhibitory polypeptide (VIP), 65
Vasopressin, *See* Antidiuretic hormone
Vegetable oils, carotenoid content, 54
Velosulin R, 465
Verbacose, 85
Very-low-calorie diet, 339–340
Very-low-density lipoproteins (VLDL), 117–120
  muscle metabolism, 353
  separation techniques, 489
  tocopherol transport, 174

Villi, 62–63
Vinblastine, 439
Vinorelbine, 439
Vioaxanthin, 371
Vision
  diabetic retinopathy, 458
  vitamin A and, 160, 165, 167
Visual pigment, 137
Vitamin A, 48, 160–167
  calcium absorption and, 227
  cellular binding proteins, 163–165
  deficiency, 167, 517
  dietary sources, 160–161, 163, 517
  digestion and absorption, 161–163
  excretion, 166
  function, 165–166
  infant requirements, 407
  normal blood values, 541
  nutrient interactions, 166
  plasma transport, 164
  pregnancy and, 400–401
  recommended intake, 40, 167
  storage of, 165–165
  structures, 161, 162
  toxicity, 167, 401, 517
Vitamin B$_1$, *See* Thiamin
Vitamin B$_2$, *See* Riboflavin
Vitamin B$_3$, 521–522
Vitamin B$_6$, 38, 48, 138, 200–206, 523–524
  antivitamin B$_6$ compounds, 201
  breast milk, 404
  deficiency, 205, 423, 523
  exercise and, 358
  glycogenolysis and, 303
  metabolism and function, 201–204
  pregnancy and, 401
  recommended intake, 41, 204
  sources, 200–201, 523
  toxicity, 205–206, 524
Vitamin B$_{12}$, 48, 138, 212–216, 524
  recommended intake, 41
  absorption, 73, 213–214
  cobalt and, 278, 530
  deficiency, 210, 212, 215, 216, 423, 524
  exercise and, 358–359
  infant requirements, 407
  protein binding, 214
  recommended intake, 216
  sources, 213, 524
  storage and retention, 214–215
Vitamin C (ascorbic acid), 48, 182, 183–186, 505, 525
  absorption, 184
  antioxidant function, 182, 185, 444
  cancer and, 444–445
  cardiovascular health and, 428–428
  deficiency, 182, 185–186, 428, 525
  diabetes and, 463
  exercise and, 357–358
  function, 184–185
  immune competence and, 444
  iron absorption and, 185, 248

isomer forms, 182
  mineral-induced deactivation, 183
  normal blood values, 541
  recommended intake, 41, 185
  sources, 183–184, 525
  toxicity, 186, 525
  vitamin E and, 176, 185
Vitamin D, 48, 167–172, 518
  absorption and transport, 169
  analogs and structures, 167–168
  calcium blood levels and, 229
  deficiency, 172, 401, 518
  function, 172
  infant requirements, 407
  magnesium and, 236, 237
  metabolism, 169–170
  osteoporosis treatment, 479
  pregnancy and, 401
  recommended intake, 40, 172
  renal metabolism, 32
  sources, 168–169, 518
  toxicity, 518
Vitamin D$_2$, 167–168
Vitamin D$_3$, 167–168
Vitamin D-binding protein (DBP), 135, 169
Vitamin D receptor, 166, 169, 170–172
Vitamin D responsive elements (VDREs), 171
Vitamin E, 48, 173–177, 510, 518
  absorption and transport, 174
  antioxidant activity, 428
  cardiovascular health and, 428
  coenzyme athletic performance system (CAPS), 376
  deficiency, 177, 518
  function, 176
  nutrient interactions, 166
  paleolithic diet, 499
  recommended intake, 40, 177
  selenium and, 271
  sources, 173–174, 518
  storage and excretion, 175–176
  toxicity, 177, 519
  vitamin C and, 185
Vitamin K, 48, 178–181, 519
  absorption and transport, 178–179
  deficiency, 181, 519
  functions, 179–181
  infant requirements, 407
  intestinal microflora and, 37, 77
  nutrient interactions, 166
  recommended intake, 40, 181
  sources, 178, 519
  toxicity, 181, 519
  vitamin E toxicity, 177
Vitamins, 159–224, 517–525, *See* specific vitamins
  classic interpretation of nutrient function, 487
  diabetes and, 463
  exercise and, 357–359
  fat-soluble, 48, 160–181, 517–519
  food sources, 48
  pregnancy requirement, 400–401

RDAs, 40–41, *See also* recommended intakes for specific vitamins
suggested readings, 224
water-soluble, 48, 159, 182–223, 517–525
Vitronectin, 478
VLDL, *See* Very-low-density lipoproteins
Von Willebrand factor, 478

W

Waist-to-hip ratio, 332
Water, 45, 151–158
   balance, 156–158
      protein and, 137
   body composition, 1, 321, 326
   content of food, 45
   dehydration, 151, 158
   digestion and, 76
   fluoridation, 273–274
   food sources, 157
   hyperhydration, 382
   intake recommendations, 157
   intoxication, 158, 243
   physiological distribution, 153–153
   solubility, 151, 159
   sports drinks and fluid replacement, 363
   sweat composition, 153–154
   urine composition, 155–156
Water softening, 419
Weight and height charts, 511–516
Weight gain, 328, *See also* Obesity
   glycogen loading and, 361
   growth charts, 511–516
   menopause and, 337
   pregnancy and, 400
Weight loss
   blood pressure control, 419
   diabetes and, 339, 459
   diet therapy, 339–340
   exercise and, 338
   pyruvate and, 385
   supplement products, 341
Weight training (or strength training)
   chromium supplementation and, 373
   muscle adaptations, 346
   ornithine and, 384–385
   thermal effect of activity, 287
   vanadium and, 388–389

Werner's syndrome, 499
Wheat proteins, 46
Whey proteins, 45
Wills factor, 206
Wilson's disease, 269
Witch hazel, 568

X

Xanthine oxidase, 193, 280
Xanthophylls, 53–54, 160
Xenical, 341
Xylans, 90
Xylitol, 85, 462, 539
Xylose, 80, 81, 89
Xyulose, 80

Y

Yellow prussiate of soda, 510
Yerba santa, 568
Yohimbe, 398
Yohimbine, 390

Z

Zeaxanthin, 54, 162, 371
Zinc, 49, 249, 254–259, 487, 533
   absorption, 254–256
   body distribution, 256
   bone health and, 479–480
   copper absorption and, 256, 265, 266
   deficiency, 166, 207, 258, 480, 533
   enzyme cofactor, 254, 256, 257
   excretion, 257–258
   function, 254
   genetic disorders of metabolism, 257
   infant requirements, 408
   iron absorption and, 255
   metabolism and function, 256–257
   pregnancy needs, 402
   recommended intake, 42, 258
   sources, 254, 533
   toxicity, 256, 257, 259, 533
Zinc carbonate, 255
Zinc fingers, 257, 487
Zinc gluconate, 255
Zinc sulfate, 255

1

6

2001

6

RI